T0257216

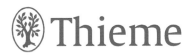

Ophthalmology Review

A Case-Study Approach

Second Edition

Kuldev Singh, MD, MPH
Professor of Ophthalmology
Director of the Glaucoma Service
Stanford University School of Medicine
Palo Alto, California

William E. Smiddy, MD
M. Brenn Green Chair in Ophthalmology
Professor of Ophthalmology
Bascom Palmer Eye Institute
University of Miami Medical School
Miami, Florida

Andrew G. Lee, MD
Neuro-ophthalmologist
Chairman
Department of Ophthalmology
Blanton Eye Institute
Houston Methodist Hospital
Houston, Texas

223 illustrations

Thieme
New York • Stuttgart • Delhi • Rio de Janeiro

Executive Editor: William Lamsback
Managing Editor: Elizabeth Palumbo
Director, Editorial Services: Mary Jo Casey
Production Editor: Sean Woznicki
International Production Director: Andreas Schabert
Editorial Director: Sue Hodgson
International Marketing Director: Fiona Henderson
International Sales Director: Louisa Turrell
Director of Institutional Sales: Adam Bernacki
Senior Vice President and Chief Operating Officer: Sarah Vanderbilt
President: Brian D. Scanlan

Library of Congress Cataloging-in-Publication Data
Names: Singh, Kuldev, 1961- editor.
Title: Ophthalmology review : a case-study approach /
  [edited by] Kuldev
    Singh Stanford University Medical Center Palo Alto, CA, USA,
    Andrew G. Lee Blanton Eye Institute Houston Methodist
    Hospital Houston, TX, USA,
    William E. Smiddy Bascom Palmer Eye Institute University of
    Miami Health System Miami, FL, USA.
Description: New York : Thieme, 2018. |
Identifiers: LCCN 2018005466 (print) | LCCN 2018005934 (ebook)
  | ISBN 9781626231771 (e-book) | ISBN 9781626231764 (print)
Subjects: LCSH: Ophthalmology--Case studies. | Eye--Diseases--
Case studies.
Classification: LCC RE69 (ebook) | LCC RE69 .O65 2018 (print) | DDC
  617.7--dc23
LC record available at https://lccn.loc.gov/2018005466
© 2019 Thieme Medical Publishers, Inc.

Thieme Publishers New York
333 Seventh Avenue, New York, NY 10001 USA
+1 800 782 3488, customerservice@thieme.com

Thieme Publishers Stuttgart
Rüdigerstrasse 14, 70469 Stuttgart, Germany
+49 [0]711 8931 421, customerservice@thieme.de

Thieme Publishers Delhi
A-12, Second Floor, Sector-2, Noida-201301
Uttar Pradesh, India
+91 120 45 566 00, customerservice@thieme.in

Thieme Publishers Rio de Janeiro, Thieme Publicações Ltda.
Edifício Rodolpho de Paoli, 25º andar
Av. Nilo Peçanha, 50 – Sala 2508,
Rio de Janeiro 20020-906 Brasil
+55 21 3172-2297 / +55 21 3172-1896
www.thiemerevinter.com.br

Cover design: Thieme Publishing Group
Typesetting by Thomson Digital, India

Printed in the United States of America by
King Publishing   5 4 3 2 1

ISBN 978-1-62623-176-4

Also available as an e-book:
eISBN 978-1-62623-177-1

Important note: Medicine is an ever-changing science undergoing continual development. Research and clinical experience are continually expanding our knowledge, in particular our knowledge of proper treatment and drug therapy. Insofar as this book mentions any dosage or application, readers may rest assured that the authors, editors, and publishers have made every effort to ensure that such references are in accordance with **the state of knowledge at the time of production of the book.**

Nevertheless, this does not involve, imply, or express any guarantee or responsibility on the part of the publishers in respect to any dosage instructions and forms of applications stated in the book. **Every user is requested to examine carefully** the manufacturers' leaflets accompanying each drug and to check, if necessary in consultation with a physician or specialist, whether the dosage schedules mentioned therein or the contraindications stated by the manufacturers differ from the statements made in the present book. Such examination is particularly important with drugs that are either rarely used or have been newly released on the market. Every dosage schedule or every form of application used is entirely at the user's own risk and responsibility. The authors and publishers request every user to report to the publishers any discrepancies or inaccuracies noticed. If errors in this work are found after publication, errata will be posted at www.thieme.com on the product description page.

Some of the product names, patents, and registered designs referred to in this book are in fact registered trademarks or proprietary names even though specific reference to this fact is not always made in the text. Therefore, the appearance of a name without designation as proprietary is not to be construed as a representation by the publisher that it is in the public domain.

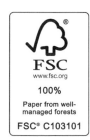

To my wife, Hilary Beaver, MD, who never ceases to be a source of motivation, inspiration, and celebration in work and in life.

Andrew G. Lee

Contents

Part XI: Orbit / Oculoplastics

Preface

The second edition of this textbook is aimed at medical students, residents, and comprehensive ophthalmologists who have an interest in general ophthalmologic problems. The format is designed to be easy to use, case-driven, and a basic introduction to clinical problems, evaluation, management, and treatment. It is not our intention to provide a complete, all-inclusive, detailed, or heavily referenced text. Instead, it is our goal to present real-world case examples of common clinical conditions and to discuss the work-up and management in a simple and easy-to-read manner.

We hope that the reader will be able to use this text in the clinic to guide the management of patients. The reader is encouraged to reference more detailed literature and texts for elements or less-common disorders that are not covered in our book.

Acknowledgments

Dr. Singh would like to thank his parents, Mandev and Kulwanti Singh as well as his wife Angele and daughter Julia Miranda Singh. He also thanks his sister Tina Singh and her children Tara and Devin. He would like to acknowledge his teachers and colleagues in the field of ophthalmology—too numerous to mention individually—who are a constant source of inspiration and guidance with particular gratitude to the late Carl Camras and Thom Zimmerman for their mentorship and innovative contributions to the profession.

Dr. Lee is deeply indebted to his wife, Hilary Beaver, M.D., who has so patiently and quietly tolerated her husband's long hours away from home and continues to be his best friend and biggest supporter. Dr. Lee thanks his parents, Alberto C. Lee, M.D. and Rosalind Go Lee, M.D., for planting the seeds of intellectual curiosity, work ethic, and a physician's calling. He is grateful to his siblings, Amy Lee-Wirts, M.D. and Richard Lee, for their love and support. Dr. Lee also thanks his daughters, Rachael and Virginia Lee whom he hopes will one day be inspired to join the long, line of white coats in the Lee family. Finally, he acknowledges the huge debt of education and academic mentoring that he owes to his friends and colleagues: Paul Brazis, M.D., Neil Miller, M.D., Tony Arnold, MD, Karl Golnik, MD, Dan B. Jones, M.D., Thomas Weingeist, M.D. And Keith Carter, M.D.

Kuldev Singh, MD, MPH
William E. Smiddy, MD
Andrew G. Lee, MD

Contributors

Thomas Albini, MD
Associate Professor
Clinical Ophthalmology
Department of Ophthalmology
University of Miami
Bascom Palmer Eye Institute
Miami, Florida

Tayyeba K. Ali, MD
Ophthalmologist
Bascom Palmer Eye Institute
Kaiser Permanente Santa Clara
Santa Clara, California

Tatyana Beketova, BS
Medical Student
McGovern Medical School at The University of
   Texas Health Science Center at Houston
Houston, TX

Elena Bitrian, MD
Assistant Professor of Ophthalmology
Mayo Clinic
Rochester, Minnesota

Donald L. Budenz, MD, MPH
Professor and Chairman
Department of Ophthalmology
University of North Carolina at Chapel Hill
Chapel Hill, North Carolina

Eitan S. Burstein, MD
Instructor
University of Virginia School of Medicine
Department of Ophthalmology
University of Virginia Health System
Charlottesville, Virginia

Sally Byrd, MD
Chair, Ophthalmology
Corvallis Clinic
Corvallis, Oregon

Andrew S. Camp, MD
Assistant Professor of Clinical Ophthalmology
Shiley Eye Institute
University of California San Diego
La Jolla, California

Thalmon R. Campagnoli, MD
PGY-2 Resident
Department of Ophthalmology
Columbia University
College of Physicians and Students
New York, NY

Brian Jen Jim Chang, MD
Ophthalmologist
Facey Medical Group
Mission Hills, California

David F. Chang, MD
Clinical Professor
Department of Ophthalmology
University of California, San Francisco
San Francisco, California

Daniel Y. Choi, MD
Ophthalmologist
Central Valley Eye Medical Group, Inc.
Stockton, California

David K. Coats, MD
Professor of Ophthalmology and Pediatrics
Baylor College of Medicine
Texas Children's Hospital
Houston, Texas

Anne L. Coleman, MD, PhD
Professor of Ophthalmology
Fran & Ray Stark Foundation
Stein Eye Institute
David Geffin School of Medicine
University of California at Los Angeles
Los Angeles, California

Scott A. Cory, MD
Ophthalmologist
Cory Eye Care Center
Portage, Indiana

Robert M. Feldman, MD
Chairman and Clinical Professor
Robert Cizik Eye Clinic
Ruiz Department of Ophthalmology and Visual Science
McGovern Medical School at the University of Texas Health
   Science Center at Houston
Houston, Texas

I. Howard Fine, MD
Clinical Professor
Department of Ophthalmology
Oregon Health & Science University
Portland, Oregon
Drs. Fine, Hoffman, & Sims, LLC
Eugene, Oregon

Nandini G. Gandhi, MD
Associate Professor
Ophthalmology
UC Davis Department of Ophthalmology
Sacramento, California

Dan S. Gombos, MD FACS
Professor and Chief
Section of Ophthalmology
Department of Head and Neck Surgery
The University of Texas MD Anderson Cancer Center
Houston, Texas

Brian E. Goldhagen, MD
Assistant Professor of Clinical Ophthalmology
Bascom Palmer Eye Institute
University of Miami School of Medicine
Miami, Florida

Alana L. Grajewski, MD
Professor of Clinical Ophthalmology
Director
Samuel & Ethel Balkan International Pediatric Glaucoma
    Center
Bascom Palmer Eye Institute
University of Miami Miller School of Medicine
Miami, Florida

Eric D. Hansen
Instructor
John A Moran Eye Center
Department of Ophthalmology
University of Utah
Salt Lake City, Utah

Weldon W. Haw, MD
Clinical Professor of Ophthalmology
University of California San Diego & Shiley Eye Institute
San Diego, California

Abigail Huang, MD
Fellow
Clinical Informatics – Oregon Health & Science University
Ophthalmology – VA Portland Healthcare System
Department of Medical Informatics
    and Clinical Epidemiology
Oregon Health & Science University
Portland, Oregon

Blake A. Isernhagen, MD
Ophthalmologist
Retina Associates of Kentucky
Lexington, Kentucky

Matthew R. Jones, MD
Ophthalmologist
Cornea and Refractive Surgery
Vantage Eye Center
Monterey, California

Robert Kule, MD
Clinical Instructor
Stanford Byers Eye Institute
Palo Alto, California

Usha Rajapuram Kumar, MD
Ophthalmologist
Kaiser Permanente
The Permanente Medical Group, Inc.
Vallejo, California

Ajay E. Kuriyan, MD, MS
Assistant Professor
Flaum Eye Institute
University of Rochester Medical Center
Rochester, New York

Byron L. Lam, MD
Professor, Robert Z. and Nancy J. Greene Chair
    in Ophthalmology
Bascom Palmer Eye Institute
University of Miami
Miami, Florida

Andrew G. Lee, MD
Neuro-ophthalmologist
Chairman
Department of Ophthalmology
Blanton Eye Institute
Houston Methodist Hospital
Houston, Texas

Bryan S. Lee, MD, JD
Private Practice, Altos Eye Physicians
Adjunct Clinical Assistant Professor of Ophthalmology,
    Stanford
Los Altos, California

Martha Motuz Leen, MD
Director, Glaucoma Division
Achieve Eye and Laser Specialists
Silverdale, Washington

John Edward Legarreta, MD
Clinical Assistant Professor of Ophthalmology
Ross Eye Institute
Department of Ophthalmology
University at Buffalo Jacobs School of Medicine
Williamsville, New York

Ella Leung, MD
Assistant Professor of Ophthalmology
Baylor College of Medicine
Houston, Texas

Charles C. Lin, MD
Clinical Assistant Professor
Byers Eye Institute
Stanford University
Palo Alto, California

Stephen A. Lin, MD
Ophthalmologist
Central Valley Eye Medical Group, Inc.
Stockton, California

Amina I. Malik, MD
Ophthalmology Specialist
Houston Methodist Hospital
Houston, Texas

Edward E. Manche, MD
Professor of Ophthalmology
Division Chief
Cornea and Refractive Surgery
Stanford University School of Medicine
Byers Eye Institute at Stanford
Palo Alto, California

Carlos A. Medina Mendez, MD
Ophthalmologist
Retinal Consultants
Sacramento, California

Mozart de Oliveira Mello Jr., MD
Opthalmologist
Ver Excelencia Em Oftalmologia Retina Vitreous
    Department
Fundaçao Banco De Olhos De Goias Retna Vitreous
    Department
Goiânia, GO, Brazil

Amir Mohsenin, MD, PhD
Assistant Professor of Ophthalmology
Ruiz Department of Ophthalmology & Visual Science
McGovern Medical School
University of Texas Health Science Center at Houston
Houston, Texas

Peter A. Netland, MD, PhD
Vernah Scott Moyston Professor and Chair
University of Virginia School of Medicine
Department of Ophthalmology
University of Virginia Health System
Charlottesville, Virginia

Bac Tien Nguyen, MD
Assistant Professor
Department of Ophthalmology
Baylor College of Medicine
Houston, Texas

Don C. Nguyen, MD
Ophthalmologist
Cataract Institute of Oklahoma
Edmond, Oklahoma

Xuan Thanh Le-Nguyen, MD
Ophthalmologist
Desert Eye Associates
Cizik Eye Center
Houston, Texas

Evelyn A. Paysse, MD
Professor
Ophthalmology and Pediatrics
Texas Children's Hospital
Baylor College of Medicine
Houston, Texas

Sarah P. Read, MD, PhD
Surgical Retina Fellow
Bascom Palmer Eye Institute
Miami, Florida

James C. Robinson, MD
Associate Professor of Ophthalmology
Medical College of Wisconsin
Milwaukee, Wisconsin

Thomas W. Samuelson, MD
Attending Surgeon
Minnesota Eye Consultants
Adjunct Professor of Ophthalmology
University of Minnesota
Minnesota Eye Consultants
Phillips Eye Institute
University of Minnesota
Minneapolis, Minnesota

Ingrid U. Scott, MD, MPH
Jack and Nancy Turner Professor of Ophthalmology
Professor of Public Health Sciences
Penn State College of Medicine
Hershey, Pennsylvania

Ruwan A. Silva, MD
Assistant Professor of Vitreoretinal Surgery
Department of Ophthalmology
Stanford University School of Medicine
Palo Alto, California

Kuldev Singh, MD, MPH
Professor of Ophthalmology
Director of the Glaucoma Service
Stanford University School of Medicine
Palo Alto, California

William E. Smiddy, MD
M. Brenn Green Chair in Ophthalmology
Professor of Ophthalmology
Bascom Palmer Eye Institute
University of Miami Medical School
Miami, Florida

Yasemin G. Sozeri, MD
Resident Physician
Medical College of Wisconsin and Froedtert Eye Institute
Milwaukee, Wisconsin

Christopher N. Ta, MD
Stanford University
School of Medicine
Palo Alto, California

Scheffer C. G. Tseng, MD, PhD
Medical Director
Ocular Surface Center, P.A.
Ocular Surface Research & Education Foundation
Chief Technology Officer
TissueTech™, Inc.
Miami, Florida

Jonathan H. Tzu, MD
Ophthalmologist
Retina and Vitreous of Texas
Houston, Texas

Aaron Wang, MD, PhD
Ophthalmology (Cornea Subspecialty)
Shiley Eye Institute
University of California San Diego
La Jolla, California

Basil K. Williams Jr., MD
Instructor
Bascom Palmer Eye Institute
Miami, Florida

Edward H. Wood, MD
Vitreoretinal Surgery Fellow
Associate Retinal Consultants
Neuroscience Center Building
Royal Oak, Michigan

Sushma Yalamanchili, MD
Associate Professor
Clinical Ophthalmology
Houston Methodist
Weill Cornell Medical College
Houston, Texas

Part I

Cornea and External Disease

I

1 Acute Follicular Conjunctivitis

Usha Rajapuram Kumar and Weldon W. Haw

Abstract

Acute conjunctivitis is a common ophthalmologic disease. Acute conjunctivitis may be caused by viruses, bacterial, chlamydia, toxins/medications, and allergic reactions. Clinical features such as history and examination can be useful in determining the etiology. In atypical cases, diagnostic examination with cultures, scrapings, direct immunofluorescence, enzyme-linked immunosorbent assays, or polymerase chain reactions may be useful in identifying the causative pathogen. In most cases of viral conjunctivitis, observation and symptomatic treatment is all that is necessary. Precaution is an important step to avoid further spread of the contagious disease. Specific therapy with anti-infective agents may be required for unusual infectious causes of conjunctivitis (i.e., bacterial, chlamydial, etc.).

Keywords: conjunctivitis, acute follicular conjunctivitis, acute conjunctivitis, viral conjunctivitis, adenoviral conjunctivitis

1.1 History

A 37-year-old female office worker has a 2-week history of photophobia, discomfort, and headache centered around her right eye. A week previously, she developed sudden onset of redness and watering of the right eye the first day back at work, having returned several days earlier from a vacation in Hawaii. She also noted swelling in front of her right ear. She saw her eye-care practitioner, who found unilateral follicular conjunctivitis with a mildly tender preauricular node. He treated her with a 2-week course of topical tobramycin–dexamethasone ophthalmic suspension drops; her node became slightly smaller, but 2 days after cessation of the topical tobramycin–dexamethasone, she had epithelial infiltrates in the cornea and persisting follicles.

Visual acuity is 20/25 and 20/20 in her right and left eyes, respectively. There is a right-sided nontender preauricular node. At penlight examination, the right eye shows a 1- to 2-mm ptosis of the upper lid and mild injection of the bulbar conjunctiva; the left eye appears quiet. Biomicroscopy reveals a moderate number of medium-sized pretarsal follicles and papillae in the right eye (▶ Fig. 1.1); the left eye demonstrates

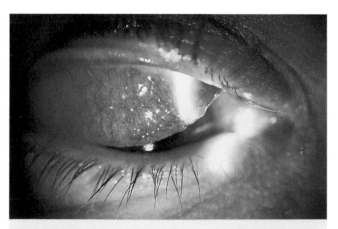

Fig. 1.1 Superior pretarsal mixed follicular and papillary conjunctivitis.

substantially fewer follicles in the inferior fornix. The right cornea shows diffuse midperipheral and a few central epithelial infiltrates, with no stromal involvement or other anterior segment findings. The left cornea and anterior segment are normal.

Differential Diagnosis—Key Points

1. Acute follicular conjunctivitis is commonly encountered in the general ophthalmologic setting. The patient's history is particularly remarkable in that she was recently on vacation, possibly increasing the risk of encountering infectious agents either from acquaintances or from fomites she may have contacted. She specifically denies any sexual contact, but stayed in hotel rooms and used swimming pool facilities.

The differential diagnosis in this case can be narrowed to include adenoviral keratoconjunctivitis, chlamydial disease (adult inclusion conjunctivitis), primary herpes simplex or Epstein–Barr (EB) keratoconjunctivitis, and molluscum contagiosum. Influenza virus, paramyxovirus, and human immunodeficiency virus (HIV) can, although rarely, cause conjunctivitis during systemic infection.[4] Toxic and allergic reactions should also be considered in previously treated or self-medicating patients, although lymphadenopathy is not a common feature.

2. Adenovirus is a leading cause of follicular conjunctivitis and can present in milder forms, such as seen in the present case, to more fulminant forms with substantial ocular morbidity. It is generally acquired by fomite—hand–eye contact or from swimming pools. These can be visually significant. Clinical symptoms and signs generally occur about 7 to 10 days after exposure to the virus.[6] Its more severe forms include epidemic keratoconjunctivitis (EKC) caused by several adenoviral serotypes including 8, 19, or 37. EKC routinely demonstrates subconjunctival or petechial hemorrhages and pseudomembranes, which may be accompanied by prominent lid edema and erythema and even preseptal cellulitis. Systemic symptoms may include fever and malaise. Pharyngoconjunctival fever (PCF) is generally a milder condition and includes an antecedent or simultaneous pharyngitis, fever, and upper respiratory symptoms, and demonstrates relatively mild or absent corneal infiltrates. PCF is most commonly caused by adenoviral serotypes 3, 5, 7, or 11.[4] In both conditions, the acute onset is in one eye, followed by the second eye a few days later; the latter eye is generally less involved with symptoms and signs.

This patient has no antecedent or concurrent systemic symptoms. She developed epithelial infiltrates only after cessation of topical tobramycin–dexamethasone; topical corticosteroid usage early in the course of acute conjunctivitis can mask this helpful diagnostic corneal finding. Typically, within a week of onset of EKC, fine diffuse punctate epithelial infiltrates develop; these coalesce into larger, coarse epithelial infiltrates about a week later. These are replaced by focal subepithelial infiltrates, which become more intense by a month after onset and typically reside in the central and paracentral cornea. These subepithelial infiltrates are thought to be a result of an immune response to viral antigens deposited in the superficial corneal stroma.[4]

Adult chlamydia inclusion conjunctivitis is caused by *Chlamydia trachomatis* serotypes D–K; it is an oculogenital disease generally found in younger, sexually active adults, but it can also be contracted from fomites including toilet seats and inadequately chlorinated swimming pools or hot tubs. Onset of first symptoms may be more difficult to pinpoint, but is likely within 1 to 2 weeks of exposure. It is commonly unilateral, and involves mild lid swelling and a minimal mucopurulent discharge. Follicles are usually predominantly located in the inferior fornices. A minimally tender preauricular node may develop as well as pseudoptosis, both features presenting with this patient. Small epithelial infiltrates as seen in this patient can develop 2 to 3 weeks after onset of the conjunctivitis. A superior micropannus may develop. Corticosteroid use again may have altered the clinical presentation of this patient. The patient denies any systemic or genital symptoms, but the clinician must remain circumspect in this regard.

Chlamydia psittaci, an infection of birds, is rarely transmitted to humans. The infection can inhabit cats, but this patient had not knowingly been exposed to birds or cats. Clinical findings are similar to inclusion conjunctivitis except that no pannus is seen; the disease is often accompanied by a mild influenzalike illness or frank pneumonia. Presentation of a Parinaud's oculoglandular syndrome, although most commonly attributed to cat-scratch disease, would also invoke another possible chlamydial condition—lymphogranuloma venereum. This is a venereal disease accompanied by lymphadenitis and occasionally systemic symptoms. The conjunctiva would classically demonstrate follicles and one or more granulomas. Newcastle disease infection (a paramyxovirus) of poultry workers may present similarly as in this patient, but the follicles are generally prominent only in the lower lid, and any epithelial infiltrates are more scant.

3. Primary herpes simplex virus (HSV) and EB virus may present as an acute follicular conjunctivitis, with possible mild conjunctival hemorrhages or even membranes. Primary herpes simplex infection in adults is often accompanied by vesicular lid lesions, with watery discharge and a preauricular node. The cornea may develop a fine punctate epitheliopathy or small fine dendritic figures. EB virus keratoconjunctivitis may manifest subepithelial infiltrates similar to adenovirus, and patients may present with no systemic manifestations or with the more classic spectrum of fever, sore throat, and lymphadenopathy of mononucleosis.

4. Molluscum contagiosum is now the most commonly encountered poxvirus and can cause a unilateral follicular conjunctivitis. The lid must be carefully examined for molluscum lesions. Punctate epithelial erosions and, rarely, a corneal pannus may develop. Corneal infiltrates are not seen. Preauricular lymphadenopathy is also not a characteristic feature, unlike the vaccinia poxvirus, which may be encountered when administered as a smallpox vaccination.

1.2 Test Interpretation

Clinical suspicion is useful in determining whether further diagnostic tests are required to confirm specific etiologies of acute follicular conjunctivitis. In most instances of typical acute conjunctivitis, simple observation for 1 or 2 weeks is reasonable if adenovirus is suspected. Her social history was unremarkable for risk behaviors for chlamydia, other than possibly through fomite exposure. Her subepithelial infiltrates were potentially consistent with chlamydia or adenovirus, although the clinical picture was possibly altered by use of prior topical corticosteroids before referral. Cultures and other tests were performed to rule out viral and chlamydial disease. Cultures may not be helpful in certain health systems or hospitals if performed infrequently.

Adenovirus can be identified by several diagnostic methods including viral cell culture, direct immunofluorescence, polymerase chain reaction (PCR), and enzyme-linked immunosorbent assay (ELISA). However, in most instances, these tests are not generally employed for various reasons, including time delay of receiving results, expense, or necessity for elaborate equipment. Recently, a rapid immunodetection assay (RPS Adeno Detector; Rapid Pathogen Screening Inc., Sarasota, FL) has been developed, which is capable of detecting 53 of the adenoviral serotypes. The assay samples regions along the palpebral conjunctiva targeting the adenovirus hexon antigen. This point-of-care testing method can be performed in the office, yields rapid results, and has a higher sensitivity and specificity compared to viral culture and PCR testing.[4,5]

HSV detection is possible through viral culture or antigen- or DNA-detection methodologies; however, these methodologies are only indicated in complex cases when the clinical diagnosis is uncertain. All cases of suspected neonatal herpes infection require laboratory testing. Scrapings from the vesicle base or conjunctiva can also be tested for HSV. For chlamydia, conjunctival scrapings for direct fluorescent antibody (DFA) testing and McCoy cell culture were performed. These tests are fairly sensitive and highly specific. These scrapings are effectively obtained with small-wire Dacron swabs.

Kits for DFA testing have an indefinite shelf life and are provided by a properly equipped laboratory with personnel properly trained to do the analysis. The conjunctiva is anesthetized with proparacaine, and the Dacron swab is rubbed across the fornix or pretarsal conjunctiva with firm strokes sufficient to harvest epithelial cells. The swab is rolled over the glass slide provided in the kit, and a smudge of material should be apparent by the naked eye when the slide is observed in reflected light. The slide is preserved with a fixative and transported to the laboratory. The same swab used for the glass slide can then be inoculated into suitable tissue culture transport medium by cutting or breaking off the top portion of the handle to allow the Dacron portion to be fully immersed in the medium. Alternatively, PCR, or nucleic acid amplification testing, is available for testing of chlamydia. Giemsa or Wright-Giemsa staining was not ordered because this test is infrequently performed now that more sensitive and specific testing is available. For this case study, test results were negative for adenovirus and herpes simplex as well as for chlamydia.

1.3 Diagnosis

Acute follicular conjunctivitis, likely adenoviral.

1.4 Medical Management

Observation and symptomatic treatment with cool compresses and unpreserved lubricants were initiated. The patient was counseled regarding the potential infectious nature of the condition: the contagious nature of the conjunctivitis and the potential for possible infectivity to others for another week or two (or longer). Strict personal hygiene including frequent hand washing, keeping personal soiled tissues, washcloths, and pillowcases isolated from others is recommended. If the patient develops conjunctival membranes or pseudomembranes, removal with a forceps or cotton swab or a self-retained amniotic membrane may provide symptomatic relief, prevent symblepharon formation, and speed resolution.

Currently, there are no FDA-approved treatments for adenoviral keratoconjunctivitis. Although controversial, a mild topical corticosteroid such as loteprednol may be considered if visually significant subepithelial infiltrates are present; the goal is to minimize visual loss related to persistent corneal scarring and maximize vision potential. It is important to note that goal of steroids is not to completely eradicate all subepithelial infiltrates. However, use of topical steroids may potentiate viral shedding.

New potential therapeutic options being evaluated include povidone iodine or a combination 0.6% povidone iodine/0.1% dexamethasone ophthalmic suspension (also known as FST-100; Shire, Lexington, MA). Antiviral agents such as trifluridine, vidarabine, and ganciclovir demonstrate only mild effectivity against adenovirus. Ganciclovir ophthalmic gel has been shown to decrease adenoviral loads experimentally; however, it has not been effective in the treatment of conjunctivitis in clinical trials. Topical cidofovir has shown benefit by reducing adenoviral titers and the formation of subepithelial infiltrates; however, in a recent clinical study, it did not demonstrate decreased duration of clinical symptoms compared to those without treatment. Several other agents which have demonstrated potential benefit, but require further investigation include 2'3'-dideoxycytidine, interferon β, interferon γ, immunoglobulin, and N-chlorotaurine.[4]

Signs of herpes epithelial keratoconjunctivitis or a positive herpes testing result would warrant initiation of topical trifluridine therapy and consideration for systemic acyclovir 400 mg five times a day for 1 to 2 weeks. Oral antivirals such as acyclovir or valacyclovir offer the advantage of reducing epithelial toxicity in an irritated eye.

Although adult chlamydial conjunctivitis often resolves spontaneously,[6] systemic therapy is recommended because of the relatively high incidence of genital and other nonocular involvement. Treatment of sexual partners is mandatory and, along with the patient, should also be evaluated for coinfection with other sexually transmitted diseases such as syphilis and gonorrhea.[6] The traditional therapy includes tetracycline 250 mg orally four times daily for 1 week, avoiding milk products and antacids, which reduce absorption. Alternatively, doxycycline, 100 mg twice a day for 7 days, can be taken with food and is usually better tolerated. Pregnant or breastfeeding women may take erythromycin, 500 mg four times daily for 1 week,[6] or sulfisoxazole, 0.5 to 1 g four times daily for 3 weeks. Azithromycin 1 g as a single dose is also effective for adult inclusion conjunctivitis.

1.5 Rehabilitation and Follow-up

The patient should be examined in 4 to 6 weeks to ensure that symptoms have improved, follicles have nearly regressed, and corneal opacities have continued to fade. If visually threatening corneal opacities or conjunctival membranes/pseudomembranes are present, then more frequent visits may be indicated. A careful history should be obtained to make certain that the prescribed medications have been taken properly. In patients with unresolved and persistent corneal opacities with residual visually significant scarring (i.e., reduced visual acuity, contrast sensitivity, or photophobia), excimer laser phototherapeutic keratectomy with low-dose mitomycin C may be considered.[4]

Suggested Reading

[1] American Academy of Ophthalmology. Conjunctivitis. Preferred Practice Pattern. San Francisco, CA: American Academy of Ophthalmology; 1998

[2] Chandler JW. Chlamydial infections. In: Krachmer JH, Mannis MJ, Holland EJ, eds. Cornea: Surgery of the Cornea and Conjunctiva. Vol. 2. New York, NY: Mosby-Yearbook Inc; 1997:779–787

[3] Stamler JF. Viral conjunctivitis. In: Krachmer JH, Mannis MJ, Holland EJ, eds. Cornea: Surgery of the Cornea and Conjunctiva. Vol. 2. New York, NY: Mosby-Yearbook Inc; 1997:773–777

[4] Jhanji V, Chan TC, Li EY, Agarwal K, Vajpayee RB. Adenoviral keratoconjunctivitis. Surv Ophthalmol. 2015; 60(5):435–443

[5] Kaufman HE. Adenovirus advances: new diagnostic and therapeutic options. Curr Opin Ophthalmol. 2011; 22(4):290–293

[6] American Academy of Ophthalmology. External disease and cornea. In: Basic and Clinical Science Course. Section 8. San Francisco, CA: American Academy of Ophthalmology; 2017–2018

2 Chronic Follicular Conjunctivitis

Brian Jem Jin Chang and Weldon W. Haw

Abstract

Most conjunctivitis symptoms will resolve within 1 to 2 weeks of onset. In some instances, conjunctivitis can be classified as chronic, or persisting beyond 16 days. Although viral conjunctivitis is the most common cause of chronic follicular conjunctivitis, the possibility of unusual infectious causes such as chlamydia must be entertained. Other causes of persisting conjunctivitis may be related to exposure to preservatives based in topical medication use (toxic) or malignancies (masquerade syndrome). Clinical examination, cultures, and suspicion for medication-induced causes may be important in identifying the cause. Treatment of the underlying cause will resolve the conjunctivitis. Removal of the offending topical agent or changing to a preservative-free alternative will resolve the toxic conjunctivitis. Failure to address toxic follicular conjunctivitis may result in significant sequelae ocular surface sequelae such as corneal/conjunctival scarring, symblepharon, and punctal stenosis.

Keywords: conjunctivitis, bacterial conjunctivitis, follicular conjunctivitis, chronic conjunctivitis, toxic conjunctivitis, medicamentosa

2.1 History

A 38-year-old female patient presents for a routine follow-up visit 15 months after penetrating keratoplasty and anterior segment reconstruction for trauma to the right eye. Her eyes are comfortable, but she complains of mild right-sided preauricular discomfort and swelling. She recalls that 6 weeks previously she developed a fever and swollen glands, particularly on the right side of her face, and her internist suspected "strep throat" or "mononucleosis." She had no ocular symptoms at that time. Throat culture and Epstein–Barr virus serology were taken and were negative. She was treated with oral penicillin for 14 days, and she recovered symptomatically except for the persisting preauricular lymphadenopathy.

The patient is otherwise healthy with a negative review of systems. Her past ocular history is also significant for medically treated traumatic angle recession glaucoma of her right eye. Her left eye is normal with no ocular history. Her ocular medications for the right eye were loteprednol etabonate 0.5% twice daily, brimonidine 0.2% twice daily, timolol gel-forming solution 0.5% twice daily, and methylcellulose at bedtime. She had last been seen 3 months previously, and no ocular inflammation was seen. Her current examination reveals a visual acuity of 20/60+ with pinhole to 20/40 in the right eye. Intraocular pressures were 28 mm Hg in the right eye and 14 mm Hg in the left eye. She has a slightly tender right preauricular lymph node. External exam reveals slight puffiness of the lids, right worse than left. Biomicroscopy of the right eye shows mild lid scurf and no other lesions. The conjunctiva reveals prominent follicles and papillae in the inferior fornix and superior pretarsal area (▶ Fig. 2.1). No granulomas are present. The keratoplasty has mild diffuse epitheliopathy. The anterior segment exam is otherwise noncontributory. The left eye shows mild pretarsal papillae, without follicles, and an otherwise normal exam.

Differential Diagnosis—Key Points

1. The patient has unilateral follicular conjunctivitis, presumed to be chronic given the associated 6-week history of preauricular lymphadenopathy with febrile illness. Chronic follicular conjunctivitis is defined as lasting more than 16 days, and is characterized by the presence of follicles in the superior and inferior tarsal conjunctiva, and less commonly the bulbar conjunctiva. It can manifest either with an acute onset of symptoms, as in this case, or with insidious onset.
2. A detailed history is necessary to elucidate the etiology of chronic follicular conjunctivitis. This should include the onset and duration of symptoms, and the presence of ocular redness, discharge, discomfort, or photophobia. The use of prescribed or over-the-counter ocular medications, lubricants, or herbal preparations must be ascertained.

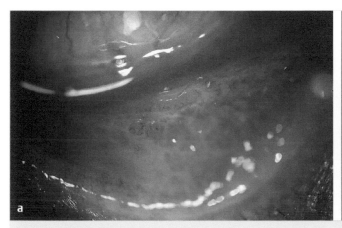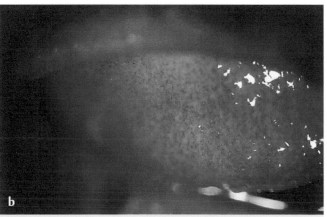

Fig. 2.1 Medium-sized "buried" pretarsal follicles in midst of papillary response. **(a)** Inferior tarsal. **(b)** Superior tarsal.

Patients frequently will not recall, or admit to, over-the-counter, herbal, or home remedies, or naturopathic or homeopathic preparations, unless directly and specifically questioned. This patient denied using any eye drops other than the prescription medications already listed. She denied close contact with animals, including cats and birds. She had not traveled to potentially endemic areas for other infectious etiologies.

3. Viral infections are common causes of chronic follicular conjunctivitis. In this case, they were high on the differential diagnosis because of the febrile prodrome and preauricular lymphadenopathy. The differential diagnosis for viral etiologies includes Epstein–Barr virus, herpes simplex virus, and adenovirus. Mitigating against these diagnoses were unilaterality and lack of corneal signs (though the latter could be masked by the use of the topical corticosteroid loteprednol). Additionally, with Epstein–Barr virus and adenovirus, at least some degree of follicular involvement is generally noted in the other eye. Another cause of chronic follicular conjunctivitis is molluscum contagiosum virus (a poxvirus). This patient had no eyelid lesions or chronic blepharitis to suggest molluscum.

4. While viral infection seemed more likely in this specific patient, it is important to consider the potential of bacterial infection. In particular, *Chlamydia trachomatis* is one of the most common causes of chronic follicular conjunctivitis. *C. trachomatis* is a sexually transmitted obligate intracellular bacterium that is responsible for two clinical forms: trachoma and adult (or neonatal) inclusion conjunctivitis. Giemsa staining with basophilic intracytoplasmic inclusions, direct immunofluorescent (DFA), and enzyme-linked immunosorbent assay (ELISA) have been developed for detection of chlamydia inclusion conjunctivitis. If indicated, treatment of the patient and partner with azithromycin 1,000 mg orally once a day, doxycycline 100 mg orally twice a day for 7 to 10 days, or erythromycin 500 mg orally four times a day for 7 to 10 days may be effective. This patient was monogamous, and she denied any gynecologic complaints, but the presence of unilateral chronic follicular disease in a sexually active adult should always raise suspicion of adult inclusion conjunctivitis. Other bacterial etiologies of chronic follicular conjunctivitis include *Moraxella* species, Lyme disease, and *Bartonella henselae*, which causes Parinaud's oculoglandular syndrome. However, the patient's presentation was not consistent with any of these.

5. Toxic follicular conjunctivitis must be considered, particularly with the patient's history of chronic topical medication usage. Also, she had hurricane epitheliopathy, a punctate keratitis with a swirling configuration inside the keratoplasty wound margin, which has been associated with toxic effect from preserved medication usage. The preservatives utilized included benzalkonium chloride and benzododecinium bromide, and may contribute to punctate keratitis and follicle formation. Timolol is rarely associated with toxic conjunctival effects but can contribute to epithelial keratitis. Brimonidine tartrate (Alphagan), a selective alpha-2-adrenergic agonist, has been reported to cause vernal-like keratoconjunctivitis with papillae and follicles. Its related product, apraclonidine hydrochloride (Iopidine), which is also an alpha-2-adrenergic agonist, is also known to cause a follicular conjunctivitis in some cases.

6. Masquerade syndromes can also present as chronic follicular conjunctivitis. Subconjunctival malignancies such as mantle cell lymphoma, B-cell non-Hodgkin lymphoma, and mucosa-associated lymphoid tissue (MALT) lymphoma should be considered for chronic, atypical follicular conjunctivitis. A noninflammatory, salmon-colored appearance and encroaching onto the globe may be typical of a lymphoma. Examination in sunlight may help accentuate and delineate the involved area of conjunctiva. There have also been case reports of ocular rhinosporidiosis and relapsing polychondritis causing chronic follicular conjunctivitis.

2.2 Test Interpretation

Pathologic examination of conjunctival scrapings reveals polymorphonuclear leukocytes and lymphocytes, with no eosinophils, suggesting a chronic inflammatory response. Viral cultures were negative for herpes simplex virus (determined by 2 days' incubation on human fibroblast cells) and adenovirus (determined by 2 weeks' incubation). Chlamydia culture on McCoy cells and conjunctival smear for direct fluorescent antibody (DFA) staining were negative. Other than *Chlamydia*, bacterial cultures were not obtained in this case given the lack of clinical suspicion of bacterial infection. Conjunctival biopsy can be considered in cases of protracted or atypical follicular conjunctivitis where masquerade syndrome is suspected.

2.3 Diagnosis

Unilateral toxic chronic follicular conjunctivitis.

2.4 Medical Management

If any cultures or stains are positive, treatment should be directed toward the specific pathogen. While cultures are pending, observation is a reasonable approach to determine the natural history of follicle development or improvement. In this case, the follicles persisted and the eye actually became more symptomatic initially, with erythema and irritation developing while culture results were pending. With negative diagnostic tests, toxic follicular conjunctivitis became the primary diagnostic possibility. Brimonidine was discontinued since it was the most likely offending agent.

In many cases, discontinuation of the offending medication is all that is required. If the specific medication is required, a preservative-free preparation should be used. Cold compresses and preservative-free artificial tears or ointments can help with irritation. Several studies have demonstrated the efficacy of topical corticosteroids, topical cyclosporine A 1%, and topical tacrolimus ointment in the treatment of chronic follicular conjunctivitis. However, it is unlikely that any of these agents would have an adequate or durable effect on the conjunctival response when the toxic agent is still being utilized.

Failure to recognize toxic follicular conjunctivitis can result in progressive punctal stenosis and subconjunctival scarring (i.e., pseudopemphigoid). This can be a self-limiting or progressive disorder. In cases of progression, conjunctival scarring, obliteration of the conjunctival fornices, symblepharon, and loss of conjunctival goblet cells will result in severe ocular surface disease. If untreated, toxic follicular conjunctivitis can result in superficial punctate keratopathy, and in severe cases, large epithelial erosions and corneal ulceration/melting.

2.5 Rehabilitation and Follow-up

Removal of the offending agent is the imperative first step. Preservative-free lubrication may be useful in comfort or symptom relief. Close observation is recommended initially for early detection of any occult infectious processes. The patient should be followed up every 2 to 3 weeks until improvement is noted. In this case, the patient's symptoms rapidly improved upon removal of brimonidine, and by 3 weeks, her follicles were improving. The follicles completely resolved by 2 months after stopping brimonidine, as did the hurricane epitheliopathy.

Toxic follicular conjunctivitis is most commonly caused by topical anesthetics, antiviral agents such as trifluridine and idoxuridine, aminoglycoside antibiotics such as gentamicin and tobramycin, and glaucoma medications such as pilocarpine, brimonidine, timolol, apraclonidine, epinephrine, and dipivefrin. Brimonidine has rarely been reported to cause follicles, and in this case, the viral prodrome may have predisposed the patient to developing this response through a subclinical irritated conjunctiva.

Suggested Reading

[1] American Academy of Ophthalmology. Conjunctivitis: Preferred Practice Pattern. San Francisco, CA: American Academy of Ophthalmology; 2013

[2] Chen HT, Chen KH, Hsu WM. Toxic keratopathy associated with abuse of low-dose anesthetic: a case report. Cornea. 2004; 23(5):527–529

[3] Feiz V, Mannis MJ, Kandavel G, et al. Surface keratopathy after penetrating keratoplasty. Trans Am Ophthalmol Soc. 2001; 99:159–168, discussion 168–170

[4] Fiore PM, Jacobs IH, Goldberg DB. Drug-induced pemphigoid. A spectrum of diseases. Arch Ophthalmol. 1987; 105(12):1660–1663

[5] García DP, Alperte JI, Cristóbal JA, et al. Topical tacrolimus ointment for treatment of intractable atopic keratoconjunctivitis: a case report and review of the literature. Cornea. 2011; 30(4):462–465

[6] Kolomeyer AM, Nayak NV, Ragam A, et al. Topical cyclosporine A 1% for the treatment of chronic follicular conjunctivitis. Eye Contact Lens. 2015; 41(4): 210–213

[7] Lindquist TD. Conjunctivitis: an overview and classification. In: Krachmer JH, Mannis MJ, Holland EJ, eds. Cornea: Surgery of the Cornea and Conjunctiva. Vol 2. New York, NY: Mosby-Yearbook Inc; 1997:745–758

[8] Shah AA, Modi Y, Thomas B, Wellik SR, Galor A. Brimonidine allergy presenting as vernal-like keratoconjunctivitis. J Glaucoma. 2015; 24(1):89–91

[9] Soparkar CNS, Wilhelmus KR, Koch DD, Wallace GW, Jones DB. Acute and chronic conjunctivitis due to over-the-counter ophthalmic decongestants. Arch Ophthalmol. 1997; 115(1):34–38

[10] Yu EN, Jurkunas U, Rubin PAD, Baltatzis S, Foster CS. Obliterative microangiopathy presenting as chronic conjunctivitis in a patient with relapsing polychondritis. Cornea. 2006; 25(5):621–622

3 Acute Bacterial Conjunctivitis

Abigail Huang and Weldon W. Haw

Abstract

Acute bacterial conjunctivitis may result in conjunctival injection associated with chemosis, papillary reaction, and purulent discharge. Gram stain and conjunctival cultures are not necessary in all cases of uncomplicated suspected bacterial conjunctivitis. Indications for Gram stain and culture include suspected bacterial conjunctivitis in neonates, immunocompromised individuals, and in cases of refractory, recurrent, or abundant purulent conjunctivitis. Treatment with a broad-spectrum topical antibiotic may shorten the symptom duration and reduce the transmissibility and the risk of rare complications. In rare situations (hyperacute conjunctivitis, gonococcal conjunctivitis, neonates), systemic antibiotics may be required to prevent complications.

Keywords: bacterial conjunctivitis, follicular conjunctivitis, acute conjunctivitis

3.1 History

A 60-year-old woman presents with complaints of decreased vision, irritation, and discharge in her right eye over the past 3 days. She reports that her eye has been stuck shut for the past 2 days, requiring a warm, wet washcloth to open the eye. She denies any trauma or surgery. She denies any contacts with ill individuals and does not have any fevers, chills, malaise, or any other ill symptoms. Her past medical history includes hypertension and a hysterectomy 10 years ago. She reports no allergies to medications and uses metoprolol for hypertension. She denies any family history of eye disease.

The patient is healthy with a negative review of systems other than her ocular complaints. She is wearing glasses. On examination, her corrected visual acuity with glasses is 20/40 OD and 20/25 OS. Manifest refraction OD is −2.50 −1.00 × 85 and corrects her to 20/30. Her manifest refraction OS is −2.00 − 0.75 × 90, which corrects her vision to 20/20. There is no afferent pupillary defect. Slit-lamp examination of the left eye is normal. The right conjunctiva is injected and edematous. There is mucopurulent discharge from the lower lid (▸ Fig. 3.1). The inferior fornix is covered with a fibrin–mucus pseudomembrane (▸ Fig. 3.2). The inferior and superior palpebral conjunctiva show a 2+ papillary reaction. The corneas are clear and with no evidence of scarring or inflammation. The anterior chambers are quiet. The right lens demonstrates mild cataractous changes. The left lens is clear. The posterior poles of the right and left eyes are normal. The cup-to-disc ratio is 0.4 in both eyes. Intraocular pressures are 18 and 15 mm Hg, respectively. Mucus from the right eye is submitted for Gram stain, and cultures are plated on blood and chocolate agar.

Differential Diagnosis—Key Points

1. Conjunctival redness with irritation and discharge is a typical feature of bacterial conjunctivitis. The presence of purulent discharge that crusts and seals the eyelids, lack of itching, and no history of conjunctivitis point to a bacterial cause of conjunctivitis. Although the absence of ill contacts and negative review of systems does not exclude the possibility of a viral etiology, it does makes it less likely. Onset of symptoms over less than 24 hours with copious purulent discharge must alert one to the possibility of more virulent genera such as *Neisseria*.

2. Rapidity of symptom onset can be useful for clinical diagnosis and for suggesting a causative organism (▸ Table 3.1).

3. Uncomplicated bacterial conjunctivitis is generally self-limited within 1 to 2 weeks of presentation. However, empiric treatment with any broad spectrum topical ophthalmic antibiotic can shorten symptom duration and decrease transmissibility.

4. Gram stain and conjunctival cultures are not necessary in cases of uncomplicated suspected bacterial conjunctivitis but should be performed in neonates, immunocompromised individuals, and in cases of refractory, recurrent, and copiously purulent conjunctivitis.

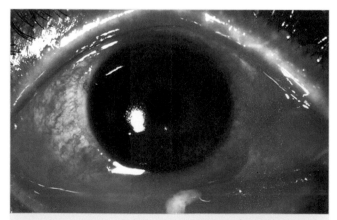

Fig. 3.1 The right eye shows hyperemia and discharge from the lower lid.

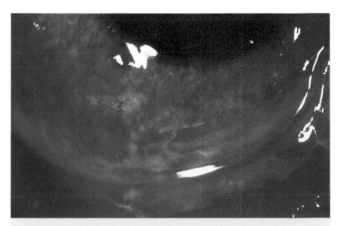

Fig. 3.2 The inferior fornix of the right eye demonstrating an inflammatory pseudomembrane covering the tarsal conjunctiva.

Table 3.1 Bacterial conjunctivitis

	Onset		
	Hyperacute (< 24 h)	**Acute (hours to days)**	**Slow (days to weeks)**
Organisms	*Neisseria gonorrhoeae*	*Haemophilus influenzae*	Enterobacteriaceae
	Neisseria meningitidis	*Staphylococcus aureus*	*Moraxella lacunata*
		Streptococcus pneumoniae	*Pseudomonas*
			Staphylococcus aureus
			Proteus spp

3.2 Test Interpretation

The Gram stain showed numerous gram-positive cocci in pairs and numerous polymorphonuclear lymphocytes. Cultures grew *Streptococcus pneumoniae* that was sensitive to penicillin, ciprofloxacin, vancomycin, and trimethoprim/sulfamethoxazole.

3.3 Diagnosis

Streptococcal pneumoniae bacterial conjunctivitis with the formation of inflammatory pseudomembranes.

Acute bacterial conjunctivitis presents as a red eye with conjunctival injection, chemosis, and purulent or mucopurulent discharge. Patients experience ocular irritation and may report that their eyelids are stuck together in the morning due to discharge. These symptoms begin in one eye and infection can spread to the other eye, often within 24 to 48 hours. Incidence of bacterial conjunctivitis was estimated at 135 in 10,000 in one study and is less common in adults than viral conjunctivitis. However, it may be responsible for 50 to 70% of conjunctivitis in children and is the eye disease most commonly seen by primary care doctors, estimated at 1% of all consultations.

When diagnosing bacterial conjunctivitis, it is important to (1) differentiate bacterial from other forms of conjunctivitis (e.g., viral, allergic) and (2) identify hyperacute bacterial conjunctivitis, which requires more intensive and systemic treatment.

It can be difficult to discern the underlying cause of conjunctivitis as symptoms are often nonspecific. Classically, a purulent/mucopurulent discharge and the presence of conjunctival papillae favor a bacterial cause, while watery discharge associated with follicles suggests a viral origin. However, a large meta-analysis found that these signs and symptoms did not correlate with underlying cause of conjunctivitis. Instead, a recent study found that the strongest predictors of bacterial conjunctivitis are a combination of three signs—lack of itching, no history of conjunctivitis, and one (and especially two) glued eyelids.

It is not necessary to perform Gram stain and conjunctival cultures in cases of suspected uncomplicated bacterial conjunctivitis. However, cultures should be performed in neonatal or immunocompromised patients and in cases of refractory, recurrent, or severe purulent conjunctivitis.

It is critical to identify hyperacute bacterial conjunctivitis (e.g., gonococcal conjunctivitis). These patients present with copious purulent discharge and decreased vision and often eyelid swelling, tenderness to palpation of the eye, and preauricular adenopathy. In such cases, there is a high risk of corneal involvement and risk of corneal perforation.

3.4 Medical Management

This patient can be managed medically with topical antibiotic drops. She was treated with trimethoprim sulfate–polymyxin B drops four times a day for 7 days. After 2 days, her symptoms had improved significantly.

Most cases of bacterial conjunctivitis are self-limiting within 1 to 2 weeks, and no differences in outcome have been observed in antibiotic treatment versus placebo groups. Thus, no treatment and immediate treatment are both reasonable approaches. However, antibiotic therapy leads to quicker recovery and return to work/school and decreases risk of transmission. All broad-spectrum antibiotic eye drops are generally effective for treating empiric bacterial conjunctivitis. Polymyxin combination drops, aminoglycosides, fluoroquinolones, and bacitracin used four times daily for a week are options for treatment. Warm compresses and artificial tears can be offered for comfort. Patients should be cautioned to avoid touching their eyes or sharing towels or washcloths while symptomatic.

Hyperacute conjunctivitis, on the other hand, mandates quick diagnosis and more aggressive therapy as serious complications such as corneal perforation can occur. A Gram stain that shows gram-negative diplococcus is highly suggestive of gonococcal conjunctivitis. Treatment consists of a one-time intramuscular dose of ceftriaxone if the cornea is not involved. If the cornea is affected, inpatient ceftriaxone intravenous therapy in combination with topical bacitracin, gentamicin, ciprofloxacin, or besifloxacin is used. In addition, frequent (every 30–60 minutes) saline irrigation of the conjunctiva is necessary. Possible chlamydial coinfection should be treated as well since up to one-third of patients with gonococcal conjunctivitis have concurrent chlamydia venereal disease.

3.5 Surgical Management

There is almost no role for surgery in acute bacterial conjunctivitis. Inflammatory membranes or pseudomembranes can be seen in several types of conjunctivitis, such as *Clostridium diphtheriae*, *Neisseria gonorrhoeae*, or beta-hemolytic *Streptococci*, viral conjunctivitis, or ligneous conjunctivitis. Pseudomembranes consisting of fibrin-rich exudate may be easily peeled from the conjunctiva, while the true membranes seen in more severe cases cause bleeding when removed. There is insufficient evidence to recommend for or against (pseudo)membrane debridement.

Suggested Reading

[1] Haimovici R, Roussel TJ. Treatment of gonococcal conjunctivitis with single-dose intramuscular ceftriaxone. Am J Ophthalmol. 1989; 107(5):511–514

[2] Limberg MB. A review of bacterial keratitis and bacterial conjunctivitis. Am J Ophthalmol. 1991; 112(4) Suppl:2S–9S

[3] McGill JI. Bacterial conjunctivitis. Trans Ophthalmol Soc U K. 1986; 105(Pt 1): 37–40

[4] Høvding G. Acute bacterial conjunctivitis. Acta Ophthalmol. 2008; 86(1):5–17

[5] Rietveld RP, ter Riet G, Bindels PJ, Sloos JH, van Weert HC. Predicting bacterial cause in infectious conjunctivitis: cohort study on informativeness of combinations of signs and symptoms. BMJ. 2004; 329(7459):206–210

[6] Rietveld RP, van Weert HC, ter Riet G, Bindels PJ. Diagnostic impact of signs and symptoms in acute infectious conjunctivitis: systematic literature search. BMJ. 2003; 327(7418):789

[7] Azari AA, Barney NP, Conjunctivitis A. Conjunctivitis: a systematic review of diagnosis and treatment. JAMA. 2013; 310(16):1721–1729

[8] AAO Corneal/External Disease Preferred Practice Pattern Panel, Hoskins Center for Quality Eye Care. Conjunctivitis PPP – 2013. Available at: http://www.aao.org/preferred-practice-pattern/conjunctivitis-ppp-2013. Published October 2013

[9] American Academy of Ophthalmology. Infectious diseases of the external eye: microbial and parasitic infections. In: Basic and Clinical Science Course (BCSC), Section 8: External Disease and Cornea. San Francisco, CA: American Academy of Ophthalmology; 2012–2013:150

4 Pterygium

Weldon W. Haw and Edward E. Manche

Abstract

A pterygium is a nonmalignant, fibrovascular overgrowth of the bulbar conjunctiva typically in the nasal interpalpebral fissure. It is often related to exposure to ultraviolet light and/or chronic dry eye disease. It is important to distinguish a pterygium from malignant conditions such as conjunctival intraepithelial neoplasia. An atypical vascular pattern, appearance, or location may increase the suspicion of a malignant lesion. In most instances, a pterygium that is not symptomatic or impacting vision can be treated conservatively with artificial tear supplementation and protection from ultraviolet light. However, surgical removal of the pterygium may be indicated in situations with progressive growth impacting vision or recalcitrant symptoms. Potential for recurrence should be discussed with the patient prior to surgical removal.

Keywords: pterygium, conjunctival intraepithelial neoplasia, pseudopterygium

4.1 History

A 32-year-old lifeguard presents with intermittent symptoms of bilateral red eye, dryness, irritation, and foreign body sensation. Visual acuity is 20/20 in both eyes. Examination reveals a fibrovascular overgrowth of the bulbar conjunctiva extending onto the cornea of both eyes (▶ Fig. 4.1).

4.2 Test Interpretation

Diagnosis is based on typical clinical presentation. Corneal topography may be useful in documenting topographic changes and identifying induced astigmatism resulting from the pterygium. Histologic examination reveals subepithelial fibrovascular tissue with disruption of Bowman's layer, increased fibroblasts, and elastoid degeneration of the underlying collagen.

4.3 Diagnosis

Pterygium, bilateral.

4.4 Medical Management

A small, nonactive, symptom-free pterygium may simply be observed. Using the slit-lamp beam to measure the horizontal and vertical dimensions of the pterygium may be useful in documenting progression on serial examinations. A small, minimally inflamed pterygium with mild symptoms may often be managed with frequent use of preservative-free artificial tears or topical nonsteroidal anti-inflammatory medications. For active exacerbation of symptoms or inflammation, a short course of a mild topical steroid may be useful in controlling the

Differential Diagnosis—Key Points

1. A pterygium is a fibrovascular overgrowth of the bulbar conjunctiva typically located in the nasal interpalpebral fissure. It is a common finding among individuals 20 to 40 years of age with exposure to ultraviolet radiation and wind. The incidence is higher in patients living closer to the equator. It occurs more commonly in males than females.

2. A pterygium in its earliest stages is indistinguishable from a pinguecula. A pinguecula is a benign, elevated, yellowish, perilimbal lesion of the interpalpebral fissure. It may arise from degenerative factors similar to pterygia. By definition, however, pingueculae do not involve the cornea. Pingueculae are believed to be precursors of pterygia.

3. A pterygium should be differentiated from a pseudopterygium. Pseudopterygia result from nonspecific inflammation from chemical injuries, trauma, burns, and infections. The resulting injury leads to a fibrovascular, bulbar conjunctival scar that extends over the cornea. A probe may be placed between the body of a pseudopterygium and the globe, whereas it may not be placed between a true pterygium and the globe. In addition, pseudopterygia differ from true pterygia as they may occur outside the interpalpebral fissure or be associated with symblepharon.

4. It is also important to distinguish a pterygium from a malignant lesion. Conjunctival intraepithelial neoplasia (CIN) may be mistaken for an atypical pterygium. CIN usually appears in the interpalpebral limbal area. It may appear as a gelatinous elevated lesion with varying degrees of keratinization, as a small elevated vascularized papillomatous lesion, or as a white plaque (leukoplakia). Although it is difficult to differentiate squamous cell carcinoma from CIN, squamous cell carcinoma tends to involve more of the limbal circumference, may be more elevated, and may be immobile or fixed to the underlying surface.

5. A pterygium may be associated with a pigmented iron line at its leading edge, the "Stocker's line," i.e., a nonspecific associated finding with no clinical value.

6. Most pterygia either grow very slowly or enter a quiescent phase. Occasionally, pterygia may either become actively inflamed or grow rapidly and progressively. Epithelial irregularity, opacification of Bowman's layer, and prominent and inflamed vessels may be predictive of an active phase.

symptoms. The topical steroid may be dosed four times daily and tapered over 2 to 3 weeks. Expected response is complete resolution of the inflammation with days of beginning the steroid. However, overly aggressive tapering of the steroids may result in recurrent inflammation. Some physicians have advocated the use of ultraviolet-blocking sunglasses and continued lubrication to limit progressive pterygium growth.

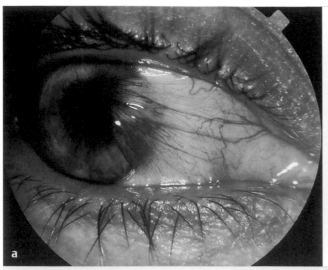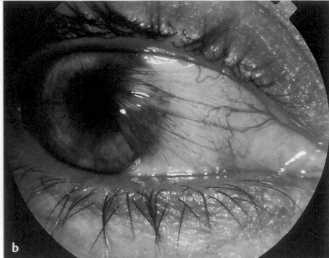

Fig. 4.1 Pterygium. Right eye.

4.5 Surgical Management

Indications for surgical pterygium excision include interference with vision from progressive growth over the visual axis, induced astigmatism, unacceptable cosmesis, and severe symptoms. Restriction of extraocular motility has also been reported. However, patients should be counseled on the published recurrence rates, which may be as high as 35 to 40%. These recurrence rates tend to be higher for fleshy, actively growing lesions. Recurrent pterygia may also demonstrate more aggressive growth as compared to the primary pterygia. Subsequent removal of recurrent pterygia may also be challenging because of fibrovascular scarring. Several techniques have been reported to diminish the recurrence rates. These include the use of irradiation, extensive removal of Tenon's capsule, application of antimetabolites such as mitomycin C, amniotic membrane transplantation, and conjunctival autografts. These adjunctive maneuvers may decrease recurrence rates to less than 5%. Complications of mitomycin C (0.02%) include persistent epithelial defects and scleral necrosis. Therefore, the concentration and duration of mitomycin C must be titrated to the appearance and aggressiveness of the pterygium, used in subconjunctival space with caution to avoid bare sclera and limbal stem cells, and used judiciously to prevent these complications.

A pterygium is usually excised under local subconjunctival anesthesia. Anesthetic infiltration with lidocaine in the correct plane will result in "tenting" up of the pterygium. This will facilitate the dissection of the pterygium and will provide adequate anesthesia for its removal. Multiple methods exist for pterygium excision. One method involves a 69 Beaver blade and Westcott scissors, which are sufficient for undermining the body of the pterygium and anterior lamellar dissection of the corneal component of the pterygium. Removal of Tenon's capsule with preservation of the overlying conjunctiva is an important step in reducing recurrence rate and optimizing postoperative results. Sending the pterygium to an appropriate ocular pathology laboratory for histopathologic examination will confirm the diagnosis. Primary conjunctival anastomosis, rotational flaps, and various conjunctival autograft or amniotic membrane transplantation techniques have been used to close the conjunctival defect created by pterygium excision. Sutures or fibrin glue can be used to secure the autologous conjunctival graft or amniotic membrane graft. Following the surgery, patients may be started on a topical antibiotic four times a day until the surface has completely re-epithelialized. A topical corticosteroid should be administered and tapered according to the severity of the postoperative inflammatory response.

4.6 Rehabilitation and Follow-up

Follow-up for medically managed pterygia is dictated by the severity of symptoms and the proximity to the visual axis. If topical steroids are used for inflammatory pterygia or during the postoperative period, earlier follow-up is indicated to assess response and to evaluate the intraocular pressure.

Suggested Reading

[1] American Academy of Ophthalmology. External disease and cornea. In: Basic and Clinical Science Course. Section 8. San Francisco, CA: American Academy of Ophthalmology;1995–1996

[2] Hoffman RS, Power WJ. Current options in pterygium management. Int Ophthalmol Clin. 1999; 39(1):15–26

[3] Leibowitz HM, Waring GO. Corneal Disorders: Clinical Diagnosis and Management. 2nd ed. Philadelphia, PA: WB Saunders Co; 1998

[4] Mutlu FM, Sobaci G, Tatar T, Yildirim E. A comparative study of recurrent pterygium surgery: limbal conjunctival autograft transplantation versus mitomycin C with conjunctival flap. Ophthalmology. 1999; 106(4):817–821

5 Recurrent Erosion/Epithelial Basement Membrane Dystrophy

Weldon W. Haw

Abstract

Epithelial basement membrane dystrophy is the most common corneal dystrophy. It can result in spontaneous episodes of recurrent erosions. Diagnosis can be made by historical features of a spontaneous recurrent erosion and evidence of the corneal dystrophy on slit-lamp examination. It is useful to evaluate for the dystrophy in both the involved and fellow eye. Treatment can be successful with pharmaceuticals (antibiotic prophylaxis, cycloplegia), bandage contact lens, or self-retained amniotic membrane grafts. Occasionally, surgical alternatives may be required. Epithelial debridement, scraping, anterior stromal micropuncture, or excimer laser phototherapeutic keratectomy can result in long-term symptom-free remissions. Hypertonic solutions are useful in maintenance therapy.

Keywords: recurrent erosion syndrome, corneal dystrophy, map-dot-fingerprint dystrophy, epithelial basement membrane dystrophy, corneal abrasion, phototherapeutic keratectomy

5.1 History

A 35-year-old woman awoke from sleep with sudden onset of unilateral pain, foreign body sensation, lacrimation, photophobia, and blurred vision immediately upon opening her eyes. The patient had a previous history of multiple similar episodes occurring in either eye. The patient's mother has also been affected with similar episodes. She had no history of prior ocular trauma.

Visual acuity is 20/400 in the involved eye and 20/20 in the fellow eye. Slit-lamp examination of the involved eye revealed a large, discrete area of epithelial sloughing (▶ Fig. 5.1). The edges of the epithelial defect were remarkable for a "heaped-up" appearance. No infiltrate was apparent. Fluorescein dye revealed pooling over the epithelial defect. Examination of the fellow eye was remarkable for diffuse, superficial gray-white opacities in a "map" and "dot" configuration (▶ Fig. 5.2).

Differential Diagnosis—Key Points

1. Onset of symptoms was sudden and noted by the patient upon opening her eyes while awakening. The prior day, the patient had not noticed any premonitory symptoms. This is the classic presentation of recurrent erosion syndrome. As the patient opens his or her eyes, the corneal epithelium that is loosely adherent to the underlying abnormal basement membrane may be pulled off, causing a discrete epithelial defect.

2. Notably, there was no acute, inciting event such as trauma. The epithelium was shed spontaneously. Also, the patient had a history of multiple spontaneous episodes. Thus, the examiner should note that the diagnosis is not a simple corneal abrasion.

3. On examination, discrete roughening of the corneal epithelium is noted with a "sloughed-off" appearance. The dislodged epithelium appears to be shed in a single large "sheet." This is also the typical appearance of a recurrent erosion resulting from pathological adherence of the epithelium to the underlying basement membrane. Occasionally, symptoms may have improved by the time the patient is examined as the epithelial changes may resolve rapidly if the defect is small.

4. Recurrent epithelial erosion is usually noted among one of two populations. The first population consists of patients with a prior history of abrading trauma or surgery in the affected eye. The second population consists of patients with an underlying corneal dystrophy. Map-dot-fingerprint dystrophy is the most common, accounting for an estimated 50% of patients with recurrent epithelial erosion syndrome. However, other basement membrane dystrophies may also present with recurrent erosions. These include Meesmann's and Reis–Bücklers dystrophies. Anterior stromal corneal dystrophies such as lattice, macular, and granular dystrophies may also cause recurrent epithelial erosion.

5. In order to differentiate between these causes, the examiner should inquire about a past history of corneal trauma or injury and whether recurrent episodes are unilateral or bilateral. Our patient denied a history of corneal injury (although the patient may often forget about a minor ocular injury in the past, as recurrent erosion may occur many years after the initial injury). Our patient also noted that her recurrent episodes occurred in either eye. These historical features suggest an underlying corneal dystrophy rather than a past traumatic event as the underlying etiology.

6. Family history may also be positive in a patient with corneal dystrophies. Our patient had a mother who reports similar episodes. Map-dot-fingerprint dystrophy may be inherited in a dominant pattern, usually with incomplete penetrance.

7. Examination of the contralateral, noninvolved eye is also important as it may reveal evidence of dystrophic changes. Examination of this patient's fellow eye demonstrated a typical pattern of map-dot-fingerprint changes. Fingerprint lines are thin concentric lines arranged in a pattern that resembles the prints on the end of a finger. Thicker geographic lines surrounded by a faint haze are called map lines. Dots are discrete, gray-white circular or oval lesions of varying sizes. These corneal changes may be variable and can change over time within the same individual. These changes may be quite subtle and may require careful examination. Map lines, dots, and fingerprint lines may be identified at the slit lamp with a broad, tangential beam or through a red reflex (▶ Table 5.1; see also the following list).

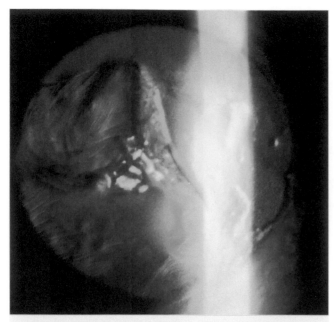

Fig. 5.1 Recurrent erosion: red reflex examination demonstrates diffuse sloughing of the epithelium as a large sheet.

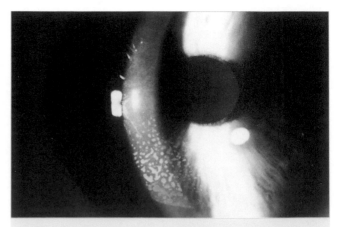

Fig. 5.2 Epithelial basement membrane dystrophy: careful slit-lamp examination reveals superficial gray-white opacities characteristic of "map" and "dot" changes.

Table 5.1 Differentiation of etiology of recurrent erosion

Traumatic	Map-dot-fingerprint
History of corneal trauma/injury in affected eye	No history of trauma
Unilateral recurrent episodes	May be bilateral recurrent episodes
No family history	May have positive family history (autosomal dominant with incomplete penetrance)
Contralateral eye—normal examination	Contralateral eye—may have evidence of map-dot-fingerprint changes

5.1.1 Summary of Epithelial Basement Membrane Dystrophy

- Most common corneal dystrophy.
- Estimated 2% of population may have dystrophy.
- May represent an estimated 50% of recurrent erosions.
- Autosomal dominant—female predominance.
- Map lines, fingerprint lines, and dots.

5.2 Test Interpretation

Diagnosis is made by careful slit-lamp examination of the involved and fellow eyes. The ocular and family history may also be useful. No ancillary tests are required for diagnosis.

5.3 Diagnosis

Recurrent epithelial erosion syndrome, basement membrane dystrophy type.

5.4 Medical Management

Medical management during the acute stage is directed at safely promoting epithelial healing while maximizing patient comfort. The application of a prophylactic topical antibiotic ointment in conjunction with a pressure patch for 24 to 48 hours may achieve both of these goals. Cycloplegia may also be useful in relieving discomfort for those patients with a significant associated anterior chamber reaction or ciliary spasm. Some clinicians have advocated the use of a soft bandage contact lens to facilitate epithelial healing. However, the use of a contact lens may lead to complications of a "tight lens syndrome" or secondary infectious keratitis. Self-retained amniotic membrane grafts are available and can be placed in the clinic setting. Both cryopreserved (Prokera) and dehydrated amniotic membrane (AmbioDisk) grafts may promote healing of the corneal epithelium.

5.5 Surgical Management

In more severe or recurrent cases, it may be necessary to pursue more aggressive therapeutic interventions. These include the use of total epithelial debridement, anterior stromal micropuncture, or excimer laser phototherapeutic keratectomy (PTK).

Epithelial debridement is most appropriately performed during the acute phase and is done by gently scraping the edge of the epithelial defect with a moist Q-tip or cellulose sponge under topical anesthesia. Performing this procedure during the acute phase is appropriate as it may cause considerable ocular discomfort. The remaining involved epithelium may then be peeled off with a nontoothed forceps. The involved eye is then managed as described earlier (antibiotic ointment, patch, bandage contact lens, or self-retained amniotic membrane graft). Since epithelial basement membrane dystrophy is a diffuse disease, gentle epithelial debridement should be performed over the entire surface of the cornea. Bowman's membrane should not be violated as this may result in subepithelial scarring. Following this procedure, patients may remain symptom-free for 1 or 2 years. However, recurrences are possible.

Anterior stromal micropuncture involves making between 15 and 25 anterior stromal micropunctures with a bent 25-gauge needle. This induces a cicatricial adhesion between the epithelium and anterior stroma. This technique is most useful in patients with posttraumatic recurrent erosions localized outside the visual axis. Following anterior stromal micropuncture, topical antibiotic ointment, cycloplegia, and a pressure patch are applied.

The newest development in the management of recurrent erosions involves the use of the excimer laser in a procedure labeled PTK or phototherapeutic keratectomy. This procedure involves removing the epithelium either manually or by laser scrape and subsequent superficial photoablation of the cornea. The entire cornea should be treated in patients with underlying anterior corneal dystrophies. This wide superficial ablation is particularly useful in the treatment of an underlying anterior corneal dystrophy associated with significant visual impairment due to scarring or recalcitrant, recurrent erosions. Complications of excimer laser PTK include delayed corneal wound healing and refractive changes.

5.6 Rehabilitation and Follow-up

Careful follow-up until resolution of the epithelial defect is recommended. It is important to be vigilant for the development of infectious keratitis. After the resolution of the epithelial defect, it may be important for patients with recurrent epithelial erosions to maintain adequate lubrication with nonpreserved artificial tears four to eight times per day and with artificial tear ointment prior to bedtime. The lubrication may prevent the lid from applying traction to epithelium loosely adherent to the underlying basement membrane. In addition, hypertonic solutions such as 5% sodium chloride have the theoretical advantage of osmotically drawing fluid from the epithelium and promoting adherence to the underlying basement membrane. Thus, 5% sodium chloride drops during the day and 5% sodium chloride ointment prior to bedtime may be useful as an alternative to artificial tears for 3 or more months following the acute episode. Vision may be impacted by irregular astigmatism or corneal haze. A corneal topography may be useful in identifying these circumstances.

Suggested Reading

[1] American Academy of Ophthalmology. External disease and cornea. In: Basic and Clinical Science Course. Section 8. San Francisco, CA: American Academy of Ophthalmology; 1995–1996

[2] Cavanaugh TB, Lind DM, Cutarelli PE, et al. Phototherapeutic keratectomy for recurrent erosion syndrome in anterior basement membrane dystrophy. Ophthalmology. 1999; 106(5):971–976

[3] Smolin G, Thoft RA. The Cornea. 3rd ed. Boston, MA: Little, Brown & Co; 1994

6 Fuchs' Corneal Dystrophy

Weldon W. Haw

Abstract

Fuchs' endothelial dystrophy is a slowly progressive dystrophy that results in cornea stromal edema associated with concurrent loss of endothelial cell density. Stromal edema may be most severe in the morning hours, and patients may notice a diurnal vision fluctuation associated with worse vision in the morning hours. Clinical features of Fuchs' endothelial dystrophy include the presence of corneal guttate with or without the presence of corneal edema. The cornea thickness may be elevated on pachymetry. Specular microscopy may be useful in qualitatively and quantitatively examining the endothelial cell layer. In mild instances, patients may be managed pharmacologically with a hypertonic ophthalmic solution. In more advanced situations, surgical management with endothelial transplantation procedures (DSAEK, DMEK, etc.) or penetrating keratoplasty (i.e., in advanced cases with corneal scarring) may be entertained.

Keywords: Fuchs' endothelial dystrophy, corneal dystrophy, endothelial dystrophy, corneal edema, cornea transplant, endothelial transplant, DSAEK, DMEK, penetrating keratoplasty

6.1 History

A 60-year-old woman presented with a history of slowly progressive loss of vision in the left greater than the right eye. Initially, her vision was worse upon awakening and gradually cleared as the day went on; more recently, however, her vision remained poor throughout the day.

Examination revealed corrected visual acuities of 20/200 in the right eye and counting fingers at 4 feet in the left eye. Intraocular pressure was 14 mm Hg in each eye. Slit-lamp examination of the cornea revealed central microcystic epithelial edema and stromal edema with folds in Descemet's membrane in the left greater than the right eye (▶ Fig. 6.1). Corneal guttatae and endothelial pigmentation extended over the central portion of the cornea in both eyes. The anterior chamber was deep and quiet, and the iris was normal in both eyes. Moderate nuclear sclerotic cataracts were present bilaterally, and dilated fundus examination revealed normal posterior poles through a hazy view. B-scan ultrasonography of the posterior poles was unremarkable.

Differential Diagnosis—Key Points

1. Corneal edema can be divided into congenital and acquired causes. Congenital causes include dystrophies such as posterior polymorphous dystrophy, congenital hereditary endothelial dystrophy, congenital glaucoma, and forceps injury. Acquired causes include pseudophakic/aphakic bullous keratopathy, Fuchs' corneal dystrophy, angle closure glaucoma, herpes simplex stromal keratitis, varicella zoster keratitis, iridocorneal endothelial (ICE) syndrome, posterior polymorphous dystrophy, hypotony, corneal hydrops (as in keratoconus), and trauma.

2. Endothelial dysfunction causes secondary stromal edema that is worse in the morning. Eyelid closure while sleeping decreases surface evaporation and maximizes corneal edema upon awakening.

3. Corneal edema is a necessary component of Fuchs' corneal dystrophy. Patients with guttata but without corneal edema are considered to have "endothelial dystrophy."

4. In addition to complaints of decreased vision, patients with advanced Fuchs' dystrophy often complain of episodes of sharp pain due to rupture of epithelial bullae. Clinical examination readily distinguishes these patients from those with recurrent erosion syndrome, who may have similar complaints.

6.2 Test Interpretation

The diagnosis of Fuchs' corneal dystrophy is usually made on the basis of the classic slit-lamp findings of epithelial and stromal edema, endothelial guttata, and endothelial pigmentation, all of which are most prominent in the central cornea.

Ultrasonic pachymetry can sometimes be helpful in detecting early subclinical corneal thickening in endothelial dystrophy and in following progression of the endothelial dystrophy. This information is useful in determining the likelihood of corneal decompensation following cataract extraction. A general rule of thumb is to proceed with cataract extraction alone if central pachymetry is less than 600 μm, and to proceed with a combined corneal endothelial transplant procedure such as Descemet's stripping automated endothelial keratoplasty (DSAEK) or Descemet's membrane endothelial keratoplasty (DMEK) in conjunction with cataract extraction if central pachymetry is greater than 600 μm. This rule of thumb is only loosely applicable, however, as trauma to the endothelium during cataract extraction varies greatly depending on the degree of skill of the

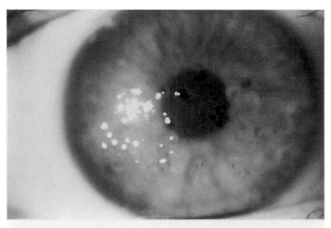

Fig. 6.1 Advanced Fuchs' corneal dystrophy with severe stromal and epithelial edema. (The image is provided courtesy of Peter R. Laibson, MD, Philadelphia, PA.)

surgeon, as well as on the density of the nucleus. If cataract surgery alone is planned, several endothelial protective measures during cataract surgery can be incorporated in order to minimize trauma to the endothelium. These include the use of a dispersive or viscoadaptive viscoelastic for endothelial protection during phacoemulsification, endocapsular and chop phacoemulsification techniques, and BSS plus (balance salt saline solution) irrigation fluid.

Specular microscopy can be useful in further elucidating the status of the endothelium in early Fuchs' corneal dystrophy. Guttata are seen as dark spots within the mosaic of endothelial cells. Increased variability in cell shape (pleomorphism) and size (polymegathism) is typically present, and overall cell density is diminished when compared to normal. As Fuchs' corneal dystrophy progresses, specular microscopy becomes more difficult to perform because of increasing corneal edema.

6.3 Diagnosis

1. Fuchs' corneal dystrophy OU.
2. Cataract OU.

6.4 Medical Management

In endothelial dystrophy, the patient is usually asymptomatic and no treatment is necessary. In early Fuchs' corneal dystrophy, "morning blur" secondary to corneal edema can be reduced through the use of hypertonic sodium chloride (e.g., NaCl 5%) drops. Initially, these may be required only upon awakening, but as the disease progresses, they may be required throughout the day. Hypertonic sodium chloride ointment at bedtime may also reduce morning blur. Another approach to reducing corneal edema involves using a hair dryer to dehydrate the cornea. The hair dryer is placed on the lowest setting and is directed toward the cornea at arm's length for several minutes. Eventually, progressive endothelial failure overwhelms such measures and corneal transplantation is necessary to rehabilitate vision.

6.5 Surgical Management

When corneal edema advances to the point where visual function is significantly affected despite conservative management, a corneal transplantation procedure is indicated. There are several surgical approaches available to a patient with Fuchs' endothelial dystrophy, including DSAEK, DMEK, or penetrating keratoplasty (PKP).

In most cases of Fuchs' endothelial dystrophy, there is pure endothelial dysfunction/corneal edema without corneal scarring. In these instances, endothelial transplantation procedures such as DSAEK or DMEK can be considered. These endothelial transplant procedures are less invasive and have more rapid visual recovery, less induced corneal astigmatism, and less graft rejection than traditional penetrating corneal transplant procedures (i.e., PKP). In DSAEK, the host endothelium is stripped and removed and the donor's endothelium and posterior corneal stroma lenticel is transplanted to the posterior cornea. Often, there is a hyperopic shift of approximately 1.0 to 1.5 D. Thus, when performed in conjunction with cataract surgery, it is important to place an intraocular lens (IOL) aiming slightly more myopic than intended correction. In DMEK, following stripping of the host Descemet's membrane, a donor's Descemet's membrane without stroma is transplanted onto the host posterior cornea. Theoretical advantages of DMEK over DSAEK include a more anatomic result with no optical interface, faster visual recovery, lower rejection rates, less hyperopic shift, and better refractive outcomes.

In instances of chronic endothelial dysfunction, bullous keratopathy associated with visually significant cornea scarring can occur. In these cases, the corneal scarring can limit the postoperative visual outcome with an endothelial (DSAEK, DMEK) transplant procedure, and this must be balanced with the risks of a PKP. As visual rehabilitation after PKP can be as long as 6 to 12 months after surgery, the patient will, for a period of time, be dependent on the less involved "better" eye for visual function in the postoperative period. Therefore, when indicated, PKP should be performed as soon as possible in the worse eye while the patient still has functional vision in the better eye.

PKP is performed using standard techniques. Simultaneous cataract extraction and IOL placement should be strongly considered if any significant lenticular opacity is present, as cataracts tend to worsen after PKP. Furthermore, cataract extraction after PKP will traumatize the endothelium and shorten graft survival. The determination of the appropriate IOL power is problematic in these patients, as postoperative keratometry cannot be predicted with great accuracy. Variations of surgical technique, the amount of oversizing of the graft, wound healing, the keratometric power of the recipient corneal rim, and donor button all contribute to the final power of the grafted cornea. Ultimately, each surgeon must develop his or her own algorithm for determining IOL power based on experience.

Suturing techniques are determined by surgeon preference and the degree of preoperative corneal edema. In cases where diffuse limbus-to-limbus edema exists, a 16-bite interrupted pattern allows for individual suture removal in the early postoperative period if necessary for suture loosening or vascularization. If the peripheral cornea is nonedematous, premature suture loosening is less of a concern, and a running or combined running–interrupted suture technique can be considered (▶ Fig. 6.2).

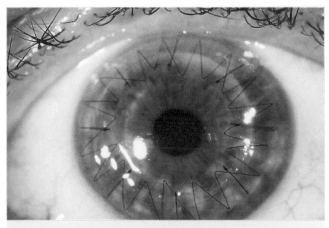

Fig. 6.2 Six weeks after penetrating keratoplasty.

6.6 Rehabilitation and Follow-up

Postoperatively, topical antibiotic and corticosteroid drops are prescribed. Ointments and/or nonpreserved artificial tears can be employed to rehabilitate the ocular surface as needed. The antibiotics are discontinued after the surface has re-epithelialized. Topical steroids are slowly tapered over 6 to 12 months. The surgeon should minimize the number and frequency of preserved topical eye drops to prevent surface toxicity. Following DSAEK or DMEK procedure, the patient should remain in the supine position until the air bubble is dissolved to allow the graft to attach. In instances of PKP, the postoperative astigmatism is managed initially by selective suture lysis and/or running suture adjustment, guided by topography. Glasses or rigid gas permeable contact lenses are prescribed when appropriate. Occasionally, high degrees of astigmatism may require surgical intervention such as astigmatic keratotomy, compression sutures, wedge resection, or, rarely, repeat PKP. Laser in situ keratomileusis (LASIK) may be useful in selected cases with large refractive errors. LASIK should be performed only after all sutures have been removed and in the presence of a secure wound.

Suggested Reading

[1] Cullom RD, Chang B, eds. Fuchs' endothelial dystrophy. In: The Wills Eye Manual: Office and Emergency Room Diagnosis and Treatment of Eye Disease. Philadelphia, PA: JB Lippincott; 1994:101–102

[2] Fuchs E. Dystrophia epithelialis corneae. Graefes Arch Clin Exp Ophthalmol. 1910; 76:478–508

[3] Roberts HW, Mukherjee A, Aichner H, Rajan MS. Visual outcomes and graft thickness in microthin DSAEK–one-year results. Cornea. 2015; 34(11):1345–1350

7 Keratoconus

Aaron Wang and Weldon W. Haw

Abstract

Keratoconus is a noninflammatory ectasia of the central cornea. Best corrected vision may be compromised from irregular corneal astigmatism and corneal scarring. Slit-lamp findings may be subtle. Corneal topography may be informative in assessing the extent of the ectasia and the severity of the disease. Treatment includes specialized rigid contact lenses, corneal cross-linking, or deep anterior lamellar or penetrating keratoplasty. We present here a case of a patient with keratoconus. The case describes typical symptoms, exam findings, differential diagnosis, testing and interpretation, and medical and surgical management for keratoconus.

Keywords: keratoconus, corneal transplant, keratoplasty, IN-TACS, hard contact lenses, pachymetry, astigmatism, corneal thinning, cornea ectasia, corneal cross-linking

7.1 History

A 19-year-old man presents with complaints of gradual decreased vision in his right eye over the past year. He has worn glasses and contacts for 9 years, and despite a recent change in his prescription and new contact lenses, he does not "see clearly." He denies any trauma, surgery, or recent eye infection. He reports his vision in both eyes was clear as a child and young adult and until last year was correctable to 20/20. His past medical history is significant for seasonal allergies. He reports allergies to penicillin and uses acetaminophen occasionally. He denies any family history of eye disease.

The patient is healthy with a negative review of systems. He is wearing contact lenses. On examination, his corrected visual acuity with contacts is 20/50 OD and 20/25 OS. Manifest refraction OD, −2.00 −7.50 × 60, only corrects him to 20/100. His manifest refraction OS is −2.25 −1.00 × 28, which corrects his vision to 20/40. There is no afferent pupillary defect. On slit-lamp examination, the lids and lashes are normal. He has an adequate tear lake and tear breakup time. The corneas are clear and with no evidence of scarring or inflammation. The anterior chamber is quiet, the lens is clear, and the posterior pole viewed after dilation is normal with a healthy foveal light reflex. The cup-to-disc ratio is 0.3 bilaterally and the intraocular pressures are 12 and 14, respectively.

On careful inspection of the cornea, mild thinning is evident centrally, Vogt's striae are visible on Descemet's membrane (▶ Fig. 7.1), and a partial Fleischer's ring is visible more prominently with cobalt blue illumination. Ultrasound pachymetry measures the corneal thickness at 450 µm in the right eye and 480 µm in the left. Computerized topography with the EyeSys system showed steepening inferiorly in the right eye (▶ Fig. 7.2). A rigid gas permeable contact lens over-refraction corrects the vision to 20/30 in the right eye.

Differential Diagnosis—Key Points

1. Individuals who present with unexplained visual deterioration must be examined carefully with attention to the cornea, anterior chamber, lens, nerve, and macula. Unexplained visual loss or deterioration must be explained by the examining ophthalmologist; otherwise, subtleties such as mild cystoid macular edema and pars planitis, a slightly swollen nerve and pseudotumor cerebri, or corneal thinning and early keratoconus will be missed.

2. There are few conditions that cause decreased vision in a young healthy patient secondary to astigmatism, ectasia, and thin corneas.

   a) Keratoconus is a disorder where the central or paracentral cornea undergoes progressive thinning, leading to irregular astigmatism and steepening where the cornea bulges out in a conelike shape. The apex of the cone is usually where the cornea is thinnest. Keratoconus is normally bilateral but usually asymmetric. Associations include atopy, Down's syndrome, eye rubbing, sleep apnea, and floppy eyelids. Hydrops, irregular corneal astigmatism, and corneal scarring can occur.

   b) Pellucid marginal degeneration may cause peripheral thinning in a quiet, uninflamed eye. It is a rare, idiopathic, bilateral condition and results in thinning inferiorly with clear overlying stroma. It can produce large amounts of irregular astigmatism usually correctable with spectacles or contacts. The apex of the cornea is usually above the area of thinning, and topography may show a crab-claw configuration.

   c) Terrien's marginal degeneration is the most common cause of peripheral thinning. It is usually seen in patients older than 40 years and causes gradual thinning and ectasia beginning superiorly. This thinning is often accompanied by lipid deposition and pannus formation. Patients have a high against-the-rule astigmatism due to flattening of the vertical meridian.

   d) Keratoglobus is a rare bilateral condition consisting of diffusely thinned corneas with ectasia and enlarged corneal diameter. It may be seen in association with connective tissue disorders. Patients with keratoglobus are prone to hydrops and perforation. Because the most pronounced thinning may be peripheral, surgical management is challenging and may require limbus-to-limbus keratoplasty.

   e) Rheumatoid arthritis may cause peripheral ulcerative keratitis in association with sclerotic processes. Central thinning, however, seen in an otherwise quiet eye, is thought to be secondary to keratoconjunctivitis sicca or upregulation of collagenases.

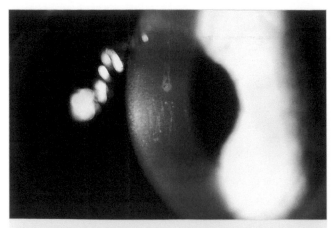

Fig. 7.1 Slit-lamp photograph of the right eye showing fine striae of Descemet's membrane, Vogt's striae, at the thinnest point in the right cornea.

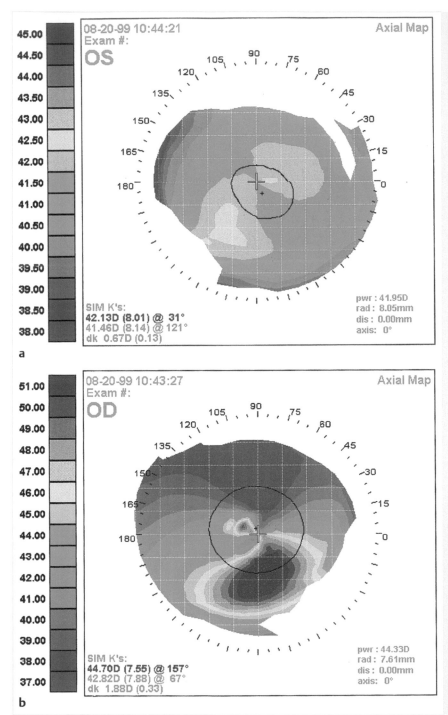

Fig. 7.2 (a) Computerized videokeratoscopy using the EyeSys system demonstrates in the right eye inferior steepening and superoinferior dioptric asymmetry. **(b)** The left eye appears relatively normal, but the cornea is thinner than average.

7.2 Test Interpretation

The major diagnostic consideration in this patient stems from unexplained visual loss in what at first appears to be a normal exam. Careful examination reveals few striae in Descemet's membrane and central thinning. Refraction demonstrates asymmetric high astigmatism with an oblique axis. Improvement with a rigid gas permeable contact lens over-refraction is suggestive of a corneal cause for the patient's abnormal best spectacle-corrected visual acuity.

The cornea is normally thickest nasally and inferiorly and thins centrally to approximately 540 µm. Corneal thickness is best measured with an ultrasound pachymeter. Using sound waves calibrated to travel in the cornea, ultrasound pachymetry gives reliable, reproducible measurements. This patient has thin corneas, more so in the right eye.

Cobalt blue illumination highlights iron deposition in the epithelium, which frequently occurs over irregular surfaces or a change in curvature. In keratoconus, hemosiderin accumulates in the epithelium around the base of a cone.

Computer-assisted videokeratoscopy or topography is one of the most helpful tests when corneal abnormalities are detected or suspected. Computerized topography most commonly employs a Placido disc nose cone and a computer-based keratoscope to capture the image and rapidly analyze the data. The computer examines topographic data points across the Placido rings and generates a color-coded map that corresponds to corneal curvature. In this case, the asymmetry between the curvature above and below the horizontal meridian is highly suggestive of keratoconus. In addition to measuring the anterior corneal curvature, optical topography units (i.e., Pentacam) can also measure the corneal thickness and posterior corneal curvature, which can also be useful in identifying corneal ectasia.

7.3 Diagnosis

Keratoconus in the right eye.

7.4 Medical Management

Keratoconus is a noninflammatory corneal ectasia of unknown etiology. Its well-described findings include thinning, iron deposition in the epithelium, and breaks in Bowman's membrane. The incidence of keratoconus is approximately 1 in 2,000 and is almost always bilateral but usually asymmetric. Cases that appear to be unilateral will often progress over time to include the other eye. Most patients, as in the case here, can be managed medically with glasses or contact lenses. If spectacle or soft contact lens correction fails to yield good visual results, then a rigid gas permeable lens or a toric lens may be used to maximize visual acuity. In more advanced keratoconus where the cornea is more protuberant, a larger hard contact lens such as a scleral lens or specialty hybrid contact lens may be needed.

This patient presented with mild keratoconus and was not correctable with glasses or soft contacts but was able to see 20/30 with rigid gas permeable lenses. Were this patient not able to see well with hard contacts and if the thinning were to progress, surgical treatment might be necessary.

7.5 Surgical Management

Keratoconus can progress and the patient may no longer benefit from contact lens wear. Ultraviolet light/riboflavin collagen cross-linking of the cornea may stiffen the cornea and slow the progression of keratoconus. Surgery would be the next step for advanced patients who have difficulty achieving a proper contact lens fit or have become intolerant of contact lens wearing, or those who have significant central corneal scarring or poor vision despite the rigid contact lens.

Surgical options include penetrating keratoplasty (PKP), deep anterior lamellar keratoplasty (DALK), or intracorneal ring segments (e.g., INTACS). INTACS can be used to flatten the cornea and address a moderate degree of myopia. With the assistance of many active eye banks, corneal transplantation has proved to be very successful for patients with advanced keratoconus and/or significant corneal scarring. Five-year success rates for PKP in patients with keratoconus approach 95%. Nonetheless, after PKP, patients are forever at risk for rejection and must be followed. Patients are treated with topical corticosteroids, which are tapered over time. Other complications include residual astigmatism, myopia, glaucoma, cataract, and mydriasis.

An alternative to PKP, DALK has some advantages. With the patient's own Descemet's membrane and the endothelium left intact, the eye is structurally more secure both during and after surgery, leading to fewer postoperative complications and more rapid visual rehabilitation. Technically, however, lamellar keratoplasty is a more challenging procedure. Recent studies found evidence that rejection is less likely to occur with DALK as compared to PKP. Best corrected visual acuity and refractive outcomes have been similar between DALK and PKP.

7.6 Rehabilitation and Follow-up

This patient has done well in a rigid gas permeable contact lens for the right eye. The left eye may eventually show changes consistent with keratoconus.

Suggested Reading

[1] Keane M, Coster D, Ziaei M, Williams K. Deep anterior lamellar keratoplasty versus penetrating keratoplasty for treating keratoconus. Cochrane Database Syst Rev. 2014(7):CD009700

[2] Kennedy RH, Bourne WM, Dyer JA. A 48-year clinical and epidemiologic study of keratoconus. Am J Ophthalmol. 1986; 101(3):267–273

[3] Krachmer JH, Feder RS, Belin MW. Keratoconus and related noninflammatory corneal thinning disorders. Surv Ophthalmol. 1984; 28(4):293–322

[4] MacIntyre R, Chow SP, Chan E, Poon A. Long-term outcomes of deep anterior lamellar keratoplasty versus penetrating keratoplasty in Australian keratoconus patients. Cornea. 2014; 33(1):6–9

[5] Maeda N, Klyce SD, Smolek MK. Comparison of methods for detecting keratoconus using videokeratography. Arch Ophthalmol. 1995; 113(7):870–874

[6] Rabinowitz YS. Keratoconus. Surv Ophthalmol. 1998; 42(4):297–319

8 Microbial Keratitis

Weldon W. Haw

Abstract

Microbial keratitis can be caused by several different bacteria. Previous contact lens wear, history of trauma, and compromised ocular surface are common contributing risk factors to the development of microbial keratitis. Diagnostic stains, culture, and sensitivities may assist in guiding directed antibiotic therapy. Aggressive treatment with broad-spectrum empiric antibiotics is warranted while waiting for identification of the causative organism. Topical ophthalmic steroids must be used with caution. Occasionally, glue or surgical alternatives may be required to maintain the integrity of the globe in cases of corneal perforation. If penetrating keratoplasty is required, it is essential to remove the infection in its entirety. Long-term graft survival may be compromised in performing a penetrating keratoplasty in an actively infected/inflamed cornea.

Keywords: corneal ulcer, keratitis, corneal infection

8.1 History

A 39-year-old woman, with a history of contact lens wear, presents with complaints of decreased vision, pain, photophobia, redness, and discharge in her left eye for the previous 48 hours.

Visual acuity was 20/20 OD and CF 3'OS. Examination of the right eye was unremarkable. Left eye external examination showed mild lid and conjunctival edema, a papillary conjunctival reaction, and a purulent discharge. The corneal stroma showed a central, dense, gray-white, necrotic-appearing infiltrate with loss of the overlying corneal epithelium (▶ Fig. 8.1). The edges of the infiltrate were indistinct and extended beyond the stromal opacity. The anterior chamber showed 2 + cell and flare and a 1-mm hypopyon. The iris, lens, and retinal examinations were unremarkable.

Subsequent examination 4 days later showed vision of 20/20 OD and 20/400 OS. Left eye examination showed minimal lid and conjunctival edema and scant purulent discharge. The cornea showed a condensing gray-white opacity with defined borders. The corneal epithelium was filling in the edges of the opacity. Examination 11 days after initial presentation showed vision of 20/20 OD and 20/400 OS. The gray-white stromal opacity had condensed further with continued corneal re-epithelialization (▶ Fig. 8.2). Subsequent examination 1 month later showed vision of 20/20 OD and 20/50 OS, and a central corneal stromal opacity.

Differential Diagnosis—Key Points

1. The differential diagnosis of a corneal ulcer is extensive including microbial, inflammatory, hypersensitive, or immune-mediated processes. The history and clinical examination in patients presenting with corneal ulcers is imperative as differentiation among etiologies can be challenging.

2. In a patient with a history of contact lens wear and the above symptoms and clinical findings, the presumptive diagnosis is microbial bacterial keratitis. It is important to identify risk factors that predispose to bacterial corneal ulcers. Contact lens wear was found to be a predisposing factor in 56% of patients in the Olmstead County study. In particular, patients should be inquired about history of any overnight wear and methods of contact lens hygiene. Other predisposing risk factors included ocular trauma (25%), lid dysfunction, ocular surface disease, conjunctival dysfunction, and lacrimal dysfunction.

3. The history of contact lens wear, lack of epithelium overlying the infiltrate, central site of the ulceration, and the presence of a suppurative reaction are all factors that point to a likely diagnosis of bacterial keratitis in this patient.

4. Bacteria that cause microbial keratitis can be divided into categories based on the clinical condition of the cornea. *Staphylococcus, Streptococcus, Pseudomonas,* Enterobacteriaceae, *Moraxella,* and *Klebsiella* have all been isolated from healthy corneal tissue. *Staphylococcus aureus, Staphylococcus epidermidis, alpha-hemolytic* and *beta-hemolytic Streptococcus, Pseudomonas,* and *Proteus* have more commonly been isolated from compromised corneas. *Pseudomonas, Staphylococcus,* and fungi have been isolated from pediatric corneas.

5. Some bacteria produce a characteristic clinical appearance. *Pseudomonas* typically has a yellowish-green discharge that sticks to the corneal surface. The gram-positive cocci, such as *S. aureus* and *Streptococcus pneumoniae,* often produce round or oval ulcers with distinct borders that are gray-white and dry in appearance. There is frequently a severe anterior chamber reaction that may include a sterile hypopyon. Gram-negative rods usually produce a wet, soupy infiltrate that may spread to involve the entire cornea and typically are associated with a severe anterior chamber reaction with hypopyon formation.

6. When bacterial keratitis is suspected, appropriate laboratory workup is indicated. This usually consists of scraping the ulcer margins and sending the specimen for bacterial (and in some cases fungal) cultures.

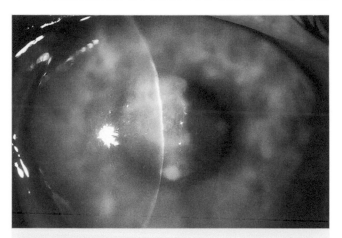

Fig. 8.1 Corneal stroma with a central, dense, gray-white, necrotic-appearing infiltrate and loss of the overlying corneal epithelium.

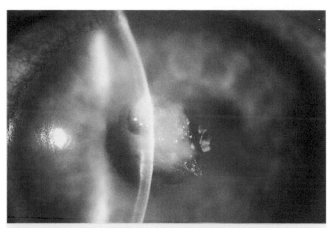

Fig. 8.2 Condensation of gray-white stromal opacity and partial corneal re-epithelialization.

8.2 Test Interpretation

The diagnosis of bacterial keratitis is generally made by taking a thorough history and performing a clinical examination. Accurate laboratory studies can aid in proper diagnosis and appropriate antimicrobial therapy. Culture swabs from the lids and conjunctivae of both eyes should be plated directly onto culture media. In addition, contact lens can be placed directly onto culture media or swabs of contact lens cases or cleaning solutions can be performed. Calcium alginate swabs that contain inert materials are preferable to cotton-tipped applicators that contain fatty acids, which may inhibit bacterial growth.

The cornea of the affected eye should then be anesthetized and a flame-sterilized spatula (Kimura) or calcium alginate swab used to take a corneal specimen. Multiple scrapings from affected areas should be performed to increase the yield of live organisms. The specimens should be plated on blood agar, chocolate agar, Sabouraud's agar, thioglycolate broth, brain-heart infusion broth, and glass slides. The bacteria typically begin to grow within 24 to 48 hours and sensitivities to antimicrobial agents can be examined usually 24 hours later. In this case, the cultures grew out a *Streptococcus* species.

8.3 Diagnosis

Streptococcal corneal ulcer, left eye.

8.4 Medical Management

The prognosis for a central *Streptococcal* corneal ulcer is fair. The mainstay of treatment is antimicrobial therapy consisting of broad-spectrum topical fortified antibiotics or topical antibiotic therapy tailored to the Gram stain. Caution should be exercised when the Gram stain is used alone, as there has been only a 60% correlation between the Gram stain and the organisms that are later cultured. The severity of the keratitis should be used as a guide to the intensity and frequency of treatment. Topical fortified antibiotics or fluoroquinolones may be used on peripheral ulcers. Central ulcers usually require a combination of topical fortified antibiotics and fluoroquinolones. Severe cases, including imminent perforation, may require subconjunctival injection of antibiotics as well as hospitalization for intravenous antibiotics.

Antibiotic choices include aminoglycosides, cephalosporins, fluoroquinolones, penicillins, synthetic penicillins, erythromycin, bacitracin, polymyxin, chloramphenicol, vancomycin, tetracycline, sulfonamides, and rifampin. Typical therapy includes gram-positive and gram-negative coverage with two topical fortified agents every hour for 36 hours. Often, a fluoroquinolone may be substituted for one of the fortified antibiotics. If there are signs of clinical improvement, then the frequency of the antibiotic may be reduced. After 48 to 72 hours, coverage may be switched to every 3 to 4 hours and to regular-strength drops after 96 hours. Once sterility has been achieved, adjunctive agents such as corticosteroids, cycloplegics, and enzyme inhibitors (doxycycline) may also be used. Corticosteroid drops may be cautiously started, with their role being to reduce damage produced by invading polymorphonuclear leukocytes and their destructive enzymes and to decrease visual loss from postinflammatory scarring. The National Eye Institute sponsored a randomized, double-masked, placebo-controlled trial looking to see if there was benefit to starting steroids in patients with culture-positive bacterial ulcers, namely called the SCUT trial (Steroids for Corneal Ulcers Trial). Participants with culture-positive bacterial ulcers were assigned to a 3-week tapering regimen of prednisolone sodium phosphate 1% beginning 48 hours after starting topical moxifloxacin 0.5%. The primary end point was best spectacle-corrected visual acuity at 3 months. Secondary end points included best spectacle-corrected visual acuity at 3 weeks, infiltrate/scar size, time to re-epithelialization, and adverse events including corneal perforation. Results showed that patients who started steroid on days 2 or 3 versus day 4 showed one line better vision at 3 months. Also, importantly, there were no serious safety concerns except in patients found to have *Nocardia*-positive ulcers in which there was a larger scar and poorer visual outcome. Subconjunctival injections of antibiotics can be used in patients with suboptimal compliance. Unfortunately, they can be associated with pain and scarring of the conjunctiva.

Other therapeutic modalities include collagen shields and bandage contact lenses. Collagen shields can be impregnated with a variety of antibiotic solutions. They can then deliver antibiotics in a sustained release fashion usually over a 24-hour time period. They can be useful in cases of noncompliance. Unfortunately, they can be dislodged and lost. Bandage contact lenses or self-retained amniotic grafts may be used in nonhealing epithelial defects once the cornea is sterile. Corneal glue with a bandage contact lens may be used to prevent total chamber collapse as the patient awaits definitive surgical intervention.

8.5 Surgical Management

Surgical management should be reserved for cases of medical failure. Structural integrity of the anterior segment should be maintained with surgical glue if possible. If a large perforation has occurred, then a penetrating corneal transplant procedure encompassing all the infected tissue can be performed to retain the structural integrity of the globe. Every attempt to sterilize the cornea should be made prior to surgical repair in order to prevent reinfection of the graft. Corneal grafts performed in actively inflamed or infected corneas are at high risk for failure. A conjunctival flap is not indicated in cases of perforation.

Corneal scarring is a common sequela of bacterial keratitis. When in the central visual axis, it can lead to significant ocular morbidity. Contact lenses (in particular, rigid gas permeable and scleral lenses) can be used to regularize the corneal surface. Phototherapeutic keratectomy can be used to remove anterior stromal scarring. Penetrating keratoplasty or deep anterior lamellar keratoplasty can be used to remove deep central or anterior stromal scarring. Healthy corneal tissue should be preserved as much as possible.

8.6 Rehabilitation and Follow-up

Once bacterial keratitis has been successfully treated, the patient should have any risk factors for the development of recurrence evaluated and corrected if possible. Discontinuation of contact lenses or modification of wearing habits may be suggested. Lid, lacrimal, or conjunctival dysfunction should be treated. In cases of severe scarring, surgical modalities may be considered.

Suggested Reading

[1] Abbott RL, et al. Bacterial corneal ulcers. In: Tasman W, Jaeger EA, eds. Duane's Clinical Ophthalmology. Philadelphia, PA: Lippincott; 1998

[2] Benson WH, Lanier JD. Comparison of techniques for culturing corneal ulcers. Ophthalmology. 1992; 99(5):800–804

[3] Erie JC, Nevitt MP, Hodge DO, Ballard DJ. Incidence of ulcerative keratitis in a defined population from 1950 through 1988. Arch Ophthalmol. 1993; 111 (12):1665–1671

[4] O'Brien TP. Bacterial keratitis. In: Krachmer JH, Mannis MJ, Holland EJ, eds. Cornea. St. Louis, MO: Mosby; 1997

[5] Srinivasan M, Mascarenhas J, Rajaraman R, et al. Steroids for Corneal Ulcers Trial Group. Corticosteroids for bacterial keratitis: the Steroids for Corneal Ulcers Trial (SCUT). Arch Ophthalmol. 2012; 130(2):143–150

9 Keratoconjunctivitis Sicca—Dry Eye

Aaron Wang, Scheffer C. G. Tseng, and Weldon W. Haw

Abstract

In this chapter, we present a case of a patient with dry eyes. The chapter describes typical symptoms, exam findings, differential diagnosis, test and interpretation, and management for dry eyes.

Keywords: dry eyes, meibomian gland, tear film, lipids, mucin, staining, Schirmer's test, osmolarity, blink, punctal plugs, Sjögren's syndrome

9.1 History

A 56-year-old man with a history of diabetes mellitus and a chief complaint of ocular irritation in both eyes was referred by an ophthalmologist for a second opinion under the impression of an unstable ocular surface due to dry eye in his right eye. He complained of burning, foreign body sensation, sandy-gritty feeling, and redness, more in his right eye. These symptoms were worse in the morning and also in the later part of the day, and made him unable to read or drive comfortably. He still has preserved emotional lacrimation. He stated that he slept on his stomach, preferring his right side.

While taking the history, it was noted that his blink rate was reduced in both eyes. His best-corrected visual acuity was 20/40 in the right eye and 20/20 in the left eye. External examination did not reveal features suggestive of rosacea. There were no palpable preauricular nodes. The lid position and relationship to the globe were normal, while the lid tension was loose and floppy. Lid tension was graded as 2+ in the right eye and 1+ in the left eye.

On slit-lamp examination, the meibomian secretion was normal as its fluid appeared clear and was easily expressible. The height of the tear meniscus was low in the upper and lower lids of both eyes. Both tarsal and bulbar conjunctivae were diffusely injected with the tarsal conjunctiva, showing a mixed papillary and follicular response. Ocular sensitivity was markedly reduced as measured by a Cochet–Bonnet esthesiometer. The tear breakup time in each eye was less than 2 seconds. Fluorescein showed superficial punctate staining and rose bengal staining was positive over the exposure zone, more prominent in the right eye. Intraocular pressure was 15 and 16 mm Hg, in the right and left eye, respectively. Fluorescein clearance test (FCT) revealed marked delayed dye clearance and decreased tear secretion (▶ Fig. 9.1) in both eyes. The lens and the fundus were unremarkable in both eyes.

Differential Diagnosis—Key Points

1. The ocular surface comprises the corneal and conjunctival epithelia extending from the upper to the lower eyelid mucocutaneous border. A healthy ocular surface requires a stable preocular tear film made by external adnexa. Through neuroanatomic feedback control, the ocular surface epithelia and the preocular tear film work as a unit to provide clear vision, maintain comfort, and serve as the first line of defense against microbial infections when the eye is open.[1]

2. The preocular tear film is composed of lipids, electrolyte- and protein-containing aqueous fluid, and mucins. Under normal circumstances, aqueous tears are primarily secreted by the main lacrimal gland, spread over the entire ocular surface by lid blinking, and then cleared from the eye into the nose through the nasolacrimal drainage system, which includes the superior and inferior puncta and canaliculi, the lacrimal sac, and the nasolacrimal duct. It has long been recognized that decreased tear secretion by lacrimal glands results in the disease state of aqueous tear deficiency (ATD), i.e., keratoconjunctivitis sicca. However, a stable tear film depends not only on necessary tear components but also on other hydrodynamic elements, including the spreading and clearance of tears. Integration of the compositional and hydrodynamic factors of the ocular surface defense occurs via a neuronal reflex involving the sensory input of the first branch of the trigeminal nerve (V_1) and the efferent output of the parasympathetic branch and the motor branch of the facial nerve (VII) (▶ Fig. 9.2).

3. ATD in the above case was aggravated by the patient's diabetes mellitus, which affects the corneal sensory nerve and thus interrupts the corneal nerve–mediated reflexes (▶ Fig. 9.2). This is essentially a neurotrophic state (as evidenced by the esthesiometer) which has led to insufficient aqueous tear secretion, low tear meniscus (less than 0.2 mm), decreased blink rate, and punctate keratitis (as seen with the rose bengal and fluorescein staining) in the exposure zone. Prolonged exposure tends to be worse in the later part of the day and during activities such as reading or driving. Thus, this patient's dry eye symptoms such as burning and foreign body sensation were more pronounced during these occasions.

4. The patient's reduced eyelid blinking also resulted in delayed tear clearance (DTC) (▶ Fig. 9.1). It has been recognized that DTC is further aggravated by floppy eyelids[2] (▶ Fig. 9.3). Floppy eyelids are known to be associated with papillary conjunctivitis and ocular inflammation, which are worse on the side the patient sleeps on; and ocular symptoms tend to be worsened upon awakening.[3] Symptoms of ocular inflammation such as redness tend to be worse in the morning due to the underlying DTC, especially in the eye corresponding with the side of sleep.[2]

5. The stimulation of lacrimation depends on the cumulative V_1 stimulation from cornea, conjunctiva, lid margin, and nasal mucosa[4] and from cortical influences, e.g., emotional lacrimation. The presence or absence of reflex tearing under maximal stimulation of V_1 has been regarded as a reliable index of the capability of the lacrimal gland to produce aqueous fluid.[5] Loss of reflex tearing is the hallmark of Sjögren's syndrome (SS)-type ATD and can be used to distinguish this from non-SS-type ATD (keratoconjunctivitis sicca). SS-type ATD also manifests more intense rose bengal staining and squamous metaplasia, indicative of severe ocular surface damage, and it correlates with the extent of lymphocyte infiltration in the lacrimal glands.[6] Given that there was preserved emotional tearing, this patient's lacrimal glands were functioning and his ATD was likely not of the SS-type.

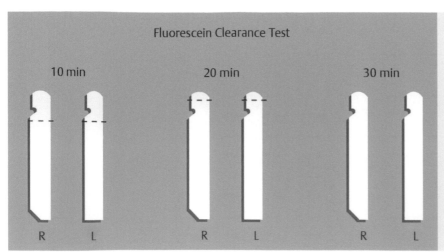

Fluorescein Clearance Test

Fig. 9.1 Fluorescein clearance test.

10 min   20 min   30 min

R   L   R   L   R   L

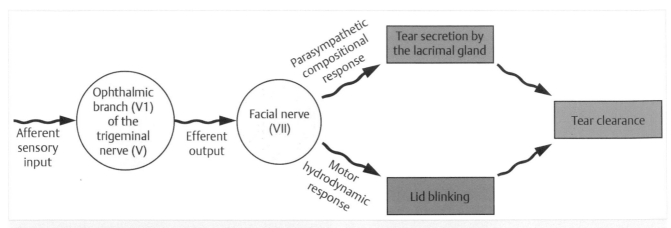

Fig. 9.2 Neuroanatomic integration.

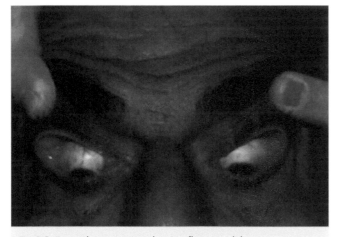

Fig. 9.3 External examination showing floppy eyelids.

Table 9.1 Interpretation of fluorescein clearance test

	Basal secretion	Reflex secretion	Tear clearance
	Wetting length of first two strips	Wetting length of last strip vs. first two strips	Dye visible after 15 minutes?
Normal	≥ 3 mm	Last strip > first two strips	No
DTC	≥ 3 mm	Last strip > first two strips	Yes
ATD with reflex	< 3 mm	Last strip > first two strips	May be delayed
ATD without reflex	< 3 mm	Last strip > first two strips	Usually delayed

Abbreviations: ATD, aqueous tear deficiency; DTC, delayed tear clearance.

9.2 Test Interpretation

The entire spectrum of tear dynamics includes secretion with or without stimulation (i.e., basal or reflex tearing), and clearance. FCT measures basal tearing, reflex tearing, and clearance, and can help diagnosis unstable tear film and DTC (see the following list and ▶ Table 9.1).[2]

9.2.1 How to Perform Fluorescein Clearance Test

- Instill one drop of 0.5% proparacaine in the fornix and then blot eye dry.
- Instill 5 µL of 0.25% Fluress with a pipette.
- Allow normal blink.

- Perform the Schirmer test for 1 minute at 10 minutes and again at 20 minutes. Insert the strip into the inferior fornix of each eye at a position two-thirds lateral to the medial caruncle. Keep the eyes closed for 1 minute, measured with a timer.
- Perform nasal stimulation with a cotton tip applicator after 30 minutes to elicit maximal sensation and repeat the Schirmer test for 1 minute.

For patients with normal tear secretion and clearance, each strip should have a wetting length equal to or greater than 3 mm. The intensity of fluorescein dye fades with time under the blue light and should no longer be seen after 15 minutes (i.e., from the second pair of strips on). After 15 minutes (i.e., the second pair of strips), the wetting length should increase because of waning of the topical anesthetics. If this does not happen, the wetting length can be further increased at the final interval of 30 minutes (i.e., the third pair of strips) by nasal stimulation. A wetting length of near zero millimeters in the first and second pairs of strips from this patient (▶ Fig. 9.1) suggested ATD. A wetting length of the last strip greater than the first two sets (▶ Fig. 9.1) also supported this diagnosis. The fact that the dye was clearly visible in the last two sets (▶ Fig. 9.1) supported the presence of DTC. The underlying cause for ATD was neurotrophic keratopathy secondary to diabetes mellitus and that for DTC was decreased blink rate and floppy eyelids.

Variations of Schirmer's testing can also be performed. Typically, Schirmer's strips are placed for 5 minutes, with eyes closed, with or without anesthetic drops, and with or without stimulation with a cotton tip applicator. A wetting length of greater than 10 mm is generally accepted as normal, keeping in mind that anesthesia would decrease reflex tearing, while stimulation would increase it.

Fluorescein, rose bengal, and lissamine green are useful stains to analyze the pattern of dryness of the ocular surface. Fluorescein is also used to determine the tear breakup time. Fluorescein is instilled and the patient is asked not to blink. The patient has an unstable tear film if a dry area appears before 10 seconds.

There are emerging technologies for the diagnosis of dry eyes.[7] Reflective meniscometry and optical coherence tomography can measure tear meniscus shape, volume, height, and thickness. Videokeratographers can analyze tear firm stability, and interferometers (e.g., LipiView, TearScience Inc., Morrisville, NC) can analyze tear lipid layer thickness and uniformity.

Tear osmolarity have been found to be increased in dry eyes and could be measured (e.g., TearLab, TearLab Corporation, San Diego, CA). Tear proteins can also be analyzed as well for proinflammatory markers (e.g., InflammaDry Detector, Rapid Pathogen Screening Inc, Sarasota, FL). High levels of inflammatory biomarkers may lead to earlier diagnosis of dry eyes. Measuring the temperature of the ocular surface (e.g., Ocular Surface Thermographer, Tomey Corporation, Japan) after opening the eyes for 10 seconds can also help diagnose dry eyes.

9.3 Diagnosis

Keratoconjunctivitis sicca due to ATD secondary to diabetes mellitus–induced neurotrophic keratitis, associated with DTC from reduced blink rate and floppy eyelids.

9.4 Medical Management

Treatments are tailored based on the underlying cause (▶ Table 9.2). For ATD, the patient will start with frequent application of artificial tears. Preservative-free tear substitutes are preferred to avoid potential medicamentosa from the preservatives. Ophthalmic gels and ointments can have a greater duration of effect than drops. Eye inserts (such as Lacrisert, Bausch & Lomb) are placed in the lower fornix, and slowly dissolve and lubricate the eye over an entire day. Because tear fluids contain complex factors, supplementation of conventional tear substitutes may not be adequate. In severe ATD, especially those with SS type, eye drops prepared from a patient's autologous serum may be necessary.[8,9] Tear-stimulating drugs include pilocarpine and cevimeline, which are cholinergics. Topical cyclosporine, a T-cell suppressant, is thought to reduce lacrimal gland lymphocyte infiltration and thereby also increase tear production, especially for SS-type ATD.

To treat dry eyes associated with DTC, it is essential to reduce ocular inflammation. Corticosteroids eye drops or ointments (e.g., prednisolone, fluorometholone, loteprednol etabonate) can be used, although they are not ideal for long-term use due to possible side effects (cataracts, glaucoma, infections, etc.). Antibiotics such as tetracyclines (oral) and macrolides (oral or topical) can help control inflammation (as well as can topical cyclosporine). These antibiotics have been reported to have anticollagenase and antimatrix metalloproteinase properties.[10]

Table 9.2 Therapeutic Management for treating dry eye

Goal	Modality	Treatment
Replace aqueous fluid	Topical treatment	Artificial tears (preferably preservative-free), autologous serum
Conserve aqueous fluid	Punctal occlusion	Punctal plugs, thermal cautery
Reduce evaporation	Cover	Eye shields or goggles, contact lens
	Reinforce lipid layer	Meibomian lipid replacement, warm compresses, lid hygiene
Reduce exposure	Reduce palpebral aperture	Tarsorrhaphy/Botox-induced ptosis
	Increase blink	Encouragement
Increase lacrimal gland secretion	Parasympathetic stimulation	Pilocarpine, cevimeline
	Suppress lacrimal gland inflammation	Cyclosporine

9.5 Surgical Management

For moderate and severe ATD, punctal occlusion with thermal cauterization or punctal plugs can be performed. The consideration of the former over the latter for punctal occlusion is based on the absence of reflex tearing. The use of permanent occlusion is generally reserved for patients with proven SS-type ATD. To maximize punctal fibrosis, the use of topical steroid preparations should be avoided immediately after treatment. With punctal occlusion, artificial tear substitutes become more effective. Intrinsic inflammatory irritation has to be eliminated first because punctal occlusion invariably induces DTC. Other surgical therapies are directed at reducing exposure by creating a conjunctival flap or by decreasing the palpebral fissure (ptosis with botulinum toxin injections or tarsorrhaphy). Repairing abnormal lids such as ectropion is also necessary to prevent exposure.

Special contact lenses (e.g., scleral or bandage contact lenses) as well as self-retained amniotic membrane tissue can also be used to protect the ocular surface and trap moisture. If meibomian gland disease is contributing to an unstable tear film, warm compresses done at home or thermal pulsations with Lipiflow (TearScience Inc., Morrisville, NC) could unblock oils to help with tear-film stability. Intense-pulse light therapy and lid massage have also been performed for people with severe dry eyes.

Suggested Reading

[1] Lemp MA. Report of the National Eye Institute/ Industry Workshop on clinical trials in dry eyes. CLAO J. 1995; 21(4):221–232

References

[1] Tseng SCG, Tsubota K. Important concepts for treating ocular surface and tear disorders. Am J Ophthalmol. 1997; 124(6):825–835

[2] Prabhasawat P, Tseng SCG. Frequent association of delayed tear clearance in ocular irritation. Br J Ophthalmol. 1998; 82(6):666–675

[3] Culbertson WW, Tseng SCG. Corneal disorders in floppy eyelid syndrome. Cornea. 1994; 13(1):33–42

[4] Jordan A, Baum J. Basic tear flow. Does it exist? Ophthalmology. 1980; 87(9): 920–930

[5] Tsubota K. SS dry eye and non-SS dry eye: what are the differences? In: Homma M, Sugai S, Tojo T, et al., eds. Sjögren's Syndrome. Amsterdam: Kugler Publications; 1994:27–31

[6] Tsubota K, Xu K-P, Fujihara T, Katagiri S, Takeuchi T. Decreased reflex tearing is associated with lymphocytic infiltration in lacrimal glands. J Rheumatol. 1996; 23(2):313–320

[7] Zeev MS, Miller DD, Latkany R. Diagnosis of dry eye disease and emerging technologies. Clin Ophthalmol. 2014; 8:581–590

[8] Fox RI, Chan R, Michelson JB, Belmont JB, Michelson PE. Beneficial effect of artificial tears made with autologous serum in patients with keratoconjunctivitis sicca. Arthritis Rheum. 1984; 27(4):459–461

[9] Tsubota K, Goto E, Fujita H, et al. Treatment of dry eye by autologous serum application in Sjögren's syndrome. Br J Ophthalmol. 1999; 83(4):390–395

[10] Li DQ, Lokeshwar BL, Solomon A, Monroy D, Ji Z, Pflugfelder SC. Regulation of MMP-9 production by human corneal epithelial cells. Exp Eye Res. 2001; 73 (4):449–459

10 Postsurgical Corneal Edema

Weldon W. Haw

Abstract

Corneal edema can occur following cataract surgery. In most cases, the edema is temporary and resolves with time. In some instances, corneal edema persists and requires management. Risk factors for persistent corneal edema include preexisting low endothelial cell density, Fuchs' endothelial dystrophy, and complicated surgery. Postoperative corneal edema may be managed medically with a combination of topical steroids, hypertonic ophthalmic solutions, and topical ophthalmic aqueous suppressants. Surgical alternatives may be used for nonresolving corneal edema refractory to medical management. In the past, penetrating keratoplasty was traditionally performed. Advances in techniques have allowed for a number of evolving endothelial keratoplasty procedures such as DMEK (Descemet's membrane endothelial keratoplasty) and DSAEK (Descemet's stripping automated endothelial keratoplasty), which allow for more rapid visual rehabilitation.

Keywords: corneal edema, Fuchs' corneal dystrophy, corneal transplant, endothelial transplant, DSAEK, DMEK

10.1 History

A 55-year-old man presented with a chief complaint of decreased vision (especially at night) in both eyes for 1 year. Past medical history was remarkable for diabetes mellitus for 10 years, which had been well controlled with oral medications. Past ocular history was unremarkable. There was no family history of systemic or ocular diseases.

Best corrected visual acuity was 20/50 in the right eye and 20/100 in the left eye. Pupillary examination and ocular motility were unremarkable. The intraocular pressures (IOPs) were 12 and 13 mm Hg in the right and left eyes, respectively. There was no visual field loss by confrontation finger counting. Slit-lamp examination was normal other than moderate nuclear sclerosis of the crystalline lens in both eyes, left worse than right. Fundus examination did not show any evidence of diabetic retinopathy. Potential acuity testing revealed a visual potential of 20/25 in each eye. A clinical diagnosis of cataract in both eyes was made and cataract surgery of the left eye was recommended for visual rehabilitation.

The patient underwent an uncomplicated phacoemulsification via temporal clear corneal incision with implantation of a posterior chamber acrylic intraocular lens in the left eye. The visual acuity was 20/100 with an IOP of 18 mm Hg on the first postoperative day. Slit-lamp examination revealed diffuse corneal edema in the central cornea as well as around the incision site (▶ Fig. 10.1), and the patient complained of persistent blurred vision without major discomfort.

Differential Diagnosis—Key Points

The patient is experiencing poor visual outcome immediately after cataract extraction secondary to corneal edema. The differential diagnosis should include the following:

1. Preexisting endothelial disease or dysfunction.
   a) Low endothelial cell density without the presence of corneal guttata can occur in a small portion of the population.
   b) Corneal guttata and Fuchs' corneal endothelial dystrophy are relatively common preexisting corneal endothelial disorders. These conditions usually occur after 50 years of age with a female preponderance. Corneal guttatae are initially evident centrally and spread toward the corneal periphery. The corneal endothelial cells of Fuchs' corneal endothelial dystrophy are larger and more polymorphic than those of normal individuals. Descemet's membrane is usually thickened. Diurnal fluctuation of vision is common in patients with advanced corneal edema.
   c) Past ocular history of an acute rise of IOP such as that seen with acute angle closure glaucoma resulting in reduction of corneal endothelial cell density should also be considered as a cause of low preoperative endothelial cell counts.
   d) Abnormality of endothelial cell morphology and function has also been reported in diabetic patients with no known corneal dystrophy.
2. Surgical trauma.
   a) Direct injury to the corneal endothelium by instruments or intraocular lens can cause diffuse or discrete patches of edema. This type of edema usually occurs in the central or temporal cornea around the incision site.
   b) Detachment of Descemet's membrane by incisional blades or misdirection of the surgical instruments intraoperatively can also cause corneal edema. It is usually most visible at the entry wound.
   c) Prolonged endothelial exposure to the ultrasound and/or irrigating solutions during phacoemulsification can also cause diffuse corneal edema. This is especially common in patients with dense/mature cataracts requiring additional phacoemulsification time, patients with miotic pupils (i.e., diabetics and pseudoexfoliation syndrome patients), shallow or hyperopic anatomic anterior chambers, or anterior placement of the phacoemulsification incision, which allow close proximity of the ultrasound tip to the endothelium.
   d) Other surgical complications, such as a vitreous strand to the wound, vitreous prolapse with corneal endothelial

contact, malpositioning of the intraocular lens, wound leaks with shallow anterior chamber, or hypotony with choroidal effusion, may result in corneal edema.

e) Thermal injury to the corneal endothelium may be caused by phaco probe or cryoprobe (in intracapsular cataract extraction).

3. Toxicity.

a) Various chemical contaminants may result in diffuse endothelial damage. This is frequently accompanied by other evidence of intraocular toxicity such as a fixed and dilated pupil.

b) Antibiotics in high concentrations are common offending agents. Errors in diluting medications may occur. Perioperative topical or subconjunctival antibiotics may enter the anterior chamber through an unsealed wound.

c) Intracameral epinephrine is occasionally used for patients with inadequate pupillary dilatation such as is seen with pseudoexfoliation syndrome. Endothelial toxicity and corneal edema may be caused by sodium bisulfite, which is used as an antioxidant for epinephrine. Preservative-free epinephrine is recommended for intracameral use.

d) Intracameral injection of lidocaine HCl, one of the anesthetic methods used for phacoemulsification, may also cause endothelial toxicity by its preservative (methyl paraben). Preservative-free preparations of lidocaine are recommended to avoid endothelial toxicity.

e) Detergents used for cleaning ophthalmic instruments, such as ethoxylated fatty acid (a cleaning solution in ultrasonic bath), benzalkonium chloride (a preservative solution), or chlorhexidine (an antiseptic used for preparing facial skin prior to surgery), can cause direct damage to the corneal endothelium. Ethylene oxide used for gas sterilization of ophthalmic instruments is also potentially toxic to the corneal endothelium.

4. Excessive postoperative inflammation.

a) Inflammation may lead to short-term endothelial dysfunction and long-term endothelial cell loss. Active inflammation can compromise endothelial cell functions, especially in older patients who may already have marginal corneal function before inflammation.

b) The degree of postoperative inflammation is dependent on many factors: preexisting conditions, surgical technique, fluids and instrumentation, intraocular lens choice, and medications used.

c) Patients with a history of uveitis such as juvenile rheumatoid arthritis, Vogt–Koyanagi–Harada disease, or recurrent granulomatous uveitis are at increased risk of excessive postoperative inflammation.

5. Postoperative IOP elevation.

a) Under normal conditions, the IOP tends to counterbalance the swelling pressure of the cornea. The difference between these two values is termed imbibition pressure. The endothelial pump plays a major role in keeping this dynamic balance of corneal hydration. If the increase of IOP postoperatively exceeds the swelling pressure in the presence of compromised endothelial function, the net flux of water is into the cornea resulting in corneal edema.

b) The use of viscoelastic substances (i.e., dispersive viscoelastic agents) for corneal endothelial protection during surgery has been associated with elevation of postoperative IOP.

c) Pupillary block glaucoma due to iris–intraocular lens adhesion can also cause postoperative IOP elevation.

6. Long-term use of topical ophthalmic medication.

a) Preoperative ocular conditions requiring long-term use of topical ophthalmic medications may be associated with compromised endothelial function. Preservatives such as benzalkonium chloride or thimerosal found in the ocular medications have been associated with progressive corneal endothelial cell damage.

10.2 Test Interpretation

1. Specular microscopy of the fellow eye.

a) This patient presented with unexpected corneal edema after apparently atraumatic cataract surgery. In the absence of preoperative specular microscopy in the operated eye, the status of the corneal endothelium in the fellow eye is the best parameter of preoperative endothelial cell function.

b) The minimum corneal endothelial cell density required to maintain corneal deturgescence varies from person to person. A cornea with endothelial density less than 1,000 cells/mm^2 is known to be at increased risk of corneal decompensation. The routine use of preoperative specular microscopic examination to screen patients for unexpected low endothelial cell counts has been controversial.

c) Noncontact specular microscopy is generally more comfortable for patients than contact microscopy. The latter, however, gives a wider field of view, though with less resolution.

d) One less expensive method of estimating endothelial cell counts is by inserting a reticule in the eyepiece of the

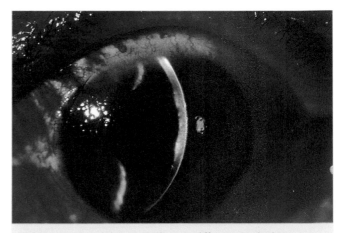

Fig. 10.1 Postsurgical corneal edema: a diffuse corneal edema was noted in the central cornea and at the temporal incision site.

slit-lamp biomicroscope and comparing the endothelial mosaics with diagrams of cells with known density. Although convenient and inexpensive, this method is difficult to master and time consuming.

2. Pachymetry.
   a) Corneal pachymetry is a useful method of estimating endothelial function.
   b) The normal cornea measures 0.52 ± 0.02 mm centrally and approximately 0.65 mm in the periphery.
   c) Corneal pachymetry can be helpful in identifying patients with a central corneal thickness greater than 0.6 mm. These patients may have marginal corneal endothelial function and are more susceptible to postoperative corneal decompensation than normal individuals.
   d) Corneal pachymetry can also be used postoperatively to monitor the recovery of endothelial function.

10.3 Diagnosis

After a detailed examination of the fellow eye, a low endothelial cell density in the absence of guttata was noted by specular microscopy in this patient. The unexpected postoperative corneal edema in the operated eye was attributed to a preexisting low endothelial density of undetermined etiology.

10.4 Medical Management

The goals of management of early postsurgical corneal edema are to maximize visual function and to minimize patient discomfort.

10.4.1 Control of Inflammation

Because persistent inflammation can have a detrimental effect on the corneal endothelial barrier functions, it is essential to control inflammation as soon as possible. Most clinicians treat patients with strong topical steroids such as prednisolone acetate 1% as often as every 1 hour for acute postoperative corneal edema. Subconjunctival corticosteroid injection may be considered for severe inflammation.

10.4.2 Control of IOP

If there is a documented elevation of IOP, topical antiglaucoma medications or systemic carbonic anhydrase inhibitors should be used to control it.

10.4.3 Topical Hypertonic Solution

Topical hyperosmotic agents can facilitate removal of fluid from the edematous cornea. A 5% sodium chloride solution or ointment is commonly used.

10.4.4 Therapeutic Hydrophilic Contact Lens

In patients with early corneal decompensation and mild edema, a thin hydrophilic lens, fitted flat to allow maximum contact between the lens and the irregular epithelium, may be helpful in restoring vision and maximizing patient comfort.

10.5 Surgical Management

10.5.1 Penetrating Keratoplasty

Prior to the routine use of endothelial keratoplasty (EK), restoration of vision in an eye with irreversible corneal edema required a penetrating keratoplasty (PK) to replace the damaged endothelial cells. A final decision about proceeding with PK should be deferred for 2 to 3 months after postoperative corneal decompensation is noted. In some patients with temporary corneal endothelial dysfunction, clarity can be regained within this time frame.

The prognosis for PK in this type of patient is generally very good with a success rate better than 85%. The long-term success of PK, however, often depends on the quality of postoperative care.

10.5.2 Postoperative Care of PK Eyes

Postsurgical Complications

The following postsurgical complications may occur following penetrating keratoplasty: wound leak, flat anterior chamber, iris incarceration in the wound, IOP, primary endothelial failure, endophthalmitis, epithelial defect, or down-growth.

Evaluation of Postoperative Astigmatism by Corneal Topography

Astigmatism is the most frequent complication of PK. Severe astigmatism can adversely affect postoperative visual outcome. Using a surgical technique that may reduce the occurrence of postoperative astigmatism should be considered. In patients with a moderate to severe degree of astigmatism, relaxing incisions or wedge corneal resection may be considered.

Differential Diagnosis of Graft Rejection versus Acute Graft Failure

Acute graft failure usually occurs shortly after PK. It may be related to poor preservation of, or surgical trauma to, the donor tissue. In this situation, corneal edema persists despite medical treatment.

Corneal allograft rejection can occur at any time after transplantation but rarely occurs within 2 weeks of surgery. One should carefully look for signs of graft rejection such as severe anterior segment inflammation, corneal stromal infiltrates or edema, keratic precipitate, or rejection line. Frequent topical corticosteroid is the mainstay of treatment for corneal allograft rejection. Periocular or systemic steroids may be considered for severe rejection or in noncompliant patients. Systemic immunotherapy with cyclosporin A may be needed in selective patients.

10.5.3 Endothelial Keratoplasty

Given the high incidence of corneal astigmatism after PK and potential for wound dehiscence, partial-thickness corneal transplants were devised as a way of diminishing these postoperative complications. These methods involve selectively transplanting the damaged endothelial layer of the cornea while leaving the majority of the corneal stromal and anterior layers intact. With the advent of EK techniques, surgical and healing time is reduced, visual rehabilitation is more rapid, and graft rejection rates are less common.

Descemet's Stripping Automated Endothelial Keratoplasty (DSAEK)

This technique involves manually stripping away host endothelium and Descemet's membrane, while leaving behind the posterior stroma of the host cornea. A graft composed of donor endothelium, Descemet's membrane, and a thin layer of posterior stromal is then transplanted onto the posterior surface of the stripped host cornea. Currently, eye banks are able to harvest and provide surgeons with precut corneal tissues for transplantation. This procedure has been extremely successful in patients with isolated corneal endothelial pathology and is now the most commonly performed procedure.

Descemet's Membrane Endothelial Keratoplasty (DMEK)

Though DSAEK has become an extremely successful procedure, there have been limitations on final visual acuity secondary to light scatter from the graft–host stromal interface. Thus, methods have been devised to try to reduce DSAEK graft thickness to help achieve better visual outcomes. The most popular current technique involves transplanting only endothelial cells and Descemet's membrane. In patient outcome studies from individuals undergoing DMEK, the visual acuity data have been excellent and often exceed acuity seen in DSAEK patients in appropriate surgical candidates. As the techniques of this procedure are further perfected, this technique has promise to further increase in popularity for individuals with endothelial pathology.

10.6 Rehabilitation and Follow-up

The patient was managed with topical corticosteroids and hypertonic saline solution four times a day for 1 week. The

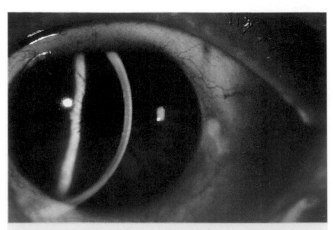

Fig. 10.2 Complete recovery of corneal edema: after 1 week of medical treatment, the cornea was clear with complete resolution of corneal edema.

corneal edema resolved completely after the treatment and the final best corrected visual acuity was 20/20 (▶ Fig. 10.2).

Suggested Reading

[1] Anders N, Wollensak J. Inadvertent use of chlorhexidine instead of balanced salt solution for intraocular irrigation. J Cataract Refract Surg. 1997; 23(6): 959–962

[2] Anderson NJ, Edelhauser HF. Toxicity of ocular surgical solutions. Int Ophthalmol Clin. 1999; 39(2):91–106

[3] Jaffe NS, Jaffe MS, Jaffe GF. Corneal edema. In: Jaffe NS, ed. Cataract Surgery and Its Complications. New York, NY: Mosby/Thieme; 1997:309–318

[4] Probst LE, Holland EJ. Intraocular lens implantation in patients with juvenile rheumatoid arthritis. Am J Ophthalmol. 1996; 122(2):161–170

[5] Feng MT, Price MO, Price FW, Jr. Update on Descemet membrane endothelial keratoplasty (DMEK). Int Ophthalmol Clin. 2013; 53(2):31–45

[6] Guerra FP, Anshu A, Price MO, Price FW. Endothelial keratoplasty: fellow eyes comparison of Descemet stripping automated endothelial keratoplasty and Descemet membrane endothelial keratoplasty. Cornea. 2011; 30(12):1382–1386

11 Dellen

Weldon W. Haw

Abstract

Dellen represents an area of peripheral, localized corneal thinning related to desiccation of the epithelial and subepithelial tissues. They occur adjacent to areas of limbal elevation resulting from filtering blebs, dermoids, chemosis etc. Dellen must be distinguished from more fulminant disease states such as inflammatory or autoimmune peripheral ulcerative keratitis. Dellen can be successfully managed with lubrication with preservative-free tears, ointment, and/or punctal occlusion. If there is persistent dellen, oral doxycycline, vitamin C, with or without a bandage contact lens, or self-retained amniotic membrane graft may be required. Further surgical intervention may be warranted in refractory dellen such as surgical removal of the offending conjunctival elevation or amniotic membrane with tarsorrhaphy.

Keywords: dellen, corneal thinning

11.1 History

A 55-year-old man with a history of glaucoma that required multiple filtration procedures in the right eye was found to have elevated intraocular pressure on maximal medical therapy. A repeat trabeculectomy procedure was performed. In order to avoid the previous surgical site, the trabeculectomy flap was established at the 7 o'clock position, which resulted in a moderately elevated filtering bleb extending from the 5 to 8 o'clock positions.

Two weeks after surgery, peripheral corneal thinning was noted adjacent to the filtering bleb (▶ Fig. 11.1). Fluorescein instillation revealed pooling with a small area of epithelial cell loss.

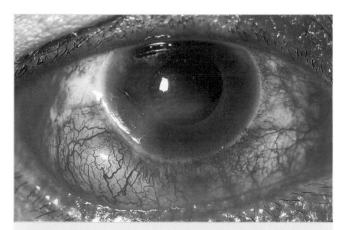

Fig. 11.1 A filtering bleb is evident extending from the 5 o'clock to the 8 o'clock positions. Note the pooling of fluorescein in the peripheral corneal delle that has developed adjacent to the filtering bleb. (This image is provided courtesy of John P. Whitcher, MD, San Francisco, CA.)

Differential Diagnosis—Key Points

1. A delle represents an area of localized corneal thinning due to desiccation of the epithelial and subepithelial tissues that results from poor tear coverage over a specific area (▶ Fig. 11.2). This localized interruption in the tear film is most commonly due to some form of limbal elevation (e.g., filtering bleb, dermoid, conjunctival elevation following muscle or scleral buckling surgery), which therefore tends to produce desiccation and delle formation at the periphery of the cornea, especially in the setting of dry eye. Because of the location, the correct diagnosis is often not considered, and inflammatory causes of peripheral corneal thinning are invoked.

2. While delle formation is a relatively benign process, inflammatory causes of peripheral corneal thinning can have disastrous consequences for the eye and might be associated with severe systemic diseases. These should therefore be considered in the differential diagnosis, along with degenerative causes of peripheral corneal thinning.

3. Inflammatory causes of peripheral corneal thinning include Mooren's ulceration, thinning associated with scleritis of various causes, and autoimmune processes such as rheumatoid arthritis, systemic lupus erythematosus, relapsing polychondritis, inflammatory bowel disease, and vasculitis syndromes such as Wegener's granulomatosis, temporal arteritis, polyarteritis nodosa, and Churg–Strauss angiitis. Systemic evaluation is required to rule out inflammatory disease in those cases that are often accompanied by significant ocular inflammation and corneal infiltration. While noninfiltrated, relatively quiet peripheral corneal melting can occur in association with disorders such as rheumatoid arthritis, systemic lupus erythematosus, or relapsing polychondritis, an epithelial defect is almost always present in active disease, and an adjacent mass that could disturb tear distribution is unlikely to be present.

4. Degenerative causes of localized peripheral corneal thinning include furrow degeneration, Terrien's marginal degeneration, pellucid marginal degeneration, and Fuchs' superficial marginal keratitis. Characteristics of furrow degeneration include an elderly patient with isolated, noninflammatory, nonprogressive, shallow peripheral thinning between the limbus and the arcus senilis. Terrien's marginal degeneration is characterized by superficial vascularization of thinned peripheral cornea preceded by a distinct lipid line. As opposed to the typically well-circumscribed area involved in dellen, pellucid marginal degeneration extends over a narrow arcuate band and is not associated with any adjacent elevation that might impede tear distribution. Fuchs' superficial marginal keratitis is characterized by intermittent, recurrent episodes of ocular irritation accompanied by marginal infiltrates that result in progressive marginal superficial stromal thinning and, in advanced cases, pseudopterygium over the area of thinning.

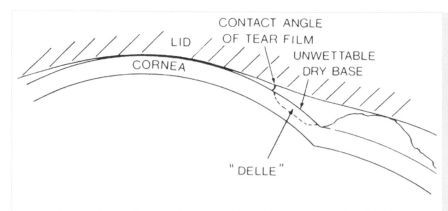

Fig. 11.2 This schematic illustrates the formation of a delle. In this case, the mass acts as a spacer that disturbs the continuity of contact between the lid and the cornea. This leads to an area consistently devoid of tear film, resulting in desiccation and thinning.

11.2 Test Interpretation

Dellen are typically associated with the following clinical characteristics. Underlying dry eye or meibomian gland dysfunction may be present. The area of thinning is usually well circumscribed, "saucerlike," with sloping edges. There is often an obvious adjacent elevation responsible for the localized interruption in tear distribution. As the patient blinks, the tear film is disrupted over the area of thinning. This can often be demonstrated more clearly by highlighting the tear film with a drop of fluorescein. If too much fluorescein is instilled, it will often pool in the depression giving the appearance that an epithelial defect is present. The epithelium, however, is usually intact along the base of the delle, and this can be demonstrated by gently removing the excess fluorescein from the excavation with a spear-tip cellulose sponge. It should be recognized, however, that due to the epithelial trauma that might accompany chronic desiccation, epithelial breakdown, scarring, and true tissue loss can occur, so that a delle evolves into a true noninfectious corneal ulcer.

The definitive diagnostic test for a delle is to rehydrate the area, which will result in thickening of the corneal stroma and resolution of the localized thinning. This is best achieved by applying a generous quantity of a viscous lubricating agent such as a 1% methylcellulose solution or ophthalmic lubricating ointment, and patching the eye shut for 15 to 30 minutes. Under these conditions, a delle should rapidly rehydrate, so that the cornea returns to near-normal thickness. Usually, because of the relative localized stromal edema, the cornea appears mildly opacified in the former area of the delle.

When perilimbal conjunctiva is removed, exposed sclera may also become thinner secondary to interference of the wetting effect of the tear film and a scleral delle may also form.

11.3 Diagnosis

Delle in right eye due to dry eye in the setting of a filtering bleb.

11.4 Medical Management

Dellen are due to inadequate tear distribution, dry eye, and lid disease such as meibomitis and blepharitis. These risk factors should be treated. Dry eye treatments include supplementation with preservative-free artificial tears, bland ophthalmic lubricating ointment, or punctal occlusion. Although rarely needed, oral doxycycline and/or vitamin C may also help further prevent keratolysis for more extreme thinning. A bandage contact lens or self-retained amniotic membrane graft can be placed within the clinic setting to enhance healing of the epithelial surface. The stability of the tear film is affected by the health of the oil layer produced by the lid's meibomian glands: lid treatments such as heat compresses and gentle massage directed to the meibomian glands might be helpful in relieving meibomian gland inspissation and reduced tear breakup time. New techniques such as LipiFlow Thermal Pulsation System (Johnson and Johnson Vision) been approved for use in patients with severe meibomian gland dysfunction.

11.5 Surgical Management

In the most severe cases, surgery may be required. Secured amniotic membrane grafting and/or a limited tarsorrhaphy may be required for progressive or nonhealing dellen unresponsive to medical management. In many cases, the localized elevation precipitating delle formation (such as with filtering blebs or following conjunctival surgery) cannot easily be resolved. Removal of the offending structure is not a reasonable option in such cases. However, a mass such as a pyogenic granuloma or dermoid may be amenable to surgical excision.

11.6 Rehabilitation and Follow-up

Since delle formation represents a relatively benign process, little is usually required in the way of visual rehabilitation. However, patients should be observed and treated over the long term for signs and symptoms of dry eye that are contributing factors to dellen formation.

Suggested Reading

[1] American Academy of Ophthalmology. Dry Eye Syndrome: Preferred Practice Pattern. San Francisco, CA: American Academy of Ophthalmology; 1998

[2] Norn MS. Desiccation of the precorneal film. II. Permanent discontinuity and dellen. Acta Ophthalmol (Copenh). 1969; 47(4):881–889

[3] Pfister R, Renner M. The histopathology of experimental dry spots and dellen in the rabbit cornea: a light microscopy and scanning and transmission electron microscopy study. Invest Ophthalmol Vis Sci. 1977; 16(11):1025–1038

[4] Robin JB, Schanzlin DJ, Verity SM, et al. Peripheral corneal disorders. Surv Ophthalmol. 1986; 31(1):1–36

12 Graft Rejection Following Penetrating Keratoplasty

Aaron Wang, Matthew R. Jones, and Weldon Haw

Abstract

In this chapter, we present a case of a patient with graft rejection after penetrating keratoplasty. The case describes typical symptoms, exam findings, differential diagnosis, and medical and surgical management for graft rejection.

Keywords: keratoplasty, graft rejection, corneal edema, keratic precipitates

12.1 History

A 30-year-old man presented with complaints of redness, photophobia, and blurred vision in his right eye for 1 week. Past ocular history included keratoconus, for which he had undergone penetrating keratoplasty (PK) in the right eye 5 months earlier. At his examination 1 month earlier, a visual acuity of 20/60 in the right eye with improvement to 20/30 with pinhole had been recorded.

Examination revealed a visual acuity of 20/400 in the right eye without improvement with pinhole. Visual acuity was 20/20 in the left eye with a rigid gas permeable contact lens. Intraocular pressure was 17 mm Hg in both eyes. Slit-lamp examination was notable for 2 + ciliary flush in the right eye. A broken, exposed interrupted suture with a surrounding infiltrate was noted in the graft at the 11 o'clock meridian. Marked stromal edema extended 2 mm into the graft from the site of the broken suture. A line of keratic precipitates demarcated the central edge of the stromal edema. The anterior chamber showed 1 + cell and flare. The left eye was quiet with a well-positioned rigid gas permeable contact lens, with thinning and mild protrusion of the central cornea. A Fleischer ring was present.

12.2 Test Interpretation

The diagnosis of graft rejection after PK is made predominantly by slit-lamp examination. Occasionally, in questionable cases, ultrasonic pachymetry can be helpful in detecting a subclinical increase in graft thickness suggestive of endothelial dysfunction. Similarly, a decrease in corneal thickness can be a useful early sign that a severe rejection episode is responding to treatment even if the edematous graft appears unchanged.

12.3 Diagnosis

OD: (1) Broken suture with suture abscess. (2) Endothelial corneal graft rejection. OS: Keratoconus.

12.4 Medical Management

Timely intervention in the management of endothelial rejection is critical to prevent irreversible endothelial damage. As such, patients must be educated to seek evaluation within 24 hours

Differential Diagnosis—Key Points

1. New symptoms in a patient with a PK (foreign body sensation, decreased visual acuity, photophobia, red eye) should be evaluated immediately. The chances of a graft-threatening problem in a patient with such symptoms are high, and successful management depends on timely presentation and intervention.
2. Broken sutures in the postoperative period after PK are common. If not removed immediately, they can lead to vascularization, suture abscess, or rejection.
3. After PK, patients may present with the signs and symptoms of iritis without signs of graft rejection. Such patients may or may not have a previous history of uveitis. Iritis should be treated as a "forme fruste" of allograft rejection.
4. Rejection after PK may take one of three major forms: epithelial rejection, subepithelial rejection, or endothelial rejection.
5. Epithelial rejection presents with a slightly elevated gray-white epithelial ridge inside the graft–host junction that stains with fluorescein and may extend for 360 degrees. The ridge represents sensitized lymphocytes that are rejecting the donor epithelium (▶ Fig. 12.1). The host stem cells replace the epithelium behind the advancing ridge. Epithelial rejection occurs most commonly within the first year after PK.

Subepithelial rejection consists of multiple round subepithelial infiltrates scattered over the graft, similar in appearance to postadenoviral subepithelial infiltrates.

Endothelial rejection may present with one or more of the following features: ciliary injection, keratic precipitates, stromal edema, anterior chamber cell, and flare. Signs of advanced rejection include superficial and deep vascularization of the graft or a linear deposit of keratic precipitates (Khodadoust's line) (▶ Fig. 12.2). Endothelial rejection is the most common cause of graft failure.

6. Risk factors for endothelial rejection include stromal vascularization, large-diameter grafts, eccentric grafts, and repeat grafts. Any cause of inflammation in the postoperative period including iritis, mild trauma, epithelial or subepithelial rejection, or broken sutures can trigger endothelial rejection.

of any new symptom of photophobia, foreign body sensation, red eye, or decreased vision.

Broken sutures should be removed at the slit lamp. If no infiltrate exists, prophylactic treatment with a broad-spectrum antibiotic in drop or ointment form should be instituted (e.g., Polytrim four times a day for 2 to 3 days; bacitracin ointment three time a day for 2 to 3 days). If a suture abscess is present, culturing should be considered and the frequent application of a broad-spectrum fluoroquinolone or other fortified antibiotic

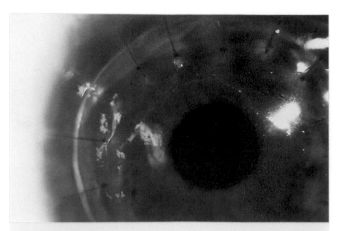

Fig. 12.1 Epithelial rejection 3 months after penetrating keratoplasty. Note centrally advancing epithelial rejection line. (The image is provided courtesy of Peter R. Laibson, MD.)

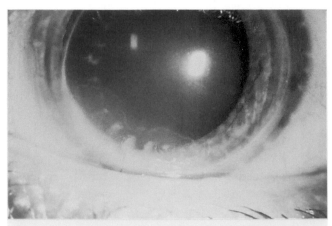

Fig. 12.2 Endothelial rejection with inferior corneal edema and Khodadoust's line. (The image is provided courtesy of Peter R. Laibson, MD.)

(e.g., ciprofloxacin every hour around the clock) may be necessary. In the presence of an abscess, topical corticosteroid frequency is typically reduced or discontinued for the first several days. After control of the abscess is achieved, the steroid can be increased judiciously to treat excessive inflammation or rejection if present.

While epithelial and subepithelial rejections do not significantly affect the health of the graft directly, they can trigger endothelial rejection if left untreated. Both epithelial and subepithelial rejections typically respond quickly to moderate doses of topical corticosteroids (e.g., prednisolone acetate 1% four times a day for 1 week, with subsequent tapering to baseline corticosteroid levels).

Endothelial rejection should be managed aggressively by using frequent topical corticosteroids. The initial frequency of topical steroid depends on the severity of the rejection episode. For mild rejection consisting of one to several keratic precipitates and a mild anterior chamber reaction, application of a topical steroid such as prednisolone acetate 1% four to six times daily and tapered over 6 weeks may be sufficient. For more severe episodes with the presence of many keratic precipitates and corneal edema, hourly application of topical steroids should be instituted. A cycloplegic agent (e.g., scopolamine 0.25% three times a day) can be used to help stabilize the blood–aqueous barrier and increase patient comfort in more severe cases. In severe or recalcitrant cases of endothelial rejection, systemic steroids (e.g., prednisone 80 mg orally daily) and/ or subconjunctival/transseptal steroids (e.g., triamcinolone 40 mg/mL) can be used to supplement topical therapy.

12.5 Surgical Management

If no improvement is noted in the amount of edema after several weeks of therapy, the steroids should be tapered and consideration given to repeat PK. Although repeat PK is often successful in these cases, repeat grafts have a higher risk of failure. This is particularly true if deep stromal vessels are present, which is often the case after severe or prolonged rejection episodes.

Descemet's stripping automated endothelial keratoplasty (DSAEK) is also an excellent option after failed PK, especially for corneas with acceptable topography and refractive outcome before failure. In DSAEK, the abnormal endothelium is stripped and replaced with a new posterior corneal lenticule (corneal stroma, Descemet's membrane, and endothelium). DSAEK has become the popular choice for isolated endothelial dysfunction. Recent studies have shown that DSAEK after failed PK provides greater wound stability, reduced suture-related complications, and similar graft survival rates and visual outcomes compared with a repeat PK. Also, graft dislocation and postoperative complication rates of DSAEK after failed PK are similar to those of primary DSAEK.

Perioperatively, prophylactic systemic steroids or, less commonly, cyclosporin A can be considered in particularly high-risk cases. Human leukocyte antigen matching of donor tissue to the recipient has not been convincingly demonstrated to reduce graft rejection in high-risk patients. There is, however, some evidence that ABO blood type matching may be of some benefit and can be considered in high-risk patients.

12.6 Rehabilitation and Follow-up

Scheduling of follow-up care during the treatment of endothelial rejection varies depending on the severity of the episode, but typically ranges from 2 to 4 days in more severe cases to 1 week in less severe cases. As it becomes apparent that the rejection process is under control, the frequency of the follow-up visits can be decreased as topical steroids are tapered. Attention can then be returned to visual rehabilitation of the eye. Residual astigmatism is addressed via suture lysis, glasses, or rigid contact lens fitting as is appropriate.

Suggested Reading

[1] Anshu A, Price MO, Price FW, Jr. Descemet's stripping endothelial keratoplasty under failed penetrating keratoplasty: visual rehabilitation and graft survival rate. Ophthalmology. 2011; 118(11):2155–2160

[2] The Collaborative Corneal Transplantation Studies Research Group. The collaborative corneal transplantation studies (CCTS). Effectiveness of

histocompatibility matching in high-risk corneal transplantation. Arch Ophthalmol. 1992; 110(10):1392–1403

[3] Cullum RD, Chang B, eds. Corneal graft rejection. In: The Wills Eye Manual. Philadelphia, PA: JB Lippincott; 1994:104–105

[4] Foulks GN. Clinical aspects of corneal allograft rejection. In: Krachmer JH, Mannis MJ, Holland EJ, eds. Cornea. St. Louis, MO: Mosby; 1997:1687–1696

[5] Jangi AA, Ritterband DC, Wu EI, Mehta VV, Koplin RS, Seedor JA. Descemet stripping automated endothelial keratoplasty after failed penetrating keratoplasty. Cornea. 2012; 31(10):1148–1153

[6] Mitry D, Bhogal M, Patel AK, et al. Descemet stripping automated endothelial keratoplasty after failed penetrating keratoplasty: survival, rejection risk, and visual outcome. JAMA Ophthalmol. 2014; 132(6):742–749

13 Blepharitis

Weldon W. Haw

Abstract

Blepharitis may be associated with staphylococcal eyelid colonization, seborrhea, and meibomian gland dysfunction. Blepharitis may result in a chronic, relapsing condition that results in significant ocular surface discomfort. Dry eye disease and rosacea are conditions often associated with blepharitis. Clinical examination of the eyelids and ocular surface is often diagnostic. Several ancillary diagnostic tests may also be informative, including tear breakup time, corneal/conjunctival staining pattern, measurements of tear osmolarity, and metalloproteinase-9 levels. Therapy includes a number of topical and oral pharmaceutical agents. Topical steroids in a short-pulse fashion may be useful for extremely symptomatic ocular surface disease. Eyelid hygiene and cleaning can be useful in maintenance and control of this chronic condition. Occasionally, more aggressive intervention may be appropriate such as LipiFlow. Suspicion for malignancy in refractory, unilateral blepharitis must be considered.

Keywords: blepharitis, meibomian gland dysfunction, staphylococcal blepharitis, seborrheic blepharitis, dry eye, ocular rosacea, ocular surface disease, LipiFlow, lid hygiene

13.1 History

A 42-year-old woman with no past ocular history presents with complaints of bilateral itching, burning, foreign body sensation, and crusting eyelids in the morning. Although she has experienced these symptoms intermittently over the last 2 years, her symptoms have recently become worse. She denies taking any ocular medications. Her symptoms are unrelated to any systemic illness including allergy, rosacea, or flulike symptoms.

Her visual acuity is 20/20 in both eyes without correction and her intraocular pressures are normal. Slit-lamp examination reveals mild erythema of the eyelid margin associated with scaling, crusting formations around the base of the eyelashes (▶ Fig. 13.1). Evidence of trichiasis (misdirected eyelashes), madarosis (loss of eyelashes), poliosis (whitening of the eyelashes), and ulceration of the eyelid is also seen (▶ Fig. 13.2). There is mild conjunctival hyperemia associated with mild papillary reaction of the inferior tarsal conjunctiva. The tear lake in both eyes is diminished. Rose bengal dye examination of the cornea was remarkable for inferior, superficial punctate epithelial erosions. A Schirmer test was performed and revealed mild aqueous tear deficiency in both eyes.

Differential Diagnosis—Key Points

1. The differential diagnosis for this set of nonspecific symptoms is extensive and includes a variety of conditions such as allergic conjunctivitis, dry eye syndrome, giant papillary conjunctivitis, pediculosis, atopic and vernal conjunctivitis, medicamentosa, and many other disease entities. Therefore, important historical features include contact lens wear, recent exposure to infected individuals, presence of dermatologic conditions (i.e., eczema, rosacea), seasonal component, unilateral versus bilateral symptoms, and use of ocular medications.

2. There are multiple classifications of blepharitis. Marginal blepharitis is most commonly classified according to etiology. This includes blepharitis from staphylococcal colonization (*Staphylococcus aureus* and *Staphylococcus epidermis*), seborrhea, meibomian gland dysfunction, or a combination of any of the above. Seborrheic blepharitis is characterized by oily, greasy deposits of the anterior eyelid usually associated with seborrheic dermatitis. There may be mild conjunctival infection and inferior punctate epithelial erosions. Patients with meibomian gland dysfunction (posterior blepharitis) have pouting or metaplastic meibomian gland orifices, prominent vasculature crossing the mucocutaneous junction, foamy or turbid meibomian secretions, eventual atrophy of the meibomian glands, and rosacea. There may be mild to moderate conjunctival infection, papillary reaction of the tarsal conjunctiva, and inferior punctate epithelial erosions with occasional scarring and neovascularization.

This patient has the characteristics of staphylococcal blepharitis. Staphylococcal blepharitis has more potential to demonstrate structural damage. There may be evidence of poliosis, madarosis, and lid ulceration. Examination of the cornea may also reveal inferior punctate epithelial erosions, infiltrates, neovascularization, thinning, and phlyctenules. Staphylococcal blepharitis may lead to several forms of keratitis including marginal infiltrates and phlyctenules. Marginal infiltrates are sterile gray-white infiltrates along the peripheral cornea at the 2, 4, 8, and 10 o'clock positions. Phlyctenules are focal, triangular, elevated, inflammatory nodules occurring on the limbus, cornea, or conjunctiva.

3. In cases of severe unilateral or asymmetric disease resistant to therapy, it is always important to consider the possibility of an underlying malignancy. Rarely, sebaceous cell carcinoma, basal cell carcinoma, or squamous cell carcinoma may masquerade as blepharitis. The presence of a nodular mass, recurrent chalazia, extensive fibrosis or ulceration, and/or loss of normal lid architecture should lead to careful reevaluation of the diagnosis. However, our patient had a history, exam, and course typical of blepharitis.

4. Multiple conditions may be associated with blepharitis. Aqueous tear deficiency is common in patients with seborrheic blepharitis or meibomian gland dysfunction and may be present in as many as 50% of patients with staphylococcal blepharitis. Seborrheic dermatitis may affect 95% of patients who also have a seborrheic blepharitis. Meibomian gland dysfunction is also associated with seborrheic dermatitis (74%) and acne rosacea (51%). These conditions should be identified and addressed during the treatment regimen. Our patient did have symptoms related to dry eyes and on clinical examination revealed evidence of an associated aqueous tear deficiency (inferior punctate keratopathy, diminished tear lake, and a positive Schirmer's test).

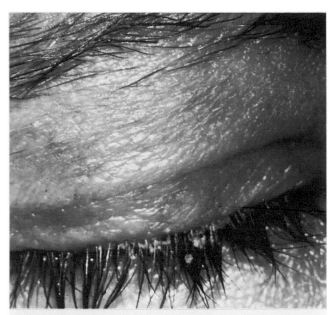

Fig. 13.1 Blepharitis. Note the crusting debris at the base of the eyelashes.

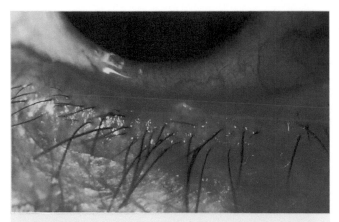

Fig. 13.2 Blepharitis. Note the disruption of normal eyelid margin architecture and the loss of eyelashes (madarosis).

13.2 Test Interpretation

Clinical examination is paramount in the diagnosis of blepharitis. However, specific diagnostic tests may be useful in selected patients. Eyelid cultures may be useful in patients with recurrent or persistent anterior inflammatory blepharitis refractory to medical management. In this same population, aqueous tear deficiency may be detected by a positive Schirmer's test or characteristic fluorescein, lissamine green, or rose bengal corneal staining pattern. An unstable tear breakup time of less than 10 seconds may help confirm meibomian gland dysfunction.

There are several clinically relevant point-of-care diagnostic modalities that may also be useful in assessing and quantifying concurrent ocular surface disease. Noninvasive, commercially available systems can quantify tear osmolarity and levels of metalloproteinase-9. These tests may be performed within the clinic setting, give immediate results, are reimbursable, and have high degree of specificity and sensitivity in diagnosing moderate to severe ocular surface disease. In addition, the dynamic tear film and anatomy of the meibomian gland can be directly assessed through imaging techniques (e.g., LipiView).

13.3 Diagnosis

Anterior blepharitis, staphylococcal type.

13.4 Medical Management

It should be emphasized to the patient that blepharitis is a chronic and relapsing condition that requires repetitious and fastidious maintenance of eyelid hygiene. The primary goals of treatment include minimizing structural damage and controlling symptoms. In staphylococcal blepharitis, the eyelid bacterial colonization may be reduced by meticulous mechanical debridement of eyelid scales with a cotton-tip applicator or lid scrub with a mild shampoo once or twice a day. Commercial and prescription-based lid cleansing solutions (i.e., hypochlorous acid 0.01%) are available and demonstrate broad-spectrum activity against microorganisms commonly found on the eyelids, including *S. epidermis* and methicillin-resistant *S. aureus*. Frequent or rough handling of the eyelids is to be avoided, as this may lead to mechanically induced lid inflammation. The application of topical antibiotic ointment before bedtime with activity against *S. aureus* may also be appropriate (i.e., erythromycin, sulfacetamide, bacitracin) in severe cases. In refractory cases, eyelid bacterial culture and sensitivity testing may be useful in directing antibiotic therapy.

A brief course of topical steroids may help reduce hypersensitivity and sterile inflammatory reactions to staphylococcal antigens (i.e., marginal keratitis and phlyctenular conjunctivitis). Preservative-free artificial tears administered four to eight times per day may be useful in treating an associated aqueous tear deficiency in these patients. Warm compresses may also help relieve discomfort during active phases and soften adherent eyelid debris.

Gentle massage of the eyelids may help mechanically express meibomian secretions in patients with meibomitis. In addition, some patients with concurrent meibomian gland dysfunction may benefit from the usage of oral omega-3 fatty acid supplementation. One to three grams per day of a high-quality omega-3 fatty acid (DHA/EPA) may improve the quality of the ocular surface. In some patients with recurrent meibomitis, the addition of topical azithromycin ophthalmic solution or erythromycin ointment, oral minocycline, doxycycline 50 to 100 mg orally twice a day, or tetracycline 250 mg orally four times a day for 4 weeks may be useful in providing symptomatic relief for severely affected patients. Indefinite use of these topical and oral antibiotics may be required to maintain control over blepharitis symptoms and should be tapered to the lowest dosage to maintain control of the patient's meibomian gland dysfunction. It should be noted that doxycycline, minocycline, and tetracycline are contraindicated in young children, as these may lead to dental staining. These medications should also be avoided in pregnant or nursing women.

13.5 Surgical Management

In cases of atypical, refractory unilateral cases, an eyelid biopsy may be indicated to evaluate for malignancy. Basal cell carcinomas and squamous cell carcinomas are the most common malignancies mistaken for blepharitis. Rarely, sebaceous cell carcinoma may masquerade as chronic, unilateral blepharitis or as a recurrent chalazion. Melanoma has also rarely been reported to masquerade as blepharitis. Patients may also require surgical management of eyelid or eyelash malposition from progressive structural damage and scarring. Point-of-care therapeutic interventions such as LipiFlow thermal pulsation system and intense pulsed light may be useful for refractory meibomian gland dysfunction.

13.6 Rehabilitation and Follow-up

Patients with mild blepharitis may be followed as needed or at their next routine visit. In more severe cases, initial follow-up may require a return visit in 3 to 6 weeks depending on the severity of the symptoms. If patients are prescribed topical steroids, earlier initial follow-up may be indicated in order to evaluate response and to assess intraocular pressure. Often, patients require a maintenance regimen of lid hygiene, artificial tears, and warm compresses. However, this regimen may be tailored to the severity of the patient's symptoms. During follow-up, it is important to emphasize to the patient the relapsing and chronic nature of the disease. Reinforcing the maintenance regimen may also prevent exacerbations in the disease process.

Suggested Reading

[1] American Academy of Ophthalmology. Blepharitis: Preferred Practice Pattern. San Francisco, CA: American Academy of Ophthalmology; 1998

[2] McCulley JP, Dougherty JM, Deneau DG. Classification of chronic blepharitis. Ophthalmology. 1982; 89(10):1173–1180

Part II

Lens

14 A Nearly Mature Cataract in a Patient with Glaucoma

I. Howard Fine and Charles C. Lin

Abstract

This chapter presents a challenging surgical case in a monocular patient with congenital glaucoma and zonular compromise. The authors present advanced surgical pearls to safely remove the cataract and prevent a dropped lens, iris trauma, and corneal decompensation.

Keywords: cataract, mature, corectopia, zonular weakness, small pupil

14.1 History

A 34-year-old Caucasian woman was referred by a glaucoma specialist for evaluation of a nearly mature cataract in her right eye. She had a complex ocular history including a phthisical left eye and congenital glaucoma status post numerous surgical procedures in the right eye including goniotomies, peripheral iridectomies, sphincterotomies, and a trabeculectomy.

On examination, visual acuity was finger counting in the right and no light perception in the left. Examination of the right eye suggested that the patient was using her superior nasal peripheral iridotomy as an entrance pupil. There was a relatively thick-walled but functioning filtering bleb in the superior nasal quadrant. Intraocular pressure (IOP) was 20 mm Hg without glaucoma medications. A few corneal guttae were observed. The anterior chamber was deep and quiet. The iris was highly atrophic throughout its entire periphery, with very little sphincter tissue. The pupil measured 3 mm and did not dilate due to 360 degrees of posterior synechiae. There were multiple sphincterotomies at the pupillary margin and a large radial cut at the 12 o'clock position (▶ Fig. 14.1). There was a dense, nearly mature cataract, an absence of zonules visible through the large superior nasal iridectomy, and questionable zonular status in the areas of broad peripheral iridectomies in two other quadrants. There was no view of the right fundus.

Differential Diagnosis—Key Points

The diagnosis was obvious, but unique challenges existed in the surgical approach to this cataract. The bleb was functional and necessary for IOP control. Corneal endothelial cell loss due to multiple previous surgical procedures indicated a risk for corneal decompensation. The pupil presented perhaps the largest surgical challenge. Any attempt to manipulate or stretch it could result in tearing of the 12 o'clock radial sphincterotomy out to the periphery with loss of entrance pupillary function. In addition, the atrophic nature of the entire iris was such that any thoughts of surgical repair seemed impossible.

There are multiple cataract surgical considerations in this case, including (1) zonular integrity with the risk for potential loss of the cataract into the posterior segment; (2) potential for postoperative inflammation and secondary glaucoma; and (3) difficult and potentially inaccurate preoperative measurements and intraocular lens (IOL) power calculations, and corneal decompensation.

14.2 Test Interpretation

The patient was unable to undergo a reliable refraction. Keratometry measurements showed 7 diopters of against-the-rule astigmatism. Corneal topography revealed 6 diopters of astigmatism that did not correlate with keratometry measurements. Axial length measured 30 mm and the horizontal white-to-white measurement was greater than 14 mm. Endothelial cell count was not performed since surgery was necessary regardless of the status of the endothelium. B-scan ultrasonography revealed that the retina was flat.

14.3 Diagnosis

Mature cataract with zonular compromise, advanced glaucoma status post multiple surgeries including a trabeculectomy with a functioning filtering bleb, atrophic iris with radial sphincterotomies, and blind phthisical fellow eye.

14.4 Medical Management

Intermittent use of glaucoma medications and massage of the bleb.

14.5 Surgical Management

The anatomical complexities of this case required unique surgical modifications. For the paracentesis and clear corneal incision, a 16-mm Fine/Thornton ring was utilized for fixation of the globe as it had a sufficiently large diameter to avoid traumatizing the bleb.

Considering the tenuous status of the cornea given the history of numerous prior intraocular surgeries, special efforts were taken to protect the endothelium. A side-port incision was made and the anterior chamber was partially filled with Viscoat, a dispersive viscoelastic solution. The cohesive viscoelastic substance Provisc was injected directly on the anterior lens capsule, forcing the dispersive Viscoat to the periphery of the anterior chamber to sequester the area of missing zonules and superiorly in a soft-shell under the endothelium.

With a combination of blunt and viscodissection, the posterior synechiae were lysed, and a Morcher iris-expander ring was inserted utilizing two hooks (▶ Fig. 14.2). This device is inserted by compression into the pupillary space, which then expands. Flanges on the top and bottom allow it to surround a pupil, much as a tire rim surrounds a tire, and holes in the flanges allow for intraocular manipulation. The expander ring maintained a broad angle of contact with the pupil as it was inserted and allowed stretching of the pupil without concentrating forces on the 12 o'clock radial sphincterotomy, thus avoiding extension of the tear. An alternative device that may be considered is the Malyugin ring, which comes in 6.2- and 7.0-mm diameters. While this device is often used in cataract surgery for mechanical pupillary dilation, because of its mechanism of action with four points of pressure, it may exert a

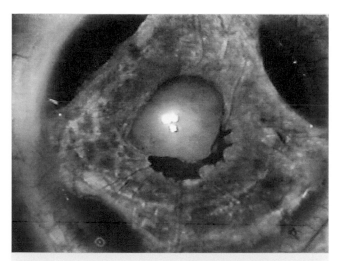

Fig. 14.1 Intraoperative surgeon's image, sitting temporally.

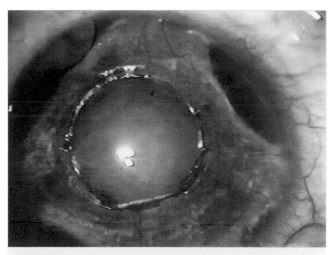

Fig. 14.2 The iris-expander ring in place.

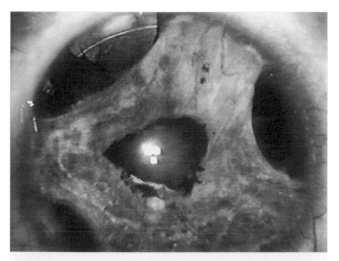

Fig. 14.3 Immediate postoperative appearance of the eye with the capsular tension ring visible in the superior nasal peripheral iridectomy.

tearing force on the sphincterotomy at 12 o'clock position, rendering it suboptimal in this case.

Following placement of the iris-expander ring, a continuous curvilinear capsulorrhexis was performed. A Morcher capsular tension ring was inserted into the capsular bag utilizing a forceps and a Lester hook. This device expands the equatorial zone of the capsule and transmits any focal force on the capsule to the entire zonular apparatus. Without the capsular tension ring, any focal force on the capsule would be transmitted only to the adjacent zonules, with much greater risk of damage. Thus, the ring adds a margin of safety when operating on cataracts in the presence of a compromised zonular apparatus. In addition, it facilitates centration of the bag and IOL postoperatively since the outward force of the ring opposes fibroses of the capsule, unopposed by compromised zonules. At this point, additional ultraviscous viscoelastic such as Healon 5 (Johnson and Johnson Vision) may be injected into the area of zonular weakness to prevent vitreous prolapse.

Cortical cleaving hydrodissection and hydrodelineation were performed. Choo choo chop and flip phacoemulsification was done. This is a uniquely safe technique for removing nuclear material because the nucleus is disassembled with mechanical forces in the form of chopping and the resulting pieces are evacuated largely by high vacuum with low-power modulation ultrasound energy. It is an endolenticular technique. Utilizing either a reverse Kelman tip or a 30-degree bevel-down straight tip enables one to approach nuclear material from above, pulling it up to the tip rather than getting underneath to mobilize and evacuate it. Ultrasound energy is concentrated at the upper levels of the endolenticular space, remote from the posterior capsule and the corneal endothelium. In addition, the technique allows for fixation of the lens between the two instruments (the chop instrument and the phaco tip) during lollipopping of the nucleus and scoring and chopping. Therefore, no downward force is exerted on the capsule or zonules during lollipopping the nucleus by the phaco tip.

Phacoemulsification took place with an effective phaco time of 6.4 seconds and an average ultrasonic energy of under 13.7%. The cortex, partially held in by the endocapsular tension ring, was carefully irrigated and aspirated. Cortex was stripped tangential to the capsulorrhexis rather than centrally in order to help pull it around the endocapsular tension ring. The capsular bag and anterior chamber were refilled with Provisc after which a bolus of the dispersive Viscoat was placed in the center of the capsulorrhexis. A 6-diopter foldable silicone IOL was injected into the capsular bag without complication.

During removal of residual viscoelastic, vitreous presented through the superior nasal iridectomy. Healon 5 was injected into the anterior chamber and the main wound was closed with a suture. A separate paracentesis was made and a split port anterior vitrectomy performed, which provides a more stable anterior chamber. Viscoelastic was injected into the anterior chamber and the iris-expander ring was removed utilizing a Lester hook. The remainder of the residual viscoelastic was removed from the anterior segment with a vitrector to avoid vitreous coming to the incision through the zonular defect in the superior nasal iridectomy. Finally, stromal hydration was performed to seal the incision and the paracentesis. The immediate postoperative appearance of the eye is seen in ▶ Fig. 14.3.

14.6 Rehabilitation and Follow-up

She was started on topical prednisolone acetate, ofloxacin, and diclofenac three times daily. Given her history of advanced glaucoma and monocular status, the patient was closely followed for an IOP spike and examined twice daily over the next 3 days. Timolol and brimonidine were started prophylactically to control her IOP, which remained below 20 mm Hg. A prostaglandin analog was avoided to minimize the risk of postoperative inflammation and macular edema. In addition, a carbonic anhydrase inhibitor was avoided to minimize the risk of exacerbating corneal edema, a known side effect of this class of medications.

By postoperative week 1, she had experienced an enormous increase in correctable acuity to 20/80. She uses a computer at work, grows flowers, and is very aware of colors and the brightness of objects. Two years postoperatively, her IOP remains in the low teens on no glaucoma medication.

Suggested Reading

[1] Fine IH. Clear corneal cataract incision with a temporal approach. In: Fine IH, Fichman RA, Grabow HB, eds. Clear Corneal Cataract Surgery & Topical Anesthesia. Thorofare, NJ: Slack Inc; 1993

[2] Fine IH. Choo choo chop and flip phacoemulsification. In: Elander R, ed. Phacoemulsification Techniques: Operative Techniques in Cataract and Refractive Surgery. Philadelphia, PA: WB Saunders Co; 1998

[3] Fine IH, Hoffman RS. Phacoemulsification in the presence of pseudoexfoliation: challenges and options. J Cataract Refract Surg. 1997; 23(2):160–165

15 Retained Lens Material after Cataract Extraction

Ruwan A. Silva and Charles C. Lin

Abstract

This chapter discusses the complications and management strategy for retained lens fragments following cataract surgery. Acute postoperative complications such as glaucoma and inflammation are addressed, along with an in-depth analysis of the need for and timing of pars plana vitrectomy and lensectomy.

Keywords: retained lens fragment, cataract, complication, lens particle glaucoma, vitrectomy

15.1 History

A 47-year-old man with a history of bungee cord trauma to the left eye had undergone a complicated cataract surgery 9 months earlier. He was lost to follow-up and presented to the retina clinic with a 2-month history of decreased vision, redness, and pain in the left eye. His visual acuity was 20/20 OD and 20/400 OS. Intraocular pressures (IOPs) were 12 and 38 mm Hg in the right and left eyes, respectively. His pupils were reactive to light with no relative afferent pupillary defect. Examination of the right eye was unremarkable aside from a mild cataract. Slit-lamp biomicroscopy of the left eye revealed mild conjunctival injection, 2 + anterior chamber cell and flare, iridodonesis, ectopia lentis, and prolapsed vitreous. Gonioscopy of the left eye demonstrated a wide open angle with lens fragments noted inferiorly. Dilated fundus examination of the left eye revealed a posterior vitreous detachment with his crystalline lens subluxated inferiorly in the anterior vitreous. His macula, retinal vessels, and optic nerve were unremarkable.

15.2 Test Interpretation

Determining the etiology of an eye with acute pain and elevated IOP involves careful assessment of the anterior chamber. Initial evaluation of all patients with glaucoma should therefore include gonioscopy to evaluate the anterior chamber angle, since the mechanism of outflow disruption often affects management. In the setting of an acute rise in IOP, this can be confounded by corneal edema. Lowering of the IOP may be required before a view of the anterior chamber angle is possible. The above case is archetypal in demonstrating the importance of gonioscopic evaluation in determining the etiology and subsequent management of a patient's elevated IOP. The finding of fluffy lens particles in the chamber angle is pathognomonic for lens particle glaucoma.

In this case, the patient's history is also invaluable as the timing of the patient's symptoms were telling and assisted in ruling out several types of glaucoma. Additionally, the distant history of trauma provided insight into the complicated nature of his cataract surgery.

15.3 Diagnosis

Lens particle glaucoma.

Differential Diagnosis—Key Points

1. Angle-closure glaucoma should be considered in any patient presenting with eye pain and blurred vision with a markedly elevated IOP on examination. Gonioscopy demonstrating an open angle in this patient, however, definitively rules out this possibility.

2. Phacolytic glaucoma typically presents with conjunctival injection, decreased vision, pain, and ocular hypertension in the presence of an open angle, similar to this case. Our patient, however, did not demonstrate the milky white aqueous humor or pseudohypopyon characteristic of phacolytic glaucoma. These putatively represent inflammatory cells and high-molecular-weight lens proteins released through the anterior lens capsule of a mature or hypermature lens.

3. Phacoantigenic glaucoma represents an acute, type III hypersensitivity reaction against lens antigens after violation of the lens capsule by penetrating lens trauma. The patient's clinical history is not consistent with this diagnosis, as the disease usually presents within 2 weeks of ocular trauma or surgery. Additionally, the hallmark granulomatous keratic precipitates of this disease were absent on physical examination.

4. Iridocyclitis must be included in the differential when a patient presents with a painful red eye, elevated IOP, and anterior chamber reaction. Typically, the IOP is lower than in the fellow eye due to inflammation of the ciliary body, but it can be markedly elevated when inflammatory debris obstructs the trabecular meshwork. Unilateral uveitis in a young male patient is commonly associated with HLA-B27. Typically, however, the IOP is reduced with HLA-B27-related anterior uveitis.

5. Angle-recession glaucoma should be considered in cases involving elevated IOP following a history of blunt trauma. Gonioscopy in angle recession shows widening of the ciliary body (which represents separation of the longitudinal and circular muscles of the ciliary body). Fortunately, only a small percentage of these patients will develop glaucoma with that risk increased if the angle recession involves over half of the patient's angle.

6. Lens particle glaucoma is the most likely diagnosis given the patient's history and physical examination. This disease usually presents several weeks after disruption of the lens capsule through surgery or ocular trauma, although it may occur months to years later. Lens particles released from the trauma are thought to obstruct aqueous outflow and increase IOP. Associated inflammation may also contribute to the elevation of IOP. The lens remnants found in the anterior chamber on gonioscopy in this case support the diagnosis of lens particle glaucoma.

15.4 Medical Management

A patient with lens particle glaucoma who presents with an acute pressure elevation must be managed aggressively. Salient issues are control of the IOP and inflammation. Initial treatment should include multiple IOP-lowering agents, frequent corticosteroids, and cycloplegics/mydriatics.

The duration and magnitude of IOP elevation that can be tolerated depends on the age of the patient, the health of the optic nerve, and the vascular perfusion of the eye. Younger patients can tolerate a markedly elevated pressure for a longer period before suffering detectable visual field loss. Patients who have known preexistent glaucomatous damage are less likely to tolerate a markedly elevated pressure, and early surgical intervention may be necessary to prevent further optic nerve damage. Microvascular disease also affects the optic nerve's tolerance to elevated IOP.

Multiple aqueous suppressants should be employed. In this case, a topical beta-blocker, an alpha-2-adrenergic agonist, and both a topical and a systemic carbonic anhydrase inhibitor were employed. Miotics should be avoided to prevent posterior synechiae formation, although in a case where the patient's lens complex has been dislocated this is of little concern. Prostaglandin analogs are typically not used in the inflamed eye. Hyperosmotic agents should be reserved for the markedly elevated pressure and are a short-term measure. Glycerin should be avoided in the diabetic patient, but isosorbide and mannitol are acceptable emergency measures to lower the pressure.

Frequent topical corticosteroids are necessary to control the inflammation. Although suppression of the immune response might delay resorption of the lens particles, their use is essential in an eye with severe inflammation. Periocular or systemic corticosteroids might also be considered. Cycloplegics/mydriatics relax the ciliary body and prevent posterior synechiae.

15.5 Surgical Management

While the incidence of retained lens fragments following cataract surgery is rare, complications including ocular hypertension and retinal detachment are not uncommon. Despite these worrisome sequelae, the majority of patients can be expected to do well, especially when a posterior chamber intraocular lens (IOL) was placed at the time of cataract surgery.

The timing of vitreoretinal surgery is controversial. While urgent intervention is recommended for uveitis, vitreous prolapse, retinal detachment, elevated IOP, or hemorrhage, the traditional approach of performing a pars plana vitrectomy and lensectomy within 1 week after cataract extraction for cases not involving the above has been questioned. Specifically, several series have shown no correlation between final visual acuity and vitrectomy timing when the surgery was performed within 1 month of cataract extraction. The risk of retinal detachment and secondary glaucoma, however, has been reported to be higher in patients in whom vitrectomy was delayed for over 1 month. The benefits of delaying immediate vitrectomy include improved corneal recovery, abatement of intraocular inflammation, and softening of lens material before secondary surgery. Delaying vitrectomy may also be a reasonable choice as it is sometimes possible to avoid a vitrectomy

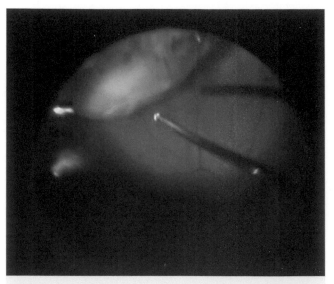

Fig. 15.1 A thorough pars plana vitrectomy is performed with care taken to remove any vitreous strands connected to the retained lens material.

altogether. Spontaneous resorption of the lens material may occur when there is minimal retained lens material or it is predominantly composed of cortex. However, complications such as chronic inflammation, disabling visual floaters, and refractory cystoid macular edema may expedite the need for vitreoretinal surgery.

When vitreoretinal surgery is pursued, surgical technique can vary widely. Adjuvant use of triamcinolone acetonide, employment of heavy liquids, and routine 360-degree prophylactic retina laser retinopexy have all been reported. While most surgeons employ microincisional vitrectomy surgery (23 gauge or smaller), use of a phacofragmatome to remove retained lens material requires at least one 20-gauge sclerotomy. Regardless of technique, several steps remain paramount. First, a thorough vitrectomy removing all vitreous adhesion to the retained lens material is critical (▶ Fig. 15.1). Because manipulation of lens material incarcerated in vitreous humor yields unwanted traction on the retina, the importance of this step cannot be overstated. Once the lens material is free from the vitreous and a peripheral vitrectomy has been completed, the retained lens material is engaged with the phacofragmatome and elevated away from the retina. Subsequent fragmentation and aspiration of the lens material is then performed in the midvitreous cavity (▶ Fig. 15.2). After larger lens material has been removed, smaller lens particles can then be removed from the eye using a vitrector (▶ Fig. 15.3). Finally, inspection of the peripheral retina for retinal breaks is performed.

15.6 Rehabilitation and Follow-up

In the case presented, the patient was initially placed on topical ocular hypotensives (timolol, dorzolamide, and brimonidine) as well as topical atropine and prednisolone acetate by the referring physician. As his pressure remained elevated and placement of an IOL was necessary, he underwent pars plana vitrectomy, lensectomy, and IOL placement 4 days after

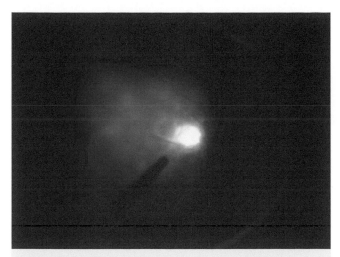

Fig. 15.2 The retained lens material is engaged, fragmented, and aspirated from the midvitreous cavity.

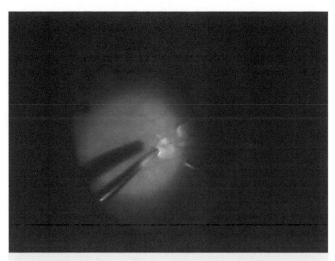

Fig. 15.3 Residual lens material is removed using the vitrector.

presentation. Postoperatively, his IOP improved to 12 mm Hg without any topical medications and his final uncorrected visual acuity was 20/30 in the left eye.

Suggested Reading

[1] Herschler J. Trabecular damage due to blunt anterior segment injury and its relationship to traumatic glaucoma. Trans Sect Ophthalmol Am Acad Ophthalmol Otolaryngol. 1977; 83(2):239–248

[2] Tönjum AM. Intraocular pressure and facility of outflow late after ocular contusion. Acta Ophthalmol (Copenh). 1968; 46(5):886–908

[3] Rofagha S, Bhisitkul RB. Management of retained lens fragments in complicated cataract surgery. Curr Opin Ophthalmol. 2011; 22(2):137–140

[4] Kim IK, Miller JW. Management of dislocated lens material. Semin Ophthalmol. 2002; 17(3–4):162–166– Review

[5] Vanner EA, Stewart MW. Vitrectomy timing for retained lens fragments after surgery for age-related cataracts: a systematic review and meta-analysis. Am J Ophthalmol. 2011; 152(3):345–357.e3

[6] Scott IU, Flynn HW. Retained lens fragments after cataract surgery. Ophthalmol Clin North Am. 2001; 14(4):675–679

16 Fibrin Deposition on Intraocular Lenses

Christopher N. Ta

Abstract

Fibrin deposition over the intraocular lens implant typically occurs 2 to 14 days following intraocular surgery. Symptoms include decreased vision, red eye, pain, and photophobia. Examination demonstrates cellular anterior chamber (AC) reaction without the presence of a hypopyon. The fibrin finding ranges from strands in the AC to dense fibrinous membrane covering the pupil. It is important to rule out endophthalmitis. Inflammation from surgery causes a breakdown of the blood–aqueous barrier, allowing fibrinogen to leak out from blood vessels into the AC. The main treatment is topical steroid, such as prednisolone. Recombinant tissue plasminogen activator (tPA) is another treatment option. This can be given by intracameral injection. Potential complications of intracameral tPA injection are AC turbidity, cornea edema, elevated intraocular pressure, bleeding, corneal toxicity, band keratopathy, and endophthalmitis.

Keywords: fibrin, anterior chamber reaction, intraocular lens, postoperative inflammation, plasminogen activator

16.1 History

A 59-year-old Caucasian woman presented to the eye clinic after intraocular surgery in the right eye, with a chief complaint of photophobia. Five days earlier, she had undergone combined cataract extraction with posterior chamber intraocular lens (IOL) implantation and trabeculectomy with mitomycin C in the right eye. Her left eye had undergone the same procedures 1 month prior to presentation. Her past medical history was significant only for hypertension. Her ocular medications were prednisolone acetate 1% every 2 hours and ofloxacin four times a day in both eyes.

Her visual acuity was 20/60 OD and 20/200 OS. Slit-lamp examination of the right eye revealed mild conjunctival injection with a low bleb. The cornea was clear. The anterior chamber had moderate cells and flare with no hypopyon. There was a meshwork of fibrin deposition on the IOL (▶ Fig. 16.1). Examination of the left eye revealed a low bleb, clear cornea, and rare cells in the anterior chamber. The IOL was in good position. Dilated fundus exam was unremarkable in both eyes except for moderate and severe glaucomatous cupping of the right and left optic nerves, respectively. The poor vision in the left eye was secondary to advanced glaucoma.

Differential Diagnosis—Key Points

1. Fibrinous reaction in the anterior chamber typically presents between days 2 and 14 after intraocular surgery. The patient may complain of decreased vision, redness, pain, and photophobia. Slit-lamp examination reveals a cellular anterior chamber reaction without the presence of a hypopyon. The fibrin can present as strands on the IOL, in the pupillary plane, or on the iris itself. In a more severe inflammatory reaction, there can also be a fibrinous membrane covering the pupil.

2. Endophthalmitis is always in the differential diagnosis, particularly if a hypopyon is present. However, patients with endophthalmitis usually have more severe symptoms, such as pain and poor vision. Examination reveals injected and chemotic conjunctiva with a severe cellular reaction in the anterior chamber and potentially a hypopyon. There may also be cells in the anterior vitreous.

3. The pathophysiology of fibrin deposition on the IOL is immune-mediated. From the surgical trauma, there is increased blood–aqueous permeability. The breakdown in the blood–aqueous barrier allows fibrinogen from blood plasma, a precursor of fibrin, to leak out of blood vessels and into the anterior chamber. In the presence of inflammatory mediators, such as prostaglandins, along with thrombin and activated coagulation factors, fibrinogen is converted to fibrin. Pathologically, fibrin appears as fine proteinaceous fibers in a meshwork. There may be associated macrophages and giant cells.

4. The incidence of fibrinous uveitis is less than 4% after normal uncomplicated cataract extraction and IOL implantation, but can be as high as 54%, depending on the patient population and study. Certain conditions that are associated with an increase in vascular permeability predispose to fibrin formation. These include diabetes, hypertension, pseudoexfoliation syndrome, uveitis, prolonged surgery, and previous intraocular surgery. Local factors that may increase the likelihood of developing a fibrinous reaction are surgical manipulation of the iris and incomplete removal of the lens cortex and epithelial cells. In addition, intraoperative use of a long-acting miotic agent, can result in posterior synechiae and pigmented membrane formation over the anterior optic. Prior history of intraocular surgery particularly in the recent past, even if done in the fellow eye, is also a risk factor for developing fibrinous uveitis.

5. Fibrin deposition indicates a severe inflammatory reaction. Complications of fibrinous uveitis are posterior synechiae, loss of iris function, membrane formation on the IOL, dislocation of the IOL, and glaucoma. The risk for developing cystoid macular edema is increased with intraocular inflammation, particularly if the posterior capsule is compromised. Posterior capsular opacification is generally due to lens epithelial migration and proliferation, but the presence of fibrin and inflammation may trigger this process.

6. The intraocular pressure (IOP) may be high due to secondary glaucoma, such as pupillary block or clogging of the trabecular meshwork from inflammatory cells. The IOP can also be low due to inflammation of the ciliary body.

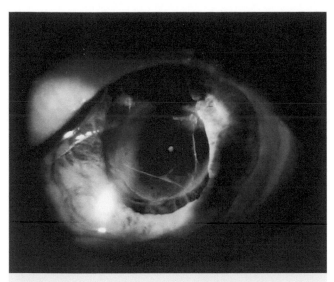

Fig. 16.1 Fibrin deposition on the IOL 5 days postoperatively.

16.2 Test Interpretation

It is important, albeit sometimes challenging, to differentiate postoperative fibrinous uveitis from endophthalmitis. The time of onset and symptoms are similar between the two diagnoses, except that more severe symptoms accompany endophthalmitis. Examination findings of ciliary injection, chemosis, severe anterior chamber reaction, hypopyon, and vitritis suggest endophthalmitis. An anterior chamber and vitreous aspirate for culture and intravitreal injection of antibiotics should be considered when endophthalmitis is suspected.

16.3 Diagnosis

Right eye: Postoperative fibrin deposition on the IOL.

16.4 Medical Management

The goal of treatment is to reduce inflammation and restore the blood–aqueous barrier. A topical steroid, such as prednisolone, is the mainstay of treatment. The usual dose is prednisolone acetate 1%, one drop four to six times a day, and up to hourly, depending on the level of inflammation. In severe cases, particularly in patients with a history of uveitis, systemic steroids may be required to control the inflammation.

In high-risk patients, preoperative topical nonsteroidal anti-inflammatory and/or topical steroid agents may prevent or minimize fibrin deposition. In addition, intraoperative subconjunctival steroid injection can minimize postoperative inflammation.

Recombinant tissue plasminogen activator (tPA) can have a dramatic effect in breaking down fibrin in severe cases of fibrin deposition. tPA converts plasminogen to plasmin, which lyses fibrin to fibrin-split products. tPA has been shown to be effective with an intracameral injection of doses as low as 3 µg. Complications with the use of intracameral tPA are rare but can include anterior chamber turbidity, corneal edema, elevated IOP, bleeding, corneal toxicity, and band keratopathy. The risk of bleeding increases with a shorter interval from the time of surgery. There is also the risk of introducing infectious microorganisms into the anterior chamber with a tPA injection.

16.5 Surgical Management

In the acute postoperative period, additional surgery in an already inflamed eye is not advisable, except when there are obvious indications for surgery, such as a dislocated IOL or intractable glaucoma. In cases when the IOL is the cause of inflammation (e.g., an anterior chamber lens that is rubbing against the iris), it is reasonable to remove the IOL. Once the acute postoperative phase has passed and the eye is quiescent, if the fibrin deposition has not resolved, an anterior chamber washout with fibrin membranectomy may be considered in cases that are particularly visually significant.

16.6 Rehabilitation and Follow-up

Medical treatment is usually successful in eliminating inflammation and fibrin deposition. However, these patients are at risk for developing infectious keratitis from topical steroid use, secondary glaucoma, and cystoid macular edema. Eye examinations should be done at a regular interval to follow visual acuity, IOP, and signs of infection or recurrent inflammation.

Suggested Reading

[1] Miyake K, Maekubo K, Miyake Y, Nishi O. Pupillary fibrin membrane. A frequent early complication after posterior chamber lens implantation in Japan. Ophthalmology. 1989; 96(8):1228–1233

[2] Baltatzis S, Georgopoulos G, Theodossiadis P. Fibrin reaction after extracapsular cataract extraction: a statistical evaluation. Eur J Ophthalmol. 1993; 3(2): 95–97

[3] Ozveren F, Eltutar K. Therapeutic application of tissue plasminogen activator for fibrin reaction after cataract surgery. J Cataract Refract Surg. 2004; 30(8): 1727–1731

17 Subluxated Crystalline Lens

David F. Chang and Bryan S. Lee

Abstract

Ophthalmologists should remember the systemic implications of bilateral lens subluxation, including the life-threatening cardiac abnormalities associated with Marfan's syndrome. Unilateral subluxation is often caused by trauma, although pseudoexfoliation may also be a cause. Bilateral subluxation is most frequently caused by hereditary systematic disorders, such as Marfan's syndrome. Glasses or contact lenses may be adequate medical management for some patients. When surgery is required, the ophthalmologist must choose between an anterior and posterior approach. Phacoemulsification requires gentle handling of the weakened zonules, and surgeons should be familiar with capsular hardware such as capsule retractors, capsule tension rings, and sutured capsule tension rings and segments. The intraocular lens (IOL) may be placed in the capsular bag or in the sulcus if the support is adequate, but a sutured lens or anterior chamber IOL may be required. Pars plana vitrectomy is more suitable for posteriorly dislocated lenses or severe vitreous prolapse.

Keywords: Marfan's syndrome, zonulopathy, lens subluxation, complex cataract

17.1 History

A 41-year-old man with Marfan's syndrome presents with complaints of variable decreased vision and bothersome glare in his left eye. The patient has a family history of Marfan's syndrome, but no history of trauma. Visual acuity is 20/70 with –5.00 D correction in the left eye, compared to 20/20 with a –0.75 D correction in the right eye. The left crystalline lens is subluxated superiorly with diaphanous zonules exposed across an area of at least six clock hours inferiorly (▶ Fig. 17.1). There is no phacodonesis and no vitreous prolapse. Dilated examination of the asymptomatic right eye revealed a very subtle inferior zonular dialysis. The intraocular pressure and fundus examination are normal.

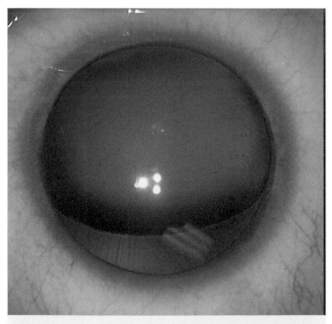

Fig. 17.1 Upward subluxation of crystalline lens in left eye of this patient with Marfan's syndrome.

Differential Diagnosis—Key Points

1. The most common cause of a unilateral dislocated or subluxated lens is trauma, and the history is usually diagnostic. Less common causes of acquired lens subluxation are pseudoexfoliation and eye rubbing associated with atopy.

2. Bilateral subluxated crystalline lenses are usually associated with a hereditary systemic disorder. The most common of these is Marfan's syndrome, which is autosomal dominant. Autosomal-recessive etiologies include homocystinuria (usually down-and-out subluxation), the Weill–Marchesani syndrome, hyperlysinemia, and sulfite oxidase deficiency. Mental retardation is usually associated with the metabolic genetic disorders. A full medical and metabolic workup should be considered with nontraumatic bilateral lens subluxation to evaluate the cause. Homocystinuria can be diagnosed by a sodium nitroprusside test of the urine. Medical and ophthalmologic examinations of family members may contribute useful information.

3. Marfan's syndrome is the most common hereditary disorder associated with lens subluxation, which occurs in 75% of affected individuals. Typical physical findings include tall stature, long, thin extremities, arachnodactyly joint laxity, pectus excavatum, kyphoscoliosis, and decreased subcutaneous fat. Establishing the diagnosis is important both for genetic counseling and because of the cardiac implications of this syndrome. Echocardiography should be performed to rule out mitral or aortic valve abnormalities and progressive dilation of the ascending aorta, since a dissecting aortic aneurism may cause sudden death. In Marfan's syndrome, the lens is usually dislocated in an upward or up-and-out direction. Aside from ectopia lentis, ocular associations may include axial myopia, glaucoma, and retinal detachment.

4. A careful ophthalmologic exam should be performed on any patient with a subluxated lens. Although a dilated exam is necessary to determine the extent of lens decentration or subluxation, phacodonesis may be more evident in the undilated eye because of associated iridodonesis. Gonioscopy may disclose a traumatic angle recession. A careful peripheral retinal exam should be performed because patients with Marfan's syndrome and homocystinuria are predisposed to retinal detachment.

17.2 Diagnosis

Lens subluxation (ectopia lentis) associated with Marfan's syndrome.

17.3 Medical Management

A subluxated lens can be managed conservatively unless significant visual symptoms or complications arise. Lens-induced optical errors such as myopic shift, lenticular astigmatism, anisometropia, and prism effect can often be corrected with spectacles or contact lenses. Lens subluxation in a pediatric patient may cause amblyopia, which must be aggressively treated and monitored.

If the crystalline lens is partially dislocated out of the pupillary axis, aphakic contact lenses might be effective. Cycloplegics can be used to increase this aphakic aperture. Conversely, miotics can be employed to minimize monocular diplopia or optical aberrations arising from the lens edge. Neodymium: yttrium-aluminum-garnet (Nd:YAG) laser zonulysis has been used to further clear the visual axis of an incompletely dislocated lens. A completely dislocated crystalline lens should be well tolerated and may remain within the eye indefinitely.

A forward shift of the crystalline lens due to zonular laxity may result in pupillary block and angle-closure glaucoma. A peripheral laser iridotomy may address this problem in the short term. More severe zonular laxity may lead to forward dislocation of the lens into the anterior chamber with resulting endothelial cell loss and corneal decompensation. The prolapsed lens can be repositioned by reclining the dilated patient so that the lens falls back behind the pupil—either spontaneously or with manual pressure applied against the cornea. Pharmacologic miosis is used to trap the mobile lens posteriorly. Recurrence of these complications would be an indication for surgical lensectomy.

17.4 Surgical Management

There are two different approaches to surgical removal of a subluxated or dislocated crystalline lens—phacoemulsification or pars plana lensectomy with vitrectomy. Phacoemulsification is done with the expectation or hope of preserving the lens capsule for intraocular lens (IOL) support. Depending on the extent of zonulopathy with an intact bag, intracapsular fixation of the IOL can be done with or without a sutured intracapsular device. Alternatively, sulcus implantation of a three-piece foldable IOL might be an option. In the absence of sufficient capsular support, a three-piece posterior chamber IOL can be implanted with iris or scleral suture fixation, or with intrascleral tunnel haptic fixation. Other options would be an anterior chamber IOL or iris-claw IOL. If the patient is left aphakic, and an aphakic contact lens is not tolerated, a secondary IOL implantation can be performed at a later stage.

17.4.1 Phacoemulsification

Depending on the severity of zonulopathy and the individual surgeon's experience, phacoemulsification may be elected with the goal of preserving the capsular bag or enough residual

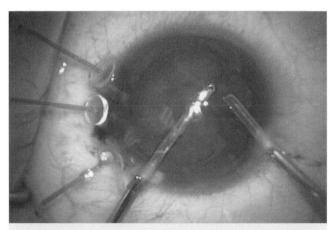

Fig. 17.2 During surgery in this case, three capsule retractors hook the capsulotomy and support the capsular bag in the meridian of the large inferior zonular dialysis. The surgeon and the microscope are oriented temporally.

capsule to support a posterior chamber IOL. However, phacoemulsification of a subluxated lens is among the most challenging of cases for an anterior segment surgeon. These eyes are highly predisposed to zonular dialysis, posterior capsule rupture, vitreous loss, and a dropped nucleus.

During phacoemulsification, care must be taken to avoid worsening the zonular dialysis. Self-retaining capsule retractors (▶ Fig. 17.2) should be inserted through limbal stab incisions after completion of a capsulorhexis. These act as artificial zonules to support and recenter a subluxated capsular bag and to restrain the equatorial capsule from being aspirated by the phaco or irrigation-aspiration tips. Capsule retractors also facilitate safe rotation of the nucleus by improving torsional counterfixation of the entire capsular bag. Although flexible iris retractors can be used for this purpose, capsule retractors are longer, sturdier, and less likely to slip off of the capsulotomy edge during phaco.

The technique of horizontal phaco chop, which utilizes inwardly directed manual forces to reduce stress on the capsular bag, is advantageous in these eyes. Regardless of the phaco technique, one should consider bringing larger sections of nucleus out of the capsular bag where they can be subchopped or emulsified within the supracapsular space. Repeatedly inflating the capsular bag with a dispersive ophthalmic viscosurgical device will restrain the flaccid posterior capsule and equatorial capsule from being inadvertently aspirated.

By employing capsule retractors, capsular tension ring (CTR) implantation can usually be delayed until after completing cortical cleanup to avoid trapping the cortex within the capsular fornices. The capsular retractors should be left in place to counter the lateral decentering forces of the CTR as it is injected. The retractors can then be removed prior to IOL implantation.

A CTR can be implanted at any point after the capsulorhexis is completed. The primary function of a CTR, however, is to resist subsequent capsular contraction, which can be concentric or asymmetric due to uneven zonular integrity. Posterior dislocation of the entire IOL–capsular bag complex may occur years later. For this reason, placing a single piece acrylic IOL without an additional capsular device may be problematic because this type of IOL is not amenable to suturing if it decenters.

There are several different surgical approaches to centering and fixating a subluxated capsular bag. The Cionni and Malyugin ring modifications incorporate a small loop with a terminal eyelet onto the CTR for scleral suture fixation of the endocapsular ring (▶ Fig. 17.3). With the Cionni ring, the loop and eyelet

emanate from one proximal section of the CTR. In contrast, one end of the Malyugin ring terminates in the eyelet, which allows this ring to be more easily injected (▶ Fig. 17.3a). With either device, the CTR is endocapsular and the small loop extends around the capsulotomy edge out of the bag so that the eyelet is located in the ciliary sulcus (behind the iris and just in front of the anterior capsule) (▶ Fig. 17.3b). The loop is normally positioned so that the sutured eyelet will anchor the ring to the sclera in the area of missing zonules. Prior to insertion of the Cionni or Malyugin CTRs, the needles of a double-armed 9–0 polypropylene (Prolene) or CV-8 Gore-Tex sutures are preplaced through the eyelet (▶ Fig. 17.3a). Passing the needles through either a Hoffman pocket or a half-thickness scleral groove will then allow scleral fixation of the eyelet in the meridian of the zonular dialysis (▶ Fig. 17.3c). After implanting and orienting the Cionni or Malyugin ring, tying the knot will recenter the ring and the capsular bag prior to placement of the IOL (▶ Fig. 17.3c).

A three-piece foldable IOL may be inserted into the capsular bag or in the sulcus, as was done in this case with optic-capsulorhexis capture (▶ Fig. 17.4a). The haptics are oriented away from the inferior zonular dialysis. Pupil constriction confirms excellent centration of the IOL (▶ Fig. 17.4b).

A second method utilizes the Ahmed capsular tension segment, which is a partial PMMA ring with the Cionni modified fixation loop for scleral fixation. The segment may be placed at any time during the surgery after capsulorhexis creation, and can be used intraoperatively as a capsular supporting device by placing an iris hook through the eyelet of the positioning loop. After the cataract has been removed, the same segment can be

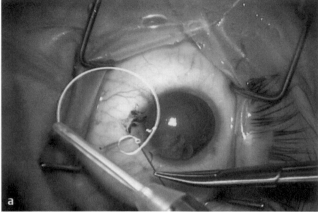

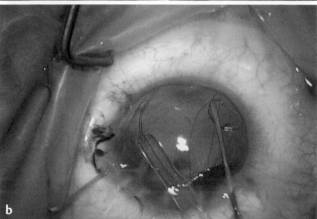

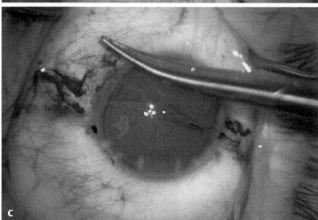

Fig. 17.3 (a) Capsular bag fixation using a Malyugin modified CTR. Prior to insertion, a double-armed 9–0 polypropylene suture is preplaced through the eyelet at the leading end of the ring. (b) As the CTR is inserted with the preloaded injector, the loop and eyelet are brought out of the capsular bag so that the eyelet is positioned within the ciliary sulcus (behind the iris and in front of the anterior capsule). After passing the two needles through a half-thickness scleral groove located inferiorly, the 9–0 polypropylene suture tips are tied resulting in centration of the updrawn capsular bag. (c) The knot falls within the half-thickness scleral groove to prevent erosion through the overlying conjunctiva.

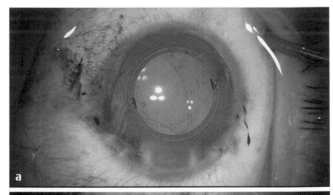

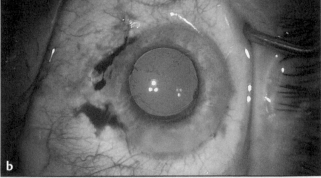

Fig. 17.4 A three-piece foldable silicone IOL has been placed in the ciliary sulcus with optic-capsulorhexis capture. (a) The haptics are in the sulcus and oriented away from the inferior zonular dialysis. (b) Pupil constriction confirms excellent centration of the IOL.

secured permanently to the sclera with a suture through the positioning loop. At this point, an additional standard CTR may also be placed inside the capsular bag to make the support more uniform.

17.4.2 Pars Plana Lensectomy and Vitrectomy

Although this approach can be used to remove any significantly subluxated lens, it is preferred if the lens descends too posteriorly while the patient is supine because of severe zonular loss or laxity. A second indication would be significant prolapse of vitreous into the anterior chamber. Under these circumstances, the goals include a complete removal of all lens material and a thorough vitrectomy carried out peripherally to the vitreous base. A separate limbal incision must then be made for the IOL implantation, which may be performed at the same time or as a second stage procedure.

17.5 Rehabilitation and Follow-up

In the absence of any randomized comparison studies, the optimal IOL to implant in a young patient lacking capsular support is very open to debate. If appropriately sized and positioned, anterior chamber IOLs have the advantage of stable long-term fixation and a predictable effective lens position. Iris-claw IOLs do not depend on precise sizing. Scleral or iris suture fixation of a posterior chamber IOL is more difficult and may be complicated by intraocular hemorrhage, pigment dispersion, optic tilt or decentration, and unintended refractive error because of its unpredictable axial position. Polypropylene knots may biodegrade or break over time, and exposed scleral knots may erode through the conjunctiva. Another approach would be intrascleral tunnel haptic fixation as first described by Scharioth and popularized by Agarwal as a "glued" IOL. Potential concerns include hemorrhage, tilting, unpredictable IOL position, hypotony, and haptic damage. This may be more difficult in patients with thin sclera, such as those with Marfan's syndrome.

Suggested Reading

[1] Rodrigo B-J, Paulina L-LE, Francesc M de R, Eduardo T-TJ, Alejandro N. Intraocular lens subluxation in marfan syndrome. Open Ophthalmol J. 2014; 8: 48–50

[2] Chandra A, Charteris D. Molecular pathogenesis and management strategies of ectopia lentis. Eye (Lond). 2014; 28(2):162–168

[3] Nahum Y, Spierer A. Ocular features of Marfan syndrome: diagnosis and management. Isr Med Assoc J. 2008; 10(3):179–181

[4] Nemet AY, Assia EI, Apple DJ, Barequet IS. Current concepts of ocular manifestations in Marfan syndrome. Surv Ophthalmol. 2006; 51(6):561–575

[5] Anteby I, Isaac M, BenEzra D. Hereditary subluxated lenses: visual performances and long-term follow-up after surgery. Ophthalmology. 2003; 110(7): 1344–1348

[6] Hoffman RS, Snyder ME, Devgan U, Allen QB, Yeoh R, Braga-Mele R, ASCRS Cataract Clinical Committee, Challenging/Complicated Cataract Surgery Subcommittee. Management of the subluxated crystalline lens. J Cataract Refract Surg. 2013; 39(12):1904–1915

[7] Siganos DS, Siganos CS, Popescu CN, Margaritis VN. Clear lens extraction and intraocular lens implantation in Marfan's syndrome. J Cataract Refract Surg. 2000; 26(5):781–784

[8] Masket S. Consultation section. Cataract surgical problem. J Cataract Refract Surg. 1998; 24(10):1289–1298

[9] Hasanee K, Butler M, Ahmed II. Capsular tension rings and related devices: current concepts. Curr Opin Ophthalmol. 2006; 17(1):31–41

[10] Hasanee K, Ahmed II. Capsular tension rings: update on endocapsular support devices. Ophthalmol Clin North Am. 2006; 19(4):507–519 Review

[11] Blecher MH, Kirk MR. Surgical strategies for the management of zonular compromise. Curr Opin Ophthalmol. 2008; 19(1):31–35

[12] Chee SP, Jap A. Management of traumatic severely subluxated cataracts. Am J Ophthalmol. 2011; 151(5):866–871.e1

[13] Cionni RJ, Osher RH. Management of profound zonular dialysis or weakness with a new endocapsular ring designed for scleral fixation. J Cataract Refract Surg. 1998; 24(10):1299–1306

[14] Moreno-Montañés J, Sainz C, Maldonado MJ. Intraoperative and postoperative complications of Cionni endocapsular ring implantation. J Cataract Refract Surg. 2003; 29(3):492–497

[15] Vasavada AR, Praveen MR, Vasavada VA, et al. Cionni ring and in-the-bag intraocular lens implantation for subluxated lenses: a prospective case series. Am J Ophthalmol. 2012; 153(6):1144–53.e1

[16] Buttanri IB, Sevim MS, Esen D, Acar BT, Serin D, Acar S. Modified capsular tension ring implantation in eyes with traumatic cataract and loss of zonular support. J Cataract Refract Surg. 2012; 38(3):431–436

[17] Wagoner MD, Cox TA, Ariyasu RG, Jacobs DS, Karp CL, American Academy of Ophthalmology. Intraocular lens implantation in the absence of capsular support: a report by the American Academy of Ophthalmology. Ophthalmology. 2003; 110(4):840–859

[18] Hirashima DE, Soriano ES, Meirelles RL, Alberti GN, Nosé W. Outcomes of iris-claw anterior chamber versus iris-fixated foldable intraocular lens in subluxated lens secondary to Marfan syndrome. Ophthalmology. 2010; 117(8):1479–1485

[19] Agarwal A, Kumar DA, Jacob S, Baid C, Agarwal A, Srinivasan S. Fibrin glue-assisted sutureless posterior chamber intraocular lens implantation in eyes with deficient posterior capsules. J Cataract Refract Surg. 2008; 34(9):1433–1438

18 Congenital Cataract

Edward H. Wood and Nandini G. Gandhi

Abstract

This chapter concisely reviews the entire approach one should take when presented with a congenital cataract. From initial diagnosis to differential diagnosis generation, workup, and ultimately medical and surgical management, this chapter includes up-to-date information and considerations for the care of patients with congenital cataracts.

Keywords: congenital cataract, leukocoria, amblyopia, cataract surgery, lens opacity

18.1 History

A pediatrician noticed white pupils in a 10-day-old infant and made the diagnosis of bilateral cataracts. The mother had had an uncomplicated pregnancy with no rash or febrile illness, the infant was born at term, and maternal serologies were all negative. There was no family history of congenital or childhood cataracts. The infant was referred to an ophthalmologist for further workup and management.

On examination, the child demonstrated a poor wince to light in both eyes, reactive pupils with no relative afferent pupillary defect, and normal extraocular movements. The globes were soft to palpation. The eyelids and conjunctiva were normal and the corneas were clear and normal in diameter. The lenses had central white opacities bilaterally (▶ Fig. 18.1). There was no view to the posterior segment in either eye. B-scan ultrasonography was performed, which revealed no retinal detachment or mass.

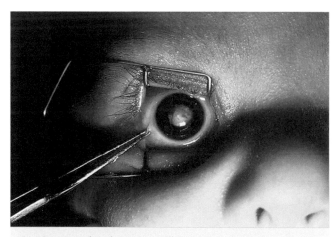

Fig. 18.1 Central nuclear congenital cataract.

Differential Diagnosis—Key Points

1. Congenital cataract is defined as a lens opacity that is present at birth or develops within the first year of life. It is a common cause of blindness in children, occurring in an estimated 1 in 10,000 live births.

2. Early detection is the most important factor in determining the eventual visual outcome. In general, the earlier the onset, the more amblyogenic the cataract will be; lens opacities that become visually significant prior to 2 to 3 months of age are the most amblyogenic.

3. The first important diagnostic distinction to make is whether the leukocoria is secondary to a cataract or another structural abnormality. While cataract is the most common cause of leukocoria, other causes such as retinoblastoma, retinopathy of prematurity, Coats' disease, retinal detachment, and persistent hyperplastic primary vitreous (PHPV) must be considered when evaluating an infant or child with a cataract. PHPV is a unilateral condition causing developmental arrest of the eye, and is the most common ocular syndrome associated with congenital cataract. This entity should be suspected in any eye that is even slightly small, and is often associated with a retrolental stalk, posterior cataract, and elongated, anteriorly rotated ciliary processes.

4. The etiology of cataracts follows the rule of thirds. One-third are idiopathic, one-third are related to a systemic syndrome or disease such as chromosomal abnormalities, metabolic disorders, and intrauterine infections, and one-third occur as an isolated inherited trait (usually autosomal dominant). Two-thirds of cases of congenital cataracts are bilateral, and the prevalence of underlying systemic disease is higher in bilateral cases. Considerations for underlying etiology are shown in ▶ Table 18.1.

5. There are a variety of morphologies of congenital cataracts that may indicate etiology and/or visual significance, as outlined in ▶ Table 18.2. The opacity may involve the entire lens or it may be localized. In general, opacities localized to the embryonic or fetal nucleus often leave the peripheral lens cortex optically clear.

Table 18.1 Underlying etiologies of congenital cataracts

	Bilateral	Unilateral
Idiopathic	50% of cases	#1 cause
Familial (hereditary)	Usually **AD**; also X-linked, AR	
Chromosomal	Trisomy 21, 13, 18, other	
Metabolic disorders	**Galactosemia**, Fabry's disease, Wilson's disease, mannosidosis, diabetes mellitus, parathyroid abnormalities	
Renal disorders	**Lowe's syndrome**, Alport's syndrome	
Intrauterine infections	Toxoplasmosis, **rubella**, cytomegalovirus, varicella, syphilis	Rarely, consider maternal history
Musculoskeletal disease	Conradi–Hünermann syndrome, Albright's syndrome, myotonic dystrophy	
Craniofacial syndromes	Hallerman–Streiff, Rubinstein–Taybi, Smith–Lemli–Opitz	
Ocular anomalies	**Anterior segment dysgenesis**, coloboma, aniridia	**Persistent hyperplastic primary vitreous (PHPV)**, retinal detachment, anterior segment dysgenesis, lenticonus, coloboma
Trauma	Less likely	Consideration, rule out child abuse

Abbreviations: AD, autosomal dominant; AR, autosomal recessive.

Table 18.2 Morphology and systemic associations of congenital cataracts

	Morphology	Associations
Nuclear	Confined to embryonic or fetal nucleus	Idiopathic, rubella (pearly white), microphthalmos
Lamellar	Affect particular lamella extending anteriorly and posteriorly, may have associated arcuate opacities, i.e., "riders"	Most common; idiopathic, AD, metabolic, infectious
Coronary	Occur in deep cortex surrounding nucleus like a crown	Idiopathic, rarely hereditary
Cerulean	Distributed blue punctate opacities	Idiopathic, Down's syndrome
Sutural	Follows anterior or posterior Y suture	Idiopathic, may occur with others
Anterior Polar	*Flat*—central, usually less than 3 mm and visually insignificant, one-third bilateral *Pyramidal*—surrounded by cortical opacity, more visually significant	Idiopathic, persistent pupillary membrane, aniridia, Peters' anomaly, anterior lenticonus, microphthalmos
Epicapsular star	Star-shaped distribution of golden flecks on anterior lens capsule	Persistent pupillary membrane
Posterior polar	Posterior centralized opacity	Idiopathic, persistent hyaloid remnants (spectrum: Mittendorf's dot to PHPV), posterior lenticonus
Membranous	Occurs when lamellar material resorbs, leaving residual chalky lens material between anterior and posterior capsule	Hallerman–Streiff
"Oil droplet"	Central round opacity	Galactosemia
"Christmas tree"	Distributed multicolored flecks	Myotonic dystrophy, hypoparathyroidism
"Sunflower"	Greenish brown discoloration of anterior lens capsule	Wilson's disease

Abbreviations: AD, autosomal dominant; PHPV, persistent hyperplastic primary vitreous.

18.2 Test Interpretation

Following a review of medical and family history, a careful examination including ophthalmoscopy with dilated pupils is the best technique for diagnosing a congenital cataract and associated abnormalities. In the event that a hand-held slit lamp is not available, either the direct ophthalmoscope or the indirect ophthalmoscope with a 20-D lens can provide a magnified view of the anterior segment. In addition, older infants can sometimes be held up to the slit lamp for examination.

After confirming the presence of a cataract, the first consideration is whether or not the opacity is visually significant. Infants younger than 2 months often do not demonstrate consistent fixation. Thus, visual significance should be expected with any of the following features: (1) central opacities greater than 3 mm in diameter or posterior opacities greater than 1 mm (if in the center of the posterior capsule), (2) significantly decreased view of the posterior pole with ophthalmoscopy, (3) strabismus associated with a unilateral cataract, or (4) nystagmus associated with bilateral cataracts. Central opacities less than 3 mm in diameter, peripheral opacities, and punctate opacities with intervening clear zones are thought to have less visual significance to varying degrees. Infants older than 2 months can undergo testing of fixation preference and behavior, objection to occlusion, tests of preferential looking (such as teller acuity cards), optokinetic nystagmus, and, in rare cases, visually evoked potentials.

The next consideration is to determine whether the cataract is an isolated finding in an otherwise healthy child or whether the cataract is part of a systemic disorder. Unilateral cataracts in a healthy baby often need no workup aside from determining the family history and that the mother did not have a febrile illness or rash during pregnancy that would point to an intrauterine infection. Infants with bilateral cataracts should be sent for laboratory testing of blood and urine. Blood tests for TORCH titers as well as levels of glucose, calcium, and phosphorus are recommended to rule out intrauterine infections and metabolic disorders. Urine tests include amino acids (to rule out Lowe's syndrome) and the reducing substances galactose-1-phosphate uridyltransferase and galactokinase (to rule out galactosemia). If the child is dysmorphic, genetic counseling is appropriate; if there is failure to thrive, a more thorough search for metabolic diseases by the pediatrician may be necessary. Our patient underwent laboratory testing and genetic consultation, which failed to reveal an underlying genetic syndrome.

An ophthalmic ultrasound examination is indicated if the cataract is so dense that there is no view of the retina. This examination allows indirect visualization of the retina and vitreous so that PHPV and other disorders of the posterior portion of the eye are seen if present.

Occasionally, it is necessary to have an examination under anesthesia. Certainly, while the child is anesthetized for cataract extraction, an examination should be performed to confirm the preoperative findings. As congenital cataracts can be associated with glaucoma, it is important to measure intraocular pressure during the exam under anesthesia if it could not be measured preoperatively.

18.3 Diagnosis

Bilateral idiopathic congenital cataract.

18.4 Medical Management

There is no medical treatment of congenital cataract. However, some children have central cataracts that allow good vision if, and only if, the pupil is pharmacologically dilated. These children can enjoy improved vision when treated chronically with mydriatics such as atropine once a day or once every other day. Because atropinic agents can cause systemic side effects in babies, a low dose is used. In addition, nonvisually significant cataracts may be observed with regular follow up, and patching therapy for amblyopia treatment is often initiated to promote optimal visual development.

18.5 Surgical Management

If the cataract is large and dense enough to interfere with visual development, surgical removal should be performed as soon as possible. If surgery is not undertaken at the appropriate time, dense amblyopia will result. However, cataract surgery prior to 4 weeks of age may increase the risk of secondary glaucoma. Therefore, it is generally suggested that unilateral cataracts undergo extraction at age 4 to 6 weeks. It is recommended that bilateral cataracts be removed by 10 weeks of life.

An important postoperative issue in these surgeries is whether an intraocular lens (IOL) is implanted or not. If chosen, the IOL power should initially target hyperopia (initially corrected with spectacles and allowing for emmetropization during the myopic shift of the growing eye) or emmetropia (potentially maximizing clear vision during critical period, with likely need for myopic correction later in life). IOLs are generally not advised in children younger than 1 year, and are reasonably well tolerated by children aged 1 to 2 years and older who have had late maturation of congenital cataracts. The disadvantages of IOLs include increased inflammation, secondary membrane/capsule opacification, and difficulty predicting the appropriate lens power in a growing eye.

Compared to cataract surgery in adults, surgery in infants is technically more difficult. Not only is the eye much smaller and therefore harder to approach, but also the anterior capsule is tough and elastic and the posterior capsule must be removed to prevent inevitable postoperative opacification. Also, the iris has a strong propensity to adhere to the posterior capsule and vitreous, requiring pupil dilation for several weeks after surgery.

Postoperative complications include posterior capsular opacification (nearly universal in cases without posterior capsulectomy/capsulotomy), secondary membrane formation (especially in microphthalmic, uveitic, or postoperatively inflamed eyes), glaucoma (occurs in 20% of eyes, higher incidence if performed prior to 4 weeks), and retinal detachment (rare, usually late complication).

18.6 Rehabilitation and Follow-Up

Excellent refractive correction together with appropriate occlusion therapy is essential in order to treat the deprivation amblyopia that results from congenital cataracts. This aspect of postoperative management requires patience and perseverance from both the ophthalmologist and the parents. If amblyopia is not aggressively treated, the child will develop severe and irreversible poor vision in the affected eye. Therefore, if there is no IOL, the child must be fitted with contact lenses or glasses immediately after the surgery. For the patient with bilateral cataracts, glasses can be a better alternative since they are much easier for the parents to manage (▶ Fig. 18.2). The power should be selected to make the patient myopic, because much of the infant's visual world is at near. For the unilateral patient, however, contact lenses are preferred, because unilateral correction by glasses produces intolerable distortion and image disparity between the operated and unoperated eyes.

Glaucoma can occur following congenital cataract surgery. Long-term follow-up of patients is necessary since glaucoma may become manifest many years after the surgery.

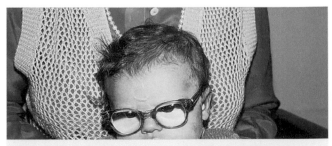

Fig. 18.2 Postoperative optical correction with aphakic spectacles.

Suggested Reading

[1] Biglan AW. Pediatric cataract surgery. In: Albert DM, ed. Ophthalmic Surgery: Principles and Techniques. Malden, MA: Blackwell Science; 1999:970–1014

[2] Buckley EG. Pediatric cataracts and lens abnormalities. In: Nelson LB, ed. Harley's Pediatric Ophthalmology. 4th ed. Philadelphia, PA: WB Saunders; 1998:258–282

[3] Lloyd IC, Goss-Sampson M, Jeffrey BG, Kriss A, Russell-Eggitt I, Taylor D. Neonatal cataract: aetiology, pathogenesis and management. Eye (Lond). 1992; 6 (Pt 2):184–196

[4] Kanski JJ, Bowling B. Clinical Ophthalmology: A Systematic Approach. 7th ed. Edinburgh: Butterworth-Heinemann/Elsevier; 2011

[5] American Academy of Ophthalmology. 2014–2015 Basic and Clinical Science Course, Section 06: Pediatric Ophthalmology and Strabismus. San Francisco, CA: American Academy of Ophthalmology; 2014

[6] Lambert SR, Buckley EG, Drews-Botsch C, et al. Infant Aphakia Treatment Study Group. A randomized clinical trial comparing contact lens with intraocular lens correction of monocular aphakia during infancy: grating acuity and adverse events at age 1 year. Arch Ophthalmol. 2010; 128(7): 810–818

19 Ocular Hypertension

Don C. Nguyen and Kuldev Singh

Abstract

This chapter goes through in detail the diagnostic and clinical considerations when encountering a patient with high intraocular pressure. A typical clinical vignette will be described, followed by analysis of other potential diagnoses in the differential. We will also discuss crucial exam features to look for when trying to discern a patient with a primary or secondary glaucoma, or solely intraocular hypertension. The chapter will also review the interpretation of different tests as well as their utility in ocular hypertension patients, including optical coherence tomography, visual field testing, and pachymetry. Important elements of the Ocular Hypertension Treatment Study (OHTS) will be reviewed. Key findings during slit-lamp exam and gonioscopy are also discussed, as well as findings seen in secondary glaucoma syndromes such as pigment dispersion and pseudoexfoliation. Lastly, we will analyze the significance of certain risk factors when determining whether or not to treat patients with ocular hypertension, as well the medical and surgical management of high intraocular pressure, and how frequent physicians should follow these patients.

Keywords: ocular hypertension, glaucoma suspect, glaucoma, pigment dispersion, pseudoexfoliation, Ocular Hypertension Treatment Study

19.1 History

A 42-year-old Caucasian man was referred to the eye clinic after being told by an optometrist that his eye pressures were high and that he might have glaucoma. Past medical history and family history were unremarkable. He was not taking any medications.

Ocular examination revealed visual acuity of 20/20 OU without correction. Pupils and motility were normal. Anterior segment biomicroscopic examination was unremarkable with a clear cornea

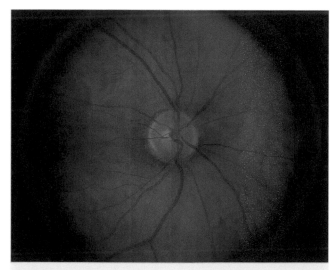

Fig. 19.1 The right optic nerve.

and lens. Intraocular pressures (IOPs) were 27 mm Hg OD and 28 mm Hg OS. Gonioscopy revealed angles open to the ciliary body band 360 degrees with moderate pigmentation of the trabecular meshwork. Dilated funduscopic examination revealed symmetric optic nerves with normal cupping (▶ Fig. 19.1, ▶ Fig. 19.2). The cup-to-disc ratio was 0.2, with an intact neuroretinal rim OU. The macula, vessels, periphery, and vitreous were normal in appearance. A 24–2 Humphrey automated perimetry was performed, which revealed no visual field defects in either eye.

Differential Diagnosis—Key Points

1. The finding of elevated IOP in the presence of normal-appearing optic nerves and visual fields makes idiopathic ocular hypertension (OHTN) the most likely diagnosis.

2. If there has been focal or generalized injury to ganglion cells related to this elevated IOP, the diagnosis of primary open-angle glaucoma (POAG) should be considered. As early injury in POAG is sometimes difficult to detect by nerve examination and visual field testing, the distinction between OHTN and POAG is not always easy to discern. In addition to stereoscopic optic nerve assessment, spectral domain optical coherence tomography (SD-OCT) can be used to assess and follow optic nerve structure which can be compromised prior to functional abnormalities noted on perimetry.

3. If gonioscopy revealed an abnormal angle (i.e., narrow, densely pigmented trabecular meshwork, peripheral anterior synechiae, neovascularization), secondary causes of elevated IOP should be investigated. Unfortunately, these secondary causes of elevated IOP are often referred to as "glaucoma" even when the optic nerve and visual field are normal.

4. Diseases such as pigmentary dispersion syndrome (PDS) and pseudoexfoliation syndrome can result in secondary IOP elevation. These diseases are associated with characteristic features that are generally visible on slit-lamp examination, such as pigmentation of the corneal endothelium (Krukenberg's spindle), heavily pigmented trabecular meshwork, and spokelike iris transillumination of the iris with PDS. Once again, patients with these conditions and elevated IOP are often referred to as having pigmentary or pseudoexfoliative glaucoma rather than OHTN.

19.2 Test Interpretation

1. Measurement of IOP is crucial in making the diagnosis. While newer measurement modalities have been introduced in recent years, Goldmann applanation tonometry remains the gold standard. Measurement by the tonopen or pneumotonometer may be more convenient or accurate in certain settings, especially in the presence of corneal disease as well as for patients with physical limitations.

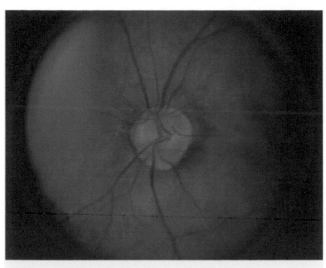

Fig. 19.2 The left optic nerve.

2. Central corneal thickness (CCT) should be measured in all ocular hypertensive patients to determine the context of each individual's IOP reading and overall glaucoma risk. The Ocular Hypertension Treatment Study (OHTS) has shown that those with greater corneal thickness are at lower risk of developing POAG. It is noteworthy that while CCT was found to be an independent risk factor for the development of POAG in OHTS, there is no validated algorithm for converting the IOP obtained from applanation tonometry to a "true" IOP. Slit-lamp examination to rule out causes of IOP elevation secondary to ocular conditions or syndromes is critical. Eyes with ocular conditions associated with transient or permanent elevated IOP may more commonly require therapy than idiopathic OHTN, even in the absence of optic nerve damage. An example of this is seen in patients with rubeosis iridis who may require panretinal photocoagulation.

3. Gonioscopy should be used to rule out a narrow or closed angle, which may be associated with IOP elevation. Transient IOP elevation is fairly commonly seen with occludable angles. Laser peripheral iridotomy may not only reverse the IOP elevation but also prevent other secondary problems associated with angle closure.

4. The optic nerve is best examined under stereoscopic magnification. The fundus contact lens is the gold standard but is sometimes cumbersome and makes subsequent fundus photography difficult. The Hruby lens approaches the contact lens in stereopsis and magnification. The 78-D and 90-D lenses, when used with the slit lamp, exaggerate stereopsis. Nevertheless, these lenses are easy to use and, in most cases, give a good estimate of the cup-to-disc ratio and other characteristics of the optic nerve. The red-free light on the slit lamp can be used to better view the neuroretinal rim and identify any defects in peripapillary nerve fiber layer. Focal cupping, thinning of the rim, nerve fiber layer dropout, or significant disc asymmetry should make one consider changing the diagnosis from ocular OHTN to POAG. SD-OCT and other imaging modalities such as scanning laser ophthalmoscopy may provide valuable additional information to help discern between these two groups of patients.

5. Automated perimetry has become the gold standard in visual field testing. Static threshold techniques can be highly sensitive in picking up even subtle visual field defects. Many patients are unable to undergo automated perimetry due to physical or nonphysical limitations and thus require manual perimetry. Although a high IOP should significantly raise your level of suspicion, the presence of focal optic nerve thinning with a correlating visual field defect alone should make one consider the diagnosis of POAG.

19.3 Diagnosis

Ocular hypertension.

19.4 Medical Management

The decision of whether and when to begin IOP-lowering therapy in a patient with OHTN is a difficult one. If structural and functional assessment reveals normal optic nerves in both eyes, you are treating a risk factor for glaucoma development (i.e., IOP elevation) and not the disease itself. Once you begin treatment, you may be committing a patient to a lifetime of unnecessary therapy. On the other hand, if you do not treat, the elevated IOP may result in undetected optic nerve damage and visual field loss. Such a delay could potentially jeopardize the patient's vision, especially as he or she ages.

Many ophthalmologists will determine an arbitrary IOP cutoff above which medical therapy is almost always initiated. Epidemiologic studies looking at this issue have failed to show a single "magic" number above which all patients should be treated. Instead of having an inflexible cutoff IOP, one should individualize each patient's treatment or observation plan based on the number of coexisting risk factors.

Factors other than thin CCT that may lead one to treat patients with IOPs in the mid to high 20 s include race and positive family history, but it should be noted that neither of these risk factors was found to be significantly related to the development of glaucoma in OHTS. Nevertheless, black populations have a higher prevalence of glaucomatous optic neuropathy than whites in most parts of the world and, thus, might be considered for treatment earlier in the course of the disease.

The age of a patient may also be important. An 80-year-old patient with normal nerves and visual fields is less likely to suffer significant vision loss over a lifetime secondary to elevated IOP than an individual in his or her 40 s. The prescriber must take into consideration the cumulative lifetime cost and added morbidity of initiating treatment for each individual patient and whether the benefits of such therapy outweigh the risks.

19.5 Surgical Management

Laser trabeculoplasty and glaucoma filtration surgery are usually not to be recommended in patients with OHTN. The potential complications, especially with filtration surgery, should not be risked in eyes with healthy optic nerves.

19.6 Rehabilitation and Follow-up

Ocular hypertensive patients, whether or not they are treated with IOP-lowering therapy, should initially be seen at least every 6 to 12 months. Yearly visual field testing and/or OCT, and dilated optic nerve examination are recommended.

Patients who are treated with IOP-lowering therapy should be seen within 4 weeks after initiation of treatment to see if the medication is effective. After the therapy has been modified and the IOP is stable, examination every 4 to 6 months is recommended for at least 2 years. If the OHTN has been stable for many years, examination every 6 to 12 months may be adequate.

Suggested Reading

[1] American Academy of Ophthalmology. Glaucoma. In: Basic and Clinical Science Course. Section 10. San Francisco, CA: American Academy of Ophthalmology; 2011–2012

[2] Kass MA, Heuer DK, Higginbotham EJ, et al. The Ocular Hypertension Treatment Study: a randomized trial determines that topical ocular hypotensive medication delays or prevents the onset of primary open-angle glaucoma. Arch Ophthalmol. 2002; 120(6):701–713, discussion 829–830

[3] Ritch R, Shields MB, Krupin T, eds. The Glaucomas. St. Louis, MO: CV Mosby Co; 1996

[4] Shields MB, ed. Textbook of Glaucoma. 6th ed. Baltimore, MD: Williams & Wilkins; 2011

20 Open-Angle Glaucoma

Bac Tien Nguyen and Sally Byrd

Abstract

To help distinguish primary open-angle glaucoma from other forms of glaucoma and other disease processes, the chapter covers both clinical findings and diagnostic testing as they are related to glaucoma. These discussion points include key features of the clinical examination, with particular focus on gonioscopy and funduscopic findings, visual field testing, optic nerve head imaging, and central corneal thickness. The numerous medical and surgical interventions used in the treatment of primary open-angle glaucoma are explored and discussed in the chapter. The surgical interventions highlighted include traditional glaucoma filtering surgery, laser procedures, modern minimally invasive glaucoma surgery, and micropulse transscleral cyclophotocoagulation.

Keywords: glaucoma, intraocular pressure, optic nerve cupping, visual field, retinal nerve fiber layer, laser trabeculoplasty, trabeculectomy, seton device, cyclophotocoagulation, minimally invasive glaucoma surgery

20.1 History

A 51-year-old African American man presented for a routine eye exam. He had no past ocular problems and no current visual complaints. Past medical history was remarkable for mild emphysema for which he used inhalers.

Examination revealed visual acuities of 20/20 in each eye, with a refraction of –3.00 + 2.25 × 110 OD and –2.25 + 2.00 × 86 OS. The pupils reacted normally with no afferent pupillary defect. Anterior slit-lamp examination was unremarkable, and pressures by applanation tonometry were 26 mm Hg OD and 32 mm Hg OS. Gonioscopy was performed and the angles were noted to be grade IV in both eyes with a clear view of the ciliary body band for 360 degrees. There was 1+ pigment of the trabecular meshwork. On funduscopic exam, the optic nerves were noted to be as pictured in ▶ Fig. 20.1a, b. There were no abnormalities of the retina or vessels. Automated visual fields were also obtained and are shown in ▶ Fig. 20.2a, b.

20.2 Test Interpretation

A careful physical exam is crucial in making the diagnosis of POAG.

1. This patient had elevated IOPs which would support a diagnosis of glaucoma, although approximately 33 to 50% of patients with POAG will present with pressures under 21 mm Hg at the time of their initial presentation. Furthermore, approximately one-sixth of patients who have other characteristic features of POAG will have IOPs consistently lower than 21 mm Hg. These patients are often classified as having normal or low tension glaucoma.
2. Careful slit-lamp examination is important to rule out other secondary causes of glaucoma. Evaluation of the

Differential Diagnosis—Key Points

1. The findings of elevated intraocular pressure (IOP), open angles, optic nerve cupping, and arcuate visual field defects put the diagnosis of primary open-angle glaucoma (POAG) at the top of the list.
2. Secondary open-angle glaucomas, such as pigmentary and pseudoexfoliation, might also be considered, but this patient did not display the corneal endothelial pigment deposits, iris transillumination defects, or heavy trabecular meshwork pigment seen in pigmentary glaucoma, nor the fibrillar deposits, anterior iris pigment dusting, or trabecular meshwork pigment often seen with pseudoexfoliation.
3. Chronic angle closure should be ruled out by careful gonioscopy.
4. Occasionally, the optic nerve atrophy that follows anterior ischemic optic neuropathy (AION) can lead to cupping which mimics that seen in glaucoma. Usually, optic nerve pallor is the more distinguishing feature, however, and the condition is not associated with elevated IOPs. Additionally, AION often occurs in nerves with very small tight cups, and the fellow or less involved eye should be assessed for this finding.
5. Congenital optic nerve findings such as an optic nerve pit, limited optic nerve colobomas, tilted discs, and disc drusen may lead to visual field findings that simulate glaucoma, and a careful examiner should keep these anomalies in mind.
6. Retinal lesions such as a retinal scar or branch retinal vein or artery occlusion may also mimic the findings of glaucoma on visual field examination.

cornea may reveal pigment deposits (Krukenberg's spindle) characteristic of pigmentary glaucoma, keratic precipitates suggestive of a secondary inflammatory glaucoma, or corneal edema seen in some variations of iridocorneal endothelial (ICE) syndrome and herpes keratitis even at lower IOPs. Cell and flare in the anterior chamber would additionally support a diagnosis of inflammatory glaucoma. Examination of the iris should look to rule out peripheral transillumination defects consistent with pigmentary glaucoma; pupillary margin atrophy; gray-white flakes around the pupil; and anterior stromal pigment dusting seen with pseudoexfoliation; the rubeotic vessels of neovascular glaucoma; and the distortion, atrophy, and corectopia characteristic of the ICE syndromes.
3. Gonioscopy is, of course, essential for diagnosis of POAG and necessary to rule out angle closure, as well as other secondary causes of glaucoma such as traumatic angle recession and the high iris insertion of juvenile glaucoma. Heavy trabecular meshwork pigmentation would be suggestive of pigmentary or pseudoexfoliative glaucoma.

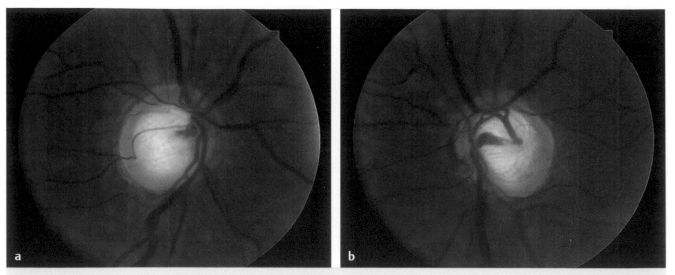

Fig. 20.1 (a) Examination of the right disc showed generalized enlargement of the cup with increased thinning of the inferior rim. (b) The left disc also shows generalized cup enlargement with more marked thinning of the inferior neural rim.

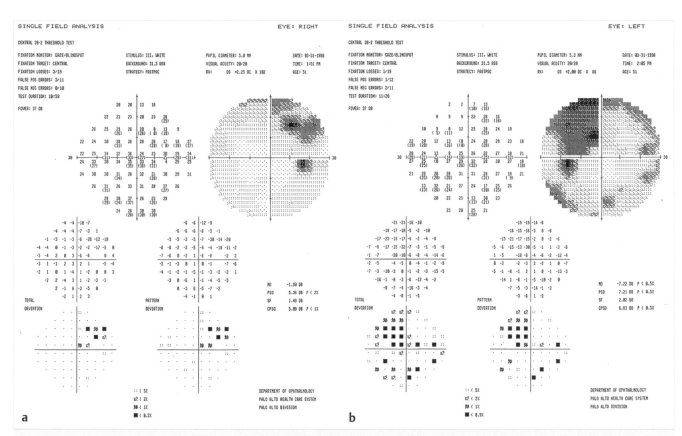

Fig. 20.2 (a) An early superior arcuate defect is noted in the right eye. (b) A more advanced superior arcuate defect is seen in the left eye.

4. Examination of the optic nerve is best done under stereoscopic magnification through a dilated pupil and should document not only the overall disc size and cup-to-disc ratio, but also evidence of focal thinning or notching of the neural rim and the presence of optic disc hemorrhages. The nerve fiber layer should be assessed with a red-free light. Other disc anomalies that could also result in visual field changes, such as disc drusen, optic pits, tilted nerves, and disc pallor, should be searched for and documented when present. The retina should also be carefully examined, particularly for lesions that might explain visual field defects found to be present.

5. Visual field testing is best measured using automatic static threshold techniques or careful manual kinetic and static testing. Glaucoma classically leads to a visual field defect in a nerve fiber bundle distribution. Examples of this include arcuate or Bjerrum's scotomas, nasal steps, paracentral scotomas, and temporal wedges. Glaucoma, however, may also lead to visual field constriction or diffuse depression that may be more difficult to recognize.

6. Central corneal thickness (CCT) measurement can typically be obtained through the use of ultrasound corneal pachymeters. Below average CCT measurements may lead to the underestimation of IOP, while above average CCT measurements may lead to an overestimation of IOP. Obtaining a CCT measurement can help stratify a patient's risk for glaucoma and subsequent progression of disease. Modern imaging technologies such as anterior segment optical coherence tomography (OCT) and certain corneal topography and tomography systems can also be used to measure CCT.

7. Retinal nerve fiber layer and optic nerve head imaging can now provide quantitative measurements of structural changes seen with glaucoma. A variety of different technologies, including confocal scanning laser ophthalmoscopy, scanning laser polarimetry, and OCT, are available to clinicians to obtain these quantitative images and measurements. These imaging modalities can aid the clinician in the diagnosis of and subsequent monitoring of glaucoma. Clinical correlation must be used when interpreting the results of these studies. The studies should be used as an adjunct to the clinical and visual field examinations.

20.3 Diagnosis

Primary open-angle glaucoma.

20.4 Medical Management

Management of glaucoma is primarily aimed at lowering the IOP below a target level felt to be safe (unlikely to cause further nerve damage) for a particular patient. Target pressures are generally set at a pressure at least 20% below the pretreatment level, but lower target pressures may be indicated depending on the pretreatment IOP levels and the degree of optic nerve damage already present. Medical agents for lowering IOP include β-blockers, both selective and nonselective, topical and oral carbonic anhydrase inhibitors, prostaglandin analogs, adrenergic agonists, and miotics. Choice of treatment is based on a number of factors including severity of the disease, the patient's age, compliance issues, known side effects, and concomitant systemic disorders. It is often prudent to start a medication in one eye only, to better separate its effectiveness from normal fluctuations in eye pressure.

20.5 Surgical Management

Surgery is indicated when medical management fails to adequately control the IOPs and there is evidence of disease progression, or in some cases as initial therapy depending on the severity of the glaucoma and other mitigating factors.

1. Laser trabeculoplasty is a commonly performed procedure in the treatment of glaucoma. It can be used as an initial therapy for certain patients, or as an alternative or adjunct to medical therapy. It is useful in patients who are unable to use medication reliably. While many of the early studies investigated the usage of argon laser trabeculoplasty (ALT), there has been a shift to selective laser trabeculoplasty (SLT). SLT is performed by using a 53- nm Nd:YAG laser, placing 400-μm spots around 360 degrees of trabecular meshwork. SLT acts by increasing aqueous outflow and results in significant IOP lowering similar to ALT, with less inflammation, less discomfort, and greater success when repeated compared to ALT. Patients should be pretreated with apraclonidine or other medications to prevent acute pressure spikes and should have their pressures rechecked 1 to 2 hours after the procedure.

2. Trabeculectomy allows for aqueous humor to leave the anterior chamber into the subconjunctival space and thus lower IOP. Trabeculectomy surgery, alone or combined with medical treatment, is reported as having an initial success rate in previously unoperated eyes of 75 to 95%. In eyes that have failed previous surgery, however, the success rate may be as low as 36%. Antimetabolite agents such as 5-fluorouracil and mitomycin C may greatly increase the success rates by preventing scarring, but must be used judiciously to prevent complications such as long-term hypotony and bleb leaks. Careful follow-up after trabeculectomy surgery is required to monitor and possibly treat potential complications, as well as to intervene if signs of early surgical failure are noted.

3. Implantation of various seton devices, such as the Baerveldt, Molteno, or Ahmed implants, uses a tube to provide a channel for aqueous humor to flow from the anterior chamber to a reservoir plate underneath Tenon's capsule. These devices are usually reserved for patients who have failed multiple filtering surgeries or those who are at high risk of trabeculectomy failure such as conjunctival scarring or certain types of glaucoma. Recent studies have investigated the use of seton device as a primary surgery prior to trabeculectomy.

4. Traditional transscleral cyclodestructive procedures using cryoablation or laser are less predictable and carry a higher risk of phthisis. They are therefore usually reserved for patients who have failed multiple other procedures, those who have extremely poor visual prognosis, and those who are otherwise too medically unstable to undergo incisional

glaucoma surgery. Endoscopic cyclophotocoagulation has been used to provide laser energy to the ciliary processes under direct visualization with less risk of phthisis and inflammation. A newer procedure using micropulse transscleral cyclophotocoagulation may be more promising procedure that also has lower risk of phthisis but longer term studies are required.

5. The use of minimally invasive glaucoma surgery is a growing field in the treatment of glaucoma. A number of new procedures and devices have been developed including trabecular meshwork micro-bypass stents, intracanalicular scaffolding devices, supraciliary microstents, ab interno trabeculotomy, ab interno canaloplasty, and subconjunctival filtering devices. The long-term efficacy and safety of these devices and procedures still under investigation

20.6 Rehabilitation and Follow-up

The frequency of follow-up examinations is generally based on severity of the disease, achievement of target IOP levels, evidence of disease progression, and duration of control. It is important at each visit to determine possible medication side effects and compliance problems and to assess visual acuity and IOP. Evaluation of the optic nerve and repeat visual field testing may be performed somewhat less frequently, again depending on the factors mentioned above. Baseline stereoscopic photos of the optic nerves are important when evaluating subtle changes in the nerves over time. Indications for adjusting therapy include failure to achieve the target IOP, evidence of progressive optic nerve damage or visual field decline, and development of side effects or compliance problems with the prescribed medications.

Suggested Reading

[1] American Academy of Ophthalmology. Primary Open-Angle Glaucoma: Preferred Practice Pattern. San Francisco, CA: American Academy of Ophthalmology; 1996

[2] American Academy of Ophthalmology. Primary Open-Angle Glaucoma: Preferred Practice Pattern. San Francisco, CA: American Academy of Ophthalmology; 2015

[3] Anderson DR. Automated Static Perimetry. St. Louis, MO: Mosby-Yearbook; 1992

[4] Ritch R, Shields MB, Krupin T, eds. The Glaucomas. St. Louis, MO: CV Mosby Co; 1996

[5] Vinod K, Gedde SJ. Clinical investigation of new glaucoma procedures. Curr Opin Ophthalmol. 2017; 28(2):187–193

21 Primary Angle-Closure Glaucoma

Peter A. Netland and Eitan S. Burstein

Abstract

In this chapter, the authors discuss the diagnostic methods, differential diagnosis, and management of acute angle-closure glaucoma.

Keywords: angle-closure glaucoma, narrow glaucoma, management, iridotomy, gonioscopy

21.1 History

A 55-year-old woman presented with a history of several hours of discomfort and blurred vision in the left eye.

Examination showed vision of 20/20 in the right eye and 20/60 in the left eye. Intraocular pressures (IOPs) were 14 and 52 mm Hg in the right and left eyes, respectively. The pupil was sluggish and middilated in the left eye. Slit-lamp examination of the left eye showed mild congestion of the episcleral and conjunctival blood vessels. There was mild corneal epithelial edema and a shallow peripheral anterior chamber (▶ Fig. 21.1). The midperipheral iris was bowed anteriorly (▶ Fig. 21.2). Examination of the lens showed mild nuclear sclerosis. Gonioscopy of the left eye revealed a marked convexity of iris contour and no visible anterior chamber angle structures (▶ Fig. 21.3). Gonioscopy of the right eye demonstrated an open, narrow anterior chamber angle. The optic nerve cups were small in both eyes.

The left eye was treated with medical therapy and laser iridotomy, which opened the anterior chamber angle and reduced the IOP to normal (▶ Fig. 21.4).

Differential Diagnosis—Key Points

1. In this patient, the IOP was elevated and gonioscopy demonstrated a closed anterior chamber angle in the left eye. The differential diagnosis should include the clinical types of angle-closure glaucoma. The most common type of primary angle-closure glaucoma in the United States is pupillary block angle-closure glaucoma. Other causes of primary angle-closure glaucoma include plateau iris configuration. In the patient described in the case history, the midperipheral iris was bowed anteriorly (iris bombé) and touched the cornea peripherally. The fellow eye had a narrow, potentially occludable anterior chamber angle. The predominant mechanism is pupillary block, although it is possible that the patient had some component of plateau iris. Reexamination and provocative testing after iridectomy would identify any plateau iris configuration. Recent evidence suggests that the physiological properties of the iris play a role in angle-closure glaucoma. Iris volume, when measured by anterior segment optical coherence tomography, has been observed to increase after dilation in eyes with narrow anterior chamber angles that are predisposed to angle closure.

2. Abnormalities of the lens may cause angle-closure glaucoma. In phacomorphic glaucoma, a cataractous and intumescent lens may cause closure of the anterior chamber angle. Trauma or hereditary disorders may cause anterior lens subluxation and angle-closure glaucoma. In rare cases, exfoliation syndrome or idiopathic factors may cause sufficient weakening of the zonules, anterior lens movement, and angle closure. Drug sensitivity to sulfonamides or other drugs may cause various problems, including acute myopia, lens swelling, and uveal effusions, which may be associated with angle-closure glaucoma. This patient was not using any of the medications associated with angle closure, nor did she have any findings associated with lens-induced angle-closure glaucoma.

3. The patient described an acute onset of her problem in the left eye. She denied repeated, brief episodes of these symptoms in the past, suggesting that she had not had intermittent angle closure. The time course described by the patient and the lack of any findings such as iris atrophy, anterior lens opacities (glaukomflecken), or peripheral anterior synechiae indicate an acute process rather than chronic angle-closure glaucoma.

4. Other disorders may cause symptoms and signs of acute angle-closure glaucoma. In neovascular glaucoma, neovascularization of the iris and angle may lead to peripheral anterior synechia formation and ultimately to closure of the angle. In uveitic glaucomas, keratic precipitates may form and anterior segment inflammation may lead to angle closure due to synechia formation, except in glaucomatocyclitic crisis, in which the angle remains open. Nanophthalmos and other congenital malformations may be associated with closure of the anterior chamber angle. Malignant glaucoma, due to posterior diversion of aqueous flow, is associated with a shallow axial and peripheral anterior chamber. Secondary causes of angle-closure glaucoma include posterior segment tumors, choroidal effusions, postsurgical changes, and other disorders. The patient described in this chapter did not have the history and physical findings associated with these other disorders.

21.2 Test Interpretation

In the history, the patient should be asked about blurred vision, colored halos around lights, pain, and eye redness. Previous episodes of similar symptoms and the duration of the symptoms should be documented. Inciting and associated factors, such as close work, emotional state, or ambient light level, may be identified. Patients with a family history of angle-closure glaucoma have a higher risk for angle-closure glaucoma compared with the general population. Epidemiologic studies have shown that certain factors may be associated with angle-closure glaucoma. The incidence of angle-closure glaucoma is highest between 55

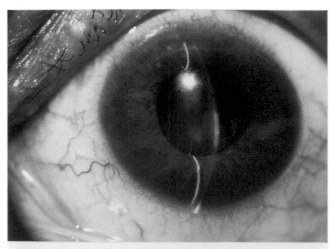

Fig. 21.1 Slit-lamp biomicroscopy of the left eye. The conjunctiva and episclera were mildly hyperemic, and the cornea was mildly edematous. The pupil was middilated and the iris had a markedly convex configuration. The IOP was 52 mm Hg.

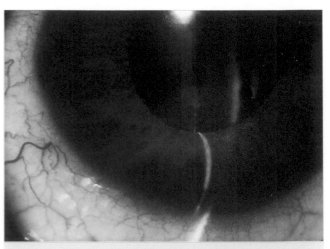

Fig. 21.2 High-power magnification view of the anterior segment of the left eye. The slit beam clearly demonstrates the marked convexity of the iris (iris bombé). The peripheral anterior chamber is absent.

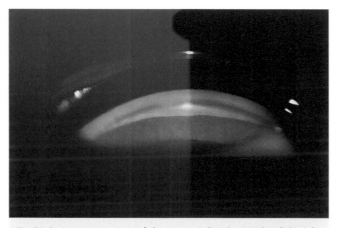

Fig. 21.3 Gonioscopic view of the anterior chamber angle of the left eye. The midperipheral iris is bowed anteriorly and the anterior chamber angle is closed.

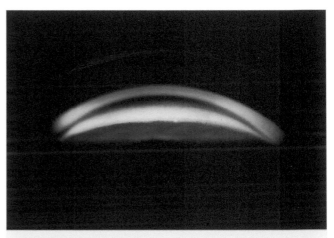

Fig. 21.4 Gonioscopic view of the anterior chamber angle of the left eye after laser iridotomy. The iris is mildly convex but has a more flat appearance compared with the preoperative configuration. The anterior chamber angle is open.

and 70 years. Although angle closure may occur in eyes with any refractive error, it is most common in hyperopic eyes. The incidence of angle-closure glaucoma varies in different ethnic groups. In the Caucasian American population, angle-closure glaucoma is about one-fifth as common as open-angle glaucoma. Compared with Caucasians, acute angle-closure glaucoma is less common in the African American population and more common in certain Asian populations.

In the physical examination, the slit-lamp biomicroscope should be used to evaluate for signs associated with angle-closure glaucoma, including conjunctival and episcleral hyperemia, corneal edema, and central and peripheral anterior chamber depth. There may be a mild anterior chamber inflammatory reaction, and the iris may have a convex configuration. The appearance of the lens should be noted. Signs of previous

episodes of angle-closure glaucoma should be documented, including iris atrophy, glaukomflecken, and peripheral anterior or posterior synechiae.

An essential part of the examination is gonioscopy, which is required to determine whether or not the patient has closure of the anterior chamber angle. In principle, high-frequency ultrasound ("ultrasound biomicroscopy") could also determine whether the angle is open or closed. Topical application of glycerin may minimize corneal edema and facilitate gonioscopy. Compression gonioscopy may be useful to determine whether the closure of the angle is appositional or synechial. Anterior segment optical coherence tomography can also be used to evaluate eyes with angle closure. In ▶ Fig. 21.5a, there is peripheral touch of the iris to the cornea, with iris bombé and a closed anterior chamber angle. In ▶ Fig. 21.5b, the patient has been

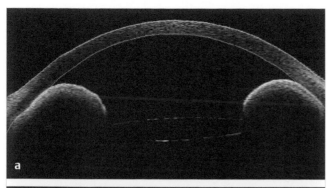

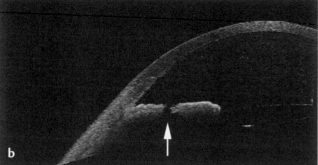

Fig. 21.5 (a) A 60 year-old man with iritis and pupillary block due to posterior synechiae. Anterior segment optical coherence tomography (OCT) before laser iridotomy shows iris bombé, with iris-corneal touch and angle closure. **(b)** Anterior segment OCT after laser iridotomy (arrow), with flattening of the iris and opening of the anterior chamber angle.

treated with laser peripheral iridotomy, which has flattened the convex configuration of the iris and opened the anterior chamber angle.

Basic elements of the eye examination should be performed, including measurement of vision and IOP. Assessment of the refractive status is helpful, because hyperopic eyes are at increased risk for developing angle-closure glaucoma. The appearance of the optic nerve should be documented when possible. The visual field should be evaluated, although this may be postponed in many cases until after the acute attack has been adequately treated. Dilation of the pupil should be deferred until after iridotomy or iridectomy.

Examination of the fellow eye usually reveals a shallow anterior chamber and a narrow angle. Although provocative testing may be helpful for certain patients considered at risk for angle-closure glaucoma, there is no need to perform provocative tests on the fellow eye in a patient who has developed angle-closure glaucoma. Approximately half of the fellow eyes in patients with acute angle-closure glaucoma will develop acute attacks within 5 years. Prophylactic iridotomy is indicated for the fellow eye, after the eye with the acute attack has been treated and is stable.

21.3 Diagnosis

Right eye: Narrow anterior chamber angle, at risk for subsequent angle-closure glaucoma. Left eye: Acute primary angle-closure glaucoma.

21.4 Medical Management

In eyes with angle-closure glaucoma, medical therapy is administered to lower the IOP rapidly and, ideally, to open the anterior chamber angle. Medical therapy usually improves the clarity of the cornea prior to definitive surgical treatment.

Osmotic drugs may be useful in the treatment of eyes with angle-closure glaucoma. Isosorbide and glycerol are administered orally and have an onset of effect within 1 hour. Isosorbide causes less nausea and vomiting compared with glycerol. In contrast with glycerol, isosorbide is not metabolized and does not have a significant caloric content. In patients with severe nausea and vomiting, intravenous mannitol may be administered. Osmotic drugs should be used with caution or avoided in patients with renal and cardiovascular disease, or those dehydrated by vomiting.

Intravenous acetazolamide may effectively and rapidly lower the IOP in eyes with angle-closure glaucoma. Acetazolamide may be administered orally, but the maximum effect occurs at about 2 hours, which is significantly later than after intravenous administration. Carbonic anhydrase inhibitors may be administered topically, but the adsorption and effect are variable because of the inflammation and edema in the setting of acute angle-closure glaucoma.

Topical cholinergic drugs may constrict the pupil and open the anterior chamber angle in some eyes with angle-closure glaucoma. Treatment may be initiated with a drop of 2% pilocarpine administered every 5 minutes for three doses. In some eyes, the pupil is unresponsive because of ischemia and paralysis of the iris sphincter due to extremely high IOP. In rare cases, paradoxical worsening of the angle-closure may occur due to forward movement of the lens and iris after treatment with cholinergic drugs.

Other topical antiglaucoma medications may be administered, including topical beta-blockers and alpha-2 agonists. These drugs are commonly used in treating angle-closure glaucoma, but their usefulness is limited by variable absorption and slow onset of action. Prostaglandin analogs are less useful in treatment of an acute attack of angle-closure glaucoma because of their slow onset of action.

Topical corticosteroids should be used to treat the marked inflammatory reaction associated with angle-closure glaucoma. Pain may be treated with analgesics, and vomiting may be treated with antiemetics. However, the focus of therapy for pain and vomiting should be on treating the underlying cause of these problems, which is the angle-closure glaucoma.

21.5 Surgical Management

Laser iridotomy is definitive therapy and the treatment of choice for angle-closure glaucoma with a component of pupillary block. When corneal clarity permits visualization of the iris, iridotomy may be performed during the attack, or the procedure may be performed after the acute attack has been treated with medical therapy when inflammation and edema have decreased. Gonioscopy determines whether the anterior chamber angle has been opened successfully after the laser iridotomy. Laser iridoplasty may be effective in opening areas of the angle that remain closed after iridotomy, even in the presence of mild to moderate corneal edema. When corneal edema resolves, laser or surgical goniosynechialysis may be performed to treat peripheral anterior synechiae that persist after the acute attack and contribute to chronically elevated IOP.

A therapeutic paracentesis can be performed, which may lower the IOP and clear the cornea for laser surgery. It is not advisable to perform a paracentesis if the patient is unable to cooperate or the risk of damage to the iris or lens is high due to severe narrowing of the anterior chamber. In eyes with a component of angle-closure due to the lens, cataract removal may deepen the anterior chamber angle.

In addition to laser treatment of the eye that has developed angle-closure glaucoma, the fellow eye should be treated with a prophylactic iridotomy if the anterior chamber angle is narrow. Without prophylactic iridotomy, approximately half of the fellow eyes in acute angle-closure glaucoma patients will develop acute attacks within 5 years.

21.6 Rehabilitation and Follow-up

At least one IOP measurement should be performed within 30 to 120 minutes of laser surgery. A follow-up examination should be performed within a week of laser surgery. If the response to treatment is inadequate, more frequent follow-up visits will be required. An additional follow-up examination should be performed 4 to 8 weeks postoperatively. Topical corticosteroids should be tapered during the postoperative period. Pupillary dilation with postdilation IOP check and gonioscopy determine whether the angle remains open after provocation. Provocative testing with inadequate iridectomy may cause pupillary block angle-closure glaucoma. Angle closure with a patent iridectomy may be due to plateau iris configuration.

Suggested Reading

[1] American Academy of Ophthalmology. Primary Angle-Closure Glaucoma: Preferred Practice Pattern. San Francisco, CA: American Academy of Ophthalmology; 1996

[2] Aptel F, Denis P. Optical coherence tomography quantitative analysis of iris volume changes after pharmacologic mydriasis. Ophthalmology. 2010; 117 (1):3–10

[3] Epstein DL, Allingham RR, Shuman JS. Chandler and Grant's Glaucoma. 4th ed. Baltimore, MD: Williams & Wilkins; 1997

[4] Hoskins HD, Kass M. Becker-Shaffer's Diagnosis and Therapy of the Glaucomas. 6th ed. Philadelphia, PA: CV Mosby; 1989

[5] Lam DS, Chua JK, Tham CC, Lai JS. Efficacy and safety of immediate anterior chamber paracentesis in the treatment of acute primary angle-closure glaucoma: a pilot study. Ophthalmology. 2002; 109(1):64–70

[6] Lam DS, Tham CC, Lai JS, Leung DY. Current approaches to the management of acute primary angle closure. Curr Opin Ophthalmol. 2007; 18(2):146–151

[7] Netland PA, Allen RA. Glaucoma Medical Therapy. Principles and Management. San Francisco, CA: American Academy of Ophthalmology; 1999

[8] Ritch R, Shields MB, Krupin T. The Glaucomas. 2nd ed. St. Louis, MO: Mosby-Year Book Inc; 1996

22 Pigmentary Glaucoma

Yasemin G. Sozeri, Scott A. Cory, and James C. Robinson

Abstract

Pigmentary glaucoma is a form of secondary open-angle glaucoma. It most commonly affects young myopic men. The pathophysiology involves an abnormal posterior bowing of the iris, which causes the posterior iris epithelium to chafe against lens zonules and liberate pigment. This pigment makes its way anterior and deposits on to the corneal epithelium (referred to as a Krukenberg spindle) as well as on to angle structures. On gonioscopy, Schwalbe's line will often appear pigmented, which is then referred to as Sampaolesi's line, and the trabecular meshwork will appear densely and evenly pigmented. Exercise can induce extra liberation of pigment and cause acute intraocular pressure spikes. Patients will often complain of blurry vision with exercise. Patients with exam findings consistent with pigmentary glaucoma without glaucomatous nerve damage are classified as pigment dispersion syndrome as opposed to pigmentary glaucoma. Treatment strategies for pigmentary glaucoma are similar to other open-angle glaucomas and include medications, laser trabeculoplasty, and incisional surgery including minimally invasive glaucoma surgeries. An additional strategy is laser peripheral iridotomy, which some believe can help reduce iris–zonule chafe and pigment liberation.

Keywords: pigmentary glaucoma, iris–zonule chafe, pigment dispersion, Krukenberg's spindle, Sampaolesi's line, laser peripheral iridotomy, laser trabeculoplasty

22.1 History

A 32-year-old myopic man presents for routine eye examination. He currently has no complaints and denies any significant past ocular or medical history. Examination revealed a best corrected visual acuity of 20/20 in each eye and no afferent pupillary defect in either eye. Intraocular pressures (IOPs) by applanation were 28 and 26 mm Hg. Slit-lamp examination disclosed vertically oriented pigment deposition on each corneal endothelium and numerous spokelike iris transillumination defects in both eyes (▶ Fig. 22.1). Gonioscopy showed fully open angles (360 degrees) in each eye with dense pigmentation of the trabecular meshwork bilaterally. On funduscopic examination, the right optic nerve had a cup-to-disc ratio of approximately 0.7 with inferotemporal thinning at the neuroretinal rim. The left eye had a cup-to-disc ratio of 0.55. Retinal examination was normal. Spectral-domain optical coherence tomography (SD-OCT) retinal nerve fiber layer (RNFL) analysis showed moderate thinning of the inferotemporal RNFL in the right eye and mild thinning in the left eye. Automated visual field testing demonstrated a moderate superior arcuate defect in the right eye and an early nasal step in the left eye.

Differential Diagnosis—Key Points

1. Elevated IOPs with pigment liberation originating from the iris, glaucomatous-appearing optic nerves, and visual field changes in a young myopic man best fits the patient profile of pigmentary glaucoma. Pigmentary glaucoma is generally a disease of the young and affects men approximately twice as often as women. Most experts agree that patients with pigmentary dispersion syndrome or pigmentary glaucoma have abnormal mechanical interaction between the posterior iris epithelium and the lens zonules, leading to the liberation of free pigment derived from the posterior iris epithelium that ultimately blocks aqueous outflow. As aqueous humor makes its way anteriorly, some of the pigment becomes attached to the corneal endothelium. The bulk of the pigment, however, eventually is filtered into the trabecular meshwork. Acute episodes of pigment liberation (such as with exercise) may cause an acute elevation of IOP, while the chronic effect of pigment deposition in the trabecular meshwork leads to sclerosis and eventual decline in function. It is often at this point when persistently elevated IOP progresses to glaucomatous optic nerve damage.

2. Although pigmentary glaucoma rarely presents a diagnostic dilemma, the differential diagnosis includes primary open-angle glaucoma with excessive pigmentation, pseudoexfoliative glaucoma, uveitis, ocular melanosis, and intraocular melanoma. A thorough and complete ocular examination is important to differentiate accurately between these various conditions.

3. Important to the diagnosis of pigmentary glaucoma is the gonioscopic examination of the trabecular meshwork. Pigmentary deposition in the trabecular meshwork due to pigmentary dispersion is often dense and evenly dispersed throughout the entire angle. In contrast, pigmentation that is pseudoexfoliative in origin is often less evenly distributed and may show dense areas of pigmentation with relatively spared areas interspersed throughout. Both pseudoexfoliative and pigmentary glaucoma may show pigmentation of Schwalbe's line, known as Sampaolesi's line. The key difference between these two diagnoses can easily be made based on careful examination of the pupillary border and anterior lens capsules. Pseudoexfoliative material is deposited on the pupillary border and anterior lens capsule, which is not characteristic of pigmentary glaucoma.

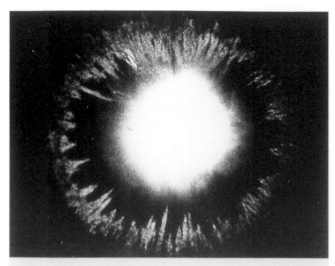

Fig. 22.1 Extensive transillumination defects in pigmentary glaucoma.

22.2 Test Interpretation

The initial examination of the optic nerve is perhaps the most critical first step in establishing whether or not a patient has glaucomatous nerve damage by the traditional methods of grading, documenting, and observing the optic disc. Cup-to-disc asymmetry, superficial nerve hemorrhages, and focal or progressive rim thinning are all useful in evaluating the severity of glaucoma. As such, baseline and sometimes serial optic nerve photos should be taken for future reference. Automated perimetry is an important diagnostic tool for evaluating the severity and progression of measurable field loss in all forms of glaucoma. Automated perimetry is based on projecting various levels of light or color stimuli into the patient's field of vision and estimating that field based on patient responses. Automated perimetry has allowed accurate and reproducible field analysis, which is critical for the long-term management of patients with glaucoma. Patients with pigmentary glaucoma tend to show glaucomatous field defects similar to patients with primary open-angle glaucoma. Most defects manifest as a diffuse decrease in sensitivity located in the peripheral field. SD-OCT has also proven to be a valuable test in evaluating, monitoring, and treating glaucoma. SD-OCT RNFL thickness analysis quantifies and qualifies glaucomatous RNFL thinning to a specific quadrant(s) and/or clock hour(s) compared to the normative database. RNFL thinning can be correlated with optic nerve head changes as well as visual field defects. RNFL thickness analysis becomes less reliable at measuring progressive thinning as the RNFL thickness decreases to 50 μm or less and thus is less useful in patients with severe disease. SD-OCT optic nerve head analysis provides objective measurements of the disc area, neural retinal rim area, cup-to-disc ratio, vertical cup, and cup area and compares these parameters to the patient's fellow eye for symmetry as well as to the normative database. Lastly, SD-OCT provides a ganglion cell analysis which measures the ganglion cell layer thickness at the macula and compares it to the fellow eye and the normative database for thinning. Along with monitoring IOP, serial optic nerve examinations, automated perimetry, and SD-OCT are useful in management of all forms of glaucoma including pigmentary glaucoma. At a minimum, adjunctive tests such as visual field testing and SD-OCT should be performed at least annually, and may often need to be repeated more frequently depending on the severity of a patient's particular disease course. It should be noted that optic nerve changes and SD-OCT-detected RNFL thinning can precede perimetry-detected visual field defects and lead to earlier detection of disease. This can be especially useful in distinguishing pigment dispersion syndrome from early pigmentary glaucoma.

22.3 Diagnosis

Right eye: Moderate-stage pigmentary glaucoma with superior arcuate defect.

Left eye: Moderate-stage pigmentary glaucoma with early nasal step defect.

22.4 Medical Management

Historically, pigmentary glaucoma was managed through the use of miotics (i.e., pilocarpine), which normalized IOP by minimizing the interaction of the iris and lens and thus limited the liberation of iris pigment. The obvious limitation of all miotic treatments is that their side effects are often poorly tolerated in the age group of patients primarily afflicted by pigmentary glaucoma. Extended release miotic therapy may decrease the degree of myopic shift and may be better tolerated. In the event that miotic therapy is intolerable or insufficient in controlling IOP, other topical agents should be initiated. IOP-lowering agents such as prostaglandin analogs, beta-blockers, carbonic anhydrase inhibitors, and alpha-adrenergic agonists are all appropriate. A desirable initial pressure reduction in IOP should be in the range of 20 to 30%. If despite this reduction there is continued visual field loss, then a multiagent regimen should be employed. When medical management fails to limit progression, or is not tolerated or is impractical, surgical alternatives should be considered.

22.5 Surgical Management

Laser peripheral iridotomy (LPI) is a treatment option that aims to directly alter the cause of pigment liberation. In pigmentary glaucoma, the origin of pigment liberation is felt to be due to an abnormal interaction between the pigment epithelium of the iris and the lens zonules, also known as a reverse pupillary block. Placement of an iridotomy is believed to decrease the potential for iris/lens interaction and thus treat the primary cause of the disease process. Unfortunately, the efficacy of LPI has yet to be adequately studied. Argon laser trabeculoplasty (ALT) is often very effective in patients with a more heavily pigmented trabecular meshwork, making it ideal as an initial treatment for patients with pigmentary glaucoma. ALT is a relatively low-risk procedure that may often provide years of effective pressure reduction. Initial treatment with ALT should be monocular, consist of a 180-degree treatment trial, and utilize the lowest effective power. If this initial treatment results in adequate pressure reduction, the other eye should be considered for treatment. Treatment of only one-half of the trabecular meshwork is often sufficient and reserves the option for future treatment. Selective laser trabeculoplasty is an alternative to ALT that has been shown to be an effective tool in lowering IOP in patients with open-angle glaucoma. It should be used with caution in patients with heavily pigmented trabecular meshwork, such as patients with pigmentary glaucoma, as there is some evidence that suggests it could lead to an IOP spike in these patients. Similar to other forms of glaucoma, if disease progression continues despite aggressive pharmacologic and laser therapy, incisional surgery should be considered. Depending on patient risk factors, disease severity, and surgeon preference, considerations may include traditional trabeculectomy, Ex-Press glaucoma mini-shunt, or glaucoma drainage implants. The role of more recently developed minimally invasive surgical options such as iStent trabecular microbypass, gonioscopy-assisted transluminal trabeculotomy, and endocyclophotocoagulation in the treatment of pigmentary glaucoma has not yet been well studied.

22.6 Rehabilitation and Follow-up

As with all forms of glaucoma, pigmentary glaucoma requires a patient-specific approach. Follow-up for pigmentary glaucoma should be based on the effectiveness of treatment, the stability of the disease process, overall severity of disease, and patient reliability.

Suggested Reading

[1] Campbell DG, Schertzer RM. Pigmentary glaucoma. In: Ritch R, Shields MB, eds. The Glaucomas. St. Louis, MO: Mosby; 1996:975–991

[2] Gandolfi SA, Vecchi M. Effect of a YAG laser iridotomy on intraocular pressure in pigment dispersion syndrome. Ophthalmology. 1996; 103(10):1693–1695

[3] Liebmann JM, Tello C, Chew SJ, Cohen H, Ritch R. Prevention of blinking alters iris configuration in pigment dispersion syndrome and in normal eyes. Ophthalmology. 1995; 102(3):446–455

[4] Sokol J, Stegman Z, Liebmann JM, Ritch R. Location of the iris insertion in pigment dispersion syndrome. Ophthalmology. 1996; 103(2):289–293

[5] Harasymowycz PJ, Papamatheakis DG, Latina M, De Leon M, Lesk MR, Damji KF. Selective laser trabeculoplasty (SLT) complicated by intraocular pressure elevation in eyes with heavily pigmented trabecular meshworks. Am J Ophthalmol. 2005; 139(6):1110–1113

[6] Hood DC, Kardon RH. A framework for comparing structural and functional measures of glaucomatous damage. Prog Retin Eye Res. 2007; 26(6):688–710

23 Neovascular Glaucoma

Daniel Y. Choi and Stephen A. Lin

Abstract

Neovascular glaucoma is a secondary angle-closure glaucoma. Diagnosis is made through a combination of the clinical history and findings on examination. Management typically consists of therapy to promptly lower intraocular pressure to a reasonable range. Glaucoma filtering surgery may be required to adequately control the intraocular pressure. A full examination to identify and treat the underlying etiology for neovascularization is required. Ultimately, the treatment for neovascular glaucoma should be customized to the patient's individual situation. As always, proper monitoring and prevention of neovascularization in high-risk patients is of utmost importance.

Keywords: neovascular glaucoma, glaucoma, angle-closure glaucoma, ocular hypertension, neovascularization

23.1 Clinical History

A 72-year-old man presents to the emergency department complaining of "a bad headache on the right side of my head." He also notes extreme redness and light sensitivity of the right eye and feels "sick to my stomach." His symptoms have developed quickly over half a day. Fearing that this may be more than "pink eye," the emergency department physician requests that an ophthalmologist evaluate the patient.

Past medical history is remarkable for hypertension, diabetes, and arteriosclerosis. A review of systems is positive for nausea and one episode of vomiting. The patient had experienced an abrupt, painless, severe decline in vision in the right eye approximately 3 months earlier. He was diagnosed at that time with an ischemic central retinal vein occlusion by his ophthalmologist.

Examination of the right eye reveals a visual acuity of hand motions. Slit-lamp examination shows severe corneal edema and conjunctival injection. A limited view of the anterior chamber reveals a small hyphema with cell and flare. The right iris does not appear to be bowed anteriorly, is minimally reactive to light, and exhibits fine and irregular branching vessels on its surface (▶ Fig. 23.1). A gonioscopic view of the drainage angle in the right eye is obscured by corneal edema. The drainage angle is wide open in the left eye. Only a dull red reflex can be appreciated on ophthalmoscopy of the right eye. The right fundus is not visible due to corneal edema and the left fundus is notable only for severe hypertensive retinopathy. B-scan ultrasonography shows an attached retina without any significant findings. The optic disc appears normal in the left eye. Intraocular pressure (IOP) is 67 mm Hg in the right eye and 19 mm Hg in the left.

23.2 Differential Diagnosis—Key Points

The differential diagnosis in this case centers on the two key examination findings of elevated IOP and iris neovascularization. It includes neovascular glaucoma (NVG), acute angle-closure glaucoma, Fuchs' heterochromic iridocyclitis, acute iridocyclitis, angle recession glaucoma, and traumatic hyphema with elevated IOP.

23.2.1 Acute, Severe IOP Elevation

An acute pressure elevation is often accompanied by corneal edema with a characteristic "steamy" appearance and conjunctival congestion. Patients complain of extreme pain and blurry vision accompanied by headache and sometimes nausea and vomiting. Corneal edema results in patient complaints of "colored halos around lights." In contrast, a chronic gradual elevation of IOP typically is associated with a relatively quiet eye with minimal symptoms.

When approaching the patient with an acute IOP elevation, gonioscopy and the slit-lamp examination to determine if the angle is open or closed is a key step to narrowing down the differential.

If the angle is closed, then the diagnosis of acute angle closure may be further subdivided into primary and secondary angle closure. Patients with primary acute angle closure classically present with pupillary block with a nonresponsive middilated pupil and iris bombé. These patients have baseline narrow iridocorneal angles that predispose them to developing pupillary block. Predisposed patients are often hyperopic with shallow anterior chambers. Gonioscopic examination of the asymptomatic fellow eye will often reveal angle narrowing. Secondary acute angle closure may result from mechanical closure due to an anterior "pulling mechanism" (e.g., NVG), a posterior "pushing mechanism" (e.g., choroidal detachment or aqueous misdirection), and a pupillary block mechanism (e.g., secluded pupil or silicone oil).

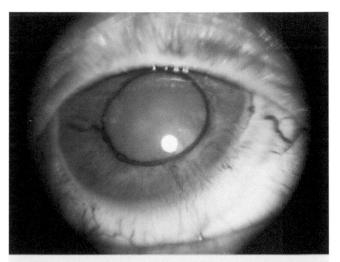

Fig. 23.1 Fine, irregular blood vessels growing over the anterior iris surface are characteristic of iris neovascularization. Growth often begins at the pupillary margin and may extend peripherally, where involvement of the drainage angle can lead to closure and elevated IOP.

If the angle is open, the underlying cause of an acute IOP elevation is likely a secondary open angle glaucoma (inflammatory, traumatic, etc.) as primary open angle glaucoma typically presents with a chronic insidious IOP elevation.

In this clinical vignette, the presence of neovascularization with an elevated IOP makes NVG the most likely diagnosis. The lack of iris bombé and the absence of a narrow angle in the fellow eye make the diagnosis of a primary angle-closure glaucoma with pupillary block unlikely. Furthermore, neovascularization and hyphema are not encountered in acute angle closure due to pupillary block. This patient had no history of trauma to suggest angle recession or a traumatic hyphema as the underlying primary etiology of the increased IOP. Although iridocyclitis can cause increased IOP, iridocyclitis rarely presents with true iris neovascularization and hyphema. Additionally, the history of a prior vein occlusion makes a primary inflammatory etiology a distant second to NVG.

23.2.2 Iris Neovascularization

Neovascularization, whether anterior or posterior, is usually associated with an underlying ocular ischemic process that results in the release of vascular endothelial growth factor (VEGF) within the eye. Diabetic retinopathy and retinal vein occlusions each account for approximately one-third of cases of iris neovascularization. Other causes of iris neovascularization include retinal artery occlusion, carotid occlusive disease, sickle cell retinopathy, chronic uveitis, intraocular tumor, and chronic retinal detachment.

Iris neovascularization usually begins with fine capillary tufts at the iris margin, which progress toward the iris root and chamber angle. Unlike iris vessels, which are uniform and radial in nature, these new vessels are irregular in caliber and direction. A fine fibrovascular membrane may be associated with these vessels and may lead to angle closure and ectropion uveae. Bleeding from neovascular growth is not uncommon and may lead to hyphema.

NVG is a secondary angle-closure glaucoma that is characterized by neovascularization of anterior segment structures that ultimately leads to angle closure, poor outflow facility, and eventual glaucomatous optic nerve damage. Iris neovascularization is invariably present prior to the invasion of the trabecular meshwork by fibrovascular membranes and ultimately permanent angle closure. Early iris neovascularization is easily overlooked on examination unless an effort is made to carefully scan the iris surface and trabecular meshwork. Any patient with risk factors for neovascularization should be thoroughly evaluated and monitored for both posterior and anterior neovascularization. Early detection, frequent monitoring, and prompt intervention may prevent the severe complications associated with extremely high IOP.

In this case, the history is extremely important. Previous vision loss and a history of a prior central retinal vein occlusion provide the reason for both the increased IOP (NVG) and also the underlying etiology for the neovascularization. The exam findings of iris and trabecular meshwork neovascularization with an elevated IOP are virtually pathognomonic for NVG. Despite this, it is always important to complete a full dilated fundoscopic examination of both eyes to rule out alternative etiologies for the neovascularization and the elevated IOP. If the view to the posterior pole is compromised due to corneal edema, a B-scan ultrasound should be obtained to rule out any significant posterior pathology.

23.3 Diagnosis

Acute ocular hypertension secondary to NVG.

23.4 Medical Management

All efforts should be made to lower IOP quickly. In general, most patients with an acutely elevated IOP due to NVG require oral carbonic anhydrase inhibitors to lower IOP to a relatively safe range. Topical aqueous suppressants including beta-blockers, alpha-2 agonists, and additional carbonic anhydrase inhibitors often should be administered. Cholinergic agents and possibly prostaglandin analogs provide a theoretical risk of further breakdown of the blood–aqueous barrier and their use is debated. Prostaglandin analogs, however, enhance uveoscleral outflow, which may play a more important role if the drainage angle is closed. Care should always be taken when using oral carbonic anhydrase inhibitors, especially in patients with renal dysfunction and/or in African American patients due to the possibility of an underlying sickle cell disorder. Hyperosmotic agents should be used with care, especially in diabetics, in the elderly, and in patients with congestive heart failure. The role of hyperosmotic agents may be limited, as osmotic gradients are weaker in the inflamed eye. Furthermore, oral agents may be difficult to administer in the setting of emesis.

Inflammation and pain may be managed with topical prednisolone and cycloplegics. Nausea and vomiting should be treated with medications delivered through a sublingual or other nonoral route.

Once the eye is stable, panretinal photocoagulation of the ischemic retina should be considered if there is a sufficient view of the posterior segment. In the acute state, an intravitreal injection (IVI) of an anti-VEGF agent should be considered once an intraocular tumor, retinal detachment, and/or significant retinal traction is ruled out. This injection will rapidly control the intraocular neovascular drive allowing for possible regression of fibrovascular membranes from the trabecular meshwork. Additionally, if filtering surgery is required to control the IOP, a prior IVI of an anti-VEGF agent may decrease intraoperative and postoperative bleeding. An anterior chamber paracentesis may be required prior to and after the IVI, given the baseline elevated IOP in NVG patients.

23.5 Surgical Management

Medical management alone is frequently inadequate for controlling the IOP in patients with NVG. Ideally, neovascularization should be inactive and/or an IVI of an anti-VEGF agent should administered prior to filtering surgery. Intraoperative bleeding is common when there is active neovascularization, and the prognosis for successful long-term control with a single surgery is often guarded. In general, first-line filtering surgery for NVG involves an aqueous shunting device (such as the Baerveldt (Johnson and Johnson Vision) and Ahmed (New World Medical) implants). If a nonvalved implant is used, venting tube incisions and/or immediate postoperative IOP-lowering medications will be required to adequately control the IOP while the capsule matures and the tube is tied off. Although trabeculectomy is another option in NVG, given the significantly high failure rate, it is rarely used acutely but remains an option after the neovascularization is completely controlled.

NVG in blind eyes may be managed more conservatively with elimination of pain as the main goal. Cyclodestructive procedures with the diode, neodymium:yttrium-aluminum-garnet (Nd:YAG) laser, or cryotherapy can alleviate pain associated with elevated pressure. Topical cycloplegics and steroid drops may also be of use. Retrobulbar alcohol or enucleation is usually reserved for refractory cases.

Suggested Reading

[1] Allen RC, Bellows AR, Hutchinson BT, Murphy SD. Filtration surgery in the treatment of neovascular glaucoma. Ophthalmology. 1982; 89(10):1181–1187

[2] Bresnick GH. Assessment of the eye at risk of neovascularisation. Eye (Lond). 1991; 5(Pt 2):198–213

[3] Kohner EM, Laatikainen L, Oughton J. The management of central retinal vein occlusion. Ophthalmology. 1983; 90(5):484–487

[4] Ritch R, Shields MB, Krupin T, eds. The Glaucomas. St. Louis, MO: CV Mosby Co; 1996:1073–1129

[5] Wand M, Dueker DK, Aiello LM, Grant WM. Effects of panretinal photocoagulation on rubeosis iridis, angle neovascularization, and neovascular glaucoma. Am J Ophthalmol. 1978; 86(3):332–339

[6] Kim M, Lee C, Payne R, Yue BY, Chang JH, Ying H. Angiogenesis in glaucoma filtration surgery and neovascular glaucoma: a review. Surv Ophthalmol. 2015; 60(6):524–535

24 Inflammatory Glaucoma

Robert Kule and Anne L. Coleman

Abstract

Intraocular inflammation or uveitis may cause a significant increase in intraocular pressure, which can lead to glaucomatous optic neuropathy. The elevation in intraocular pressure may result from various mechanisms, including reduced trabecular meshwork outflow and peripheral anterior synechiae formation. Identifying the underlying etiology of the inflammation is important in order to manage the disease effectively. Accurate diagnosis may be achieved with a thorough history, complete eye examination, and secondary testing, such as serologic workup and body imaging. Treatment of inflammatory glaucoma is achieved using topical and oral ocular hypertensive drugs, as well as surgical intervention, such as filtering surgery and implantation of glaucoma drainage devices. If the uveitis is active, treatment of the underlying systemic disease and control of the inflammation are essential.

Keywords: glaucoma, inflammation, uveitis, corticosteroid, herpes simplex, peripheral anterior synechiae, secondary open-angle glaucoma, secondary closed-angle glaucoma

24.1 History

A 38-year-old Caucasian man presented with a 2-day history of blurry vision, photophobia, tearing, and pain involving his left eye. His ocular history is notable for one episode of herpes simplex keratitis involving the left eye, which occurred 12 months ago and which resolved after treatment with trifluridine eye drops.

Examination showed vision of 20/20 in the right eye and 20/60 in the left eye, which improved to 20/40 with pinhole. Intraocular pressures (IOP) were 12 and 46 mm Hg, respectively. Slit-lamp examination of the right eye was unremarkable. The left cornea revealed fine, stellate keratic precipitates (KPs) scattered in a diffuse pattern. The anterior chamber was deep centrally and peripherally, with 2 + cells and aqueous flare. Patchy atrophy of the iris pupillary sphincter was noted on transillumination (▶ Fig. 24.1). No iris nodules, heterochromia, or posterior synechiae were observed. The lens was clear. Gonioscopy demonstrated angles open to the ciliary band in both eyes with moderate pigmentation of the trabecular meshwork and prominent iris processes but no peripheral anterior synechiae (PAS). On funduscopic exam, the vitreous appeared clear, and optic discs were symmetric with healthy rims.

Differential Diagnosis—Key Points

1. IOP can be elevated, stable, or reduced in response to inflammation. The main cause of IOP rise associated with uveitis, where the majority of eyes have open angles, is thought to be increased resistance to aqueous outflow. Several mechanisms have been proposed, including obstruction of the trabecular meshwork by inflammatory precipitates, swelling of the trabecular lamellae and endothelium, and alteration of aqueous dynamics by the breakdown in the blood–aqueous barrier. Less commonly, angle closure can result from pupillary block, PAS, or forward rotation of the ciliary body.

2. Large, "mutton-fat" KPs are found in granulomatous forms of uveitis, such as sarcoidosis and sympathetic ophthalmia. Fine, fibrillar KPs in a stellate pattern, as described in this case, are associated with herpetic or Fuchs' heterochromic uveitis.

3. Iris atrophy is characteristic of herpetic inflammation. Segmental atrophy due to occlusive vasculitis of the iris stromal vessels occurs with herpes zoster, whereas patchy atrophy around the pupillary sphincter is seen in herpes simplex.

4. The risk of developing herpes simplex iridocyclitis increases with recurrent episodes of keratitis, especially stromal keratitis. Herpetic uveitis can occur, however, in the absence of noticeable keratitis. The risk of associated glaucoma in cases of herpes simplex uveitis is estimated at 28 to 40%.

5. Many conditions can produce intraocular inflammation and elevated IOP (see the following list). The differential diagnosis in this case includes Fuchs' heterochromic iridocyclitis (typically unilateral, rarely bilateral, insidious onset, rarely symptomatic for ocular irritation, cataract formation, heterochromia), HLA-B27-associated uveitis (asymmetrically bilateral, arthritic conditions, synechiae formation), and glaucomatocyclitic crisis (unilateral, minimal inflammation, diagnosis of exclusion).

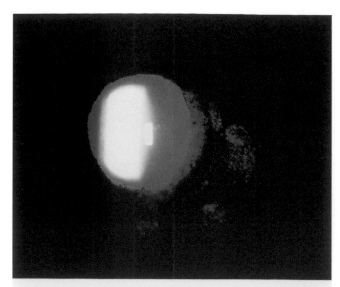

Fig. 24.1 Transillumination of this eye makes it easy to see the patchy iris atrophy associated with herpetic uveitis. (The image is provided courtesy of Drs. Gary N. Holland and Thomas H. Pettit, Los Angeles, CA.)

24.1.1 Inflammatory Conditions Associated with Glaucoma

1. Anterior uveitis:
   a) HLA-B27-positive uveitis (Reiter's, ankylosing spondylitis, etc.).
   b) Juvenile rheumatoid arthritis.
   c) Fuchs' heterochromic iridocyclitis.
   d) Lens-induced uveitis.
   e) Herpetic keratouveitis (simplex and zoster).
   f) Posner–Schlossman syndrome.
2. Intermediate uveitis (pars planitis).
3. Panuveitis:
   a) Sarcoidosis.
   b) Toxoplasmosis.
   c) Syphilitic uveitis.
   d) Behçet's syndrome.
   e) Sympathetic ophthalmia.
   f) Vogt–Koyanagi–Harada syndrome.
4. Masquerade syndrome (intraocular neoplasm).

24.2 Test Interpretation

A detailed history and review of system is essential in approaching the patient with inflammatory glaucoma. Key points include onset and duration of symptoms, unilateral or bilateral involvement, race, age, prior ocular conditions, risk factors for immune suppression or sexually transmitted diseases, and history of travel or trauma. A family history of rheumatological or ocular disease is especially important, as is a review of systems for arthritic, dermatological, or pulmonary symptoms.

Slit-lamp examination of the cornea may reveal epithelial or stromal scarring caused by herpetic or syphilitic keratitis, epithelial edema suggesting an acute rise in IOP, and KPs, which may differentiate granulomatous from nongranulomatous inflammation. The iris should be carefully evaluated for the presence of nodules (seen in sarcoidosis), heterochromia (classic for Fuchs' iridocyclitis), and posterior synechiae formation (which can cause acute angle closure from pupillary block). An anterior chamber reaction consisting of cells and aqueous flare is the hallmark of anterior uveitis. Glaucomatocyclitis crisis (Posner–Schlossman syndrome) typically presents with mild, recurrent, unilateral inflammation, whereas severe bilateral reactions with hypopyon formation can be seen in Behçet's disease and HLA-B27-related uveitis. Masquerade syndromes from an intraocular neoplasm may also present as apparent severe inflammation.

Careful visualization of the angle, by means of gonioscopy, is critical in the evaluation of all patients with elevated IOP. The configuration of the angle should be noted, and anatomically narrow angles that may be predisposed to closure must be identified. Heavy pigmentation of the trabecular meshwork can be seen in pseudoexfoliation, pigmentary dispersion syndromes, and uveitis. In the last case, the pigment is usually heaviest in the inferior angle, overlying the pocket formed by the iris root and scleral spur. The formation of PAS is an important feature of chronic inflammation, and PAS can lead to elevated IOP and secondary angle closure. PAS can be distinguished from normal iris processes by two features: (1) PAS appear more solid or sheetlike, and (2) PAS obliterate the angle recess. Iris processes tend to be open and lacy, follow the normal curve of the angle, and reveal normal angle structures in the open spaces between processes. Neovascular vessels in the angle, which differ from normal iris vessels in that they extend anteriorly over the scleral spur to reach the trabecular meshwork, can be seen in Fuchs' iridocyclitis. In the case of an apparently closed angle, a small lens (such as the Zeiss gonioscopy lens) should be used to indent the central cornea. This maneuver (indentation gonioscopy) helps differentiate between an appositionally closed angle that opens with aqueous pressure and an angle that is permanently closed by PAS.

Dilated funduscopic examination is essential in determining whether inflammation involves the posterior segment. The collection of white cellular aggregates in the vitreous ("snowballs") or inferior pars plana ("snowbank") suggests intermediate uveitis. Inflammatory changes of the retina, retinal vessels, or choroid, with concomitant iridocyclitis, suggest conditions that can cause panuveitis, such as sarcoidosis, toxoplasmosis, sympathetic ophthalmia, or Vogt–Koyanagi–Harada syndrome. Detailed attention should be paid to the optic nerve to look for glaucomatous changes such as asymmetry, excavation, notching, disc hemorrhage, or nerve fiber layer defects.

Based on the history and physical exam, diagnostic laboratory testing may be helpful. Special effort should be aimed at identifying infectious etiologies that can be treated with antibiotics. Commonly ordered tests include RPR/FTA-ABS to look for syphilis, serum or aqueous titers for toxoplasmosis, and skin PPD (purified protein derivative) or QuantiFERON-TB Gold test for tuberculosis. HLA (human leukocyte antigen) haplotype testing is helpful for suspected HLA-B27 uveitis and Behçet's disease. ANA (antinuclear antibody) testing is frequently positive in juvenile rheumatoid arthritis. Herpetic keratouveitis can usually be identified by the clinical picture alone.

24.3 Diagnosis

Herpes simplex anterior uveitis.

Secondary open angle glaucoma (inflammatory glaucoma).

24.4 Medical Management

The medical management of inflammatory glaucoma should generally be directed at two main objectives: controlling inflammation and reducing IOP.

Corticosteroids constitute the mainstay of therapy for most causes of ocular inflammation. Topical administration is preferred for anterior uveitis, and commonly used agents include prednisolone 1% and dexamethasone 0.1%. Initial dosing may require frequent, every-hour treatment, which can then be tapered based on the clinical response. A newer generation of steroids, such as rimexolone and loteprednol, is reported to be less likely to cause a steroid-induced rise in IOP and may be considered for patients on chronic therapy. Nonsteroidal anti-inflammatory agents such as flurbiprofen, ketorolac, and diclofenac can also help control ocular inflammation. In severe cases or those with associated extraocular involvement, systemic therapy with immunosuppressive medications such as methotrexate or azathioprine may be necessary.

Aqueous suppressants are generally considered the drugs of choice for control of elevated IOP in inflammatory glaucoma. Topical agents in this category include beta-adrenergic antagonists, such as timolol and levobunolol, and the carbonic anhydrase inhibitors, dorzolamide and brinzolamide. Adrenergic agonists, such as apraclonidine and dipivefrin, may provide additional pressure lowering. Miotics are not usually used in the inflamed eye, as they aggravate the breakdown of the blood–aqueous barrier and potentiate the formation of posterior synechiae. Latanoprost and other prostaglandin analogs (PGAs) have classically been avoided due to possible risks of exacerbating the uveitis, causing cystoid macular edema (CME), and reactivating herpes simplex keratouveitis; however, recent evidence suggests that these complications are rare, and PGAs may be used in patients with uveitic glaucoma, particularly when the IOP is not controlled with aqueous suppressants alone. Uveitis caused by infectious agents, such as syphilis or toxoplasmosis, must be treated with appropriate antibiotics. Topical trifluridine is effective against herpes simplex keratitis with epithelial involvement and for prophylaxis against recurrence of epithelial disease in patients on topical steroids. Topical antivirals penetrate poorly into posterior stroma and anterior chamber, however, and oral acyclovir has been reported to be helpful against herpetic keratouveitis, both in the acute setting and for prophylactic maintenance therapy.

Cycloplegic agents, including atropine or cyclopentolate, can aid in relieving pain from ciliary muscle spasm, in preventing formation of posterior synechiae, and in stabilizing the aqueous–blood barrier.

24.5 Surgical Management

In general, glaucoma surgery should be deferred, if possible, until active inflammation has been brought under control.

Surgery is indicated if, despite maximal medical therapy, the IOP remains dangerously elevated, or glaucomatous visual field defects and disc changes develop.

Laser peripheral iridotomy should be performed for acute angle closure due to pupillary block, which may be caused by posterior synechiae. The main complication is transient anterior chamber inflammation and increased IOP, which may be ameliorated by premedication with steroids and apraclonidine. If laser iridotomy is unsuccessful, a surgical iridectomy may be required. Laser peripheral iridotomy should be avoided, however, in narrow angle patients with near-360-degree posterior synechiae, as the shunting of aqueous through the iridotomy may cause seclusio pupillae, precipitating iris bombé.

Laser trabeculoplasty is ineffective and contraindicated in eyes with active inflammation. The risk of an acute rise in IOP is greatly increased, as is formation of PAS leading to secondary angle closure.

For inflammatory glaucoma with open angle, or chronic angle closure, a trabeculectomy can be performed to lower IOP. The use of an antimetabolite such as 5-fluorouracil or mitomycin C significantly improves success rates. The risk of bleb failure is higher in younger patients and those with uncontrolled inflammation. Surgery to place an aqueous drainage device, such as an Ahmed valve or Molteno implant, has also been shown to be effective. Laser cyclophotocoagulation may be associated with an intense inflammatory response postoperatively and should be used with caution.

24.6 Rehabilitation and Follow-up

Frequent follow-up is essential for patients with uveitic glaucoma, as many of these conditions have a waxing and waning course. Attention must be paid to the presence of inflammation, and steroids should be used to control inflammation despite the risk of steroid-induced pressure elevation. Problems associated with chronic intraocular inflammation, such as band keratopathy and CME, should be actively sought and treated.

In addition to monitoring IOP, optic nerve examination and visual field testing are required to detect the development or progression of glaucoma. In addition, the angle should be closely evaluated with gonioscopy at each visit to look for evidence of neovascularization or PAS formation, which may lead to secondary angle closure. The development of glaucomatous damage often occurs well after the initial presentation of acute inflammation, and one should remain vigilant for glaucoma even after the apparent resolution of uveitis.

Suggested Reading

[1] Herpetic Eye Disease Study Group. Acyclovir for the prevention of recurrent herpes simplex virus eye disease. N Engl J Med. 1998; 339(5):300–306

[2] Moorthy RS, Mermoud A, Baerveldt G, Minckler DS, Lee PP, Rao NA. Glaucoma associated with uveitis. Surv Ophthalmol. 1997; 41(5):361–394

[3] Shields BM. Textbook of Glaucoma. 4th ed. Baltimore, MD: Williams & Wilkins; 1998:308–322

[4] Horsley MB, Chen TC. The use of prostaglandin analogs in the uveitic patient. Semin Ophthalmol. 2011; 26(4–5):285–289

25 Primary Congenital Glaucoma

Elena Bitrian and Alana L. Grajewski

Abstract

This chapter reviews the clinical findings, differential diagnosis and unique challenges in the treatment of Primary Congenital Glaucoma.

Keywords: glaucoma, pediatric, childhood, congenital, goniotomy, trabeculotomy, drainage device

25.1 History

A 3-month-old female infant was referred after her mother noted "cloudy eyes and tearing" for 3 to 4 weeks. The child was the product of a full-term uneventful pregnancy and delivery with no use of forceps. There was no known family history of glaucoma and she had a 3-year-old brother without any ocular problems.

On examination in the office, the child was photophobic and was more comfortable in dim illumination. Both eyes had a diffuse corneal haze, the right more than the left. Estimated corneal diameters measured in the office were 12 mm in her right eye and 11 mm in her left eye (► Fig. 25.1). Intraocular pressure (IOP) measurements were taken with iCare while the infant nursed on a bottle, and were 45 and 36 mm Hg for the right and left eyes, respectively.

Differential Diagnosis—Key Points

1. Cloudy corneas, tearing, and photophobia with high IOPs are highly suggestive of childhood glaucoma. In this particular clinical presentation, primary congenital glaucoma (PCG) is the most likely diagnosis. However, other ocular conditions that can present with a "cloudy cornea" cannot be excluded until an examination under anesthesia is performed.

PCG is the most common nonsyndromic glaucoma in childhood, and it usually presents within the first 2 years of life. Generally, the younger the presentation, the more serious the disorder and the more guarded the prognosis. It is most often bilateral (75% of the cases), but unilateral and asymmetric cases are seen, such as with this particular infant. Males are slightly more commonly affected than females. PCG is usually inherited in an autosomal recessive manner, and in 10 to 40% of cases, there is a reported family history of glaucoma. It is more common in consanguineous populations and there are families with multiple siblings with glaucoma from birth.

The most common clinical presentation includes corneal enlargement with clouding, epiphora, and photophobia, all of which were present in this child. These symptoms are secondary to ocular abnormalities caused by elevated IOP.

2. Other causes of corneal haze or opacity include birth trauma (forceps), sclerocornea, congenital hereditary endothelial dystrophy, posterior polymorphous dystrophy, numerous metabolic diseases, uveitis, and various forms of anterior segment dysgenesis such as Peter's anomaly. Each of these has certain unique characteristics that help distinguish it from primary infantile glaucoma.

3. Glaucoma in children is characterized by elevated IOP and characteristic optic nerve cupping. In addition, ocular enlargement (buphthalmos) is often seen. Ocular enlargement secondary to childhood glaucoma should not be confused with megalocornea or increased axial length seen in myopia, and those two entities do not have elevated IOP and corneal edema.

4. Nasolacrimal duct obstruction is the most common cause of epiphora in this age group. Photophobia, corneal haze, and corneal enlargement are not associated with this problem. A mucopurulent discharge is often present and tends to respond quickly to standard treatment.

5. Ocular tumors in infancy can also mimic childhood glaucoma. Some ocular tumors may be associated with a secondary elevated IOP that can produce some of the same signs and symptoms of PCG. As the treatment is distinctly different, it is imperative that this be considered in each child in whom the view to the posterior segment is obscured. Intraoperative ultrasound at the time of the initial examination under anesthesia is, in this circumstance, essential.

6. Finally, elevated IOP can also be associated with various systemic syndromes such as Sturge–Weber, Rubinstein–Taybi, and Lowe's syndromes, rubella, and trisomy 13.

25.2 Test Interpretation

The testing for primary infantile glaucoma can be thought of as those examinations with or without anesthesia. An office examination is typically without anesthesia. Very young infants can often be pacified with a bottle for obtaining an initial pressure measurement in the office. The ICare is the preferred method to check IOP in clinic since it does not require anesthetic eye drops for pressure care and there is minimal contact with the corneal surface for the reading.

A full examination under anesthesia is usually performed initially in the operating room and requires general anesthesia with laryngeal mask or endotracheal intubation. Brief examinations can be safely performed under anesthesia supervision without intubation using an inhalational anesthetic by mask with an oral airway. The examination under anesthesia consists of pressure measurement, corneal diameter measurements, ultrasonography (axial length and biomicroscopy if needed), anterior segment examination, and gonioscopy. The dilated fundus examination with optic disc photos can be done if surgery is not planned. If surgery is planned, the pupils are not dilated.

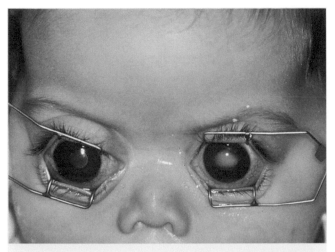

Fig. 25.1 Examination under anesthesia. Both corneas are enlarged, the right more than the left. The left cornea demonstrates a moderate central corneal haze; the right cornea has a more subtle epithelial edema seen best with the microscope.

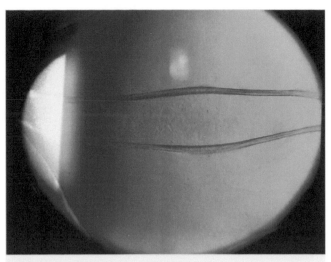

Fig. 25.2 Horizontal break in Descemet's membrane, Haab's striae, right eye.

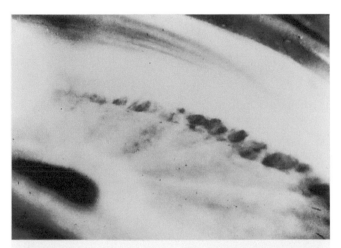

Fig. 25.3 Gonioscopy demonstrates the high flat insertion with peripheral anterior stromal thinning typical of primary congenital glaucoma.

25.3 Diagnosis

The diagnosis of PCG depends on several factors, with IOP measurement being only one. Anesthetic agents as well as facial compression from the mask can influence IOP measurements. Because of this, it is best to obtain two sets of measurements: the first under light anesthesia as soon as the child is quiet, and the second measurement once the airway is secured. Any consistent method to measure IOP is acceptable. In the operating room, the most common method to check IOP is Tonopen, as well as hand-held applanation instruments (Perkins). The normal IOP in infants is slightly lower than that found in adults. This is because the ciliary body does not reach the capacity for full aqueous production until several months after birth. Asymmetric IOPs are often helpful in distinguishing bilateral from unilateral or asymmetric cases.

Normal neonatal corneal diameters are 10 to 10.5 mm horizontally and increase 0.5 to 1.0 mm over the first year. Any corneal diameter ≥ 11.5 mm in a newborn is almost certainly pathologic. With respect to ocular enlargement, measurement of axial length by A-scan ultrasonography is extremely useful for diagnosis and follow-up. A child younger than 3 years can suffer stretching of the tissues due to elevated IOP. This stretching can produce Descemet's breaks (also known as Haab's striae) and increased axial length. After 3 years of age, elevated IOP does not cause those changes. On occasions, the anterior segment examination can be limited by corneal edema and opacity. Nevertheless, one should record the corneal breaks in Descemet's membrane as these become useful for comparison in follow-up (▶ Fig. 25.2). On gonioscopy, the iris appears stretched with thinning of the anterior stroma and a high flat insertion into the trabecular meshwork (▶ Fig. 25.3). If surgery is not planned, dilated retina examination and optic disc stereo photographs are performed. Stereoscopic disc photographs are clinically one of the most useful tools for long-term follow-up.

25.4 Medical Management

PCG is a surgical disease. Medications can be used in the preoperative period to minimize any further damage from elevated IOP and to decrease the corneal edema. Medical treatment prior to surgery facilitates a better examination of the anterior and posterior segments and often allows to perform angle surgery through an ab interno approach. Topical glaucoma agents that can be used include carbonic anhydrase inhibitors (brimonidine and dorzolamide) and selective beta-blockers. Beta-blockers must be used with caution in children and usually 0.25% dose is used on younger children. The use of topical alpha-2 agonist in small children is associated with profound sedative effects. In addition, these agents prolong the effect of anesthesia and these are contraindicated in infants. Oral acetazolamide can be administered in a syrup suspension of acetazolamide at 5 to 10 mg per kg every 6 to 8 hours.

25.5 Surgical Management

Prompt surgery is essential in most cases of childhood glaucoma. Damage from elevated IOP is more likely the longer IOP remains elevated and the higher the IOP is. In the case we presented, with the presumptive diagnosis of PCG made at the time of the office examination, the child should be placed on medication (topical or oral carbonic anhydrase inhibitor) until the pediatrician and anesthesiologist give clearance for general anesthesia. In order to minimize the time until treatment as well as limit exposure to anesthesia, surgery should be planned for the same time as the initial full examination under anesthesia if the diagnosis is confirmed. For this reason, the initial examination should be performed by a surgeon familiar with angle surgery for childhood glaucoma. The surgical procedure of choice for PCG is angle surgery, either goniotomy or trabeculotomy. Both procedures have high success and low complication rates. These procedures work equally well. The preferred approach is to treat the angle of 360 degrees with either of these methods before moving on to other surgery. The success rate of this procedure is between 80 and 90% with initial angle surgery, thus making the need for a second procedure rare. If IOP remains uncontrolled following 360 degrees of surgical treatment of the angle, without other factors complicating the clinical picture (e.g., hyphema or anterior chamber inflammation), the temporary use of topical medications can be tried. After a sufficient time from surgery and if medical therapy is not adequate, a glaucoma drainage device such as a Baerveldt shunt is placed. This style of drainage device is preferred in infants as its low contour better conforms to the globe and so it is less likely to displace the globe. There have been reports of success with trabeculectomy; however, these rarely function without the use of an antimetabolite. Mitomycin C enhances the success rate of filtering surgery in children. Given the long-term risks of a mitomycin bleb in a child, however, traditional angle surgery and/or a drainage implant is preferred. Cyclodestructive procedures are reserved for those cases that fail filtration procedures.

25.6 Rehabilitation and Follow-up

After completion of a full examination under anesthesia and angle surgery, the child should be placed on topical cycloplegics and steroids for 1 to 2 weeks. A second examination under anesthesia is performed at 8 to 10 weeks postoperatively. All measurements are repeated. If the IOP is acceptable, the baby is dilated for disc photography and fundus examination. Follow-up examinations under anesthesia can be performed about every 2 to 3 months, until it is certain that the IOP is stable or the child is able to be examined in clinic. At that point, examinations can be every third to fourth month and then reduced to every 6 months, when the patient is stable. By the age of 3 or 4 years, the child can generally be examined in the office.

Suggested Reading

[1] Weinreb RN, Grajewski AL, Papadopoulos M, Grigg J, Freedman S. Childhood Glaucoma: Consensus Series - 9. Amsterdam: Kugler Publications; 2013

[2] al-Hazmi A, Zwaan J, Awad A, al-Mesfer S, Mullaney PB, Wheeler DT. Effectiveness and complications of mitomycin C use during pediatric glaucoma surgery. Ophthalmology. 1998; 105(10):1915–1920

[3] Anderson DR. Trabeculotomy compared to goniotomy for glaucoma in children. Ophthalmology. 1983; 90(7):805–806

[4] Dickens CJ, Hoskins HD Jr. Diagnosis and treatment of congenital glaucoma. In: Ritch R, Shields MB, Krupin T, eds. The Glaucomas. St. Louis, MO: CV Mosby Co; 1989:773–785

[5] Eid TE, Katz LJ, Spaeth GL, Augsburger JJ. Long-term effects of tube-shunt procedures on management of refractory childhood glaucoma. Ophthalmology. 1997; 104(6):1011–1016

26 Ocular Hypotony

Thomas W. Samuelson

Abstract

Ocular hypotony is a relatively common adverse event following filtration surgery. Hypotony can present at any time postoperatively, ranging from the immediate postoperative period to many years later. The causes of hypotony following filtration surgery are numerous and varied. The workup of this condition should be systematic utilizing history to ensure proper adherence to pharmacologic therapy including discontinuation of aqueous suppressants, the Seidel test to assess for wound leaks, fundoscopy to assess for choroidal effusion, and gonioscopy to rule out cyclodialysis cleft formation. Once the cause of hypotony has been identified, appropriate treatment is initiated. Common treatment modalities include observation, discontinuation of all aqueous suppressants, cycloplegia, and treatment of wound leaks as needed utilizing direct closure with sutures when necessary. In cases of anterior chamber shallowing, reformation with viscoelastic material may be warranted. In cases of primary overfiltration, use of a bandage contact lens to tamponade the filtration site, autologous blood patches, and/or bleb compression sutures may be useful. Finally, when more conservative measures fail, returning to the operating room to place additional scleral flap sutures may be necessary.

Keywords: glaucoma, low pressure, overfiltration, choroidal effusion, maculopathy

26.1 History

A 45-year-old woman was referred for surgical management of inflammatory glaucoma in her aphakic right eye. Her left eye had had only light perception since birth due to persistent hyperplastic primary vitreous.

The preoperative visual acuity with aphakic correction was 20/20. The intraocular pressure (IOP) was 40 mm Hg on maximum medical therapy including oral agents. Central corneal thickness was 535 μm in each eye. There was 1+ cell and flare in the anterior chamber (AC) with scattered, fine, keratic precipitates. There was vitreous at the pupillary plane. The optic disc was markedly excavated with a cup-to-disc ratio of 0.9 and a notch inferiorly. The visual field had a superior altitudinal defect.

A trabeculectomy with mitomycin C and subtotal vitrectomy was performed without incident. Postoperatively, the visual acuity remained 20/20. The IOP was well controlled in the range of 9 to 12 mm Hg for the first postoperative year. However, 1 year after surgery, the patient presented with a complaint of worsening vision.

The visual acuity was 20/60. An increase in hyperopic correction of + 1.50 diopters improved the visual acuity to 20/20. The bleb was highly elevated, avascular, and cystic. The remainder of the examination was unchanged from baseline with the exception of moderate chorioretinal folds involving the posterior pole and macula. The IOP was 3 mm Hg.

Differential Diagnosis—Key Points

This patient has hypotony with maculopathy. The differential diagnosis of hypotony in this case includes several disorders.

1. **Primary overfiltration.** This disorder is most common in the early postoperative period following trabeculectomy when the eye is still recovering from chronic pharmacologic aqueous suppression and the conjunctiva has yet to contract in the region of the filter. Hypotony related to overfiltration is a diagnosis of exclusion. Primary overfiltration implies that the basic problem relates to excessive outflow rather than to an abnormally low production of aqueous. Clinically, the bleb is generally exuberant and highly elevated. Primary overfiltration must be distinguished from secondary overfiltration that may result from a wound leak or cyclodialysis cleft. These conditions are discussed below.

2. **Underproduction (hyposecretion) of aqueous.** Hyposecretion of aqueous is an important cause of ocular hypotony. Hyposecretion may occur when aqueous suppressants are not discontinued following filtration surgery. Pharmacologic hyposecretion of aqueous is diagnosed by obtaining the appropriate history. Hyposecretion may also occur in response to inflammation. Clinically, there may be significant flare in the AC due to decreased clearance of proteins and altered blood–aqueous barrier. The bleb is generally lower and more vascularized in such eyes. Hyposecretion may also result from ciliary detachment or ocular ischemia; these conditions are addressed below.

3. **Bleb leak.** A bleb leak can result in hypotony and may occur at any time following glaucoma filtration surgery. A Seidel test is mandatory in any postsurgical patient with hypotony. The entire bleb and incision line should be painted with fluorescein; the leak is apparent where the dye is displaced. In general, a bleb leak will result in a lower bleb. However, bleb morphology may be variable in eyes with leaks and should not be relied on for the diagnosis. The diagnosis and management of bleb leaks are discussed in Case 28.

4. **Cyclodialysis cleft.** A cyclodialysis cleft is a relatively uncommon condition that may result in profound hypotony. It is most common following cataract surgery utilizing a scleral tunnel incision. However, a cleft may also occur following glaucoma filtration surgery when the block excision is too posterior and the ciliary body is disinserted from the scleral spur. Additionally, a cleft may also occur following trauma. Hypotony results from increased outflow facility as aqueous is diverted from the AC into the suprachoroidal space. The diagnosis is made by careful gonioscopy. If the AC is too shallow to visualize the angle, viscoelastic material may be injected to deepen the AC to improve visualization.

5. **Retinal detachment**. Retinal detachment may cause hypotony by increasing uveal scleral outflow or by decreasing aqueous production. The diagnosis is made by fundus examination or by ultrasound in the event that media opacity precludes a view of the posterior pole.

6. **Choroidal effusion**. This is not typically a primary cause of hypotony but rather a result of hypotony. However, the presence of fluid in the suprachoroidal space may result in ciliary detachment that in turn may decrease aqueous production, which may exacerbate hypotony. The diagnosis of choroidal effusion is made by indirect biomicroscopy and identification of smooth, dome-shaped, lobular elevation of the retina. Characteristically, the AC is shallow.

7. **Ocular ischemia**. Ocular ischemia–related hypotony results from decreased aqueous production due to underperfusion of the ciliary body. Associated findings may include rubeosis iridis, low-grade AC reaction, and scattered blot hemorrhages in the retina. Carotid artery blood flow studies or fluorescein angiography will provide the definitive diagnosis.

8. **Occult globe perforation**. This disorder is a rare cause of ocular hypotony. Most commonly, globe perforation occurs during retrobulbar injection or during placement of the rectus traction suture used to stabilize the globe during surgery. The diagnosis is made by fundus examination.

26.2 Test Interpretation

The slit-lamp and fundus examination generally provide the necessary information to correctly identify the etiology of ocular hypotony (▶ Table 26.1). Once the visual acuity and IOP are measured, the bleb is examined carefully. The elevation, vascularity, and extent of the bleb should be noted (▶ Fig. 26.1). The presence or absence of microcyst formation within the bleb should be noted. Examination of the bleb should include a Seidel test to rule out a bleb leak. A Seidel test is best accomplished by using a moistened strip of fluorescein and directly painting the bleb and incision line. A wound leak is identified by detecting a stream of bright green aqueous using cobalt blue light at the slit lamp (▶ Fig. 26.2). It is important to realize that an intermittent leak may not be apparent if hypotony is profound and there is no flow gradient. In such cases, gentle pressure may be applied to the globe under direct visualization at the slit lamp. The increased pressure gradient may reveal an occult leak.

Slit-lamp biomicroscopy is used to document the AC depth. The AC may be shallow or of normal depth. A shallow AC is a nonspecific sign and, unlike the bleb appearance, does not help discern the etiology of the low IOP. Finally, the presence of intraocular inflammation should be noted. This inflammation is a nonspecific sign, but pronounced AC flare may be a sign of decreased aqueous production.

Table 26.1 Differential diagnosis of postoperative hypotony

Diagnosis	Test results/exam features[a]
Overfiltration	Seidel (−)
	Bleb high on exam
Bleb leak	Seidel (+)
	Bleb variable—generally low
Decreased production—pharmacologic	History of aqueous suppression therapy
	Seidel (−)
	Bleb low
Decreased production—nonpharmacologic	Seidel (−)
	Increased Inflammation, increased flare fundus exam/ultrasound
	R/O retinal detachment
	Ciliary detachment
	Choroidal effusions
	Bleb low
Cyclodialysis cleft	Gonioscopy confirms presence of cleft bleb low
Retinal detachment	Fundus exam/ultrasound
Ocular ischemia	Peripheral retinal hemorrhage
	Angle neovascularization
	Carotid studies
Globe perforation	Fundus exam detects perforation or vitreous hemorrhage

[a]A Seidel test is mandatory on every patient with hypotony.

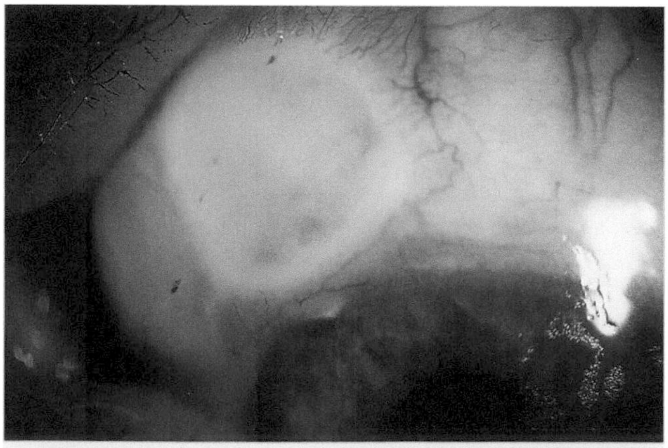

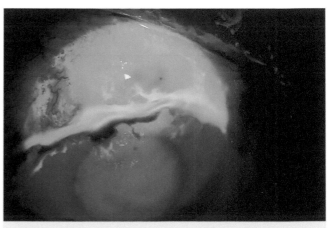

Fig. 26.1 Typical appearance of an overfiltering bleb in a patient with hypotony.

Fig. 26.2 Positive Seidel's test in a patient with hypotony.

The fundus examination will rule out retinal detachment, an uncommon but important cause of low IOP. Additionally, fundus examination may document the presence of choroidal effusion. Occasionally, a very anterior or annular choroidal effusion may be occult and not visible on standard fundus exam with indirect biomicroscopy. Such cases may be detected by ultrasound biomicroscopy. Finally, the macula should be examined for striae, which may result from hypotony. The macular striae characteristic of hypotonous maculopathy do not typically have an exudative component. Fluorescein angiography is generally not helpful. Finally, the fundus exam may reveal a swollen or hyperemic optic disc, another nonspecific sign of hypotony.

Gonioscopy is useful to rule out a cyclodialysis cleft or excessively large sclerostomy site. Additionally, gonioscopy is necessary to rule out angle neovascularization in cases of ocular ischemia.

Refraction is useful in cases of reduced visual acuity associated with hypotony. Relative myopia may result from shallowing of the AC and forward displacement of the lens or intraocular lens. Conversely, relative hyperopia may result when profound hypotony causes contraction of the globe and decreased axial length. An axial length measurement may confirm reduced axial length relative to baseline values or compared to the fellow eye. Reduced axial length is a common finding in patients with hypotonous maculopathy (▶ Fig. 26.3). In general, choroidal effusions are more common in elderly patients with rigid sclera, while globe contraction is more common in younger patients with less rigid sclera.

The patient in this case discussion had hypotony associated with a large, avascular, Seidel-negative bleb. Slit-lamp examination found the eye to be quiet and noninflamed. Gonioscopy excluded a cyclodialysis cleft. The axial length was 0.75 mm shorter and refraction 1.5 diopters more hyperopic than baseline readings. Maculopathy was detected by fundus exam. There was no retinal or choroidal detachment. Finally, a careful patient history confirmed that the patient was not taking any topical or systemic medications that could suppress aqueous production.

26.3 Diagnosis

Hypotony due to primary overfiltration.

26.4 Medical Management

For mild hypotony early in the postoperative period, pharmacologic treatment may stabilize the eye until the overfiltration spontaneously resolves. Cycloplegic agents may help deepen the AC and stabilize the blood–aqueous barrier. While aqueous suppressants are often administered to treat bleb leaks, they are not helpful in cases of hypotony related to overfiltration. Topical corticosteroids may quiet the eye and maximize aqueous production. However, they may also make the bleb thinner and less vascular, preventing bleb contraction. As such, the benefit of topical corticosteroids on aqueous production must be weighed against the potential negative effect on an overfiltering bleb.

26.5 Surgical Management

When hypotony is profound and persistent, surgical intervention may be necessary. Several procedures have been advocated to treat overfiltration including compression shells or sutures, inflammation-inciting measures such as trichloroacetic acid, autologous blood patch (▶ Fig. 26.4), and bleb remodeling with Nd:YAG laser. As a rule, mild cases may respond to these measures. However, more profound and protracted hypotony often requires surgical revision such as resuturing of the scleral flap with either transconjunctival scleral flap sutures or bleb revision performed by dissection down to bare sclera and directly resuturing the scleral flap (▶ Fig. 26.5, ▶ Fig. 26.6). Mattress sutures have also been described to compress the bleb externally (▶ Fig. 26.7).

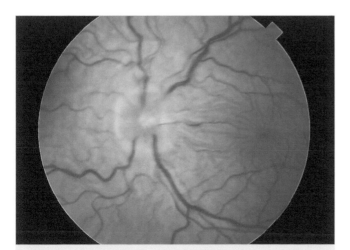

Fig. 26.3 Typical fundus appearance of a hypotonous eye with disc swelling and chorioretinal folds.

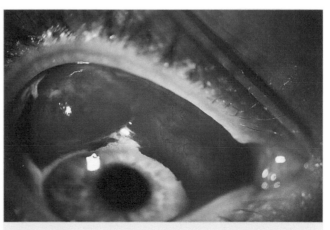

Fig. 26.4 Mild cases of overfiltration hypotony may be successfully managed with an autologous blood patch.

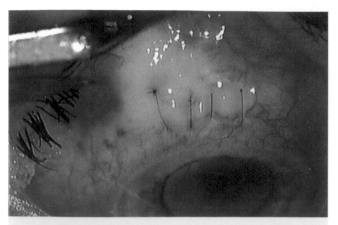

Fig. 26.5 Transconjunctival scleral flap sutures to treat hypotony related to excess filtration. (The image is provided courtesy of Marlene Moster, MD.)

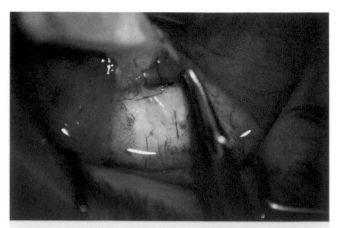

Fig. 26.6 Resuturing the scleral flap is often effective in treating hypotony related to overfiltration when more conservative measures fail.

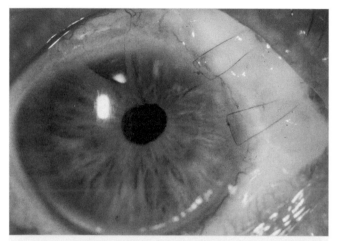

Fig. 26.7 Horizontal mattress "compression" suture often helps with bleb dysesthesia and/or hypotony. (The image is provided courtesy of Paul Palmberg, MD.)

26.6 Rehabilitation and Follow-up

Cycloplegic agents and conservative observation failed to reverse the hypotony. An autologous blood patch also failed. The patient was then taken to the operating room where two additional sutures were placed in the scleral flap (▶ Fig. 26.6).

The bleb was not excised. The patient responded well with increased IOP into the 20 s. The axial length, refraction, and visual acuity returned to normal. One month postrevision, suture lysis was performed resulting in IOP of 13 mm Hg. Six years later, the IOP has remained in the low teens with no recurrent hypotony.

Suggested Reading

[1] Leen MM, Moster MR, Katz LJ, Terebuh AK, Sc, hmidt CM, Spaeth GL. Management of overfiltering and leaking blebs with autologous blood injection. Arch Ophthalmol. 1995; 113(8):1050–1055

[2] Lynch MG, Roesch M, Brown RH. Remodeling filtering blebs with the neodymium:YAG laser. Ophthalmology. 1996; 103(10):1700–1705

[3] Samuelson TW, Pederson JE. Resolution of mitomycin-C associated overfiltration hypotony following resuturing of the scleral flap. Invest Ophthalmol Vis Sci. 1993; 34:816

[4] Stamper RL, McMenemy MG, Lieberman MF. Hypotonous maculopathy after trabeculectomy with subconjunctival 5-fluorouracil. Am J Ophthalmol. 1992; 114(5):544–553

[5] Wise JB. Treatment of chronic postfiltration hypotony by intrableb injection of autologous blood. Arch Ophthalmol. 1993; 111(6):827–830

[6] Palmberg P, Zacchei A. Compression sutures-a new treatment for leaking or painful filtering blebs. Invest Ophthalmol Vis Sci. 1996; 37:S444

[7] Shirato S, Maruyama K, Haneda M. Resuturing the scleral flap through conjunctiva for treatment of excess filtration. Am J Ophthalmol. 2004; 137(1):173–174

[8] Richman J, Moster MR, Myeni T, Trubnik V. A prospective study of consecutive patients undergoing full-thickness conjunctival/scleral hypotony sutures for clinical ocular hypotony. J Glaucoma. 2014; 23(5):326–328

27 Posttrabeculectomy Wound Leak

Xuan Thanh Le-Nguyen and Robert M. Feldman

Abstract

This chapter discusses the initial evaluation, diagnosis, and treatment options for bleb leaks associated with hypotony after trabeculectomy.

Keywords: hypotony, trabeculectomy, treatment of hypotony, bleb leaks, glaucoma

27.1 History

A 59-year-old woman with advanced primary open-angle glaucoma underwent a limbus-based trabeculectomy with intraoperative application of mitomycin C in the right eye. The scleral flap was closed with two 10–0 nylon sutures. Tenon's capsule was closed with a running locking 8–0 dissolvable suture (Vicryl, Ethicon, Inc., Somerville, NJ), and the conjunctiva was closed with a running, nonlocking 8–0 dissolvable suture.

Five months postoperatively, the patient presented for examination because of a dramatic decrease in vision in the right eye. On examination, the best-corrected visual acuity was 20/100 in the right eye and 20/30 in the left eye. The anterior chamber of the right eye was very shallow, and the intraocular pressure (IOP) was 2 mm Hg (▶ Fig. 27.1).

Differential Diagnosis—Key Points

The causes of postoperative shallow anterior chamber and low IOP can be divided into two major groups depending on the timing of the complication.

1. **Early postoperative (less than 4 weeks).** Early postoperative shallowing of the anterior chamber associated with low IOP may be due to overfiltration, reduced aqueous production, wound leak, or choroidal effusion or hemorrhage (▶ Fig. 27.2).
   a) Bleb overfiltration occurs when there is an excessive outflow of aqueous. Early postoperative cases may be due to intraoperative surgical limitations and imprecision, such as a large ostium with a small flap, the presence of an ostium in close relation to the edge of the scleral flap, and loose sutures. Ultimately, excessive flow is due to a relative lack of resistance to aqueous outflow. The incidence of early postoperative shallowing and hypotony might be reduced by tighter scleral flap sutures with sequential suture release by argon laser suture lysis or releasable suture techniques. Overfiltration is initially managed by external tamponade. However, surgical correction to tighten the scleral flap may be required. Usually, this problem will correct itself within 2 weeks of surgery if there are no intervening complications.
   b) Causes of postoperative aqueous hyposecretion include the postoperative use of topical aqueous suppressants or systemic carbonic anhydrase inhibitors, excessive postoperative use of topical phenylephrine, and detachment of the ciliary body. Cyclodialysis clefts may

lead to hypotony initially by increased outflow, which may continue or be superimposed by choroidal effusions and decreased aqueous production.
   c) A wound leak is one of the most common causes of early shallowing of the anterior chamber with hypotony. A Seidel test is necessary to localize the leak (▶ Fig. 27.3). Causes include conjunctival buttonholes, wound dehiscence, or a traumatized thin filtering bleb. The management of wound leak depends on the character and location of the filtering bleb. Initial treatment may be a pressure patch with aqueous suppression and withholding of topical corticosteroids until resolved. Use of a Simmons shell or an oversized bandage contact lens may be useful. Definitive therapy is surgical closure.
   d) Choroidal effusion is a common complication following filtering surgery and usually associated with hypotony. The effusion is usually transient, and the management is mainly topical or systemic corticosteroids combined with cycloplegics. Systemic corticosteroids should be reserved for cases of "kissing" choroidals. Surgical drainage is indicated if there is persistent shallowing of the anterior chamber, corneal decompensation, or synechial formation. These will generally resolve with conservative treatment by 2 weeks, after which drainage and reformation of the anterior chamber should be considered.

2. **Late Postoperative (Greater than 4 Weeks).** The most common causes of late postoperative anterior chamber shallowing with low IOP are chronic hypotony and late bleb leaks.
   a) Chronic hypotony (IOP less than 5 mm Hg) might be a manifestation of overfiltration, aqueous hyposecretion, cyclodialysis cleft, undetected retinal detachment, or bleb leaks. Postoperative chronic hypotony is more common after trabeculectomy with antifibrotics (5-fluorouracil or mitomycin C) as compared to trabeculectomy alone.[1],[2],[3] The most common sequela is hypotony maculopathy, which is more common in young males and in high myopes.[4],[5] Clinical manifestations of hypotony include choroidal and retinal folds, optic disc swelling, and engorgement and tortuosity of the retinal vasculature.

   The management of chronic hypotony is mainly directed at eliminating the underlying cause. The goal is to decrease excessive aqueous outflow and eliminate the choroidal effusion. Aqueous suppression should be discontinued, including stopping beta-blockers in the other eye as a crossover effect exists.[6] Large overfiltering blebs can be reduced in size by placement of compression sutures, cryotherapy, argon or Nd:YAG laser, or injection of autologous blood. Oddly enough, needle revision can be successful in reshaping blebs and reducing hypotony. If the previous measures fail, more invasive surgical bleb revision, including resuturing the scleral flap, might be required.

b) Late bleb leak is a well-documented complication of filtering surgery with antimetabolite usage and may develop months or years after the initial surgery.[2,7] This condition is more common with cystic, thin-walled, avascular blebs. In contrast to early leaks, late bleb leaks carry a high risk of developing infections, such as blebitis or endophthalmitis.[5] Chronic hypotony maculopathy can also occur and may result in permanent reduction of central vision. Typically, stopping a late leak is not adequate in the long term as it will likely recur. Some form of bleb recovering or resurfacing is required to treat late bleb leaks definitively.

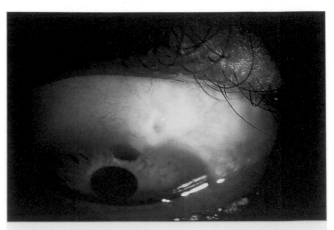

Fig. 27.1 Slit-lamp photograph of the right eye demonstrating a low filtering bleb.

27.2 Test Interpretation

The clinical examination should include characterization of bleb appearance and assessment of the leak. A moistened sterile fluorescein strip should be applied to the bleb under cobalt blue slit-lamp illumination. A leak is defined as a spontaneous focal-point source of aqueous leakage from an area of interrupted conjunctival tissue. Anterior chamber depth should also be assessed (▶ Fig. 27.3 and ▶ Table 27.1).

27.3 Diagnosis

Late bleb leak.

27.4 Medical Management

With the advent of antimetabolites, the success rates of glaucoma filtering procedures have drastically improved.[2] However, the improved pressure-lowering effect has increased postoperative complications including bleb leaks (both early and late), hypotony, and hypotony-induced maculopathy.[1] Although many treatment options have been proposed, successful closure of bleb leaks following trabeculectomy remains difficult, and the best method of repair is controversial.

If left untreated, hypotony with a flat anterior chamber can have many complications such as cataract, corneal decompensation, synechiae, choroidal effusions, or macular edema.[4,8]

Management of bleb leaks is challenging. Typically, initial treatment is aqueous suppression and observation (with or without a bandage contact lens). Suppression of aqueous production slows the flow through the leak, allowing epithelial proliferation and healing with closure of the defect. This is often inadequate as a long-term solution, as these leaks may spontaneously resolve and reappear elsewhere within the ischemic bleb.

Other techniques include the following.

27.4.1 Autologous Blood Injections

Autologous blood has been used in the medical field for many established applications including its use as a "patch"; examples include closure of spinal tap leaks or pulmonary air leaks.

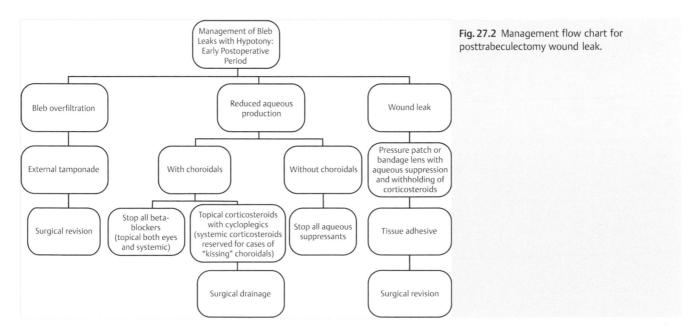

Fig. 27.2 Management flow chart for posttrabeculectomy wound leak.

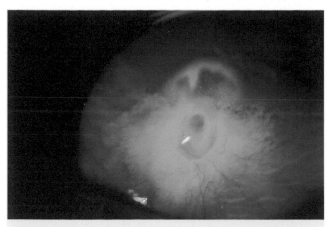

Fig. 27.3 Cobalt blue filter slit-lamp photograph of the right eye. Leaking aqueous can be seen after the application of fluorescein dye.

Table 27.1 Grading system for anterior chamber depth

Grade 1	Peripheral iris–cornea touch
Grade 2	Iris sphincter–cornea touch
Grade 3	Lens–cornea or vitreous–cornea touch

conjunctiva, thin sclera, and/or melted sclera, etc.). These approaches include excision of the bleb with advancement of adjacent conjunctiva, revision of the bleb with autologous conjunctival graft, patch material over the ostium/sclera (materials include clear cornea, amniotic membrane, or scleral patch grafts), Tenon's capsule pedicle plugs, glue, and rotational conjunctival-Tenon's flap grafts.[12,13,14,15] A technique of free conjunctival patching over ischemic blebs has been reported to have excellent results.[14]

Autologous blood can be injected into the bleb or into the surrounding subconjunctival tissue. The procedure can be performed with topical anesthesia at the slit lamp. The underlying hypothesis is that whole blood contains factors, blood cells, and other proteins that may initially cause obstruction of flow. Some of these components may also contribute to fibroblastic transformation to replace inactivated Tenon's capsule fibroblasts. Complications of the procedure include hyphema, bleb perforation, very high IOPs, and infection. This procedure is often ineffective, and multiple injections might be necessary.[9]

27.4.2 Argon Laser

The mechanism behind how argon laser closes a conjunctival leak is not entirely understood. It is thought that there may be a mechanical effect caused by the shrinking of the conjunctiva (possibly bringing the ends of a tear together) or a thermal effect characterized by the coagulation of epithelial cells to form a seal over the break. The application of laser may also cause a release of inflammatory products that can promote healing. Unfortunately, this technique is plagued with complications such as fenestration and pitting of the conjunctiva, corneal stromal opacities, and need for retreatment.[10]

27.4.3 Continuous-Wave Nd:YAG Laser

This laser is not readily available to most surgeons and is expensive. Disadvantages include iatrogenic bleb leaks, pupillary retraction toward the bleb, pigmentation precipitation by the laser that can affect future laser treatment, and pupil flattening or peaking. The mechanism by which Nd:YAG laser remodels filtering blebs is not readily explained, and the long-term results have been disappointing.[11]

27.5 Surgical Management

Various surgical approaches to repair leaking blebs have been described. The decision on which approach to use will depend on the cause of the leak (bleb cyst structure, weak overlying

27.6 Rehabilitation and Follow-up

Once the leak is closed, the patients are to be followed closely for recurrent leaks if an ischemic bleb remains. If definitive surgical intervention was successful, the bleb will no longer be ischemic, and the risk of recurrence will be low.

References

[1] The Fluorouracil Filtering Surgery Study Group. Five-year follow-up of the Fluorouracil Filtering Surgery Study. Am J Ophthalmol. 1996; 121(4):349–366

[2] Greenfield DS, Liebmann JM, Jee J, Ritch R. Late-onset bleb leaks after glaucoma filtering surgery. Arch Ophthalmol. 1998; 116(4):443–447

[3] Beckers HJ, Kinders KC, Webers CA. Five-year results of trabeculectomy with mitomycin C. Graefes Arch Clin Exp Ophthalmol. 2003; 241(2):106–110

[4] Villarrubia HJ, Bell NP. Hypotony. In: Feldman RM, Bell NP, eds. Complications of Glaucoma Surgery. New York, NY: Oxford University Press; 2013:85–91

[5] Kangas TA, Greenfield DS, Flynn HW, Jr, Parrish RK, II, Palmberg P. Delayed-onset endophthalmitis associated with conjunctival filtering blebs. Ophthalmology. 1997; 104(5):746–752

[6] Tanna AP. Late hypotony without leak. In: Feldman RM, Bell NP, eds. Complications of Glaucoma Surgery. New York, NY: Oxford University Press; 2013:171–178

[7] Karolina C, Baril C, Bourret-Massicotte D, et al. Risk factors for a severe bleb leak following trabeculectomy: a retrospective case-control study. J Glaucoma. 2015; 24(7):493–497

[8] Stamper RL. Hypotony maculopathy. In: Feldman RM, Bell NP, eds. Complications of Glaucoma Surgery. New York, NY: Oxford University Press; 2013:181–186

[9] Smith MF, Magauran RG, III, Betchkal J, Doyle JW. Treatment of postfiltration bleb leaks with autologous blood. Ophthalmology. 1995; 102(6):868–871

[10] Hennis HL, Stewart WC. Use of the argon laser to close filtering bleb leaks. Graefes Arch Clin Exp Ophthalmol. 1992; 230(6):537–541

[11] Geyer O. Management of large, leaking, and inadvertent filtering blebs with the neodymium:YAG laser. Ophthalmology. 1998; 105(6):983–987

[12] Bochmann F, Kaufmann C, Kipfer A, Thiel MA. Corneal patch graft for the repair of late-onset hypotony or filtering bleb leak after trabeculectomy: a new surgical technique. J Glaucoma. 2014; 23(1):e76–e80

[13] O'Connor DJ, Tressler CS, Caprioli J. A surgical method to repair leaking filtering blebs. Ophthalmic Surg. 1992; 23(5):336–338

[14] Panday M, Shantha B, George R, Boda S, Vijaya L. Outcomes of bleb excision with free autologous conjunctival patch grafting for bleb leak and hypotony after glaucoma filtering surgery. J Glaucoma. 2011; 20(6):392–397

[15] Sethi P, Patel RN, Goldhardt R, Ayyala RS. Conjunctival advancement with subconjunctival amniotic membrane draping technique for leaking cystic blebs. J Glaucoma. 2016; 25(2):188–192

28 Failing Filtering Bleb

Xuan Thanh Le-Nguyen and Robert M. Feldman

Abstract

This chapter reviews the clinical findings, differential diagnosis, and treatment for a failed filtering bleb.

Keywords: failed bleb, flat bleb, surgical management of failed blebs, glaucoma

28.1 History

A 53-year-old African American woman with advanced primary open-angle glaucoma and a target intraocular pressure (IOP) of 15 mm Hg underwent a limbus-based trabeculectomy with intraoperative application of mitomycin C in the right eye. At the 1-year postoperative visit, the IOP was at target, and a moderately elevated diffuse ischemic bleb was present with microcysts.

Three months later, the patient presented with an IOP of 28 mm Hg. The anterior chamber was deep; the filtering bleb, however, was almost flat (▶ Fig. 28.1).

28.2 Differential Diagnosis—Key Points

Modern techniques for performing trabeculectomy have led to very high success rates.[1] However, late failure can occur, and the surgeon must be prepared to manage these cases.

Elevated IOP in the setting of a *deep anterior chamber* in the postfiltration eye may be classified based on the appearance of the filtering bleb and the timing of the elevated IOP. When associated with a high bleb, the most likely cause is an encapsulated filtering bleb (Tenon's capsule cyst), which typically does not occur as late as this case. When associated with a low bleb, the most likely causes are tight scleral flap sutures, occlusion of the sclerostomy site potentiating filtration failure, or fibrosis within the bleb.

Risk factors for filtration failure include young age, race, inflammatory conditions such as uveitis, a history of prior failed

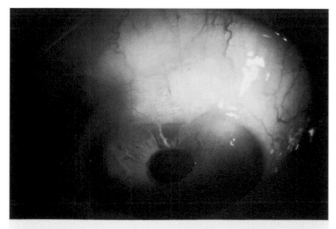

Fig. 28.1 Slit-lamp photograph demonstrating a flat filtering bleb.

filtering procedure or other conjunctival procedure, neovascular glaucoma, and aphakia. Older patients typically have a less robust propensity toward scar formation than younger patients. One also has to consider that iatrogenic surgical techniques, such as excessive cautery, failure to adequately control hemorrhage, or excessive intraocular manipulation, may also lead to failure of the filtering bleb.[2,3]

28.2.1 Elevated IOP Associated with High Bleb

Encapsulated Filtering Bleb (Tenon's Cyst) (Early)

The most common cause of filtering surgery failure is encapsulation of the filtration bleb, typically causing failure during the first 6 weeks after surgery. Clinically, the encapsulated bleb appears as an elevated, dome-shaped structure at the site of the filtration bleb. Histopathologically, the cyst consists of dense subconjunctival connective tissue, few cells, and no cellular lining. The aqueous becomes entrapped within the cystlike cavity of hypertrophied Tenon's capsule.[4,5,6]

Many encapsulated blebs will eventually resolve spontaneously without intervention. However, digital compression can be applied to encourage filtration, and topical anti-inflammatory agents might be used to inhibit further fibrosis. If conservative treatment fails to reduce IOP, surgical intervention might be indicated (see below).

28.2.2 Elevated IOP Associated with Low Bleb (Early)

Tight Scleral Flap Sutures

In the early postoperative period, elevated IOP in the setting of a low bleb can indicate that the scleral flap sutures are too tight. While in the operating room, each surgeon has his or her own technique on how to titrate the tightness of the knots as well as the placement and number of sutures to try to control bleb formation. Postoperatively, however, the management is often done using an argon laser or releasing releasable sutures if placed. A suture lysis lens can be used on a topically anesthetized eye to lyse sutures per surgeon preference. The procedure should be followed by a gentle digital ocular massage to facilitate the egress of aqueous if necessary. One suture at a time should be cut, and the procedure should not be done during the first 3 postoperative weeks to avoid overfiltration and hypotony. Unfortunately, the procedure may be associated with hypotony due to excessive flow, conjunctival burns, or buttonholes.

Occlusion of the Sclerostomy Site

In the early postoperative period, the internal sclerostomy may become obstructed (tissue incarceration), causing elevation of IOP. Although this is uncommon, incarceration can be ruled out by gonioscopy. Possible causes of obstruction include incompletely excised Descemet's membrane, iris, ciliary body, lens capsule, vitreous, or coagulated blood. Late in the postoperative period, progressive growth of the fibroblasts might lead to membrane proliferation over the internal ostium.

Episcleral Fibrosis (Late)

A bleb may be inadequate due to fibrosis at the scleral flap, which occurs from the episclera. It also can be due to loculations within the bleb or a "ring of steel" limiting outward extension of the bleb and limited filtration. A bleb may appear "perfect" but still have inadequate filtration.

28.3 Test Interpretation

A filtering bleb can be evaluated at the slit-lamp exam. It should be evaluated for height, vascularity, microcysts, localization (focal vs. diffuse), and the presence of encapsulation or a "ring of steel." Gonioscopic examination is an integral part of assessing the patency of the internal ostium. The failing bleb is typically low to flat and heavily vascularized.

Other methods can also be used to assess the trabeculectomy if needed. Ultrasound biomicroscopy can be useful to evaluate the ostomy and flap. Newer imaging modalities, such as anterior segment optical coherence tomography, can give the clinician important information about bleb morphology that would affect the management course.[7]

28.4 Diagnosis

Late filtration failure.

28.5 Medical Management

When evaluating a patient with the above presentation, high IOP after filtering surgery with a deep anterior chamber, the clinician should follow a logical approach as outlined in ▶ Fig. 28.2. Medical management alone is limited to cases of encapsulation and cases where the filter cannot be salvaged surgically.

28.6 Surgical Management

Surgical management generally consists of needle revision, but more aggressive revision may be required to salvage a failing bleb[7,8] (▶ Fig. 28.2).

28.7 Rehabilitation and Follow-up

Once the IOP is controlled, patients are to be followed closely for any signs of recurrent failure. IOP-lowering medication might be necessary to maintain low IOP, even if surgical revision was successful.

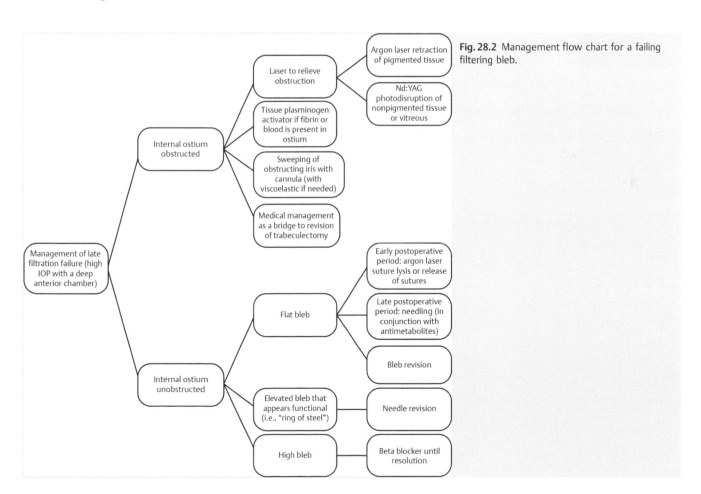

Fig. 28.2 Management flow chart for a failing filtering bleb.

References

[1] Mankiewicz KA, Seibold LK, Kahook MY, Sherwood MB. Wound healing in glaucoma. In: Feldman RM, Bell NP, eds. Complications of Glaucoma Surgery. New York, NY: Oxford University Press; 2013:33–41

[2] Baik AK, Brandt JD. Elevated IOP with a deep anterior chamber. In: Feldman RM, Bell NP, eds. Complications of Glaucoma Surgery. New York, NY: Oxford University Press; 2013:100–106

[3] Van Buskirk EM. Mechanisms and management of filtration bleb failure. Aust N Z J Ophthalmol. 1992; 20(3):157–162

[4] Feldman RM, Gross RL, Spaeth GL, et al. Risk factors for the development of Tenon's capsule cysts after trabeculectomy. Ophthalmology. 1989; 96(3):336–341

[5] Ophir A. Encapsulated filtering bleb. A selective review–new deductions. Eye (Lond). 1992; 6(Pt 4):348–352

[6] Van Buskirk EM. Cysts of Tenon's capsule following filtration surgery. Am J Ophthalmol. 1982; 94(4):522–527

[7] Feldman RM, Tabet RR. Needle revision of filtering blebs. J Glaucoma. 2008; 17(7):594–600

[8] Anand N, Khan A. Long-term outcomes of needle revision of trabeculectomy blebs with mitomycin C and 5-fluorouracil: a comparative safety and efficacy report. J Glaucoma. 2009; 18(7):513–520

29 Flat Anterior Chamber

Martha Motuz Leen

Abstract

Aqueous misdirection is a secondary angle-closure glaucoma. Diagnosis is suspected when a flat (or very shallow) central and peripheral anterior chamber is observed, and other causes of flat anterior chamber have been ruled out. This rare condition typically occurs in eyes with short axial lengths that are predisposed to angle-closure glaucoma and have undergone prior laser or incisional surgery. Also known as "ciliary block" or "malignant" glaucoma, treatment consists of initially reversing the aqueous misdirection medically, followed by surgical intervention if necessary.

Keywords: aqueous misdirection, ciliary block, malignant glaucoma, angle-closure glaucoma, secondary glaucoma, flat anterior chamber, shallow anterior chamber

29.1 Clinical History

A 53-year-old woman with a history of bilateral chronic angle-closure glaucoma presented with a shallow anterior chamber in the right eye 1 day after a mitomycin trabeculectomy.

Examination revealed a visual acuity of 20/400 in the right eye and 20/40 in the left eye. Intraocular pressures (IOPs) were 34 mm Hg in the right eye and 12 mm Hg in the left eye. Slit-lamp examination of the right eye showed a moderately elevated filtration bleb that was negative for Seidel's testing. The anterior chamber was shallow with iridocorneal contact extending from the periphery to within 1 mm of the pupillary margin. Central shallowing was also present with a posterior chamber intraocular lens located 0.5 mm posterior to the corneal endothelium. Anterior chamber cells were graded 3+. A surgical iridectomy was confirmed to be patent since ciliary processes were easily visible. Slit-lamp examination of the left eye showed a filtration bleb, deep anterior chamber, patent surgical iridectomy, and pseudophakia.

Fundus examination demonstrated a poor view with an excellent red reflex in the right eye and moderate glaucomatous cupping with an otherwise unremarkable retina in the left eye. B-scan ultrasonography of the right eye revealed a flat retina and absence of choroidal effusions.

Differential Diagnosis—Key Points

1. *Shallowing or flattening of the anterior chamber* after filtration surgery is common, especially in the early postoperative setting. It is useful to identify those clinical features that are typical of each of the potential causes of shallowing (▶ Table 29.1). For instance, if the IOP is low, overfiltration or choroidal effusions are suspected. If the IOP is normal or high, pupillary block, choroidal hemorrhage, and aqueous misdirection are considerations. It is also useful to classify whether shallowing of the anterior chamber involves the periphery only or both central and peripheral areas (▶ Fig. 29.1a, b). Using bleb height as a criterion for differentiating diagnoses is not as helpful, since the bleb may be either high or low with each of these entities. In addition to these features, the response to a surgical confirmatory intervention, an iridectomy, can point to the correct diagnosis.

2. *Overfiltration* is the most common cause of shallow anterior chamber after filtration surgery. In the early postoperative period, overfiltration may occur through a large bleb or loose scleral flap with little resistance to outflow, a conjunctival buttonhole, a conjunctival wound leak, or a cyclodialysis cleft. In the later postoperative period, overfiltration may occur by transudation or leak from a bleb that is avascular and very thin, especially if antimetabolites were used. Chronic overfiltration itself without hypotony is not expected to shallow the anterior chamber as the hydrostatic pressure in the anterior chamber and vitreous cavity equalize. However, when overfiltration is associated with a low IOP, the ciliary body and choroid tend to become diffusely edematous. This results in an anterior rotation of the ciliary body, leading to shallowing of the anterior chamber centrally and peripherally in phakic and pseudophakic eyes. A patent iridectomy is identified. Choroidal effusions are not present on fundus examination, but overfiltration is often a precursor for their development.

3. A choroidal effusion is an accumulation of serous fluid in the suprachoroidal space, most commonly in eyes that are severely hypotonous in the early postoperative period. Although the suprachoroidal space may be considered one continuous area, firm connections of the choroid to the sclera at the vortex veins and optic nerve head lead to a lobulated appearance of choroidal effusions. This results in an anterior rotation of the ciliary body with shallowing of the anterior chamber both centrally and peripherally in phakic and pseudophakic eyes. The presence of this fluid contributes to a vicious cycle of reduced aqueous production and possibly enhanced uveoscleral outflow, in turn aggravating hypotony and the tendency for more choroidal effusion. Overfiltration is often identified as the initial cause of hypotony. A patent iridectomy is present. Smooth light-brown or tan choroidal elevations are seen on funduscopy. In some cases, choroidal effusions are very low and cannot easily be discerned without ultrasonography. In severe cases, surgical drainage of straw-colored suprachoroidal fluid reverses the cycle.

4. Pupillary block occurs when there is apposition of the iris to the lens in phakic or pseudophakic eyes, or to the anterior vitreous face in aphakic eyes. The aqueous is unable to flow anteriorly and accumulates just beneath the iris, causing a convex bowing of the iris (iris bombé). Peripheral anterior chamber shallowing results in appositional closure of the angle. It is important to recognize that the central chamber tends not to be as shallow. The IOP may be normal initially and then progressively elevated. A patent iridectomy is not present. Although creation of an iridectomy is a routine part of most glaucoma filtration surgery, a complete opening

may not always be present, with underlying iris pigment epithelium still intact or iris incarceration into the sclerotomy. The iridectomy may also become obstructed with ciliary processes, blood, or vitreous, or become bound down by synechiae in an inflamed eye. If the surgical wound was dissected too posteriorly, ciliary body tissue rather than iris may have been excised. The anterior chamber will readily deepen after an iridotomy is created. If there is any doubt about its patency, another iris opening should be created.

5. A choroidal hemorrhage is an accumulation of blood that occurs in the suprachoroidal space in either the early or the late postoperative period, usually acutely and in association with severe pain. The ciliary body rotates anteriorly, shallowing the anterior chamber peripherally and centrally in phakic and pseudophakic eyes. Since the choroidal circulation is not subject to autoregulation, hypertensive patients with fragile vessels may be unable to accommodate the increased choroidal blood flow when the IOP is lowered, increasing the risk of choroidal hemorrhage. Aphakic eyes may also be at higher risk. Unlike choroidal effusions, the IOP tends to be normal or high. A patent iridectomy is present. Smooth dark-brown or red choroidal elevations are seen on funduscopy, sometimes requiring ultrasonography for confirmation when small in size. In severe cases, surgical drainage of red or dark-brown suprachoroidal fluid is required.

6. Aqueous misdirection occurs when aqueous is unable to flow anteriorly past a relative block at the junction of the ciliary processes, lens equator (when present), and anterior vitreous face. Subsequently, aqueous is diverted posteriorly within or adjacent to the vitreous body (▶ Fig. 29.2). As the aqueous accumulates, the vitreous is displaced forward, causing anterior ciliary body rotation and shallowing of the anterior chamber peripherally and centrally. This can lead to a vicious cycle as the aqueous volume continues to increase in the space behind the vitreous, the permeability of the compressed vitreous body decreases further, and the apposition of the anterior hyaloid face with the ciliary processes and lens equator worsens. The IOP may be normal initially and become progressively elevated as the cycle continues. The presence of a patent iridectomy must be confirmed, and choroidal elevations are generally not present. Aqueous misdirection can occur in the early postoperative period or later when cycloplegics are discontinued. It most commonly occurs after surgery on phakic eyes with chronic angle-closure glaucoma. Terms that have been used synonymously with aqueous misdirection include *ciliary block* and *malignant glaucoma*.

A wide spectrum of presentations is possible with each of these diagnoses, and more than one can occasionally occur as a sequence of events. For example, an eye with chronic angle-closure glaucoma may have developed a wound leak resulting in hypotony with initial choroidal edema, then progressing to a small anterior choroidal effusion. As the ciliary body rotates forward and the anterior chamber shallows, greater apposition occurs between the anterior hyaloid, ciliary processes, and lens equator. This leads to misdirection of aqueous posteriorly with progressive shallowing of the anterior chamber and elevation of the IOP. Therefore, presence of a choroidal effusion does not entirely eliminate the possibility of aqueous misdirection. In this example, drainage of the choroidal effusion alone might result in reversal of aqueous misdirection.

29.2 Test Interpretation

Slit-lamp examination of anterior chamber depth may reveal shallowing in the periphery only with an iris bombé configuration, features that would be suggestive of a pupillary block mechanism. If the anterior chamber is shallow both centrally and peripherally, choroidal thickening, choroidal effusion, choroidal hemorrhage, or aqueous misdirection would be more likely.

The bleb is inspected and checked for pinpoint leaks and for slow transudation, especially if the tissue is very thin. A Seidel test can be performed to identify an area of leakage or transudation by painting a bleb or incision site with a fluorescein strip and viewing the area with a cobalt blue light. Although a pinpoint leak can usually be seen immediately, delineation of an area of bleb transudation may require several seconds of observation. If present, overfiltration with choroidal thickening, or choroidal effusion, is suspected.

Determination should be made if an iridectomy exists and is patent. Even with a previously patent iridectomy, it may become blocked with iris, vitreous, or blood or become bound down to the underlying lens. If a patent iridectomy is confirmed, pupillary block can be ruled out, but not the other entities. If ciliary processes are seen through a patent iridectomy and appear to be anteriorly rotated, or in apposition against the vitreous, aqueous misdirection is suspected. If there is any question of the patency of the iridectomy, it should be opened or a new iridotomy created with laser. If shallowing readily reverses as a result, a diagnosis of pupillary block is made.

Table 29.1 Causes of shallow anterior chamber

Diagnosis	Shallowing	IOP	Relief with iridectomy	Common features
Overfiltration	Peripheral only, or central and peripheral	Low	No	Bleb leak often present
Choroidal effusion	Central and peripheral	Low	No	Light-brown choroidals
Pupillary block	Peripheral only	Normal or high	Yes	Iris bombé
Choroidal hemorrhage	Central and peripheral	Normal or high	No	Dark-brown choroidals; acute pain
Aqueous misdirection	Central and peripheral	Normal or high	No	History of chronic angle-closure glaucoma

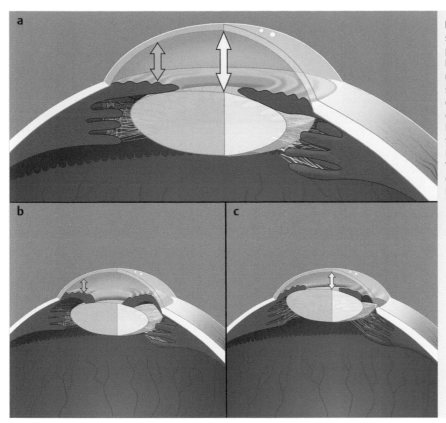

Fig. 29.1 (a) normal anterior chamber depth should be distinguished from (b) which shows peripheral shallowing alone characteristic of iris bombe commonly seen with pupillary block and (c) where the anterior chamber is more uniformly shallow despite a patent iridectomy. The configuration illustrated in (c) may be seen with overfiltration, serous choroidal effusion, choroidal hemorrhage or aqueous misdirection. (Adapted from Skuta GL. The angle closure glaucomas. In: Kaufman PL, Mittag TW, assoc eds. Glaucoma. Vol. 7. In: Podos SM, Yanoff M, eds. Textbook of Ophthalmology. Philadelphia, PA: Mosby-Year Book; 1994:8–23.)

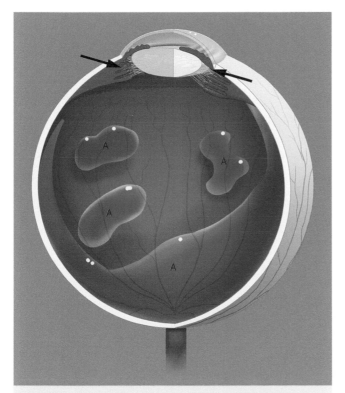

Fig. 29.2 Aqueous misdirection in a phakic eye. Apposition of anteriorly rotated ciliary processes, lens, and anterior hyaloid (arrows) predisposes to posterior misdirection of aqueous (A) into the vitreous cavity. The lens and iris become progressively displaced anteriorly, closing the angle, and increasing the IOP. (Adapted from Skuta GL. The angle closure glaucomas. In: Kaufman PL, Mittag TW, assoc eds. Glaucoma. Vol. 7. In: Podos SM, Yanoff M, eds. Textbook of Ophthalmology. Philadelphia, PA: Mosby-Year Book; 1994:8–21.)

If the iridectomy is patent, the pupil should be dilated. When choroidals are larger, they are easily identified on fundus examination, appearing smooth and dome-shaped and varying from one to four in number. The convex choroidals may occasionally be extensive enough that they meet in the midvitreous, often referred to as "kissing" choroidals. Serous choroidal effusions tend to have a tan or light-brown appearance, whereas choroidal hemorrhages tend to have a dark-brown or red appearance. If choroidals are not seen, careful evaluation of the vitreous may suggest optically empty pockets indicative of fluid accumulation typical of aqueous misdirection.

A small pupil may prohibit adequate visualization of the posterior pole. In such cases, conventional B-scan ultrasonography is useful to identify choroidal elevation or choroidal thickening. Ultrasound can also help differentiate between a serous choroidal effusion that is echolucent and choroidal hemorrhage that is echogenic. Ultrasound can be used to inspect the vitreous for pockets of fluid that may be seen with aqueous misdirection. Sometimes, a choroidal edema that is very anterior can be too subtle to identify despite funduscopy with a large pupil or conventional B-scan ultrasonography. In this instance, high-frequency ultrasound biomicroscopy can prove useful to better visualize the anterior choroidal edema, as well as to identify the ciliary block that is characteristic of aqueous misdirection.

29.3 Diagnosis

In the case study described, a patent peripheral iridectomy is present with central as well as peripheral shallowing and there is no iris bombé. These features exclude pupillary block as a mechanism. There is no bleb leak or wound leak and the eye is not hypotonous, making overfiltration less likely. Funduscopy and ultrasound demonstrate no choroidal elevation, excluding serous choroidal effusion or choroidal hemorrhage. The ciliary processes are noted to be easily visible through the iridectomy. The diagnosis is aqueous misdirection in the right eye.

29.4 Medical Management

The first line of therapy for aqueous misdirection is medical management. A cycloplegic–mydriatic combination of atropine 1% and phenylephrine 2.5% is instilled four times a day to maximally rotate the ciliary body and lens posteriorly, attempting to break the ciliary block. Topical aqueous suppressants as well as an oral carbonic anhydrase inhibitor are used to reduce aqueous production and slow down fluid collection within the vitreous body. An oral or intravenous osmotic agent can be considered to actually reduce the volume of aqueous in the vitreous cavity in an effort to break the cycle of fluid accumulation. Miotics are to be avoided since instillation results in an anterior rotation of the ciliary body, exacerbating the ciliary block. Prompt recognition and treatment of aqueous misdirection can abort the process earlier in its course.

29.5 Surgical Management

If the aqueous misdirection is not corrected medically and the condition continues to worsen, then vitreous disruption by laser treatment or surgery may be attempted. Neodymium:YAG laser disruption of anterior hyaloid face and posterior capsule through the pupil, when accessible in pseudophakic and aphakic eyes, or through an iridectomy, can be performed to allow trapped pockets of fluid to move anteriorly with more ease. Argon laser shrinkage of the ciliary processes through a peripheral iridectomy can also be attempted to break the apposition between the ciliary processes and lens or vitreous.

If there is lenticular–cornea contact and the IOP is not yet elevated, intracameral viscoelastic injection may have a therapeutic effect by deepening the anterior chamber, rotating the ciliary body posteriorly, and temporarily reversing the vicious cycle of misdirected aqueous. Even a small amount of viscoelastic injection can rapidly raise the IOP and should therefore be performed with careful monitoring.

If laser modalities are ineffective, then a core pars plana vitrectomy with reformation of the anterior chamber is recommended. Surgical disruption of the vitreous helps to reestablish anterior flow of trapped aqueous as well as to prevent the recurrence of the cycle by eliminating the potential for intact vitreous gel to act as a diaphragm across the globe. In pseudophakic and aphakic eyes, the vitrectomy is extended anteriorly to remove anterior hyaloid, lens zonules, or capsule in the vicinity of the iridectomy. In phakic eyes, anterior removal is more challenging since the integrity of the lens must be maintained. For this reason, recurrence of aqueous misdirection after vitrectomy in phakic eyes may be more common due to less complete removal of anterior hyaloid. It is useful to place a sclerotomy within reach of the iridectomy to facilitate removal of the vitreous in its vicinity.

29.6 Rehabilitation and Follow-up

Cycloplegia, such as with atropine 1% daily, may need to be maintained indefinitely. In cases where the aqueous misdirection is broken pharmacologically or with laser treatment, recurrence can occur when cycloplegia is discontinued, even months later. Instillation of miotics can trigger a recurrence by rotating the ciliary body and lens anteriorly, starting the cycle of misdirection. If a vitrectomy was required for reversal of aqueous misdirection, cycloplegia can often be stopped, though caution should be exercised in phakic eyes, which may be at higher risk of recurrence. In the fellow eye, prophylactic laser iridotomy, avoidance of miotics, and anticipation of possible aqueous misdirection with any future surgery are recommended protective measures.

Suggested Reading

[1] Byrnes GA, Leen MM, Wong TP, Benson WE. Vitrectomy for ciliary block (malignant) glaucoma. Ophthalmology. 1995; 102(9):1308–1311

[2] Givens K, Shields MB. Suprachoroidal hemorrhage after glaucoma filtering surgery. Am J Ophthalmol. 1987; 103(5):689–694

[3] Lieberman MF. Diagnosis and management of malignant glaucoma. In: Higginbotham EJ, Lee DA, eds. Management of Difficult Glaucomas. Cambridge: Blackwell Scientific Publications; 1994:183–194

[4] Tello C, Chi T, Shepps G, Liebmann J, Ritch R. Ultrasound biomicroscopy in pseudophakic malignant glaucoma. Ophthalmology. 1993; 100(9):1330–1334

[5] Wirbelauer C, Karandish A, Häberle H, Pham DT. Optical coherence tomography in malignant glaucoma following filtration surgery. Br J Ophthalmol. 2003; 87(8):952–955

[6] Quigley HA, Friedman DS, Congdon NG. Possible mechanisms of primary angle-closure and malignant glaucoma. J Glaucoma. 2003; 12(2):167–180

[7] Ruben S, Tsai J, Hitchings RA. Malignant glaucoma and its management. Br J Ophthalmol. 1997; 81(2):163–167

[8] Harbour JW, Rubsamen PE, Palmberg P. Pars plana vitrectomy in the management of phakic and pseudophakic malignant glaucoma. Arch Ophthalmol. 1996; 114(9):1073–1078

[9] Quigley HA. Angle-closure glaucoma-simpler answers to complex mechanisms: LXVI Edward Jackson Memorial Lecture. Am J Ophthalmol. 2009; 148 (5):657–669.e1

30 Persistent Choroidal Detachment

Donald L. Budenz

Abstract

Choroidal effusions are not uncommon after glaucoma filtration surgery. They are present in up to 30% of cases immediately postoperatively in carefully controlled studies in which investigators look for them. They are often confused with retinal detachments or suprachoroidal hemorrhages but are easily distinguishable on careful clinical exam or ultrasound. They are usually benign but may precede suprachoroidal hemorrhages and block the visual axis. Conservative management usually results in resolution. Surgical management is not difficult for the anterior segment surgeon to perform and is recommended when vision is affected for a prolonged period.

Keywords: choroidal effusion, glaucoma surgery, complications, management

30.1 History

An 80-year-old woman with a 20-year history of glaucoma presented for consultation 8 months following combined cataract extraction, intraocular lens implant, and trabeculectomy with mitomycin C in the right eye. She complained of a "shadow" since her surgery, which was blocking her temporal vision. This was so debilitating that she almost ran over a small boy with her car.

The visual acuity was 20/30 in the affected eye and the intraocular pressure (IOP) was 7 mm Hg. A large, ischemic filtering bleb was present with a negative Seidel's test. The cornea was clear, the anterior chamber deep and quiet, and the cup-to-disc ratio was 0.8. The peripheral fundus was not visible due to a small and fibrotic pupil. A B-scan ultrasound was performed, which showed 360-degree ciliochoroidal detachments with serous fluid inside the detachments. There was a large nasal choroidal detachment that measured 8 mm (▶ Fig. 30.1). There was no retinal detachment overlying the choroidal detachment.

Differential Diagnosis—Key Points

1. Most patients with persistent choroidal effusions are asymptomatic. They present with a low or low-normal IOP as the only presenting sign. Vision may be reduced if the pressure is very low, causing corneal, retinal, or choroidal folds. Also, if the effusions are large, they may block the visual axis, causing profound visual loss.

2. The differential diagnosis of low IOP after filtering surgery includes overfiltration, filtering bleb leak, retinal detachment, cyclodialysis cleft, iridocyclitis, and choroidal effusion. Overfiltration is a diagnosis of exclusion and typically presents with a large and/or ischemic filtering bleb, which has no leak by Seidel's testing. The posterior pole may have choroidal effusions, which are due to the low pressure from overfiltration. Late bleb leaks may also cause low IOP and choroidal detachments and are diagnosed by demonstrating a positive Seidel's test. Occasionally, a provocative Seidel's test, using gentle pressure on the globe, may reveal an occult leak. Serous retinal detachments are a rare postoperative complication of filtering surgery but should always be excluded as a possible cause of hypotony in any patient. Retinal detachment may be diagnosed on fundus examination and/or ultrasound (▶ Fig. 30.2). A cyclodialysis cleft may result from surgical trauma and this should be ruled out on gonioscopy. This may be occult and difficult to diagnose without the aid of high-resolution ultrasound (ultrasound biomicroscopy). Iridocyclitis may cause hypotony and typically presents in uveitics or following tapering of topical steroid medications.

3. Suprachoroidal hemorrhage (▶ Fig. 30.3) may cause choroidal detachment, but the IOP is generally high and the patient usually has considerable pain associated with this.

4. Choroidal effusions have a bullous appearance, similar to retinal detachment and choroidal hemorrhage. Unlike those conditions, the bullous detachments of serous choroidal effusions have the normal orange fundus appearance, rather than being translucent (retinal detachment) or dark red/brown (suprachoroidal hemorrhage). Both serous and hemorrhagic choroidal detachments typically have four bullous lobes, one in each quadrant. This is because the choroid is firmly attached to the exit site of the four vortex veins, as well as being attached to the optic nerve posteriorly and scleral spur anteriorly. Transillumination with a muscle light may help distinguish serous from hemorrhagic choroidal detachments; hemorrhagic detachments will block the transillumination better than serous detachments. When in doubt, standard B-scan echography is the definitive way to differentiate these three entities (see Test Interpretation below).

5. Annular ciliochoroidal detachment is an underdiagnosed condition in which the anterior-most choroid becomes separated from the sclera. The fundus typically appears normal. and diagnosis is made by ultrasound biomicroscopy or conventional resolution ultrasound performed through a water bath. These patients may have a closed anterior chamber angle on gonioscopy due to forward rotation of the ciliary body. In this circumstance, the IOP may be normal or elevated.

6. Choroidal effusions are common after glaucoma filtration surgery due to surgically induced hypotony. Low IOP results in the leakage of protein-rich serum from the choroidal vasculature into the suprachoroidal space. The ciliary body often becomes detached and intraocular inflammation may result. These factors may decrease aqueous production, contributing to hypotony. Alternatively, choroidal effusion may promote increased uveoscleral aqueous outflow, contributing to hypotony. The condition can be viewed as a pathologic cycle, whereby profound hypotony leads to ciliochoroidal effusion, which in turn causes hypotony.

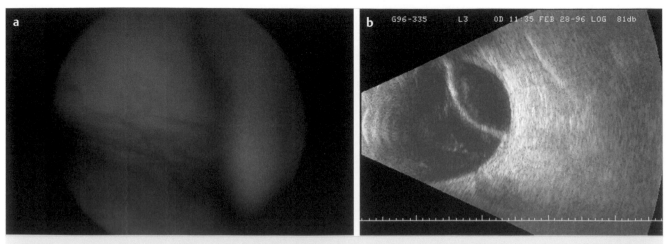

Fig. 30.1 Serous choroidal effusions. **(a)** The typical appearance of serous choroidal effusion. Smooth, orange, bullous detachments are seen. **(b)** The typical B-scan echographic appearance of serous choroidal detachments. The wall is generally thicker and smoother than that seen in a retinal detachment. The inside of the detachment is echographically clear due to the serous nature of the interior, unlike hemorrhagic choroidal detachment. (▶ Fig. 30.1a is provided courtesy of Albert M. Maguire, MD, Philadelphia, PA. ▶ Fig. 30.1b is provided courtesy of Sarah Keene, Philadelphia, PA.)

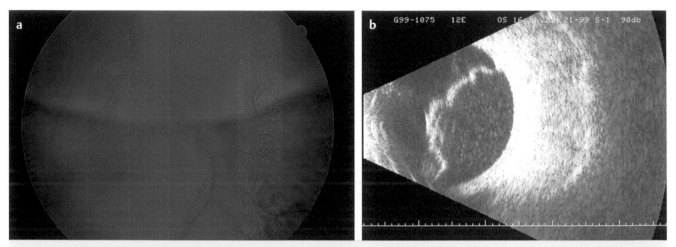

Fig. 30.2 Retinal detachment. **(a)** The clinical appearance of a retinal detachment. The surface is bullous but more translucent and lacks the typical orange color of the retinal pigment epithelium usually seen in a choroidal effusion. **(b)** B-scan ultrasound of a retinal detachment. The wall is generally thinner and the surface is less regular than that seen in choroidal detachment. (▶ Fig. 30.2a is provided courtesy of Albert M. Maguire, MD, Philadelphia, PA. ▶ Fig. 30.2b is provided courtesy of Randall Hughes, Miami, FL.)

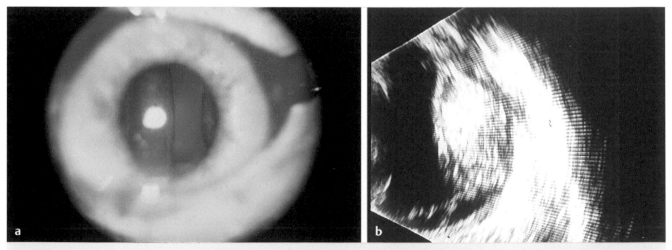

Fig. 30.3 Hemorrhagic choroidal detachment. **(a)** Photograph of a hemorrhagic choroidal detachment. The color, ranging from dark-red to brown, is diagnostic of this entity. **(b)** The B-scan ultrasound shows the echographically dense cavity of suprachoroidal blood, easily distinguished from a serous detachment of the retina or choroid. (▶ Fig. 30.3a is provided courtesy of Albert M. Maguire, MD, Philadelphia, PA. ▶ Fig. 30.3b is provided courtesy of Sarah Keene, Philadelphia, PA.)

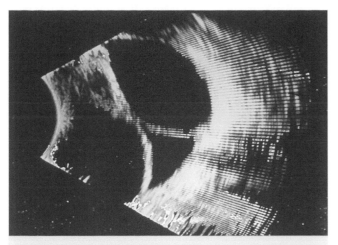

Fig. 30.4 Kissing choroidal detachments. In severe cases, the serous detachments of the choroid may be so elevated that the contralateral retinal surfaces become apposed centrally. These have been termed "kissing" choroidals. While visually debilitating, kissing choroidal detachments have the same excellent prognosis as nonkissing detachments. The B-scan echographic appearance is shown in this figure.

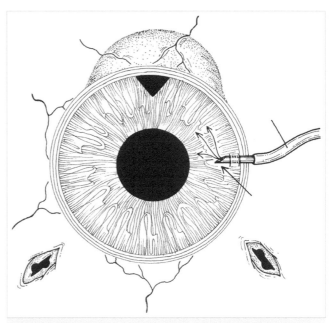

Fig. 30.5 Drainage of choroidal effusions. See text for description of technique.

30.2 Test Interpretation

In serous choroidal effusion, B-scan ultrasound reveals an echographically clear space between the detached choroid and the sclera, distinguishing this from choroidal hemorrhage. Additionally, the choroid is thicker than the retina, which helps distinguish choroidal effusion from retinal detachment. The clinical and echographic appearance of choroidal effusion, retinal detachment, and choroidal hemorrhage are shown in ▶ Fig. 30.1, ▶ Fig. 30.2, and ▶ Fig. 30.3.

30.3 Diagnosis

Right eye: Persistent serous choroidal detachment.

30.4 Medical Management

Observation usually results in complete resolution of ciliochoroidal effusions without sequelae. Elevation of IOP may hasten the spontaneous drainage of the serous fluid by driving proteins out through the sclera. The water component of the fluid may drain via the sclera as well, or perhaps gets reabsorbed into the choroidal capillary system. Discontinuation of systemic carbonic anhydrase inhibitors and topical aqueous suppressants in the affected eye may aid in this resolution. Discontinuation of topical beta-blocker in the contralateral eye is also recommended, since this may contribute to reduced aqueous production in the affected eye.

The benefit of topical steroid and cycloplegic therapy has not been well established, but there is little to argue against trying this treatment. We do not use systemic steroids, as advocated by some, because their effectiveness has not been established and the potential risk of systemic side effects outweighs the potential benefit. Oral carbonic anhydrase inhibitors have been used with varied success. We believe these drugs more likely potentiate the problem, although dramatic resolution of choroidal effusions has been reported following initiation of oral acetazolamide.

30.5 Surgical Management

The indications for drainage of serous choroidal effusions include lenticulocorneal touch, nonresolving effusions blocking the visual axis, hypotony causing corneal or retinal folds, failing filtering bleb due to poor aqueous production, overlying serous retinal detachment, or serous choroidal detachment accompanying a bleb leak. The presence of "kissing" choroidal detachments (▶ Fig. 30.4) is not necessarily an indication for immediate intervention as there seem to be no particular sequelae that accompany apposition of the retinal surfaces. However, insofar as these are accompanied by profound visual loss due to blocking of the visual axis, we prefer to drain them if they do not resolve in short order. The anxiety related to the visual loss associated with choroidal detachments that block the visual axis is substantial, and drainage of choroidal effusions is a simple and effective procedure with very few potential complications.

The technique for drainage of choroidal effusions is illustrated in ▶ Fig. 30.5. A paracentesis is made through the temporal peripheral cornea and the anterior chamber is reformed with balanced salt solution (BSS) or a viscoelastic if it is shallow. An anterior chamber maintainer, which is attached to a BSS infusion line, is inserted. This obviates the need to constantly reform the anterior chamber as the choroidal space is drained. A radial conjunctival incision is made in the inferotemporal or inferonasal quadrant, extending 3 to 4 mm posterior to the corneoscleral limbus. Inferior locations are chosen to permit continued drainage of fluid from superior choroidal detachments via gravity postoperatively. A 2- to 3-mm radial sclerostomy is then fashioned using a supersharp blade until the suprachoroidal space is entered. The location of this incision need only be just posterior to the limbus since the choroid is detached up to the scleral spur. While making the sclerostomy incision, it is helpful for the surgeon and assistant to retract each side of the incision as the cut-down is made to aid in visualization. The critical point comes when the incision reaches the level of the suprachoroidal space and straw-colored serous fluid gushes out. The incision is opened to an adequate length to allow a sclerostomy punch to fit into it on either side. A single punch is then performed on each side of the incision to allow continued drainage of the choroidal fluid postoperatively. Also, leaving the sclera open may prevent reformation of choroidal effusions if the postoperative IOP remains low, since the pressure in the suprachoroidal space will be equivalent to atmospheric pressure. The conjunctival incision is then closed with an absorbable suture and the same procedure performed in the contralateral inferior quadrant. The anterior maintainer is removed and a suture is oftentimes needed to close the paracentesis track. If a filtering bleb leak or cyclodialysis is present, these may be addressed at this time. Subconjunctival injections of antibiotics and steroids are employed.

30.6 Rehabilitation and Follow-up

The patient is examined 1 day postoperatively and placed on a brief course of a topical steroid, antibiotic, and cycloplegic agent (if phakic). Persistent effusion and/or drainage may be noted, but complete resolution of the serous effusion is usually prompt. Visual recovery is generally dramatic if the choroidal effusion involved the visual axis.

Suggested Reading

[1] Bellows AR, Chylack LT, Jr, Hutchinson BT. Choroidal detachment. Clinical manifestation, therapy and mechanism of formation. Ophthalmology. 1981; 88(11):1107–1115

[2] Brubaker RF, Pederson JE. Ciliochoroidal detachment. Surv Ophthalmol. 1983; 27(5):281–289

[3] Burney EN, Quigley HA, Robin AL. Hypotony and choroidal detachment as late complications of trabeculectomy. Am J Ophthalmol. 1987; 103(5):685–688

[4] Liebmann JM, Weinreb RN, Ritch R. Angle-closure glaucoma associated with occult annular ciliary body detachment. Arch Ophthalmol. 1998; 116(6):731–735

[5] Vela MA, Campbell DG. Hypotony and ciliochoroidal detachment following pharmacologic aqueous suppressant therapy in previously filtered patients. Ophthalmology. 1985; 92(1):50–57

IV

31 Nonproliferative Diabetic Retinopathy

Thalmon R. Campagnoli and William E. Smiddy

Abstract

The staging of nonproliferative diabetic retinopathy remains an important tool for directing follow-up regimens and estimating prognosis. Until recently, maximal systemic glucose control was the only treatment option, and that was generally considered to be for prevention of progression to more severe stages, especially proliferative retinopathy. The Early Treatment Diabetic Retinopathy Study (ETDRS) recommended consideration of panretinal laser before the appearance of proliferative retinopathy. Association with macular edema is still the most important determinant of treatment, but recent studies of the DRCR Network have demonstrated improvement in the degree of nonproliferative retinopathy, and might be a more important treatment goal in the future.

Keywords: diabetes, nonproliferative retinopathy, microaneurysms, laser

31.1 History

A 53-year-old man with a 10-year history of type II diabetes mellitus presented with a 2-month history of blurred vision OU. Medical history is positive for hypertension, peripheral neuropathy, and a history of hepatitis C. Best corrected visual acuity was 20/20 OU. Slit-lamp examination was unremarkable. The intraocular pressure was 11 mm Hg in the right eye and 12 mm Hg in the left eye. Funduscopic examination on the right showed a normal disc, no macular edema, macular lipid, or neovascularization. Intraretinal hemorrhages in two quadrants and a mild degree in the other two quadrants were present in both eyes. There was a cotton-wool spot superior to the right macula (▶ Fig. 31.1). Fluorescein angiography demonstrated microaneurysms with mild perifoveal capillary dropout, but no neovascularization (▶ Fig. 31.2).

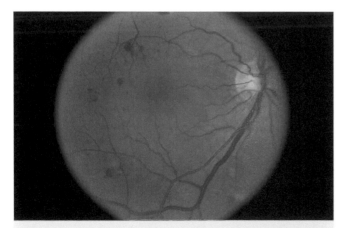

Fig. 31.1 Normal funduscopic appearance of the right eye with a normal disc. There is no macular edema or macular lipid. Temporal through the macula can be seen a moderate number of intraretinal hemorrhages with microaneurysms.

Differential Diagnosis—Key Points

1. It is estimated that over 25 million Americans aged 20 years or older have diabetes mellitus. The Los Angeles Latino Eye Study (LALES) found a prevalence of 56% of diabetic retinopathy in individuals with 5 to 9 years of diabetes duration. A previous study had shown a 78% prevalence of diabetic retinopathy after a 10-year duration of systemic disease. The 14-year follow-up study of the Wisconsin Eye Survey of Diabetic Retinopathy (WESDR) demonstrated a 96% incidence of developing new retinopathy, an 86% progression rate, and 26% incidence of diabetic macular edema.

2. It is common that diabetic patients present with blurred vision that they attribute to refractive problems rather than complications from diabetic retinopathy. This may delay the correct diagnosis and treatment.

3. Microaneurysms and intraretinal hemorrhages may be clinical findings in other retinal vascular conditions such as branch and central retinal vein occlusion, radiation retinopathy, perifoveal retinal telangiectasia, and Eales' disease. Usually, the medical history yields evidence of the diabetic condition, but screening for diabetes should be performed in patients with the ophthalmoscopic features of diabetic retinopathy. The more generalized distribution in diabetes usually distinguishes nonproliferative diabetic retinopathy (NPDR) from cases of branch retinal vein occlusion, which have a segmental distribution; predominance of venular changes and unilateral presentation also increase the likelihood of branch or central vein occlusion diagnosis.

31.2 Test Interpretation

The most important aspect of evaluating diabetic retinopathy is the clinical examination. The most important examination tool is magnified observation of the macula and posterior pole—accomplished most effectively with a fundus contact lens.

Fundus photography may increase the sensitivity of assessing NPDR severity and differentiate it from early proliferative diabetic retinopathy. Formal grading of the level of retinopathy was determined from photographs in the Early Treatment Diabetic Retinopathy Study (ETDRS). While detailed grading may not be clinically necessary, photographic slides may guide follow-up schedules or treatment. Fluorescein angiography may define surprisingly large areas of ischemia, which, when perifoveal, may explain decreased vision. Eyes with large areas of nonperfusion may indicate a poorer prognosis. Early neovascular complexes are easily recognized by fluorescein leakage.

Electrophysiologic studies are not part of a standard evaluation, but have been shown to demonstrate early and characteristic changes with increased degrees of ischemia.

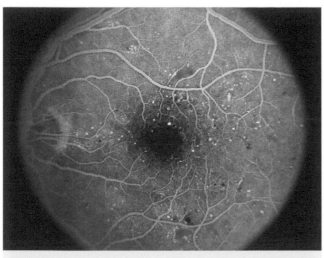

Fig. 31.2 Angiographic appearance of the left eye showing somewhat more microaneurysms than were apparent from clinical examination. Notice the foveal vascular zone with a somewhat irregular distribution. Notice small areas of capillary nonperfusion one disc diameter inferior and superior to the foveal vascular zone and also temporal to the macula.

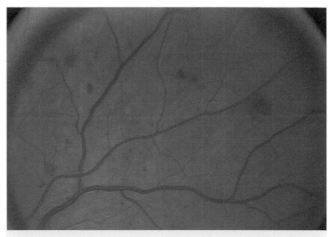

Fig. 31.3 ETDRS standard photograph 2A, the standard for microaneurysms.

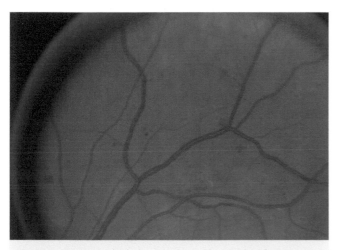

Fig. 31.4 ETDRS standard photograph 6A, the standard for venous beading.

The use of spectral-domain optical coherence tomography (SD-OCT) is not recommended for minimal diabetic retinopathy screening. SD-OCT is commonly indicated in diabetic retinopathy to help in detecting the cause of unexplained visual acuity loss, identify areas of vitreomacular interface abnormalities, ensure presence or absence of macular edema, and assess other possibly associated macular diseases (e.g., age-related macular degeneration).

31.3 Diagnosis

Moderately severe nonproliferative diabetic retinopathy, OU.

31.4 Medical Management

Numerous studies including the Diabetes Complications Control Trial, the United Kingdom Prospective Diabetes Study, the ETDRS, and the WESDR have identified baseline clinical characteristics associated with a more rapid or a higher rate of progression of retinopathy. These consistently include severity of baseline retinopathy, duration of disease, and degree of glycemic control. Some studies have shown that accompanying systemic features such as hypertension and hypercholesterolemia may also increase the risk of progression. Perhaps, more importantly, some of these studies have also shown that control of blood glucose and hypertension may lower these risks. Doxycycline, a substance known to carry retinal anti-inflammatory and neuroprotective effects, has been used in attempts to induce regression or reduce progression of mild and moderate NPDR, but no success was achieved. A study evaluating eyes treated for diabetic macular edema suggested decreased progression of retinopathy after intravitreal steroid or anti–vascular endothelial growth factor injection; however, the optimal control of medical conditions continues to be of major importance in eyes diagnosed with diabetic retinopathy.

The ETDRS has demonstrated efficacy in instituting laser treatment even before proliferative diabetic retinopathy develops. Type II diabetics show a larger treatment benefit compared to type I patients. The threshold for considering scatter laser treatment is the presence of severe NPDR. This patient's right eye approaches that threshold. The "4–2–1" rule has been developed to assist the clinician in making this determination by simplifying the definition of severe NPDR into a clinically useful algorithm. The definition of severe NPDR includes four quadrants of microaneurysms and intraretinal hemorrhages equal to or greater than standard photograph 2A (▶ Fig. 31.3), two quadrants of venous beading equal to or exceeding the degree present in standard photograph 6A (▶ Fig. 31.4), and one quadrant of intraretinal microvascular abnormality equal to or exceeding the degree present in standard photograph 8A (▶ Fig. 31.5). When two or three of these features are present, "very severe NPDR" is defined, which carries a 50% risk of

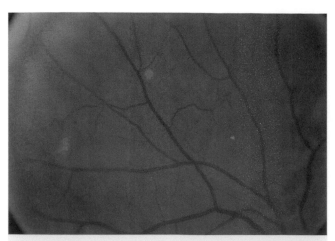

Fig. 31.5 ETDRS standard photograph 8A, the standard for intraretinal microvascular abnormalities.

developing high-risk characteristics (severe proliferative diabetic retinopathy and its incumbent risk of visual loss) within 1 year. This risk is diminished by approximately 50% with laser treatment.

31.5 Rehabilitation and Follow-up

Patients with diabetic retinopathy require careful follow-up examinations with a frequency dependent on the severity of the retinopathy. An annual examination is recommended for patients with minimal or absent NPDR. An examination is recommended every 6 to 12 months for patients with mild to moderate (more than microaneurysms only, but less than severe NPDR) nonproliferative disease if there is no macular edema, but every 4 to 6 months if there is nonclinically significant edema present, and 1 to 2 months if clinical significant macular edema (see Chapter 32, Diabetic Macular Edema) is present. Patients with severe or very severe NPDR should be reexamined every 2 to 4 months.

Suggested Readings

[1] The Wisconsin Epidemiologic Study of Diabetic Retinopathy. XVII. The 14-year incidence and progression of diabetic retinopathy and associated risk factors in type I diabetes. Ophthalmology. 1998; 105:1801–1815

[2] Varma R, Torres M, Peña F, Klein R, Azen SP, Los Angeles Latino Eye Study Group. Prevalence of diabetic retinopathy in adult Latinos: the Los Angeles Latino eye study. Ophthalmology. 2004; 111(7):1298–1306

[3] Early Treatment Diabetic Retinopathy Study Research Group. Early photocoagulation for diabetic retinopathy. ETDRS report number 9. Ophthalmology. 1991; 98(5) Suppl:766–785

[4] Nathan DM, Bayless M, Cleary P, et al. DCCT/EDIC Research Group. Diabetes control and complications trial/epidemiology of diabetes interventions and complications study at 30 years: advances and contributions. Diabetes. 2013; 62(12):3976–3986

[5] United Kingdom Prospective Diabetes Study (UKPDS) VIII. UK Prospective Diabetes Study (UKPDS). VIII. Study design, progress and performance. Diabetologia. 1991; 34(12):877–890

[6] Scott IU, Jackson GR, Quillen DA, Klein R, Liao J, Gardner TW. Effect of doxycycline vs placebo on retinal function and diabetic retinopathy progression in mild to moderate nonproliferative diabetic retinopathy: a randomized proof-of-concept clinical trial. JAMA Ophthalmol. 2014; 132 (9):1137–1142

[7] Bressler SB, Qin H, Melia M, et al. Diabetic Retinopathy Clinical Research Network. Exploratory analysis of the effect of intravitreal ranibizumab or triamcinolone on worsening of diabetic retinopathy in a randomized clinical trial. JAMA Ophthalmol. 2013; 131(8):1033–1040

[8] Ismail-Beigi F, Craven T, Banerji MA, et al. ACCORD trial group. Effect of intensive treatment of hyperglycaemia on microvascular outcomes in type 2 diabetes: an analysis of the ACCORD randomised trial. Lancet. 2010; 376(9739): 419–430– Erratum in: Lancet 2010;376:1466

[9] Ferris F. Early photocoagulation in patients with either type I or type II diabetes. Trans Am Ophthalmol Soc. 1996; 94:505–537

[10] American Academy of Ophthalmology Retina/Vitreous Panel. Preferred Practice Pattern® Guidelines. Diabetic Retinopathy. San Francisco, CA: American Academy of Ophthalmology; 2014. Available at: www.aao.org/ppp

32 Diabetic Macular Edema

Thalmon R. Campagnoli and William E. Smiddy

Abstract

Treatment of diabetic macular edema has been transformed during the past decade with the advent of anti-vascular endothelial growth factor therapy. While laser has not been totally removed from the treatment armamentarium, it plays a small role in current therapy algorithms. There are specific associated features such as proliferative disease, initial visual acuity, and systemic control that can influence the treatment approach. Indications for treatment have changed little, but optical coherence tomography imaging studies now play the dominant role in diagnosing and monitoring treatment, with diminishing roles for fluorescein angiography. Surgical management of diabetic macular edema remains controversial, and probably should best be considered in cases with demonstrable preretinal traction.

Keywords: diabetes, retinopathy, macula, edema, intravitreal injection, laser

32.1 History

This 58-year-old man with a 20-year history of type I diabetes, recent-onset hypertension, and chronic hypercholesterolemia sought consultation because of blurred vision of several weeks' duration.

Examination disclosed best corrected visual acuity of 20/30 in each eye. There was no afferent pupillary defect. Slit-lamp examination showed only trace nuclear lens opacity. Tensions were 20 in each eye.

Funduscopic examination showed moderate microaneurysms scattered about all quadrants of both eyes. In the right eye, there was clinically significant diabetic macular edema with a circinate lipid ring surrounding the center of the macula (▶ Fig. 32.1). No neovascular changes were seen. In the left eye, in addition to the microaneurysms and macular edema, there was early neovascularization at the disc (NVD) (▶ Fig. 32.2). Fluorescein angiography demonstrated macular leakage OU and NVD in the left eye (▶ Fig. 32.3). Optical coherence tomography (OCT) confirmed macular edema OU.

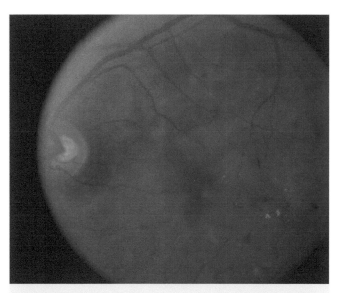

Fig. 32.2 Appearance of left eye is similar to right with lipid and macular thickening temporal to macula. Early NVD is present at the inferior part of the disc.

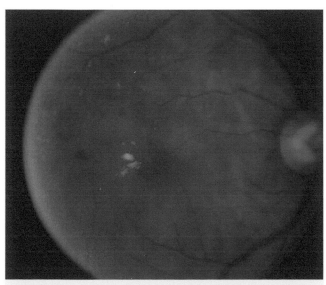

Fig. 32.1 Funduscopic appearance of right eye demonstrating the diabetic macular edema temporal to fovea. This approaches the center and accounts for visual loss.

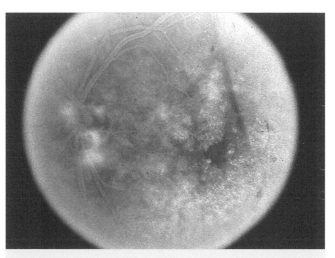

Fig. 32.3 Fluorescein angiogram shows macular edema leakage, but also confirms the NVD as evidenced by late leakage.

The patient underwent bilateral macular edema treatment with intravitreal anti-vascular endothelial growth factor (anti-VEGF) injection in OU. He was scheduled for follow-up examination in 1 month to reevaluate the early neovascularization of the disc in OS and repeat anti-VEGF therapy for persistent macular edema in OU. The patient returned for a third office visit 1 month after the second anti-VEGF treatment, when a decision for a third anti-VEGF injection and focal laser treatment in OD was made in virtue of unresolved edema. OS demonstrated 20/20 visual acuity and normal macular contours on OCT, and no further treatment was recommended at the time.

Differential Diagnosis—Key Points

1. The patient meets the criteria for clinically significant macular edema in each eye. The Early Treatment Diabetic Retinopathy Study (ETDRS) defines clinically significant diabetic macular edema as macular thickening within 500 µm of the center, lipid within 500 µm of the center associated with macular thickening that may be present greater than 500 µm of the center, and macular thickening of 1 disc area, any portion of which is within 1 disc diameter of the center of the fovea. It is imperative to evaluate the involvement or noninvolvement of the macular 1-mm center by the diabetic macular edema (DME), given that the risk of visual loss and the need for treatment are greater when the center is involved.

2. Visual acuity is not part of the definition of clinically significant macular edema, and is of less importance compared to the clinical examination in deciding whether or not to recommend treatment. When the visual acuity is in the 20/20 range, treatment with laser may be recommended if there is clinically significant diabetic macular edema not involving the macular center. In case the macular center is involved, anti-VEGF therapy is advocated as a better initial treatment strategy. In selected cases, treatment may be deferred provided close follow-up examination may be obtained, but usually the presence of center-involving clinically significant macular edema (CSME) implies need for immediate treatment.

3. This patient presented with possible early proliferative disease in the left eye. It is generally believed that panretinal photocoagulation (PRP) may exacerbate macular edema. This was a leading cause of what was termed "early persistent visual loss" following PRP in the Diabetic Retinopathy Study (DRS). Accordingly, it was recommended that macular edema be treated first with prompt attention to PRP following laser treatment. For patients with high-risk characteristics as defined by the DRS (which this patient did not yet have), PRP and macular edema treatments were usually offered simultaneously or within a couple of weeks.

The introduction of anti-VEGF therapy for CSME minimized the concerns regarding the occurrence of "early persistent visual loss" phenomena, considering the action of inflammatory molecules released after PRP is commonly suppressed by the anti-VEGF effect. For patients with severe nonproliferative disease or early proliferative changes, PRP is considered, but this may be deferred once it is not uncommon to notice retinopathy stabilization and regression of early proliferation

after anti-VEGF therapy for DME; careful follow-up is crucial in allowing assessment of further treatment need.

4. Optimal control of systemic conditions is important in optimizing the natural course and even the response to treatment. Patients with hypercholesterolemia or systemic hypertension tend to respond poorer to treatment. Accordingly, medical consultation for optimal treatment of the systemic condition is recommended before reevaluating for macular edema treatment.

5. In a patient with diabetes and at least moderate retinopathy and macular thickening, the diagnosis is hardly questionable. However, hypertensive retinopathy and cystoid macular edema following cataract surgery, or radiation retinopathy, are two entities which may mimic the appearance in this patient.

32.2 Diagnosis

Clinically significant diabetic macular edema, center-involving (ci-CSME) OU.

Early proliferative diabetic retinopathy, OS.

32.3 Test Interpretation

The clinical examination forms the basis for diagnosis and is the primary factor in deciding if treatment is recommended for patients with diabetic macular edema. Fluorescein angiography may be useful by defining degrees of nonperfusion (and therefore assigning the cause of visual loss to an entity other than macular edema) and in localizing areas of maximal microaneurysm leakage, which may be helpful in guiding treatment. In some cases, stereoscopic fundus photography may also be of value in confirming the presence or absence of macular thickening. These modalities have been largely supplanted by spectral domain OCT (SD-OCT). SD-OCT provides superior quantitative and qualitative assessment of retinal thickening areas, and has especial reproducibility, allowing precise change(s) detection.

32.4 Medical Management

Medical treatment therapies are necessary to maximize treatment of hypercholesterolemia or systemic hypertension. Optimal control of blood sugar is a long-term goal to be pursued, but is rarely valuable in effecting the short-term improvements in retinopathy.

32.5 Surgical Management

Anti-VEGF therapy with bevacizumab, ranibizumab, or aflibercept has mostly replaced laser treatment in DME, and is the first-line therapy for center-involving DME. Intravitreal corticosteroids are considered a good alternative for poor-responsive, pseudophakic eyes with no history of elevated intraocular pressure. A sequence of three intravitreal injections with the same initial drug within 4- to 6-week intervals is usually necessary before considering other therapies.

Laser treatment was previously established by the ETDRS as the cornerstone treatment for diabetic macular edema; nowadays, its benefit is that it might avoid long-term injection-based therapy. The treatment technique involves the use of 50- or 100-µm spot sizes, with 0.1- to 0.2-second burn durations (generally, the argon laser treatment is used). The burn-intensity end point is some whitening of the retina, but not as intense as for PRP. The ETDRS technique involved direct treatment of microaneurysms, but allowed for a grid treatment of the thickened area. Many utilize a modified grid treatment whereby the initial treatment is aimed at obvious microaneurysms, with a filling in of the thickened area which yields, effectively, a grid treatment.

The ETDRS modified grid treatment has been widely adopted by retina specialists in association with anti-VEGF therapy. Multiple recent trials demonstrated better results when anti-VEGF drugs are combined to laser therapy for center-involving CSME. In cases of non–center involving CSME, laser monotherapy following the ETDRS technique (modified or not modified) is still the best option.

Rare patients will present with macular edema that appears to be due to traction induced by a taut, thickened posterior hyaloid. Such cases are easily identified preoperatively by SD-OCT, but may respond only to surgical removal of the thickened posterior hyaloid.

32.6 Rehabilitation and Follow-up

Generally, after patients are treated for diabetic macular edema with an anti-VEGF agent with or without focal laser, they are followed up in 4 to 6 weeks. If there is clinical evidence of persistent visual loss attributable to remnant or recurrent edema, then the patient is retreated in this time frame. A sequence of anti-VEGF intravitreal injections is sometimes needed for the complete edema regression and best visual acuity achievement. Switching to another anti-VEGF drug might be beneficial for patients with persistent edema, especially if poor response is noticed after three consecutive attempts with the same drug in 4- to 6-weeks intervals. Intravitreal corticosteroids are a good alternative in some cases, and it might offer greater benefit in eyes with severe edema. Repeated laser treatment can also be considered 3 to 6 months following initial treatment. Care is taken not to overtreat in patients who have had multiple treatments, since it may not be possible to eliminate the macular thickening and recover the vision despite successive anti-VEGF/corticosteroids and laser therapy, and after a point those treatments may become visually counterproductive.

Suggested Readings

[1] Lewis H, Abrams GW, Blumenkranz MS, Campo RV. Vitrectomy for diabetic macular traction and edema associated with posterior hyaloidal traction. Ophthalmology. 1992; 99(5):753–759

[2] Harbour JW, Smiddy WE, Flynn HW, Jr, Rubsamen PE. Vitrectomy for diabetic macular edema associated with a thickened and taut posterior hyaloid membrane. Am J Ophthalmol. 1996; 121(4):405–413

[3] Early Treatment Diabetic Retinopathy Study, Report #2: Treatment techniques and clinical guidelines for photocoagulation of diabetic macular edema. Ophthalmology. 1987; 94:761–774

[4] Early Treatment Diabetic Retinopathy Study, Report #1: Photocoagulation for diabetic macular edema. Arch Ophthalmol. 1985; 103:1796–1806

[5] Diabetic Retinopathy Study Report #12: Macular edema in Diabetic Retinopathy Study patients. Ophthalmology. 1987; 94:754–760

[6] Elman MJ, Bressler NM, Qin H, et al. Diabetic Retinopathy Clinical Research Network. Expanded 2-year follow-up of ranibizumab plus prompt or deferred laser or triamcinolone plus prompt laser for diabetic macular edema. Ophthalmology. 2011; 118(4):609–614

[7] Rajendram R, Fraser-Bell S, Kaines A, et al. A 2-year prospective randomized controlled trial of intravitreal bevacizumab or laser therapy (BOLT) in the management of diabetic macular edema: 24-month data: report 3. Arch Ophthalmol. 2012; 130(8):972–979

[8] Do DV, Nguyen QD, Boyer D, et al. da Vinci Study Group. One-year outcomes of the da Vinci Study of VEGF Trap-Eye in eyes with diabetic macular edema. Ophthalmology. 2012; 119(8):1658–1665

[9] American Academy of Ophthalmology Retina/Vitreous Panel. Preferred Practice Pattern® Guidelines. Diabetic Retinopathy. San Francisco, CA: American Academy of Ophthalmology; 2014. Available at: www.aao.org/ppp

[10] Wells JA, Glassman AR, Ayala AR, et al. Diabetic Retinopathy Clinical Research Network. Aflibercept, bevacizumab, or ranibizumab for diabetic macular edema. N Engl J Med. 2015; 372(13):1193–1203

33 Proliferative Diabetic Retinopathy

Thalmon R. Campagnoli and William E. Smiddy

Abstract

Proliferative diabetic retinopathy might be encountered less frequently, or be diagnosed at an earlier stage, currently but remains an important and moderately common cause of visual loss in a diabetic patient. The dichotomy of high-risk versus non-high-risk characteristics is probably only important as an impetus for urgency, but not determination of treatment in current practice. The mainstay of treatment is probably still panretinal laser photocoagulation, but intravitreal injection of anti-vascular endothelial growth factor (anti-VEGF) agents is playing a larger role currently, as evidenced by recent results of Protocol S from the DRCR Network. Anti-VEGF injections are especially important when there is concurrent macular edema, and are also unequivocally valuable in the setting of vitreous hemorrhage severe enough to prevent laser application. Diagnostic modalities are generally unnecessary, but fluorescein angiography can still be helpful for the diagnosis of early proliferative disease.

Keywords: diabetes, retinopathy, proliferative, neovascularization, laser, photocoagulation, intravitreal injections, anti-VEGF treatment

33.1 History

A 50-year-old man with a 5-year history of type II diabetes mellitus presented for a second opinion from an ophthalmologist regarding the possibility of diabetic retinopathy. The patient was asymptomatic upon initial presentation.

His examination showed vision of 20/20 in each eye. Pressures were 12 and 13 mm Hg, in the right and left eyes, respectively. Slit-lamp examination was unremarkable. The lens was perfectly clear. On funduscopic examination of the right eye, there was a mild degree of hard exudates scattered about the posterior pole, but there was no definite macular thickening. Questionable neovascularization elsewhere was seen at the distal portion of both temporal arcades. Most prominent, however, was definite neovascularization at the disc that was in excess of one disc area in extent (▸ Fig. 33.1). In the left eye, there were intraretinal hemorrhages with microaneurysms in all four quadrants, but this exceeded the standard photograph 2A for hemorrhages in only two quadrants (▸ Fig. 33.2).

33.2 Risk Factors for Severe Visual Loss in Diabetic Retinopathy Study

1. Any neovascularization.
2. Neovascularization at the disc (as compared to neovascularization elsewhere).
3. Severe neovascularization:
   a) Neovascularization within one disc diameter of the optic disc exceeding one-quarter to one-third disc area in size—DRS standard photograph 10A.
   b) Neovascularization elsewhere exceeding one-half disc area in extent.
4. Vitreous hemorrhage.

Differential Diagnosis—Key Points

1. In the setting of a patient with diabetes mellitus with bilateral retinopathy, it is quite clear that the diagnosis is diabetic retinopathy. Of principal importance is understanding the staging of each eye so that proper treatment recommendations may be determined. The classification of diabetic retinopathy is simplified to "nonproliferative" diabetic retinopathy and "proliferative" diabetic retinopathy. This classification system is based on the findings of numerous multicentered studies of natural history and responses to treatment. The right eye has proliferative diabetic retinopathy (PDR), whereas the left eye has nonproliferative diabetic retinopathy.

   PDR is defined by the presence of neovascularization and/or vitreous hemorrhage (presumed neovascularization), and is typically subdivided into early (non-high-risk) PDR or high-risk PDR. The Diabetic Retinopathy Study (DRS) identified four high-risk features and defined as high-risk eyes the ones containing three or four of these features (see list below).

2. Other causes of retinal neovascularization should also be considered in the differential diagnosis, but given this medical history they are extremely unlikely. Neovascularization due to branch retinal vein occlusion usually does not produce neovascularization directly at the disc and thus would most commonly be in the differential diagnosis of neovascularization elsewhere. However, the appearance of collateral vessels at the disc as sometimes occurs after branch or central retinal vein occlusion may mimic neovascular vessels at the disc. These are more characteristically of larger caliber ("loopy") and are nonprogressive. Unlike neovascularization, collateral vessels pose no threat of vitreous hemorrhage. Other causes of neovascularization typically share the ischemic state and may be seen in uveitis, in various forms of occult vasculitis, Eales' disease, proliferative sickle retinopathy, and radiation retinopathy.

3. Other causes of nonproliferative retinopathy mimicking the findings in this patient's left eye include radiation retinopathy and hypertensive retinopathy.

4. Diabetic retinopathy, particularly proliferative phases, may occur asymptomatically. It is for this reason that many patients commonly go undiagnosed until more severe complications have ensued (i.e., vitreous hemorrhage or tractional retinal detachment). Thus, a careful, complete, dilated funduscopic examination with some form of high-magnification fundoscopy should be performed on a regular basis.

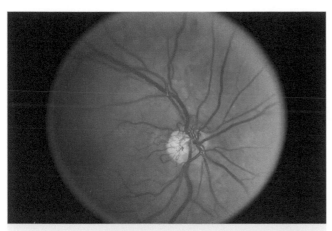

Fig. 33.1 Examination of the right disc showed neovascularization involving over one disc area, extending beyond the temporal and superior margins of the disc. Stereoscopic view showed this clearly to be elevated over the retinal surface. No vitreous hemorrhage was present.

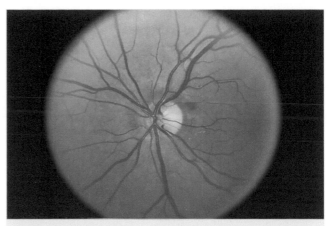

Fig. 33.2 The left eye showed a moderate number of microaneurysms and intraretinal hemorrhages with occasional hard exudates. No intraretinal microvascular abnormalities or venous beading were noted. A moderate degree of hemorrhage was noted only in two quadrants.

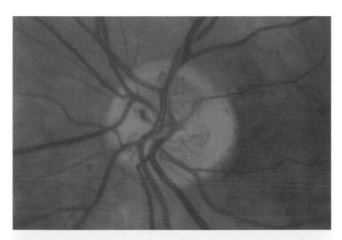

Fig. 33.3 Standard photograph 10A from the Diabetic Retinopathy Study showing neovascularization involving one-third to one-half of the disc area.

33.3 Test Interpretation

Usually, the staging of retinopathy, either proliferative or nonproliferative, is achieved by clinical examination. While the direct ophthalmoscope may be suitable for the purposes of staging the condition, slit-lamp biomicroscopy with a precorneal lens is more accurate. The use of the 60- or 90-diopter lens gives an inverted, indirect image; however, it typically sacrifices some degree of stereopsis and, accordingly, some sensitivity. The contact lens evaluation allows optimal stereoscopic evaluation, but may be limited by media opacities in many patients.

Fluorescein angiography is usually not a diagnostic modality. However, in questionable vascular lesions, the fluorescein angiogram may demonstrate leakage from neovascular vessels, whereas other vascular malformations such as intraretinal microvascular abnormalities may not show leakage. Another use of fluorescein angiogram is for detection of retinal nonperfused areas and treatment guidance which might prompt treatment even before PDR is manifest in selected cases. A clinically useful tool is to obtain high-quality stereoscopic fundus photographs in all fields. Examination of these photographs is the most sensitive means of evaluating the fine details of the fundus vasculature. Strictly speaking, neovascularization is typically seen as fine vessel outgrowth from the venous side of the circulation, which most characteristically leads to slightly elevated vascular frond. This is in contrast to the intraretinal microvascular abnormalities which are within the retina and, therefore, flat.

Spectral-domain optical coherence tomography is especially useful in order to noninvasively demonstrate and quantify associated macular edema and/or vitreomacular traction leading to decreased vision in PDR eyes (▶ Fig. 33.3), and also assess other possible vision-threatening macular diseases.

33.4 Diagnosis

Right eye: Proliferative diabetic retinopathy with high-risk characteristics.

Left eye: Moderately severe nonproliferative diabetic retinopathy.

33.5 Medical Management

The DRS defined a poor prognosis for patients with neovascularization, and especially for those with high-risk characteristics as defined by eyes containing three or four of the characteristics as listed in section 33.2 Risk Factors for Severe Visual Loss in Diabetic Retinopathy Study.[1] The mainstay of treatment for PDR is panretinal laser photocoagulation (PRP). PRP is typically performed under topical anesthesia with the use of a pan-fundus contact lens and is at least minimally uncomfortable, or using a laser indirect delivery system. A significant proportion of patients will require retrobulbar anesthesia because of pain incurred with laser treatment. Commonly, PRP is delivered in two or more sessions to avoid either severe pain or choroidal detachment from excessive treatment. Usually, a relatively short burn duration (0.1 second or less) is the best way to minimize patient discomfort. Spot size ranging from 200 to 500 μm is usually utilized. A total of approximately 1,500 laser spots are aimed for, but probably more important is the area of retina lesioned by the laser. That is, fewer spots are necessary when larger spot sizes are used. Usually, a 1- to 2-week interval between laser sessions is recommended, but this is accelerated with more severe neovascularization.

Complications of panretinal photocoagulation include an almost universal finding of some degree of pain in the immediate posttreatment period, which usually responds to over-the-counter analgesics. Vitreous hemorrhage may occur following laser photocoagulation; it is unclear whether that is the coincidence or whether it is due to laser-induced remodeling of the neovascular complexes during initial stages of regression. Most patients will recognize diminished illumination in an eye undergoing the procedure, most distinctly noticed as a decrease in night vision. Although peripheral visual field loss has been documented, it is not usually clinically significant. Exacerbation of preexisting (even nonclinically significant) diabetic macular edema may follow PRP. For this reason, treatment of diabetic macular edema with focal photocoagulation and/or anti-VEGF therapy is recommended either before or at least during PRP treatment. The DRS documented a 20% incidence of early persistent visual loss (≥ 2 lines) following PRP, mostly due to this phenomenon.

The Early Treatment Diabetic Retinopathy Study[2] and, to a lesser degree, DRS[1] defined potential efficacy for patients even before proliferative retinopathy ensues. This is discussed in a previous chapter.

The results of the DRS showed that for patients with high-risk characteristics the rate of severe visual loss (5/200) after 2 years decreased from 27 to 10%. Long-term follow-up studies have documented the relative stability of eyes following an initially successful response to panretinal photocoagulation. While a treatment benefit was seen in the DRS for early proliferative cases, the magnitude of the response was not sufficient to support a strong treatment recommendation. Nevertheless, consideration could be given to laser treatment in these cases.

Recently, adjunctive anti-VEGF therapy has been reported to be beneficial for PDR, especially when accompanying vitreous hemorrhage limits amenability to treatment. This is also potentially useful in the PDR eye that is associated with macular edema. Another role for anti-VEGF treatment is an eye with aggressive neovascularization for which surgical intervention has been recommended, to mitigate intraoperative bleeding. Its role in the treatment of very severe NPDR and early PDR without macular edema is currently under investigation.

33.6 Surgical Management

The indications and surgical treatment of patients with severe complications of diabetic retinopathy are beyond the scope of this chapter. Patients with vitreous hemorrhage or fibrovascular proliferation leading to traction that threatens the macula (with or without detachment) are considered for vitrectomy. Typically, earlier vitrectomy is considered for patients with vitreous hemorrhage and type I diabetes. Patients with type II diabetes are commonly observed for spontaneous improvement of vitreous hemorrhage. The results of vitrectomy are best for patients with vitreous hemorrhage and worse for patients with severe degrees of traction or retinal detachment.

33.7 Rehabilitation and Follow-up

After completion of a course of PRP, the patient should be observed within a few weeks. If the retinopathy progresses, vitrectomy must be considered. If the retinopathy regresses completely, then a conservative, observational follow-up regimen may be pursued, contingent upon the stability of the retinopathy and visual acuity. Follow-up PRP and/or anti-VEGF therapy is considered when there are multiple recurrent vitreous hemorrhages or when the regression of the neovascularization is incomplete, particularly when the morphology of the neovascularization is feathery, with fine caliber vessels.

Suggested Readings

[1] The Diabetic Retinopathy Study Research Group. Four risk factors for severe visual loss in diabetic retinopathy. The third report from the Diabetic Retinopathy Study. Arch Ophthalmol. 1979; 97(4):654–655

[2] Early Treatment Diabetic Retinopathy Study Research Group. Early photocoagulation for diabetic retinopathy. ETDRS report number 9. Ophthalmology. 1991; 98(5) Suppl:766–785

[3] Moss SE, Klein R, Kessler SD, Richie KA. Comparison between ophthalmoscopy and fundus photography in determining severity of diabetic retinopathy. Ophthalmology. 1985; 92(1):62–67

[4] American Academy of Ophthalmology Retina/Vitreous Panel. Preferred Practice Pattern® Guidelines. Diabetic Retinopathy. San Francisco, CA: American Academy of Ophthalmology; 2014. Available at: www.aao.org/ppp

34 Retinal Arterial Occlusion

Amir Mohsenin and William E. Smiddy

Abstract

Retinal arterial occlusion, whether it be branch or central, is the characteristic cause of sudden, mostly irreversible loss of vision. It is most important as a potential warning signal of systemic vascular disease, and referral for a systemic medical workup has long been the recommended consequence of the diagnosis. Atherosclerosis is the most common medical association, but a more thorough evaluation for carotid plaque or arrhythmias would be the suggested focus for the internist's workup. The classic finding of a Hollenhorst plaque and retinal whitening appearing within hours of the loss of vision with fading during the following week remain the classic presentation. Optical coherence tomography imaging of later cases can demonstrate the inner retinal atrophy that follows from the ischemic injury.

Keywords: retina, vascular occlusion, thrombus, ischemia, cholesterol

34.1 History

A 69-year-old woman presented 4 weeks after sudden visual loss in the right eye. Medical history included a 6-year history of systemic hypertension and a 1-year history of diabetes mellitus. Examination showed visual acuity of 20/30 and 20/25 in the right and left eyes, respectively. There was no afferent pupillary defect. Intraocular pressures were 16 mm Hg in each eye. Slit-lamp examination was remarkable only for early nuclear sclerosis of the lens in both eyes. On funduscopic examination of the right eye, the inferotemporal retinal artery appeared sclerotic and attenuated with a glistening yellow cholesterol embolus (Hollenhorst's plaque) at its proximal part (▶ Fig. 34.1). There was an area of superficial retinal whitening, most prominent in the posterior pole along the distribution of the obstructed artery. Funduscopic examination of the left eye was normal.

Fluorescein angiography demonstrated a corresponding filling defect in the inferior branch retinal artery distribution (▶ Fig. 34.2).

Differential Diagnosis—Key Points

1. The hallmarks of arterial occlusion are sudden, dense loss of vision corresponding to a zone of retinal whitening and arterial attenuation. The retinal whitening is due to edema but is transient; after a few days, it resolves and the diagnosis may be more difficult. The characteristic cherry-red spot of central retinal artery occlusion (CRAO) is due to the retinal pigment epithelium and choroidal coloration remaining visible through the central, thin foveola—made more prominent because the thicker, surrounding macular tissues are translucent due to the acute ischemic edema (▶ Fig. 34.3).

2. Approximately 57% of retinal arterial occlusions involve the central retinal artery, 39% involve the branch retinal artery, and 5% involve the cilioretinal artery.

3. Branch retinal artery occlusion (BRAO) results from embolic or thrombotic occlusion of the affected vessel. The temporal retinal arteries are involved in 90% of cases. Three main varieties of emboli include cholesterol emboli arising in the carotid arteries, platelet-fibrin emboli associated with large vessel arteriosclerosis, and calcific emboli arising from diseased cardiac valves. These are not commonly able to be differentiated clinically. Rare causes of emboli include cardiac myxoma, fat emboli from long bone fractures, septic emboli from infective endocarditis, and migraine (in patients younger than 30 years).

4. CRAO is often caused by atherosclerosis-related thrombosis occurring at the level of the lamina cribrosa. Other causes include emboli, spasm, and dissecting aneurysm. Emboli are seen in the retinal arterial system in about 20% of eyes with CRAO. Patients with atherosclerotic CRAO are at increased risk of early death from systemic vascular disease.

5. Systemic workup of patients with arterial occlusions is usually deferred to the internist, but might include a complete physical examination, carotid evaluation (e.g., Doppler flow studies or angiography) as indicated, electrocardiogram, and echocardiography. Systemic hypertension (70%) and diabetes (25%) are also commonly associated with retinal arterial occlusions.

34.2 Test Interpretation

Diagnosis of most cases of acute retinal artery occlusion (CRAO or BRAO) may be achieved by clinical examination of the fundus with the indirect ophthalmoscope or slit-lamp biomicroscopy. Acute occlusions are more obvious due to the characteristic edema.

Intravenous fluorescein angiography may be useful in showing the details of the abnormal circulation of central or branch artery occlusion. The principal abnormality is delayed appearance of the dye in the arterial circulation. Cilioretinal artery sparing may be demonstrable. Late staining of the optic nerve head may also occur. The filling of the retinal arteries is often abnormal, with the fluorescein partially filling an artery. Venous filling is usually slowed, and occasionally the dye will not progress beyond laminar flow. Leakage of the dye from the vessel wall is not normally seen except at the site where an embolus lodges within a retinal artery. Delayed choroidal filling occurs in about 10% of CRAO cases and suggests ophthalmic artery occlusion. The occlusion frequently recanalizes within a few weeks of obstruction and, accordingly, the angiogram may show only subtle changes in more chronic cases.

Visual field testing may also be helpful in making a diagnosis in nonacute cases of BRAO. The characteristic finding is a

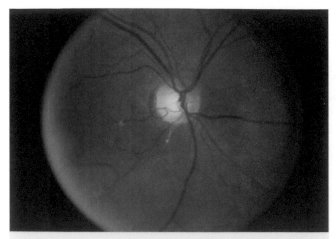

Fig. 34.1 Photograph of the right fundus showing inferotemporal branch artery occlusion with prominent Hollenhorst's plaques.

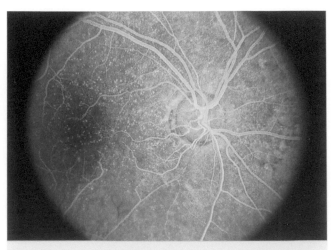

Fig. 34.2 Fluorescein angiogram of the same eye showing limited filling of the inferotemporal retinal artery and its branches. Numerous drusen are also apparent, scattered about the posterior pole.

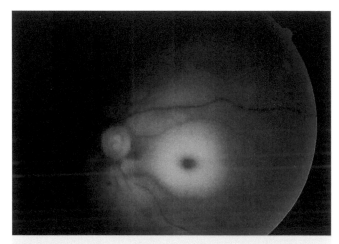

Fig. 34.3 Funduscopic appearance of a different patient 3 days after sudden visual loss. Retinal edema indicative of CRAO is apparent, with classic foveal "cherry-red spot" in evidence.

sectoral, or even hemifield, abnormality that has a distinct border respecting the horizontal midline.

Electroretinography is not usually necessary, but characteristically reflects inner retinal ischemia by a decrease in B-wave amplitude.

34.3 Diagnosis

Branch retinal artery occlusion, right eye.

34.4 Medical Management

The visual prognosis in BRAO is much better than for CRAO; 80% of eyes with BRAO eventually improve to 20/40 or better. Possibly, the most important aspect of medical management is diagnosing systemic conditions.

No specific ocular therapy has been proven to improve the visual prognosis. Systemic vascular disease may contribute to the arterial occlusion and predispose the patient to avoidable future stroke or heart attack. Indeed, in one study, CRAO patients had twice the mortality rate (56% 9-year survival) of age-matched controls. In acute cases, digital pressure on the globe for 15 seconds, followed by a sudden release, may dislodge or advance an embolus. Lowering the intraocular pressure with intravenous acetazolamide, topical intraocular pressure–lowering drops, or anterior chamber paracentesis, if less than 24 hours old, may also dislodge or advance an embolus. Augsburger and Magargal noted at least a three-line improvement in vision in 35% of eyes at 1 month after the acute event, when paracentesis was performed early. Inhalation of a mixture of 5% carbon dioxide and 95% oxygen (carbogen) or retrobulbar or systemically administered calcium channel blockers to promote vasodilation have been advocated, but the results are generally disappointing.

Retinal neovascularization may develop after BRAO, particularly in patients with diabetes mellitus. Iris neovascularization secondary to BRAO is extremely rare, but develops in up to 20% of eyes with CRAO within 12 weeks, especially when also associated with central vein occlusion. Full-scatter panretinal photocoagulation is effective in eradicating the new iris vessels in about two-thirds of cases. Ipsilateral carotid artery stenosis may also be present and be a cause of rubeosis iridis.

There is no good evidence that anticoagulation enhances prognosis in an isolated retinal arterial occlusion.

Studies using fibrinolytic agents have been reported, but have found limited use, presumably due to the need for prompt treatment, specialized catheterization techniques, or limited visual recovery.

34.5 Rehabilitation and Follow-up

The most important reason for follow-up examination is to monitor for subsequent neovascularization. Reinforcement of regimens prescribed by the patient's internist should be provided.

Rehabilitation efforts are not specific to arterial occlusive disease, and low vision aids as indicated may be sought. Prism glasses for patients with dense hemifield defects have been described, but are of limited general benefit.

Suggested Readings

[1] American Academy of Ophthalmology. Arterial Occlusive Disease. San Francisco, CA: American Academy of Ophthalmology; 1998

[2] Brown GC. Retinal arterial obstructive disease. In: Schachat AP, Murphy RB, Patz A, eds. Medical Retina. St. Louis, MO: CV Mosby; 1989

[3] Augsburger JJ, Magargal LE. Visual prognosis following treatment of acute central retinal artery obstruction. Br J Ophthalmol. 1980; 64(12):913–917

[4] Brown GC, Reber R. An unusual presentation of branch retinal artery obstruction in association with ocular neovascularization. Can J Ophthalmol. 1986; 21(3):103–106

[5] Kraushar MF, Brown GC. Retinal neovascularization after branch retinal arterial obstruction. Am J Ophthalmol. 1987; 104(3):294–296

[6] Brown GC, Shields JA. Cilioretinal arteries and retinal arterial occlusion. Arch Ophthalmol. 1979; 97(1):84–92

[7] Richard G, Lerche R-C, Knospe V, Zeumer H. Treatment of retinal arterial occlusion with local fibrinolysis using recombinant tissue plasminogen activator. Ophthalmology. 1999; 106(4):768–773

35 Central Retinal Vein Occlusion

William E. Smiddy

Abstract

Central retinal vein occlusion presents with a broad spectrum of severity. The most common systemic association in older patients is hypertension or its long-term sequelae, but the classic association with oral contraceptives in younger patients should be remembered. Other hypercoagulability conditions have also been associated. The diagnostic hallmark is intraretinal hemorrhage in all four quadrants, with collateralization at the disc being more prominent a bit later in the course. The degree of induced ischemia is usually the most important determinant of visual acuity, but the secondary macular edema may also play an important role in the visual acuity. Most important is that the macular edema represents a frequently reversible component for which intravitreal anti-vascular endothelial growth factor (anti-VEGF) or corticosteroid injection therapy may target. Similar to macular edema due to diabetic retinopathy, various treatment algorithms have been demonstrated to be beneficial in high proportions of patients. Optical coherence tomography plays a major role in directing the course of treatment. Neovascular glaucoma still occurs, and represents a source of catastrophic ocular demise, but in some cases may be controlled with anti-VEGF treatment in conjunction with panretinal photocoagulation especially if iris neovascularization can be detected early.

Keywords: central retinal vein occlusion, retina, venous occlusive disease, intravitreal injections, anti-VEGF, macular edema, neovascularization

35.1 History

A 45-year-old woman presented with a 3-week history of decreased vision in the right eye. Her only medications were oral contraceptives and did not have hypertension. The vision had gradually diminished during the first week after onset and then stabilized. Examination disclosed best corrected visual acuity of 20/100 OD and 20/20 OS. There was a right afferent pupillary defect. Slit-lamp examination showed no signs of iris neovascularization; the patient was pseudophakic with a clear posterior capsule. Intraocular pressures were 12 and 14 mm Hg, respectively. Funduscopic examination on the right showed intraretinal hemorrhage distributed throughout each quadrant with mild disc edema, but no definite collaterals (▶ Fig. 35.1). Macular edema was evident over about a disc area at the fovea. The cup-to-disc ratio was 0.3. Examination of the left eye was normal.

Fluorescein angiography showed good perfusion in the midperiphery and late dye leakage at the fovea. The optical coherence tomography (OCT) showed marked central macular edema (▶ Fig. 35.2).

Intravitreal triamcinolone was administered. The macular edema resolved, and remained resolved 3 months later (▶ Fig. 35.3) with improvement of vision to 20/30. However, the edema and visual loss recurred at 6 months at which time a second intravitreal triamcinolone was administered with similar resolution, but with recurrence only 3 months later. She has been maintained on intravitreal bevacizumab now about every 3 months with a stable OCT and visual acuity of 20/30.

Differential Diagnosis—Key Points

Acute visual loss typically suggests a vascular event. As in this case, acute visual loss may be followed by continued deterioration. Other abnormalities based on these historical features such as optic neuropathies must be considered but are usually distinguished by clinical examination features.

1. The pattern of intraretinal hemorrhages in this case markedly narrowed the differential diagnosis. Extensive intraretinal hemorrhages in all quadrants is a characteristic finding of central retinal vein occlusion (CRVO), and only in cases with less extensive hemorrhage does diagnostic confusion exist. The distribution of intraretinal hemorrhages in all quadrants distinguishes a CRVO from branch or hemiretinal vein occlusion. Diabetic retinopathy or advanced radiation retinopathy with diffuse intraretinal hemorrhage may mimic this entity, but those histories were lacking.

2. Confluent, extensive intraretinal hemorrhage may mimic subhyaloid or subretinal hemorrhage. Subretinal and subhyaloid hemorrhages are almost always consolidated rather than scattered, typically in the posterior pole.

3. The most common systemic disease associated with CRVO is hypertension. A majority of patients have hypertension, cardiovascular disease, or diabetes. CRVOs are unilateral in at least 95% of cases. This patient was taking oral contraceptives, which have been etiologically implicated as a risk factor for CRVO. Patients with bilateral CRVO more commonly have other systemic medical conditions such as hyperviscosity syndromes (e.g., multiple myeloma, macroglobulinemia, coagulation defects, or polycythemia vera). Systemic defects are found frequently enough in bilateral cases that systemic evaluation is recommended. Systemic evaluation in unilateral cases is usually limited to referral to a general medical doctor for a complete physical examination, especially for younger patients such as in this case. Cessation of the oral contraceptives was recommended. Patients with isolated unilateral CRVOs have such a low incidence of these systemic diseases that the medical workup is left to the discretion of the patient's ophthalmologist and internist.

35.2 Test Interpretation

The ophthalmoscopic appearance is typically characteristic and diagnostic. Fluorescein angiography may demonstrate retinal nonperfusion, which may provide prognostic information for the development of neovascular glaucoma. Lower visual acuity

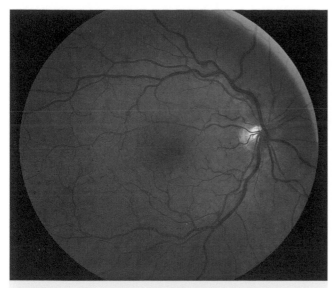

Fig. 35.1 Fundus photograph OD demonstrating intraretinal hemorrhage in all four quadrants and tortuous vessels. There are no collaterals. The visual acuity is 20/100.

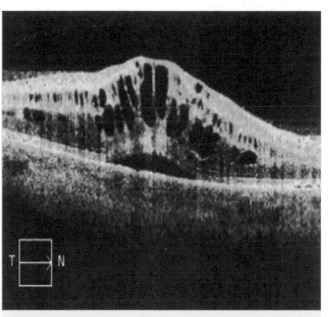

Fig. 35.2 The OCT OD marked intraretinal edema, consistent with the visual loss.

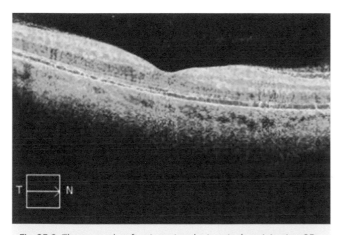

Fig. 35.3 Three months after intravitreal triamcinolone injection OD, the OCT shows resolution of the macular edema and visual acuity improvement to 20/30.

35.3 Diagnosis

CRVO, with secondary macular edema, OD.

35.4 Medical Management

The first step in the treatment of a patient with CRVO is identification and treatment of systemic disorders in concert with the patient's primary care physician; in this case, cessation of oral contraceptives was recommended due to its implication as a risk factor for venous thrombosis. Aspirin or other anticoagulants have been shown to decrease the risk of subsequent thrombotic events in systemic thrombotic conditions. This is the rationale behind aspirin therapy (80 mg daily) after CRVO. However, it is not infrequent that an incident patient was already taking aspirin or anticoagulants at the time of the vascular event, for other systemic vascular disorders. Thus, anticoagulants do not completely prevent vaso-occlusive disease, and since some side effects may occur, their use should be considered carefully for CRVO.

Management of patient with CRVO is in two categories: neovascularization of the anterior segment and macular edema.

Neovascularization, as in other retinal vascular disorders, is a response to ischemia. CRVOs have historically been divided into ischemic (complete, nonperfused) versus nonischemic (incomplete, well-perfused, or partial) vein occlusions. Approximately 30% of eyes with CRVO are nonperfused, and approximately half of these cases will develop neovascular glaucoma. Typically, the visual acuity is more profoundly diminished in such patients. The Central Vein Occlusion Study (CVOS) evaluate the role of prophylactic PRP in ischemic CRVO, finding that when severe retinal ischemia (at least 5 disc areas of nonperfusion) or rubeosis iridis should be treated with PRP. Eyes with vitreous hemorrhage or other media opacities that prevent laser treatment can

implies a higher risk group for more severe visual loss and poorer response to treatment.

Most useful, especially for assessing response to therapy, is OCT.

The electroretinogram may yield valuable information—the B wave arises in the inner nuclear layer of the retina (probably the Müller cells), and the A wave arises in the photoreceptors. A decreased B/A wave amplitude measuring less than 1.0 indicates ischemia and an increased risk of neovascular glaucoma. Cases with B/A ratios greater than 1.0 indicate that the ischemic injury has not disproportionally affected the portion of the retina subserved by the retinal versus choroidal circulation. Accordingly, such patients usually do not develop neovascular glaucoma.

be considered for cryopexy or vitrectomy, but carry a poor prognosis

Macular edema is the more common sight-threatening complication of CRVO that is encountered. The CVOS found grid photocoagulation not to be efficacious in patients with macular edema; although macular edema could be reduced, the visual outcomes were the same in control groups. However, intravitreal triamcinolone and anti-vascular endothelial growth factor agents have been found to be effective in ameliorating vision loss by decreasing macular edema. As with their use in other retinal vascular disorders, an initial period of more frequent injections (perhaps 4–6 weeks) can usually be followed by less frequent injections once the macular edema has resolved.

Laser treatment has been used and advocated to create a chorioretinal anastomosis, but its role is not well established. Pilot studies of intravenous or intravitreal fibrinolytic agents have been reported but, also, do not have proven efficacy.

35.5 Surgical Management

The role for surgical management is currently established only for media opacities preventing photocoagulation or for control of intraocular pressure in eyes with some visual potential. Glaucoma surgery is commonly done in conjunction with laser or retinal cryopexy. The most effective means of controlling the pressure in cases with neovascular glaucoma is placement of a shunt device.

35.6 Rehabilitation and Follow-up

The CVOS and other studies have found development of rubeotic glaucoma occurs 3 to 6 months after the onset of the CRVO. Thus, the recommended interval for follow-up examinations (if injection therapy is not instituted) is monthly for 6 months after diagnosis. After 1 year, the incidence of rubeosis is extremely low unless a previously perfused case converts to a nonperfused case. This transition is usually heralded by a decrease in visual acuity.

Suggested Reading

[1] Central Vein Occlusion Study Group. Argon laser photocoagulation for macular edema in branch vein occlusion. Arch Ophthalmol. 1997; 115:486–491

[2] Fekrat S, Goldberg MF, Finkelstein D. Laser-induced chorioretinal venous anastomosis for nonischemic central or branch retinal vein occlusion. Arch Ophthalmol. 1998; 116(1):43–52

[3] Lloyd MA, Heuer DK, Baerveldt G, et al. Combined Molteno implantation and pars plana vitrectomy for neovascular glaucomas. Ophthalmology. 1991; 98 (9):1401–1405

[4] McAllister IL, Douglas JP, Constable IJ, Yu DY. Laser-induced chorioretinal venous anastomosis for nonischemic central retinal vein occlusion: evaluation of the complications and their risk factors. Am J Ophthalmol. 1998; 126(2): 219–229

[5] Sabates R, Hirose T, McMeel JW. Electroretinography in the prognosis and classification of central retinal vein occlusion. Arch Ophthalmol. 1983; 101 (2):232–235

[6] Haller JA, Bandello F, Belfort R, Jr, et al. OZURDEX GENEVA Study Group. Randomized, sham-controlled trial of dexamethasone intravitreal implant in patients with macular edema due to retinal vein occlusion. Ophthalmology. 2010; 117(6):1134–1146.e3

[7] Jonas JB, Kreissig I, Degenring RF. Intravitreal triamcinolone acetonide as treatment of macular edema in central retinal vein occlusion. Graefes Arch Clin Exp Ophthalmol. 2002; 240(9):782–783

[8] Wu L, Arevalo JF, Berrocal MH, et al. Comparison of two doses of intravitreal bevacizumab as primary treatment for macular edema secondary to central retinal vein occlusions. Retina. 2010; 30:1002–1011

[9] Ip MS, Scott IU, VanVeldhuisen PC, et al. SCORE Study Research Group. A randomized trial comparing the efficacy and safety of intravitreal triamcinolone with observation to treat vision loss associated with macular edema secondary to central retinal vein occlusion: the Standard Care vs Corticosteroid for Retinal Vein Occlusion (SCORE) study report 5. Arch Ophthalmol. 2009; 127(9):1101–1114

[10] Brown DM, Campochiaro PA, Singh RP, et al. CRUISE Investigators. Ranibizumab for macular edema following central retinal vein occlusion: six-month primary end point results of a phase III study. Ophthalmology. 2010; 117(6): 1124–1133.e1

[11] Brown DM, Heier JS, Clark WL, et al. Intravitreal aflibercept injection for macular edema secondary to central retinal vein occlusion: 1-year results from the phase 3 COPERNICUS study. Am J Ophthalmol. 2013; 155(3):429–437.e7

36 Branch Retinal Vein Occlusion

William E. Smiddy

Abstract

Branch retinal vein occlusion has a wide spectrum of involvement, but is usually less severe than central retinal venous occlusive disease. While systemic hypertension is more common in patients with this condition, it is not universal and is more commonly spontaneous and unassociated with systemic diseases. Retinal neovascularization may occur, but is not common. Sectoral scatter laser photocoagulation has been demonstrated long ago to be a useful modality to prevent progressive fibrovascular proliferation and vitreous hemorrhage, and is still an important treatment in such cases. The more common vision-threatening aspect is macular edema. While focal laser has been proven beneficial to prevent additional visual loss, its role has mostly been supplanted by intravitreal therapy with corticosteroids or anti-vascular endothelial growth factor therapy. Treatment protocols have been defined through many clinical trials, but generally parallel those for macular edema due to other etiologies such as central retinal vein occlusion and diabetic macular edema. Similarly, optical coherence tomography monitoring is the mainstay of determining how to modify or to direct ongoing treatment.

Keywords: branch retinal vein occlusion, retinal occlusive disease, macular edema, neovascularization, intravitreal injection, anti-VEGF

36.1 History

A 66-year-old man had a 2-month history of decreased vision OS characterized by a central scotoma that was centered superatemporally. He had a 20-year history of hypertension that he reported was well controlled on medications. The visual acuity was 20/200 at first presentation, OS. A branch retinal vein occlusion (BRVO) was diagnosed.

The right eye had previously incurred a central retinal vein occlusion (CRVO) that responded to several injections of several anti-vascular endothelial growth factor (anti-VEGF) agents, as well as a couple of intravitreal triamcinolone injections. The visual acuity OD had improved from 20/400 to 20/80 after resolution of the macular edema.

The intraocular pressures were 15 mm Hg in each eye. Funduscopic examination OD showed a dry macula with collateral vessels at the optic nerve head. In the left eye, there was an anomalous arterial venous crossing along the inferotemporal arcade with dot-and-blot hemorrhages extending from the midportion of the inferotemporal arcade posteriorly into the macula. There was moderate to marked macular edema (▶ Fig. 36.1).

Intravitreal bevacizumab was administered without improvement, followed by aflibercept which had a better effect and has been applied for about a year every 6 weeks. The visual acuity has stabilized at 20/70 (▶ Fig. 36.2).

Differential Diagnosis—Key Points

This patient presented initially with intraretinal hemorrhages and macular edema that involved the fovea. Although neovascularization and vitreous hemorrhage were absent, these can be additional features of a BRVO. Intraretinal hemorrhage, macular edema, and retinal neovascularization with or without vitreous hemorrhage have distinct differential diagnoses.

1. The most common cause of intraretinal hemorrhage is diabetic retinopathy. Characteristically, this is associated with microaneurysms in a distribution that involves many if not all quadrants and, importantly, usually both eyes, generally to a similar degree. More severe diabetic retinopathy is accompanied by intraretinal microvascular abnormalities, lipid exudates, venous beading, and other signs of ischemia including neovascularization. Less common causes of intraretinal hemorrhage include radiation retinopathy and various forms of uveitis. CRVO is characterized by intraretinal hemorrhages in all quadrants. In this case, the intraretinal hemorrhages were present segmentally in the distribution of the inferotemporal branch retinal vein.

2. Retinal neovascularization is a response to ischemia. This, too, is commonly associated with diabetic retinopathy, but may be difficult to distinguish from patients with BRVOs. However, as with intraretinal hemorrhages, other features of diabetic retinopathy are usually more prominent in a more generalized distribution in contrast to the segmental distribution seen with BRVOs. A vitreous hemorrhage may accompany any disease process with retinal neovascularization. Other causes of retinal neovascularization and/or vitreous hemorrhage include the sickle cell retinopathies and various forms of uveitis.

3. With chronicity, there may be vascular collateralization, commonly prominent at the nerve head. These collaterals may mimic retinal neovascular vessels. The fluorescein angiogram may be valuable in differentiating between the two entities, as neovascularization classically displays fluorescein leakage.

36.2 Test Interpretation

Clinical examination is the most important diagnostic test in making the diagnosis. However, ancillary tests include fundus photography, fluorescein angiography, and optical coherence tomography (OCT) may confirm the clinical diagnosis but are most helpful in monitoring and directing therapy. Fundus photography may allow easier detection of diabetic retinopathy and, consequently, earlier detection of neovascularization.

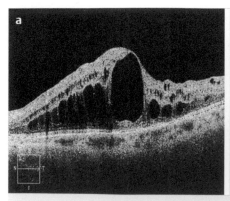
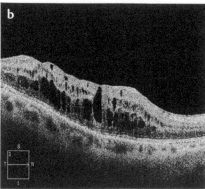
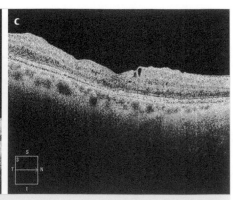

Fig. 36.1 (a) OCT appearance of the left eye with substantial macular edema distributed inferonasally, but spreading into the center. Vision was 20/200. (b) OCT appearance of the right eye at presentation and (c) after treatment with many intravitreal agents for a central retinal vein occlusion. The marked intraretinal edema has resolved with vision OD of 20/80.

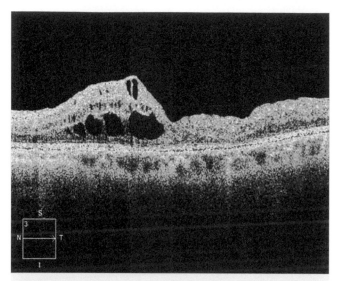

Fig. 36.2 OCT appearance 6 months later, OS, after intravitreal bevacizumab and, subsequently, aflibercept that has been required every 6 weeks to maintain regression of the edema. The vision has stabilized at 20/70.

Fluorescein angiography is valuable in assessing the retinal perfusion status. Although this does not direct treatment, it may influence the frequency of follow-up examinations to look for the onset of retinal neovascularization. The fluorescein angiogram may also depict a characteristic segmental pattern of retinal vascular leakage. While this may confirm the presence of the macular edema, it does not necessarily diagnose its cause. Relying solely on clinical examination, the macular edema may be mimicked by zones of nonperfusion or ischemia, causing diagnostic uncertainty; the angiogram usually clarifies this and may disclose unsuspected areas of retinal neovascularization and distinguish neovascularization (which is characterized by dye leakage) from collateral vessels (which do not leak dye).

36.3 Diagnosis

BRVO with macular edema, OS.

36.4 Medical Management

Systemic hypertension is a risk factor for the development of a vein occlusion, but it does not appear to be an independent risk factor for the severity of the course once a vein occlusion occurs. However, the ophthalmologist should encourage maximal control of hypertension in all patients. Other risk factors that are less firmly established include patients with diabetes, other cardiovascular disease, glaucoma, increased body mass at age 20, hyperopia, higher serum cholesterol, lower high-density liquid protein levels, a variety of less clinically apparent coagulation disorders, and alcohol consumption. Systemic evaluation for an isolated BRVO is probably only warranted for a younger patient or with bilateral disease, but the ophthalmologist is encouraged to notify the patient's primary care physician of such an occurrence.

The mainstay of medical management was laser photocoagulation for many years, and may still be employed in selected cases. The Branch Vein Occlusion Study (BVOS) studied laser photocoagulation in patients with complications due to BRVO. The most common complication of BRVO is macular edema which may be self-limited with a fair degree and frequency of spontaneous resolution. However, the BVOS established that when the visual acuity is 20/40 or worse for at least 3 months, then a focal grid photocoagulation pattern is recommended in the area of edema; 63% of treated eyes gained two lines or more of vision compared to 36% of untreated control eyes after 3 years of follow-up.

The BVOS also recommended scatter laser photocoagulation be performed in the quadrant of the vein occlusion when neovascularization ensues. While the exact pathogenesis of retinal vein occlusion is uncertain, occlusion of the vein typically occurs at the crossing point of an artery where the artery and vein share a common adventitial sheath, suggesting a role for endothelial damage due to chronic turbulence of flow. Furthermore, the artery usually passes anterior to the vein, in contrast to a random distribution in unaffected eyes. It has been observed that the neovascularization commonly occurs in front of the vein, rather than from the arteries. It was found that the incidence of vitreous hemorrhages decreased from approximately 60% in controls to 30% of laser-treated patients with neovascularization.

Prophylactic laser treatment in patients with fluorescein angiographically defined retinal capillary nonperfusion (larger than 5 disc diameters in width) was also evaluated by the BVOS, with the conclusion the frequency of neovascularization was too infrequent to be justified.

The advent of intravitreal therapy for retinal vascular disease has prompted many controlled clinical trials which have demonstrated that intravitreal triamcinolone as well as the gamut of anti-VEGF agents generally offers better final visual acuity and resolution of macular edema compared to focal laser, and are now the mainstay of treatment of macular edema secondary to BRVO. As with their use in treating other retinal vascular conditions, the frequency of treatment can often be extended after initial control of the edema.

Anticoagulant treatment has not been shown to be beneficial in the prevention or management of BRVO. However, as with the treatment of other nonocular vaso-occlusive disorders, aspirin therapy is often prescribed.

36.5 Surgical Management

The role of vitrectomy in eyes with BRVO is limited to nonclearing vitreous hemorrhage or tractional and/or rhegmatogenous macular detachment from fibrovascular proliferation in more severe cases. In some cases, an epiretinal membrane may occur. Usually, an epiretinal membrane induces minimal visual loss, but if the vision decreases below about 20/60, vitrectomy with membrane peeling may be considered. Surgical decompression of the common adventitial sheath at the block site should still be considered experimental.

36.6 Rehabilitation and Follow-up

Patients presenting with BRVO and vision better than 20/32 should be followed every 3 to 6 months initially, as laser and intravitreal drug trials usually studied patients with at least this degree of visual loss. Treatment is generally recommended for patients presenting macular edema causing visual loss at and below these visual acuity levels.

While there are various treatment frequency regimens studied by clinical trials, generally the clinician institutes intravitreal therapy initially (perhaps every 4–6 weeks), followed by less frequent injections depending on the clinical response. Studies comparing the results of the various agents have not been published for BRVO patients. Switching to other agents is considered if there is inadequate response after a course of initial treatment.

Segmental scatter photocoagulation to the affected zones is recommended if retinal neovascularization is detected. Vitrectomy is an option for nonclearing vitreous hemorrhage or for progressive fibrovascular proliferation causing visually important traction retinal detachment. Some have advocated optic nerve sheath decompression or lysis of the common adventitial sheath at the occlusion site in selected cases.

Suggested Reading

[1] The Branch Vein Occlusion Study Group. Argon laser photocoagulation for macular edema in branch vein occlusion. Am J Ophthalmol. 1984; 98(3):271–282

[2] Branch Vein Occlusion Study Group. Argon laser scatter photocoagulation for prevention of neovascularization and vitreous hemorrhage in branch vein occlusion. A randomized clinical trial. Arch Ophthalmol. 1986; 104(1):34–41

[3] Finkelstein D, Clarkson J, Diddie K, et al. Branch Vein Occlusion Study Group. Branch vein occlusion. Retinal neovascularization outside the involved segment. Ophthalmology. 1982; 89(12):1357–1361

[4] Duker JS, Brown GC. Anterior location of the crossing artery in branch retinal vein obstruction. Arch Ophthalmol. 1989; 107(7):998–1000

[5] The Eye Disease Case-control Study Group. Risk factors for branch retinal vein occlusion. Am J Ophthalmol. 1993; 116(3):286–296

[6] Ikuno Y, Ikeda T, Sato Y, Tano Y. Tractional retinal detachment after branch retinal vein occlusion. Influence of disc neovascularization on the outcome of vitreous surgery. Ophthalmology. 1998; 105(3):417–423

[7] Opremcak EM, Bruce RA. Surgical decompression of branch retinal vein occlusion via arteriovenous crossing sheathotomy: a prospective review of 15 cases. Retina. 1999; 19(1):1–5

[8] Osterloh MD, Charles S. Surgical decompression of branch retinal vein occlusions. Arch Ophthalmol. 1988; 106(10):1469–1471

[9] Smiddy WE, Isernhagen RD, Michels RG, Glaser BM, de Bustros SN. Vitrectomy for nondiabetic vitreous hemorrhage. Retinal and choroidal vascular disorders. Retina. 1988; 8(2):88–95

[10] Scott IU, Ip MS, VanVeldhuisen PC, et al. SCORE Study Research Group. A randomized trial comparing the efficacy and safety of intravitreal triamcinolone with standard care to treat vision loss associated with macular Edema secondary to branch retinal vein occlusion: the Standard Care vs Corticosteroid for Retinal Vein Occlusion (SCORE) study report 6. Arch Ophthalmol. 2009; 127(9):1115–1128

[11] Haller JA, Bandello F, Belfort R, Jr, et al. OZURDEX GENEVA Study Group. Randomized, sham-controlled trial of dexamethasone intravitreal implant in patients with macular edema due to retinal vein occlusion. Ophthalmology. 2010; 117(6):1134–1146.e3

[12] Campochiaro PA, Heier JS, Feiner L, et al. BRAVO Investigators. Ranibizumab for macular edema following branch retinal vein occlusion: six-month primary end point results of a phase III study. Ophthalmology. 2010; 117(6):1102–1112.e1

[13] Wu L, Arevalo F, Berrocal MH, et al. Comparison of two doses of intravitreal Bevacizumab as primary treatment for macular edema secondary to branch retinal vein occlusions (PACORES Group). Retina. 2009; 29:1396–1403

37 Nonexudative Age-Related Macular Degeneration

John Edward Legarreta

Abstract

The hallmark of nonexudative (or atrophic) age-related macular degeneration (AMD) is drusen, which frequently coexists with a variable degree of atrophy of the retinal pigment epithelium (RPE) in the macula. The size of the drusen and degree of atrophy are generally related to degree of visual loss, and form the basis for consideration of the efficacy of preventative vitamin therapy. Nonexudative maculopathy is distinguished from exudative AMD by the lack of exudation on imaging studies such as fluorescein angiography or optical coherence tomography. Fundus autofluorescence might demonstrate more widespread atrophic RPE changes than color photographs or clinical examination suggests, and may be an important parameter for evaluating future therapies directed at atrophic AMD. At the present time, the only established treatment strategy is the prophylactic benefit of vitamin supplementation as defined in the Age-Related Eye Disease Study. Patients with more severe degrees of visual loss may benefit from a low vision evaluation resulting in low vision aids strategically targeted to their needs, but this is generally palliative in extent. A key importance in recognizing the eye with atrophic AMD is to prompt awareness on the part of the patient and monitoring by the physician for the development of exudative AMD.

Keywords: drusen, autofluorescence, AREDS, metamorphopsia

37.1 History

A 68-year-old man presented for follow-up retina evaluation for nonexudative macular degeneration in both eyes. Vision was stable per patient and the patient had no prior history of laser or intravitreal injections. Visual acuity was 20/50 on the right and 20/60 on the left. Pupil examination was normal and intraocular pressures were within normal limits in both eyes. Slit-lamp examination showed mild to moderate nuclear sclerotic lens opacities in both eyes. Funduscopic examination showed cup-to-disc ratios of 0.3 in the right eye and 0.5 in the left eye without glaucomatous atrophy. The macular examination was notable for marked retinal pigment epithelium (RPE) depigmentation with drusen and central macular atrophy in both eyes (▶ Fig. 37.1). There was no subretinal or intraretinal fluid, blood, or exudate.

Optical coherence tomography (OCT) was performed in both eyes and showed drusen and central RPE atrophy in both eyes (▶ Fig. 37.2). There was no evidence of macular fluid. Fundus autofluorescence (FAF) was performed which showed central hypo-autofluorescence in both eyes (▶ Fig. 37.3).

Observational follow-up was recommended and the patient was instructed to continue to use the Amsler grid daily, to continue AREDS2 vitamin supplementation, and to have a diet with sufficient green, leafy vegetables.

Differential Diagnosis—Key Points

1. Correlating the degree of visual loss to the ophthalmoscopically evident degree of RPE depigmentary change in patients with bilateral drusen and atrophy may be inaccurate. Confluent, geographic atrophy of the RPE involving the central macula and fovea is associated with visual loss, but there may be a large degree of variability to the vision loss depending on the degree of atrophy of the outer retina. A disparity in the visual acuity from substantial visual loss out of proportion to the degree of pigmentation raises the possibility of occult exudative disease or coexisting diagnoses. Common coexisting disease processes include nuclear sclerotic cataract, vascular occlusive disease, amblyopia, or optic neuropathies. The normal clinical history, pupillary responses, and the normal-appearing optic nerve head seem to rule these out.

2. OCT was obtained which ruled out choroidal neovascularization. Typically, with choroidal neovascularization, there is subretinal or intraretinal fluid and/or sub- or intraretinal hemorrhage. These findings were lacking in this case. Additionally, the central macular thickness was thin in both eyes, but the remaining retinal thickness appears to be normal, and it is likely that the photoreceptors are not as atrophic as on the appearance on OCT, which can explain why the patient has better than expected vision given the appearance on clinical exam and imaging.

3. Pattern dystrophies, inflammatory-induced changes, trauma-induced RPE changes, or other degenerations such as Stargardt's or cone dystrophy may mimic atrophic, nonexudative age-related macular degeneration (AMD). The pattern of symmetry or clinical history of onset of visual loss, as well as OCT features, usually allows a distinction between atrophic AMD and these other entities.

37.2 Diagnosis

Nonexudative age-related macular degeneration, OU.

37.3 Test Interpretation

OCT has replaced fluorescein angiography as the first-line test for determining whether or not exudative disease is present as well as determining the extent of geographic atrophy. FAF may enhance the assessment of the extent of RPE pigmentary changes in atrophic disease, since the contrast between depigmented RPE and relatively normal RPE may be less obvious ophthalmoscopically, especially in lightly pigmented patients.

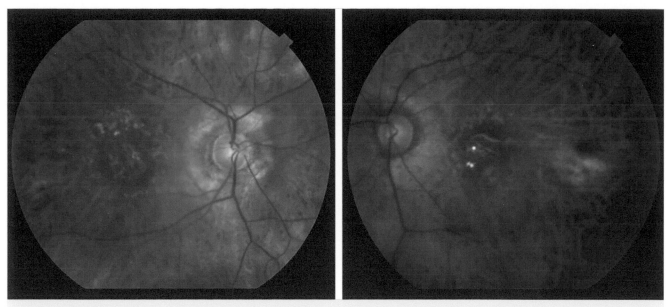

Fig. 37.1 Funduscopic appearance of patient with nonexudative AMD in both eyes. No subretinal fluid was detected, but there is moderate to amount of depigmentary changes, drusen, and macular atrophy in both eyes.

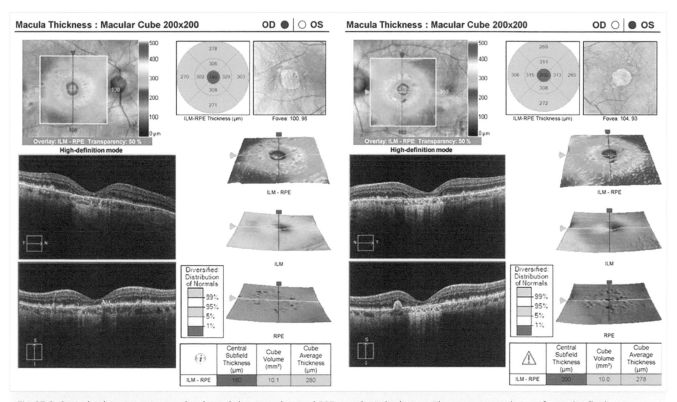

Fig. 37.2 Optical coherence tomography showed drusen and central RPE atrophy in both eyes. There was no evidence of macular fluid.

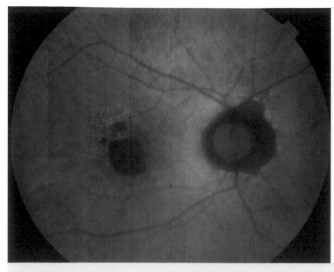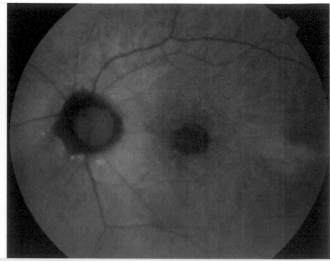

Fig. 37.3 Fundus autofluorescence showed central hypo-autofluorescence in both eyes.

Other testing that might be pertinent in such patients includes tests to rule out other causes of potential visual loss such as a visual field test, color vision, and potential acuity meter testing. Potential acuity meter testing may yield falsely better result in patients with exudative disease.

Another test that is sensitive, but not specific, is Amsler grid testing. This is a semi-quantitative way of ascertaining whether the quality of vision is decreased in a manner consistent with an alteration in the RPE or subretinal space. Although it is only a minority of cases in which the Amsler grid test detected transition to exudative disease, it remains a useful tool if applied as a means of monitoring a patient at risk of developing exudative maculopathy.

37.4 Medical Management

At the current time, individuals with intermediate nonexudative AMD or advanced nonexudative AMD or exudative AMD in the other eye should have dietary supplementation with AREDS2 vitamins. Studies have shown that vitamin supplementation has some benefit in slowing the progression to advanced AMD in about 25% of patients. Additionally, patients are encouraged to avoid tobacco smoking. At the time of this publication, several clinical trials are under way targeting several pathways involving the pathogenesis of nonexudative AMD; however, no treatment has been proven efficacious to date.

37.5 Rehabilitation and Follow-up

Low vision aids are the primary rehabilitative tools for patients with substantial visual loss. These usually restore a marginal degree of visual function, but may be helpful for specific tasks. The key component in the patient with limited macular function is identifying the most convenient and effective means of providing magnification and delivering light to the subject material. Frequently, patients find that focused light is helpful, whereas bright overhead lights tend to be too diffuse to be of benefit. For distance vision, a variety of telescopic aids are available, but magnification comes at the expense of constricting the visual field. Patients considering low vision evaluation must be counseled candidly as to the limits of potential benefits. Still, low vision aids offer at least a modest degree of satisfaction in a majority of patients.

Patients with nonexudative macular degeneration are routinely counseled to use the Amsler grid test for optimal diagnosis of transition to exudative disease. In addition, they are encouraged to evaluate each eye's perception independently for deviation of straight lines such as those in doorways, light poles, and building edges.

Examination every 3 to 12 months is generally recommended by most clinicians, depending on the stability of the exam and testing. It is emphasized to the patient that any changes in visual symptoms, especially increased metamorphopsia, should prompt immediate reevaluation.

Suggested Reading

[1] American Academy of Ophthalmology. Comprehensive Adult Eye Evaluation, Preferred Practice Pattern. San Francisco, CA: American Academy of Ophthalmology; 1997

[2] American Academy of Ophthalmology. Rehabilitation: The Management of Adult Patients with Low Vision, Preferred Practice Pattern. San Francisco, CA: American Academy of Ophthalmology; 1994

[3] Cho E, Hung S, Seddon JM. Age-related macular degeneration: nutrition. In: Berger JW, Fine SL, Maguire MG, eds. Age-Related Macular Degeneration; Philadelphia, PA: Mosby; 1999:57–67

[4] Klein R, Klein BEK, Jensen SC, Meuer SM. The five-year incidence and progression of age-related maculopathy: the Beaver Dam Eye Study. Ophthalmology. 1997; 104(1):7–21

[5] Smiddy WE, Fine SL. Prognosis of patients with bilateral macular drusen. Ophthalmology. 1984; 91(3):271–277

[6] Lim LS, Mitchell P, Seddon JM, Holz FG, Wong TY. Age-related macular degeneration. Lancet. 2012; 379(9827):1728–1738

[7] Jager RD, Mieler WF, Miller JW. Age-related macular degeneration. N Engl J Med. 2008; 358(24):2606–2617

[8] Age-Related Eye Disease Study 2 Research Group. Lutein + zeaxanthin and omega-3 fatty acids for age-related macular degeneration: the Age-Related Eye Disease Study 2 (AREDS2) randomized clinical trial. JAMA. 2013; 309 (19):2005–2015

[9] Fung AE, Lalwani GA, Rosenfeld PJ, et al. An optical coherence tomography-guided, variable dosing regimen with intravitreal ranibizumab (Lucentis) for neovascular age-related macular degeneration. Am J Ophthalmol. 2007; 143 (4):566–583

38 Exudative Age-Related Macular Degeneration

John Edward Legarreta

Abstract

The definitional features of exudative age-related macular degeneration (AMD) include hemorrhage and exudation of fluid or exudate into the intraretinal, subretinal, and subretinal pigment epithelial (retinal pigment epithelium [RPE]) spaces, in the setting of an eye with other atrophic RPE findings such as drusen. The source of these sight-threatening features is choroidal neovascularization (choroidal neovascular membrane [CNVM]), which may form either under the retina or RPE. Symptoms include loss of central vision and metamorphopsia. Imaging modalities include fluorescein angiography and, more so, optical coherence tomography. The mainstay of treatment has become intravitreal injections of anti-vascular endothelial growth factor agents—bevacizumab, ranibizumab, and aflibercept. There is a variety of strategies for the frequency of application of these agents. These have demonstrated unprecedented efficacy compared to those previously available for quenching the growth of the CNVM, yet still there is a large unmet need for preserving or restoring lost vision. Furthermore, these injections typically require long-term, repetitive therapy. The previous distinction between classic and nonclassic CNVM characteristics is of less therapeutic importance than previously delineated. Other causes of CNVM that might mimic the diagnosis of exudative AMD include the presumed ocular histoplasmosis syndrome, myopic degeneration, and idiopathic CNVM. Each of these is generally treated in a similar fashion.

Keywords: choroidal neovascularization, optical coherence tomography, anti-VEGF, intravitreal injection

38.1 Case Report

An 87-year-old woman presented complaining of decreased vision in her right eye. She had a prior history of nonexudative age-related macular degeneration (AMD) in both eyes.

Examination showed vision of 20/40 in the right eye and 20/50 in the left eye. There was no definite afferent pupillary defect. Slit-lamp examination showed the patient to be pseudophakic in both eyes. Intraocular pressures were within normal limits in each eye. Funduscopic examination on the right showed drusen with retinal pigment epithelium (RPE) changes in the macula with new subretinal fluid and pigment epithelial detachment. No hemorrhage was noted. On the left, there were drusen with RPE changes in the macula but no hemorrhage was noted.

Optical coherence tomography (OCT) was performed (▶ Fig. 38.1), and in the right eye, it showed a pigment epithelial detachment with adjacent subretinal fluid. The left eye showed drusen with no evidence of macular fluid. Fluorescein angiography (FA) (▶ Fig. 38.2) was performed, and in the right eye, it showed delayed stippled hyperfluorescence with late leakage, consistent with an occult choroidal neovascular membrane (CNVM). The patient underwent an intravitreal injection of bevacizumab and was instructed to follow up in 4 weeks.

Differential Diagnosis—Key Points

1. Decreased vision in a patient with nonexudative AMD must always be evaluated for the possible conversion to an exudative process. The presence of macular fluid with or without the presence of hemorrhage is typical of a CNVM and can be confirmed with OCT and/or FA imaging.

2. Subretinal hemorrhage is typically a consequence of subretinal choroidal neovascularization. However, in rare instances severe intraretinal hemorrhages from retinal vascular disease, trauma, or a retinal tear may also lead to subretinal hemorrhage. Subretinal hemorrhages may extend substantially, even after initial onset. Usually, with choroidal neovascularization, there is relatively localized hemorrhage, but in rare cases a massive subretinal hemorrhage may affect the entire macula or be even more extensive.

3. The differential diagnosis of subretinal hemorrhage and subretinal fluid is, for the most part, the differential diagnosis of subretinal choroidal neovascularization. The most common cause of choroidal neovascularization is AMD. The hallmark of macular degeneration is the RPE changes with drusen. These should be demonstrable either within the same eye or in the fellow eye. The presumed ocular histoplasmosis syndrome is another common cause of choroidal neovascularization, but is usually accompanied by other stigmata such as atrophic "punched-out" choroidal scars ("histo spots"). A third cause of subretinal neovascularization, hemorrhage, and fluid association is myopic degeneration with widespread RPE depigmentary changes or staphyloma formation. A fourth category is so-called idiopathic neovascularization. Other causes are much rarer.

38.2 Diagnosis

Occult choroidal neovascularization with subretinal fluid and pigment epithelial detachment secondary to a new conversion to exudative AMD in the right eye.

38.3 Test Interpretation

OCT is the gold standard for determining the presence or absence of macular fluid in the retina, and thus defining the presence or absence of choroidal neovascularization. FA, though no longer the gold standard or primary test in most patients, still has utility in helping define the type choroidal neovascularization and in cases where the clinical presentation and OCT imaging are unable to determine a clear diagnosis. A classic CNVM on FA demonstrates filling in the early frames, with leakage of the membrane in the later frames. Such features are used to define either "classic" or "nonclassic" portions of the membrane. The terms "poorly defined" and "occult choroidal neovascularization" describe membranes that are more extensive

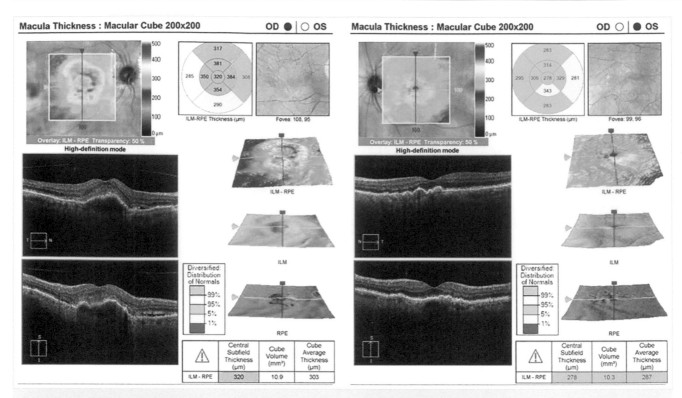

Fig. 38.1 Optical coherence tomography in the right eye showed a pigment epithelial detachment with adjacent subretinal fluid. The left eye showed drusen with no evidence of macular fluid.

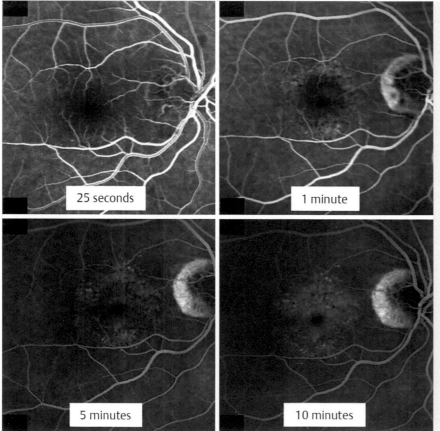

25 seconds

1 minute

5 minutes

10 minutes

Fig. 38.2 Fluorescein angiographic appearance in the right eye showed delayed stippled hyperfluorescence with late leakage, consistent with an occult choroidal neovascular membrane.

than the area of apparent dye leakage, as in the example in this case.

38.4 Medical Treatment

The first established treatment of choroidal neovascularization was thermal laser photocoagulation; photodynamic therapy (commonly called "cold laser") was an important advance that utilized a photosensitizing agent to target the abnormal vessels. However, the advent of intravitreal antiangiogenic (anti-vascular endothelial growth factor [anti-VEGF]) therapy has surpassed all other treatment modalities and is the first choice of treatment for patients with exudative AMD. Pegaptanib, bevacizumab, ranibizumab, and aflibercept are the four antiangiogenic agents that can be injected intravitreally but, presently, pegaptanib is rarely used and bevacizumab, ranibizumab, and aflibercept are the three commonly used medications.

As for the treatment strategy, three treatment algorithms have emerged:
1. Monthly: An anti-VEGF agent is injected every 4 weeks. The goal of this approach is to prevent the accumulation of blood and fluid due to the underlying exudative process. This approach was initially used in many of the early clinical trials, but has now become the least popular approach compared with the other two techniques.
2. Pro re nata or "as needed": An anti-VEGF agent is injected every time fluid or blood is present, as detected on exam and imaging. The primary goal with this approach is to minimize the number of injections and to only give injections when exudation is present.
3. Treat-and-extend: An anti-VEGF agent is injected when fluid or blood is present. The patient is then brought back at a set interval, and if there is no blood or fluid on the follow-up exam, the patient is given another injection and the interval between follow-up visits (time between injections) is lengthened. The typical increment for lengthening between exams is usually 1 to 2 weeks. If, on a follow-up exam, there is blood or fluid present, the patient is injected and the interval between visits decreases to the last interval where the patient did not have blood or fluid on exam. The primary goal with this approach is to extend a patient to the maximum interval of visits before blood or fluid reappears.

38.5 Rehabilitation and Follow-up

Macular degeneration is the most common cause of significant, irreversible visual loss in the elderly population. Low vision rehabilitation, including magnifiers and focused lights, should be considered in these cases. However, before embarking on the purchase of such equipment, the patient must be counseled as to the limitations and expense involved.

Suggested Reading

[1] Macular Photocoagulation Study Group. Argon laser photocoagulation for ocular histoplasmosis. Results of a randomized clinical trial. Arch Ophthalmol. 1983; 101(9):1347–1357

[2] Macular Photocoagulation Study Group. Recurrent choroidal neovascularization after argon laser photocoagulation for neovascular maculopathy. Arch Ophthalmol. 1986; 104(4):503–512

[3] Macular Photocoagulation Study Group. Argon laser photocoagulation for neovascular maculopathy. Three-year results from randomized clinical trials. Arch Ophthalmol. 1986; 104(5):694–701

[4] Wood WJ, Smith TR. Senile disciform macular degeneration complicated by massive hemorrhagic retinal detachment and angle closure glaucoma. Retina. 1983; 3(4):296–303

[5] de Juan E, Jr, Machemer R. Vitreous surgery for hemorrhagic and fibrous complications of age-related macular degeneration. Am J Ophthalmol. 1988; 105 (1):25–29

[6] Macular Photocoagulation Study Group. Krypton laser photocoagulation for neovascular lesions of age-related macular degeneration. Results of a randomized clinical trial. Arch Ophthalmol. 1990; 108(6):816–824

[7] Macular Photocoagulation Study Group. Argon laser photocoagulation for neovascular maculopathy. Five-year results from randomized clinical trials. Arch Ophthalmol. 1991; 109(8):1109–1114

[8] Macular Photocoagulation Study Group. Laser photocoagulation of subfoveal neovascular lesions in age-related macular degeneration. Results of a randomized clinical trial. Arch Ophthalmol. 1991; 109(9):1220–1231

[9] Merrill PT, LoRusso FJ, Lomeo MD, Saxe SJ, Khan MM, Lambert HM. Surgical removal of subfoveal choroidal neovascularization in age-related macular degeneration. Ophthalmology. 1999; 106(4):782–789

[10] Thomas MA, Kaplan HJ. Surgical removal of subfoveal neovascularization in the presumed ocular histoplasmosis syndrome. Am J Ophthalmol. 1991; 111(1):1–7

[11] Lambert HM, Capone A, Jr, Aaberg TM, Sternberg P, Jr, Mandell BA, Lopez PF. Surgical excision of subfoveal neovascular membranes in age-related macular degeneration. Am J Ophthalmol. 1992; 113(3):257–262

[12] Berger AS, Kaplan HJ. Clinical experience with the surgical removal of subfoveal neovascular membranes. Short-term postoperative results. Ophthalmology. 1992; 99(6):969–975, discussion 975–976

[13] Ormerod LD, Puklin JE, Frank RN. Long-term outcomes after the surgical removal of advanced subfoveal neovascular membranes in age-related macular degeneration. Ophthalmology. 1994; 101(7):1201–1210

[14] Lopez PF, Grossniklaus HE, Lambert HM, et al. Pathologic features of surgically excised subretinal neovascular membranes in age-related macular degeneration. Am J Ophthalmol. 1991; 112(6):647–656

[15] American Academy of Ophthalmology. Indocyanine green angiography. Ophthalmology. 1998; 105(8):1564–1569

[16] Scott IU, Smiddy WE, Schiffman J, Feuer WJ, Pappas CJ. Quality of life of low-vision patients and the impact of low-vision services. Am J Ophthalmol. 1999; 128(1):54–62

[17] Lewis H, Kaiser PK, Lewis S, Estafanous M. Macular translocation for subfoveal choroidal neovascularization in age-related macular degeneration: a prospective study. Am J Ophthalmol. 1999; 128(2):135–146

[18] Miller JW, Schmidt-Erfurth U, Sickenberg M, et al. Photodynamic therapy with verteporfin for choroidal neovascularization caused by age-related macular degeneration: results of a single treatment in a phase 1 and 2 study. Arch Ophthalmol. 1999; 117(9):1161–1173

[19] Ciulla TA, Rosenfeld PJ. Anti-vascular endothelial growth factor therapy for neovascular age-related macular degeneration. Curr Opin Ophthalmol. 2009; 20:158–165

[20] Solomon SD, Lindsley K, Vedula SS, Krzystolik MG, Hawkins BS. Anti-vascular endothelial growth factor for neovascular age-related macular degeneration. Cochrane Database Syst Rev. 2014; 29(8):CD005139

[21] Fung AE, Lalwani GA, Rosenfeld PJ, et al. An optical coherence tomography-guided, variable dosing regimen with intravitreal ranibizumab (Lucentis) for neovascular age-related macular degeneration. Am J Ophthalmol. 2007; 143 (4):566–583

39 Myopic Degeneration

Amir Mohsenin and William E. Smiddy

Abstract

Myopic degeneration parallels age-related macular degeneration in the categorization into atrophic versus neovascular forms and in treatment of neovascularization. The pathophysiology seems similar in that visual loss follows from progressive retinal pigment epithelium atrophy and may culminate in the egress of choroidal neovascular vessels through attenuated areas of Bruch's membrane. Although the neovascularization is commonly more self-limited than in exudative AMD, mitigation strategies can preserve somewhat better vision than natural history. Recently, anti-vascular endothelial growth factor (anti-VEGF) treatment with ranibizumab has been approved, and efficacy with other anti-VEGF agents has been reported; these are now the mainstays for treatment of neovascular forms. There is still no treatment for atrophic forms, despite many investigators over the years experimenting with limiting staphylomata, but this is an area where stem cells or even gene therapy might prove useful in the future.

Keywords: choroidal neovascularization, myopia, macula, anti-VEGF, intravitreal injections

39.1 History

A 38-year-old urologist presented with a 1-year history of visual loss in the right eye. He had been told that he had a choroidal neovascular membrane (CNVM) in the right eye that was not amenable to any treatment. At the time of presentation, he had a 1-month history of distortion with a paracentral scotoma in his left eye. The patient was noted to be a high myope with a spherical equivalent refraction of –10 diopters.

Examination disclosed vision of 20/200 in the right eye and 20/20 in the left eye. The slit-lamp examination was unremarkable. The funduscopic examination showed a tilted (myopic) disc and a pigmented CNVM surrounded by pigment epithelial atrophy (▶ Fig. 39.1). In the left eye, there was a similar tilted myopic disc with a prominent lacquer crack extending across the superior aspect of the fovea with some hemorrhage on the nasal side of the fovea (▶ Fig. 39.2). The fluorescein angiogram confirmed the large subfoveal CNVM in the right eye (▶ Fig. 39.3). However, it also showed a smaller, extrafoveal CNVM superior to the left fovea.

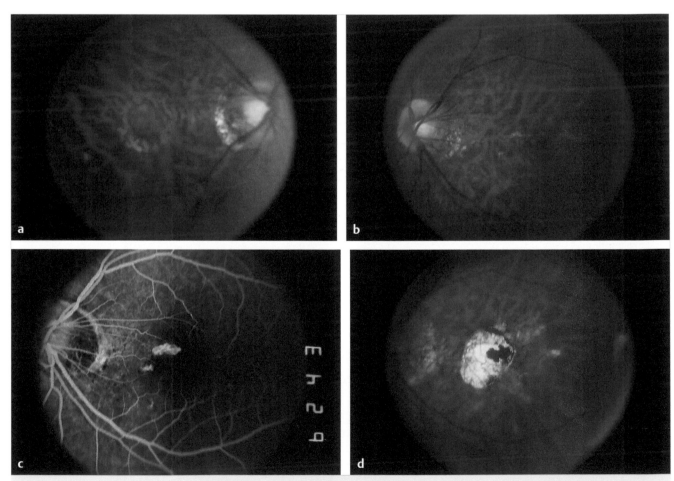

Fig. 39.1 Funduscopic appearance of right eye at presentation. A rim of retinal pigment epithelial atrophy surrounds a central area of choroidal neovascularization. The optic nerve head is tiled with some peripapillary atrophy. The vision was 20/200.

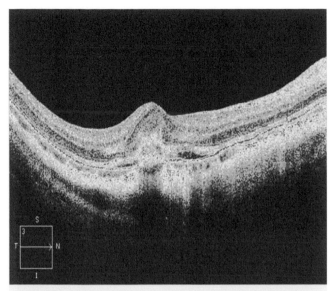

Fig. 39.2 Funduscopic appearance of left eye. A lacquer crack is evident coursing across the superior macula. Along the nasal aspect of this is slight subretinal fluid consistent with a choroidal neovascular membrane.

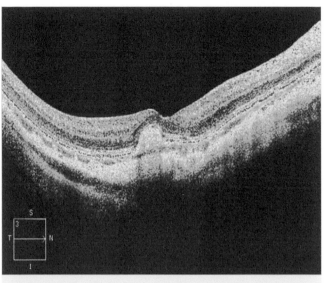

Fig. 39.3 Fluorescein angiographic appearance of the right eye at initial presentation. It shows a large subfoveal choroidal neovascular membrane. The broad margin of a chorioretinal atrophy surrounds the area of choroidal neovascularization.

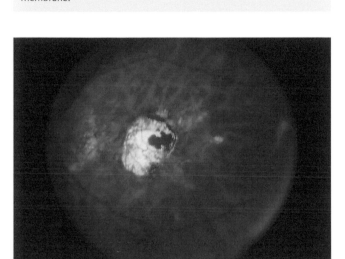

Fig. 39.4 Fluorescein angiographic appearance 6 years after treatment confirms a juxtafoveal recurrence of the choroidal neovascularization inferior and temporal to the original scar.

No treatment was recommended for the right eye. Argon blue-green laser treatment was recommended and performed for the CNVM in the left eye. The patient maintained 20/20 vision in the left eye without recurrent neovascularization for 6 years.

He then returned with a 1-month history of decreased central vision in the left eye. He characterized the loss of vision as finding everything to be cloudy. The visual acuity was 20/200 in the right eye and 20/30 in the left eye. The slit-lamp examination was unremarkable. The funduscopic examination of the right eye showed a somewhat enlarged area of retinal pigment epithelium atrophy approximately three times the size of the original (untreated) CNVM. There were signs of chronic leakage. In the left eye, there was a nearly one-disc-area region of retinal pigment epithelial atrophy corresponding to the previous laser treatment scar. However, along the inferior and temporal (foveal side) of this there was evidence of recurrent CNVM (▶ Fig. 39.4).

Laser treatment was performed utilizing the krypton laser in the left eye. The patient returned to Peru for further follow-up examination locally.

The patient had a history of glaucoma for which he was using Propine drops OU initially. Upon presentation, his glaucoma regimen had been changed to a beta-blocker OU. The intraocular pressures were 14 mm Hg in the right eye and 13 mm Hg in the left eye on second presentation and 9 mm Hg in the right eye and 12 mm Hg in the left eye upon initial presentation. Also, retinal lattice degeneration was noted in the periphery of both eyes, although no atrophic holes were seen in association with this.

Differential Diagnosis—Key Points

1. Pathologic myopia with CNVM. The patient was a high myope (−10 D). Myopic degeneration characteristically occurs only in patients with high myopia (> 6 diopter refractive error).
2. Fundus characteristics of pathologic myopia can include a tilted optic nerve head, posterior staphyloma, lacquer cracks, and retinal lattice degeneration. Peripapillary retinal pigment epithelial atrophy is often present and can make assessment of glaucomatous optic nerve changes difficult.
3. The patient also had retinal lattice degeneration, without atrophic holes. Prophylactic treatment of such lesions is probably not indicated at this stage. If the fellow eye (especially if highly myopic) developed a retinal detachment, then the patient would be at a higher risk for developing a retinal detachment in the fellow and prophylactic laser or retinocryopexy treatment should be considered, but many would still not recommend treatment.

4. The fluorescein angiogram and clinical features show characteristic features of CNVM. There are several conditions that may be the cause of choroidal neovascularization. Most common is age-related macular degeneration, but this is unlikely in this young patient. Other causes of choroidal neovascularization include presumed ocular histoplasmosis syndrome, which is usually accompanied by atrophic chorioretinal scars ("histo spots") distributed throughout the retina, typically most prominently in the midperiphery. These were not present in this case. Any chorioretinal scar, whether it is from previous inflammatory or from infectious chorioretinitis, may ultimately give rise to choroidal neovascularization.

5. A trauma-induced choroidal rupture may also be the site of choroidal neovascularization, and should be considered in the differential diagnosis.

39.2 Diagnosis

Subretinal choroidal neovascularization and recurrence secondary to myopic degeneration, OU.

39.3 Diagnostic Tests

Aside from clinical examination, the fluorescein angiogram remains the gold standard for the diagnosis and delineation of a CNVM. Indocyanine green (ICG) angiography may also contribute information regarding the nature and location of more poorly defined CNVM. Optical coherence tomography (OCT) has become an essential tool in both the diagnosis and management of macular edema associated with CNVMs. In addition, OCT can aid in the diagnosis of myopic macular schisis. Combined A- and B-scan ultrasonography may demonstrate the increased axial length or a staphyloma that commonly accompanies patients with myopic degeneration.

39.4 Medical Treatment

Intravitreal injection of anti-vascular endothelial growth factor (anti-VEGF) agents is the mainstay treatment for myopic CNVM. The safety and efficacy profile of intravitreal anti-VEGF injections has largely been established from studies investigating their role in the treatment of neovascular macular degeneration. Anti-VEGF injections have been shown to be effective as monotherapy for myopic CNVM and studies comparing bevacizumab to ranibizumab have shown similar efficacy.

Other treatment modalities have also been tested. Prior to the advent of anti-VEGF agents, photodynamic therapy (PDT) with verteporfin was a commonly used therapy. Studies comparing anti-VEGF to PDT have shown anti-VEGF to be superior while the benefit of combining anti-VEGF and PDT has not been well established. Laser photocoagulation has also been utilized as primary treatment for selected neovascular membranes.

Choroidal neovascularization is seen in about 5% of patients with axial length > 26.5 mm, is bilateral in 12% of those cases, and is often represented as a Fuchs' spot—a subfoveal dark spot generally accepted to represent a late, self-limited stage of neovascularization. There may be two types of neovascularization, with elderly patients having a more progressive form of vessel growth and younger patients frequently having a more focal, self-limited form that causes less visual loss. Lacquer cracks (characteristic breaks in Bruch's membrane) appear to represent the point of entry for choroidal neovascularization, as they have been found to be more frequent in cases with neovascular membranes. Frequently, the patient will present with focal, well-defined choroidal neovascularization surrounded by retinal pigment epithelial atrophy. Such cases (as in this patient's right eye) are characteristically not accompanied by significant subretinal fluid.

39.5 Surgical Management

Surgical intervention for myopic CNVM has fallen to the wayside largely in favor of medical management. Pars plana vitrectomy with excision of subretinal CNVMs carries significant risks including but not limited to retinal detachment and endophthalmitis. Visual acuity gains after surgery are modest at best and inferior to anti-VEGF monotherapy.

39.6 Rehabilitation and Follow-up

Patients with nonexudative myopic degeneration may commonly suffer visual symptoms just as severe as those with exudative complications. Specifically, a loss of central vision from a moderate-to-severe degree is extremely common. Patients are typically recommended for follow-up examinations twice annually; however, patients should monitor their central visual acuity with an Amsler grid. New distortion or central metamorphopsia should prompt ophthalmological consultation.

In cases of myopic CNVM, follow-up examinations are typically performed 4 weeks following initial anti-VEGF treatment. The follow-up interval can later be extended based on response to treatment and stability. OCT is usually performed at each visit in order to identify subclinical CNVM or for the development of macular schisis.

Rehabilitation efforts include the use of low vision aids. Typically, with the loss of macular function, the need for magnifiers and focal delivery of light are the general strategies. These may take the form of high plus lenses in a spectacle, magnifying loupes, telescopic magnification lenses, or closed circuit video instruments. There is some promise in the possible use of implantable microchip technology, but this technology is still in its infancy.

Suggested Readings

[1] Avila MP, Weiter JJ, Jalkh AE, Trempe CL, Pruett RC, Schepens CL. Natural history of choroidal neovascularization in degenerative myopia. Ophthalmology. 1984; 91(12):1573–1581

[2] Hera R, Chiquet C, Romanet JP. Surgical removal of subfoveal choroidal neovascularization in pathologic myopia: a 12-year follow-up study. Int Ophthalmol. 2013; 33(6):671–676

[3] Hotchkiss ML, Fine SL. Pathologic myopia and choroidal neovascularization. Am J Ophthalmol. 1981; 91(2):177–183

[4] Rabb MF, Garoon I, LaFranco FP. Myopic macular degeneration. Int Ophthalmol Clin. 1981; 21(3):51–69

[5] Soubrane G, Pison J, Bornert P, Perrenoud F, Coscas G. Néo-vaisseaux sous-rétiniens de la myopie dégénérative: résultats de la photocoagulation. Bull Soc Ophtalmol Fr. 1986; 86(3):269–272

[6] Wang E, Chen Y. Intravitreal anti-vascular endothelial growth factor for choroidal neovascularization secondary to pathologic myopia: systematic review and meta-analysis. Retina. 2013; 33(7):1375–1392

40 Idiopathic Central Serous Chorioretinopathy

Ella Leung

Abstract

Central serous chorioretinopathy (CSCR) is characterized by the detachment of the neurosensory retina from the underlying retinal pigment epithelium. Risk factors include steroids, type A personality, and pregnancy. Most CSCRs resolve spontaneously within 3 months. Treatment for persistent cases includes photodynamic therapy.

Keywords: central serous chorioretinopathy, neurosensory detachment, subretinal fluid, macular detachment, photodynamic therapy

40.1 Case History

A 35-year-old engineer presented with blurriness in his left eye for 3 weeks. He denies any past medical history, trauma, diabetes, hypertension, steroids, or previous surgeries. On examination, the visual acuity was 20/20 in the right eye and 20/50 in the left eye. With a +2.00 lens, the vision in the left eye improved to 20/30. Anterior segment examination and intraocular pressures were unremarkable in both eyes. A dilated fundus examination of the right eye was normal. The left eye had an elevated, circumscribed neurosensory detachment of the retina.

There were no retinal tears, hemorrhages, or exudates. The patient noted central metamorphopsia on Amsler grid testing of his left eye. On optical coherence tomography (OCT), there was subretinal fluid under the fovea in the left eye. Fluorescein angiography (FA) of the left eye revealed an expanding area of leakage in the macula (▶ Fig. 40.1).

The patient was observed closely. One month later, the subretinal fluid completely resolved, and the vision returned to 20/20.

Table 40.1 Risk factors associated with central serous chorioretinopathy

Pharmacologic	Systemic	Other
Corticosteroids	Hypertension	Idiopathic
Psychotropic medications	Systemic lupus erythematosus	
	Pregnancy	
	Cushing's disease	
	Helicobacter pylori infection	

Differential Diagnosis—Key Points

1. Albrecht von Graefe first described a central serous detachment of the retina in 1866, calling it recurrent central retinitis. Others have named it capillarospastic central retinitis, central angiospastic retinopathy, and chorioretinopathia centralis serosa.[1] In the 1960s, Donald Gass introduced the term "central serous chorioretinopathy" (CSCR). The range of names reflect the hypothesized etiologies and differential diagnoses for the disease.

2. The pathophysiology of CSCR is unclear. It may be related to increased aldosterone causing an upregulation of potassium channels in the choroidal endothelial cells, leading to fluid leakage, choroidal thickening, increased hydrostatic pressure, defects in the retinal pigment epithelium (RPE), and subsequent accumulation of subretinal fluid.[2,3] Steroids can precipitate or exacerbate the condition. Other reported risk factors include male gender, type A personalities, excess stress, psychotropic medications, Cushing's disease, hypertension, and pregnancy (▶ Table 40.1).[1,4]

3. The differential diagnoses of CSCR include serous retinal detachments due to vascular, inflammatory, neoplastic, and anatomic abnormalities of the macula (▶ Table 40.2). A thorough history and appropriate imaging can help determine the diagnosis.

4. CSCR typically causes serous detachments in young to middle-aged men, while choroidal neovascular membranes (CNVMs) from exudative age-related macular degeneration appear as gray or yellow-green plaques in older individuals.[1] Eyes with CNVMs from primary ocular histoplasmosis have peripapillary atrophy and punched-out chorioretinal lesions. Polypoidal choroidal vasculopathy features grapelike clusters of dilated vessels that are most characteristically imaged with indocyanine green angiography. Isolated cavernous or capillary hemangiomas appear as collections of dilated, tortuous blood vessels. Diffuse choroidal hemangiomas in Sturge–Weber syndrome cause the fundus to appear red-orange "ketchup" in color.

5. Local or systemic inflammation may result in cystoid macular edema and subretinal fluid. Patients with posterior scleritis have pain, thickened sclera, and a possible "T sign" on echography. Sympathetic ophthalmia has a preceding history of trauma or surgery. Patients with Vogt–Koyanagi–Harada disease may have

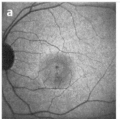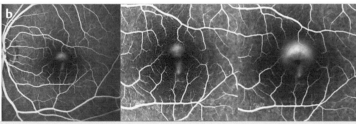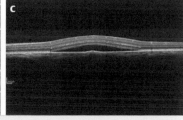

Fig. 40.1 (a) A red-free photo of the patient with central serous chorioretinopathy in the left eye. (b) Fluorescein angiography demonstrated leakage in the macula. (c) Heidelberg OCT showed subretinal fluid under the fovea. (The images are provided courtesy of Luiz Roisman, MD.)

Table 40.2 Differential diagnoses of neurosensory retinal detachment involving the macula

Vascular	Inflammatory	Neoplastic	Anatomic
Age-related macular degeneration	Posterior scleritis	Choroidal melanoma	Optic nerve pit
Choroidal neovascular membrane	Sympathetic ophthalmia	Choroidal nevus	
Choroidal hemangioma	Vogt–Koyanagi–Harada disease	Leukemia	
Polypoidal choroidal vasculopathy		Metastatic carcinoma	

systemic manifestations such as poliosis, vitiligo, tinnitus, and a positive family history. CSCR, on the other hand, is painless without signs of intraocular inflammation.

6. Benign and malignant neoplasms, such as choroidal melanomas and atypical choroidal nevus, may cause serous retinal detachments. Choroidal melanomas are classically elevated, dome-shaped brown masses and may have orange pigment. Leukemia and carcinoma can present as yellow-white choroidal infiltrates or vitritis. Congenital abnormalities such as optic disc pits may result in fluid extending from the optic nerve margin to the macula. CSCR is not due to other ocular pathologies.

40.2 Imaging and Workup

The diagnosis of CSCR is based on the appropriate clinical setting, physical examination, and exclusion of other causes of neurosensory detachments. CSCR can be visualized on fundus examination as a circumscribed neurosensory detachment of the macula. There may be a hyperopic shift, metamorphopsia, mild dyschromatopsia, reduced contrast sensitivity, and decreased visual acuity. Retinal pigment epithelium mottling may indicate areas of prior leakage.

On OCT, there is fluid between the neurosensory retina and RPE. Enhanced depth imaging OCT may show a thickened choroid with increased choroidal vascular diameters.[3] FA or indocyanine green angiography may demonstrate midphase hyperfluorescent plaques. The pathognomonic "smokestack" on FA is found only in a minority of patients; more commonly, "ink-blots" or expanding pinpoint leakages from focal RPE defects are seen.[3] Diffuse leakage may occur in cases of bullous CSCR.[3] Hyperautofluorescent areas of leakage and fluid tracts on fundus autofluorescence can become hypoautofluorescent over time. Scotomas on microperimetry may develop and correlate with the affected areas.[1] Multifocal electroretinograms can demonstrate depression beyond the areas of serous detachment.[3]

40.3 Diagnosis

Central serous chorioretinopathy.

40.4 Treatment

40.4.1 Medical Management

CSCR is usually a self-limited disease that resolves spontaneously within 3 months. Treatment may be considered in chronic cases or for occupational purposes. Stopping systemic corticosteroids may lead to faster resolution of CSCR, while increasing corticosteroids may exacerbate the disease.

Systemic treatments that have been investigated include oral rifampin, methotrexate, carbonic anhydrase inhibitors, adrenergic receptor antagonists such as metoprolol and propranolol, and aldosterone or mineralocorticoid receptor antagonists such as ketoconazole, mifepristone, eplerenone, spironolactone, and finasteride.[1] These treatments have yet to be shown in prospective, randomized-controlled trials to significantly improve visual acuity.[5] Although *Helicobacter pylori* has been associated with CSCR, treating the infection has not been shown to have a beneficial effect on vision.[6]

In chronic cases, photodynamic therapy (PDT) or focal argon laser applied to the point of leakage may lead to fluid resorption. The laser may stimulate the RPE to increase resorption of subretinal fluid, or it may cause temporary vascular hypoperfusion with subsequent remodeling.[7] A meta-analysis found that PDT was superior to focal laser photocoagulation and anti-vascular endothelial growth factor injections in resolving subretinal fluid.[8] Indirect laser may also be used to barricade the area of leakage. Potential complications include scotomas, subretinal neovascularization, and expansion of the laser burns.[3] Other treatments currently being investigated include subthreshold micropulse laser and transpupillary thermotherapy.

40.4.2 Surgical Management

There are no surgical treatment options for CSCR.

40.5 Rehabilitation and Follow-up

CSCR resolves spontaneously in 60 to 80% of patients within 3 months, although there may be residual mottling of the retinal pigment epithelium.[3] CSCR can recur in 18 to 50% of patients, and 20% of patients may develop CSCR in the contralateral eye.[3]

References

[1] Nicholson B, Noble J, Forooghian F, Meyerle C. Central serous chorioretinopathy: update on pathophysiology and treatment. Surv Ophthalmol. 2013; 58 (2):103–126
[2] Salz DA, Pitcher JD, III, Hsu J, et al. Oral eplerenone for treatment of chronic central serous chorioretinopathy: a case series. Ophthalmic Surg Lasers Imaging Retina. 2015; 46(4):439–444
[3] Liegl R, Ulbig MW. Central serous chorioretinopathy. Ophthalmologica. 2014; 232(2):65–76
[4] Yannuzzi LA. Type-A behavior and central serous chorioretinopathy. Retina. 1987; 7(2):111–131
[5] Shulman S, Goldenberg D, Schwartz R, et al. Oral Rifampin treatment for longstanding chronic central serous chorioretinopathy. Graefes Arch Clin Exp Ophthalmol. 2015
[6] Dang Y, Mu Y, Zhao M, Li L, Guo Y, Zhu Y. The effect of eradicating Helicobacter pylori on idiopathic central serous chorioretinopathy patients. Ther Clin Risk Manag. 2013; 9:355–360
[7] Watzke RC, Burton TC, Woolson RF. Direct and indirect laser photocoagulation of central serous choroidopathy. Am J Ophthalmol. 1979; 88(5):914–918
[8] Ma J, Meng N, Xu X, Zhou F, Qu Y. System review and meta-analysis on photodynamic therapy in central serous chorioretinopathy. Acta Ophthalmol. 2014; 92(8):e594–e601

41 Epiretinal Membrane

Ajay E. Kuriyan

Abstract

Epiretinal membranes (ERMs) are commonly seen patients and can be visually significant. Clinical exam and optical coherence tomography are used to diagnose ERMs. Vitrectomy and ERM peel, with or without internal limiting membrane peel, is employed in cases of visually significant ERMs.

Keywords: epiretinal membrane, macular pucker, cellophane maculopathy, vitrectomy

41.1 History

A 73-year-old woman presented with an 18-month history of progressively decreasing vision in the right eye. She had metamorphopsia and best corrected Snellen visual acuity of 20/200. A retinal detachment was repaired with a primary pars plana vitrectomy, endolaser, and gas 2 years previously. Funduscopic examination of the right eye showed a prominent epiretinal membrane (ERM) with moderate vascular distortion (▶ Fig. 41.1). Optical coherence tomography (OCT) demonstrated an ERM with an abnormal foveal contour (▶ Fig. 41.2)

Differential Diagnosis—Key Points

1. There are relatively few entities to consider in the differential diagnosis of an appearance such as this one. Cystoid macular edema may give the appearance of a more diffuse preretinal membrane, probably because of the altered reflection created by a stippling of the internal retinal surface induced by the edema. A diagnostic subset of an ERM is the vitreomacular traction formation that follows a zone of incomplete posterior vitreous separation. Folds in the retina associated with current or previous hypotony retinopathy may also simulate the clinical appearance of an ERM, but the OCT usually distinguishes it by virtue of lacking preretinal tissue. Additionally, the OCT of a patient with choroidal folds from hypotony will have folds in the retinal pigment epithelium (RPE) layer on OCT, which would not be present in patients with ERMs.
2. The classification of ERMs is generally based on morphology or etiology. Morphology runs a full spectrum from mild cellophanelike changes (cellophane maculopathy or surface wrinkling retinopathy) to a more severe distortion of the macular components (macular pucker). All of these terms describe ERMs. The etiologic groups are idiopathic or secondary ERMs. Posterior vitreous separation may be a stimulating factor for the formation of idiopathic membrane. As a general rule, the clinical appearances of idiopathic and secondary ERMs are the same, although membranes following retinal tear or detachment may be prominently pigmented; it is the history and other associative features that may allow one to distinguish between these diagnoses. Entities that cause secondary ERM include a retinal break formation (as in this patient) with or without retinal detachment, inflammatory disorders, retinal vascular disorders, trauma, or previous surgery.
3. The classic symptomatology includes a subacute onset of decreased vision most commonly characterized by metamorphopsia. The visual loss may be biphasic; not infrequently, the first phase of visual loss may be more generalized and attributable to debris in a separated vitreous. Usually, the ERM has formed maximally by 3 to 6 months and its appearance or effect on vision changes little thereafter. Associated features include the distortion of the macular vessels, which may in turn cause a vascular leakage (▶ Fig. 41.3, not the patient in this case) and cystoid edema (▶ Fig. 41.4, not the patient in the case), obstructed axoplasmic flow, and, in the most severe cases, a low-lying tractional retinal detachment. Cases secondary to previous retinal detachment may have a pigmented component to the ERM, but the vast majority of idiopathic and secondary cases are translucent.

41.2 Test Interpretation

The principal test that is routinely utilized to evaluate ERM is OCT, which allows visualization of the hyperreflective membrane on the surface of the retina. Distortion of the foveal contour, increased foveal thickness, and, in some patients, cystoid edema can be seen using OCT. Additionally, hyporeflective changes in the outer retinal structures (e.g., ellipsoid zone disruption) can be visualized with OCT. However, this can be due to shadowing artifact from inner retina hyperreflective changes secondary to the ERM. Shadowing artifact can be detected by assessing relative hyporeflectivity of the RPE layer on OCT.

Although rarely performed for ERMs, fluorescein angiography demonstrates mild diffuse retinal vascular leakage seen throughout the distribution of the ERM. This is in contrast to cases of diabetic macular edema, in which the leakage is typically more focal in areas of leaking microaneurysm, or cases of cystoid macular edema, in which the leakage is centered on the fovea. The vascular distortion may be more apparent on fluorescein angiography than on clinical examination. Ultrasound is rarely used in this diagnosis, but may show a high posterior vitreous separation that may be of some value in distinguishing this from an impending or full-thickness macular hole in which the posterior vitreous separation may not yet have occurred.

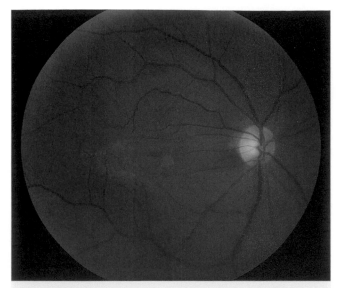

Fig. 41.1 Clinical appearance immediately before epiretinal membrane peeling. The epiretinal membrane can be seen most prominently temporal to the fovea. There is vascular distortion that is most apparent temporally.

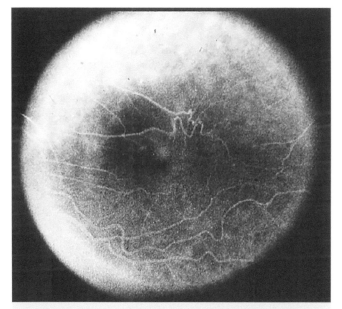

Fig. 41.3 Fluorescein angiography of a different patient, which demonstrates more prominent vascular distortion superotemporal to the fovea. There are several areas of focal leakage in association with these distorted vessels. Most prominent is an area of focal leakage superior to the fovea.

41.3 Diagnosis

ERM secondary to previous peripheral retinal break and retinal detachment, right eye.

41.4 Medical Management

Medical management may involve treatment of an underlying inflammatory disorder. There is no known medical treatment

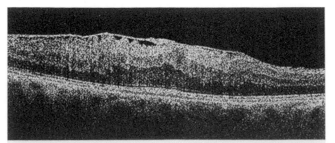

Fig. 41.2 Optical coherence tomography immediately before epiretinal membrane peeling. The hyperreflective epiretinal membrane can be seen on the surface of the retina. There is foveal contour distortion and thickening of the retina.

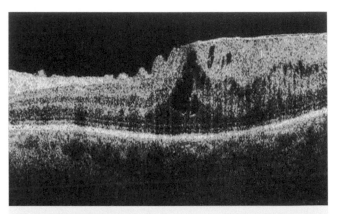

Fig. 41.4 Optical coherence tomography of a different patient who presented with an epiretinal membrane shows cystoid macular edema.

for ERMs secondary to peripheral retinal breaks or idiopathic membranes. Observational follow-up examination is recommended when the visual acuity loss and symptoms are minimal. ERMs normally form over a few months, but usually do not cause any additional visual loss after their formation. Thus, a patient may be reassured that visual acuity, once stable, will likely not decline further.

41.5 Surgical Management

Once the attributable best corrected visual acuity reaches the 20/40 to 20/60 range or worse, or in selected cases in which the visual acuity is better but the metamorphopsia is more severe and out of proportion to the visual acuity, surgical treatment may be considered. Surgical treatment includes vitrectomy, which is typically facilitated by a preexisting posterior vitreous detachment. Next, the ERM is engaged with a vitreoretinal pick. If there is not an edge under which the pick can be safely placed, a sharp instrument such as a barbed MVR blade is used to cut down and create an edge in the macula. Typically, the thickest part of the ERM is sought in such cases. Naturally, the center of the fovea should be avoided whenever possible in developing such an edge. The membrane is then gently raised from the retinal surface, ideally releasing any adhesions from the macula first. Once approximately half of the circumference

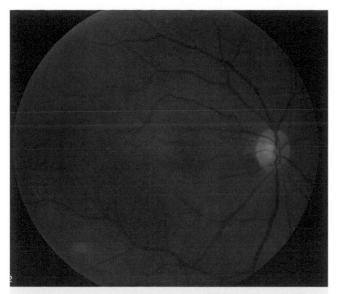

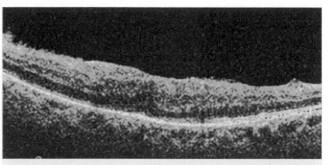

Fig. 41.6 Optical coherence tomography 6 weeks after epiretinal membrane peeling surgery. The hyperreflective epiretinal membrane is no longer seen on the surface of the retina. There is greatly improved foveal contour distortion and thickening of the retina.

Fig. 41.5 Clinical appearance 6 weeks following the removal of the epiretinal membrane. Vision is improved to 20/60 and the distortion and surface opacities are markedly improved.

of the membrane has been released, intraocular forceps are used to complete the removal of the membrane in one large piece. Often, the internal limiting membrane is removed along with this. When the ERM is thinner, it may be necessary to remove it in multiple pieces.

The patient in this case underwent a vitrectomy with removal of the ERM. By 3 months postoperative, the visual acuity had improved to 20/60 and her metamorphopsia had markedly improved. The appearance of the macula showed no evidence of ERM formation (▶ Fig. 41.5). The postoperative OCT showed decreased foveal thickness and improvement of the foveal contour (▶ Fig. 41.6).

41.6 Rehabilitation and Follow-up

Postoperative treatment typically involves topical corticosteroid and antibiotic drops. The visual acuity improves most rapidly during the 6 weeks following surgery and is usually maximally improved by 3 to 6 months postoperatively. There may be small degrees of improvement even after this. The surgical complication rate is acceptably low with less than 5% of patients developing any complication (the most common complication is retinal detachment). Phakic patients have an extremely high rate of progressive nuclear sclerosis, as do all eyes after vitrectomy, but cataract surgery may be performed in an uncomplicated fashion. Most series of ERM report visual acuity improvement of a magnitude of approximately 50 in 80% of cases. The recurrence of ERMs is very rare, with less than 3% developing a clinically significant recurrence. The most important prognostic factor associated with best overall final vision is good preoperative vision.

Suggested Reading

[1] Michels RG. Vitrectomy for macular pucker. Ophthalmology. 1984; 91(11): 1384–1388

[2] Song SJ, Kuriyan AE, Smiddy WE. Results and prognostic factors for visual improvement after pars plana vitrectomy for idiopathic epiretinal membrane. Retina. 2015; 35(5):866–872

[3] Smiddy WE, Maguire AM, Green WR, et al. Idiopathic epiretinal membranes: ultrastructural characteristics and clinicopathologic correlation. 1989. Retina. 2005; 25(5) Suppl:811–820, discussion 821

[4] Gao Y, Smiddy WE. Morphometric analysis of epiretinal membranes using SD-OCT. Ophthalmic Surg Lasers Imaging. 2012; 43(6) Suppl:S7–S15

42 Vitreomacular Traction

Thalmon R. Campagnoli and William E. Smiddy

Abstract

Vitreomacular traction has become recognized as a more common and more varied condition with the advent of spectral-domain optical coherence tomography (OCT) testing. However, OCT testing must be used in conjunction with clinical assessment of symptoms and clinical course to determine if any intervention is necessary. Only cases that are symptomatic, seemingly progressive, and causing enough visual loss to be inducing more than a minimal degree of visual loss should even be considered for intervention. Intervention classically was limited to surgical intervention, but intravitreal injection of ocriplasmin has now become available as an approved treatment modality; however, cases with a limited zone of vitreofoveal attachment, those without associated epiretinal proliferation, and younger, phakic patients are probably the ideal candidates. Even more recently, there has been a resurgence of interest and good reported results with using simply an expansile intravitreal gas injection in such cases ("pneumatic maculopexy"). In addition, expectant observation has been demonstrated to be a suitable approach, especially for cases with minimal or no symptoms. The OCT is invaluable as an adjunct for diagnosis and monitoring.

Keywords: vitreomacular traction, vitreous detachment, macular hole, ocriplasmin, intravitreal injection, vitrectomy

42.1 History

A 78-year-old woman presented with a 3-month history of progressively worsening blurred vision and metamorphopsia in the right eye interfering with driving and reading abilities. The vision was 20/60 OD and 20/40 OS. Slit-lamp examination demonstrated clear cornea, absence of cataract, and intraocular pressure of 13 mm Hg in both eyes (OU). Fundoscopic examination showed focal areas of adherent posterior vitreous to the macula associated with raised retinal tissue, OD, and a nonspecific loss of foveal reflex, OS. Optical coherence tomography (OCT) in OD demonstrated a hyperreflective layer correspondent to the posterior hyaloid partially attached to the macula, leading to elevation and distortion of the retina (▶ Fig. 42.1). The OCT OS also showed focal vitreomacular attachment with distortion of the inner foveal layers.

An intravitreal ocriplasmin injection was performed OD, without improvement in vision or OCT appearance after 1 month (▶ Fig. 42.1b). A pars plana vitrectomy (PPV) was performed OD with release of the vitreomacular traction (VMT) and improvement of the foveal contour (▶ Fig. 42.2). The vision was 20/30 OD 1-month postoperatively. The OS has remained unchanged with vision of 20/40 without clinically important or progressive symptoms, so it has been observed.

Differential Diagnosis—Key Points

1. This patient developed VMT. VMT is a vitreoretinal interface abnormality originated by the elevation of the posterior cortical vitreous when it is incompletely separated from the macular region, generating retinal traction and distortion in the area where it remains attached, leading to vision changes (decreased vision, metamorphopsia, photopsia, diplopia). It is essential to distinguish it from a full-thickness macular hole (FTMH) and an epiretinal membrane (ERM), as the treatment urgency and approach would be very different. Also, myopic traction maculopathy should be distinguished from VMT since surgical approach, if decided upon, would entail differences.

2. VMT prevalence ranges between 1 and 2% depending on the diagnostic modality and population ethnicity. Age is a major risk factor for VMT occurrence, and its incidence can be as high as 60 to 65% in eyes with ERM. Uveitis, retinal breaks, and retinal vascular diseases (vein occlusions, diabetic retinopathy, macular telangiectasia) are also correlated to increased VMT formation.

3. OCT is the most definitive method to diagnose VMT, and to distinguish it from the other entities on the differential diagnosis listed above (▶ Fig. 42.1). A history of slowly and progressive visual loss, metamorphopsia, photopsia, or diplopia over several months should prompt investigation. Ophthalmic examination with fundus contact lens at the slit lamp provides ideal visualization of the vitreomacular interface anatomy due to its superior magnification and stereoscopic view; however, a suspended precorneal fundus lens is also helpful for diagnosis, but does not offer as much objective detail as OCT.

4. Spontaneous resolution of VMT can occur, especially in cases in which the vitreoretinal attachment involves a diameter less than 1,500 μm of the macular surface on OCT. However, persistence of VMT can lead to worsening visual acuity and major complications such as cystoid macular edema, foveal neurosensory detachment, and lamellar or FTMH formation.

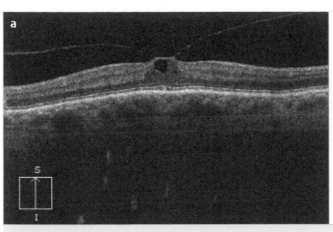
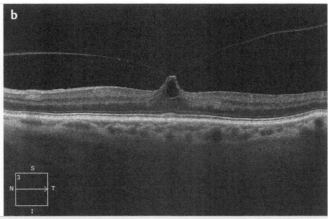

Fig. 42.1 Optical coherence tomography Image showing **(a)** vitreomacular attachment at the fovea with evidence of slight traction which **(b)** progressed to more evident traction over the ensuing month.

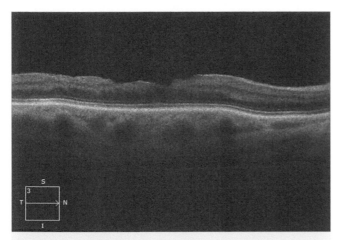

Fig. 42.2 Optical coherence tomographic appearance after surgery, showing no residual vitreous attachment and a virtual normalization of the inner retinal layers.

42.2 Test Interpretation

OCT is the most accurate method to diagnose VMT. The appearance of a thin, hyperreflective layer focally attached to a distorted macular surface and concurrently detached from the perifoveal region ("gull wing" or "pagoda sign") best characterize VMT. An OCT-based classification subdivide VMT into (1) focal (total extension of vitreofoveal adhesion ≤ 1,500 µm) or (2) broad (total adhesion > 1,500 µm). Intraretinal pseudocysts are usually seen in the area of vitreoretinal attachment, and neurosensory retinal detachment may also ensue, especially if the traction is significant and/or the attachment is broad.

In cases of generalized macular thickening, fluorescein angiography (FA) may demonstrate vascular leakage associated with areas of intraretinal pseudocysts. However, the widespread use of OCT and its superior imaging quality to identify architectural changes involving the retinal layers and surface limit the role of FA for diagnosis and/or monitoring of VMT and its associated retinal changes, even though FA may be helpful in diagnosing and/or monitoring retinal vascular diseases known to coexist with VMT.

42.3 Diagnosis

1. VMT OD.
2. VMT OS, nonprogressive.

42.4 Management

Management of VMT depends mostly on the patient's symptoms.

Observation is preferred when the patient's symptoms and vision loss are minimal. Thirty to forty percent of VMT cases present spontaneous release of the traction and stabilization or resolution of symptoms within 1 to 2 years, especially when the attachment is focal. However, approximately 60 to 65% of eyes may present worsening visual acuity according to some reports, particularly when there is broad attachment and important intraretinal cystoid changes.

PPV used to be the only surgical treatment available for VMT. The necessary mechanical changes for traction release are usually obtained by the removal of the vitreous gel with special attention to extricating the focal foveal attachment so as to avoid creating a macular hole. While many surgeons advocate for the internal limiting membrane peeling, there is no clear answer regarding the benefit of its removal in VMT. Most recently, ocriplasmin was approved as a pharmacologic option to treat VMT. Ocriplasmin, a recombinant protease, targets the adhesive components of the vitreoretinal adhesion resulting in its separation from the retina in some cases. A cornerstone study evaluating the efficacy of ocriplasmin intravitreal injection for VMT treatment in comparison to placebo (saline injection) demonstrated benefit in more than double of cases treated with ocriplasmin (26.5% resolution of adhesion vs. 10.1%). It appears that the best use of ocriplasmin is in younger patients (< 65 years old), phakic eyes, eyes without an ERM, eyes with an associated FTMH, and in cases of focal VMT; however, the relatively small number of studies evaluating ocriplasmin and reports of complications such as dyschromatopsia, electroretinographic changes, and ellipsoid layer disruption may be concerning for its widespread use.

The use of intravitreal injection of expansile gas has also been demonstrated to be beneficial for VMT resolution; however, there is no controlled, randomized study that could definitively prove its efficacy and safety.

42.5 Rehabilitation and Follow-up

The rate of visual improvement after PPV for VMT is around 80%, but most others gain stabilization of their vision.

In cases in which a decision for observation is taken, it is recommended that patients can be educated to self-monitor for worsening metamorphopsia, decreased vision, or development of scotoma through periodic evaluations with Amsler grid testing.

Suggested Reading

[1] Duker JS, Kaiser PK, Binder S, et al. The International Vitreomacular Traction Study Group classification of vitreomacular adhesion, traction, and macular hole. Ophthalmology. 2013; 120(12):2611–2619

[2] Meuer SM, Myers CE, Klein BE, et al. The epidemiology of vitreoretinal interface abnormalities as detected by spectral-domain optical coherence tomography: the beaver dam eye study. Ophthalmology. 2015; 122(4):787–795

[3] Tzu JH, John VJ, Flynn HW, Jr, et al. Clinical course of vitreomacular traction managed initially by observation. Ophthalmic Surg Lasers Imaging Retina. 2015; 46(5):571–576

[4] Gonzalez MA, Flynn HW, Jr, Bokman CM, Feuer W, Smiddy WE. Outcomes of pars plana vitrectomy for patients with vitreomacular traction. Ophthalmic Surg Lasers Imaging Retina. 2015; 46(7):708–714

[5] Stalmans P, Benz MS, Gandorfer A, et al. MIVI-TRUST Study Group. Enzymatic vitreolysis with ocriplasmin for vitreomacular traction and macular holes. N Engl J Med. 2012; 367(7):606–615

[6] Jackson TL, Nicod E, Angelis A, et al. Pars plana vitrectomy for vitreomacular traction syndrome: a systematic review and metaanalysis of safety and efficacy. Retina. 2013; 33(10):2012–2017

[7] Folk JC, Adelman RA, Flaxel CJ, Hyman L, Pulido JS, Olsen TW. Idiopathic Epiretinal Membrane and Vitreomacular Traction Preferred Practice Pattern(®) Guidelines. Ophthalmology. 2016; 123(1):152–181

43 Vitreous Hemorrhage

William E. Smiddy and Thalmon R. Campagnoli

Abstract

Vitreous hemorrhage is most commonly associated with retinal vascular disease, usually indicating a proliferative retinopathy, but an important cause not to miss is when it occurs secondary to a new retinal tear. Proliferative diabetic retinopathy frequently heralds its presence in this way, prompting appropriate treatment aimed at reversing and controlling the retinal neovascularization. Other proliferative retinopathies that may present with a vitreous hemorrhage include branch retinal vein occlusion, sickle retinopathy, or proliferations due to other syndromes or ischemia. Choroidal vascular diseases, most commonly choroidal neovascularization due to wet age-related macular degeneration, may manifest as vitreous hemorrhage through a retinal "breakthrough" mechanism. Most important due to the opportunity to treat during a window of opportunity is vitreous hemorrhage in association with a posterior vitreous detachment, especially when secondary to a retinal tear which might be treatable before the onset of retinal detachment. The mainstay of diagnostic modalities (when the vitreous hemorrhage is so severe as to prevent direct visualization) is B-scan ultrasound. Close follow-up is the paradigm of clinical follow-up, especially if the ultrasound test has not shown definite tear or detachment. Mimicking conditions include vitreous opacities due to inflammatory disease.

Keywords: vitreous hemorrhage, retinal tear, retinal detachment, posterior vitreous detachment, ultrasound

43.1 History

This 90-year-old woman presented with a 3-month history of sudden decreased vision in the left eye. Her visual acuity was 20/40 OD and 2/200 OS. Intraocular pressures were 12 mm Hg in each eye. Slit-lamp examination showed a well-positioned posterior chamber lens implant on the right. There was vitreous adherent to the wound superiorly. In the left eye, she had 2 + nuclear sclerosis. There was a very dense vitreous hemorrhage in the left eye precluding a view posteriorly.

Past ocular history was pertinent for vision of 20/50 on the right and 20/200 on the left 3 years previously due to atrophic age-related macular degeneration OD and a previously treated, subfoveal choroidal neovascular membrane OS. Medical history was negative for diabetes or hypertension.

B-scan/A-scan ultrasonography showed vitreous hemorrhage with posterior vitreous detachment (PVD) OS. There was no retinal tear or detachment, and a disciform scar could not be resolved in the left macula.

She was observed without treatment for 3 months. On follow-up, the visual acuity improved to 20/400 and a subfoveal laser scar with contiguous subretinal hemorrhage extending inferiorly to the midperiphery was visible.

Differential Diagnosis—Key Points

1. Spontaneous vitreous hemorrhage in an elderly patient, especially with the history of previously treated macular degeneration, suggests the possibility of breakthrough bleeding into the vitreous cavity from a subretinal hemorrhagic process. Extension of subretinal hemorrhage before breakthrough bleeding occurs may compound sightimpairing tissue damage from the underlying neovascularization process.

2. The most common causes of vitreous hemorrhage in nondiabetic patients are PVD, retinal tear (with or without avulsed retinal vessel syndrome), and retinal detachment. Other less common or historically obvious causes include blunt trauma, Terson's syndrome, choroidal melanoma, penetrating trauma, and macroaneurysms.

3. Prompt diagnosis and treatment may prevent further or permanent visual loss. Vitreous hemorrhage at the time of PVD is associated with a higher risk of retinal tear (23–45%) than PVD without hemorrhage (3–12%). Untreated proliferative retinopathies should also be considered in all cases.

4. Vitreous hemorrhage often occurs in proliferative retinopathies. The most common cause of vitreous hemorrhage in a patient with diabetes mellitus is proliferative diabetic retinopathy. Other proliferative etiologies include branch retinal vein occlusion, sickle cell retinopathy, or choroidal neovascularization. Often, the possibility of these entities is apparent from the previous history or examination of the fellow eye.

5. It may be difficult to differentiate vitreous blood, especially when chronic, from vitreous opacities due to inflammatory disorders. Conditions such as toxoplasmosis, pars planitis, or other forms of intermediate and posterior uveitis may present with vitreous opacities. In such cases, careful examination for granulomatous signs in the anterior segment may betray the diagnosis. Pars planitis may lead to neovascularization and vitreous hemorrhage directly. Clues may sometimes be obtained from careful examination of the fellow eye and careful delineation of the previous history.

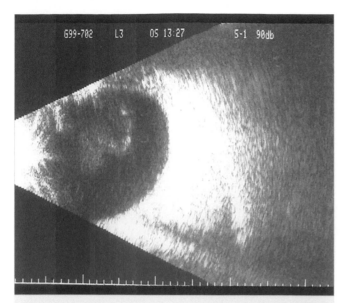

Fig. 43.1 Ultrasonographic appearance showing vitreous opacities and posterior vitreous detachment. No retinal detachment is in evidence. This slice through the macula does not show macular elevation.

43.2 Test Interpretation

One key element of the clinical examination is the presence or absence of an afferent pupillary defect. More extensive disease, such as retinal detachment or extensive subretinal hemorrhage with breakthrough bleeding, often manifests with an afferent pupillary defect. Indirect ophthalmoscopy with scleral depression may allow a view of the peripheral retina despite substantial degrees of blood in the midvitreous. Seeing the peripheral retina intact at or near the ora serrata for 360E lends some confidence in ruling out associated retinal detachment.

The most important ancillary test to rule out progressive causes for vitreous hemorrhage is echography (▶ Fig. 43.1). It is generally possible to rule out retinal detachment with echography. In some selected cases, a peripheral retinal tear may be detectable by ultrasound. Proliferative retinopathies may frequently be able to be diagnosed by echography as the vitreoretinal attachment of the retinal neovascularization may be evident.

If it is uncertain whether the vitreous opacities may represent inflammatory cells rather than red blood cells, laboratory testing (such as toxoplasmosis titers, TB skin testing, syphilis serologies) or even diagnostic vitrectomy may be indicated.

43.3 Diagnosis

Vitreous hemorrhage due to breakthrough bleeding associated with choroidal neovascularization, OS.

43.4 Medical Treatment

There are no known medical treatments to hasten the clearance of vitreous hemorrhage. Having the patient sleep in a slightly inclined position does not hasten the clearance of the hemorrhage, but it may allow the blood to settle inferiorly and facilitate examination of the patient. The temporary, partial visual improvement is reassuring to the patient.

Laser treatment, when possible, is the mainstay of treatment for most proliferative retinopathies.

43.5 Surgical Treatment

Vitrectomy for cases of nonclearing vitreous hemorrhage in eyes with acceptable visual potential is the mainstay of surgical treatment. The appropriate timing and indication for surgery are controversial. In patients with known proliferative retinopathies, such as diabetic retinopathy, surgical intervention is dependent on a variety of factors, including the chronicity of the hemorrhage, the presumed severity of the existing proliferation, and the degree of previous laser photocoagulation applied. Generally, type I diabetics undergo earlier vitrectomy compared to type II diabetics, with vitrectomy usually being recommended for patients with nonclearing vitreous hemorrhage of 2 to 6 months' duration.

Patients with vitreous hemorrhage not associated with proliferative retinopathies, retinal detachment, or retinal tears are generally observed. If there are no signs of spontaneous clearing within 3 to 6 months, vitrectomy can be recommended. However, it is important to attempt to assess the visual potential in such cases. In patients with macular degeneration, the visual potential is understandably limited. A special case is vitreous hemorrhage due to penetrating trauma or a globe rupture. Usually, further vitreous surgery, which may include vitrectomy, scleral buckling, and other maneuvers, is recommended within 2 weeks of onset to preempt irreversible cicatricial changes.

43.6 Rehabilitation and Follow-up

In this patient, the visual acuity was improving 2 months after presentation. The visual potential was 20/200, and there was good vision in the fellow eye. Surgical intervention therefore was deferred. However, even in patients in whom the vitreous hemorrhage is noted to be due to breakthrough bleeding from macular degeneration, vitrectomy can be considered. The most common setting in which vitrectomy is offered despite limited visual potential would be in a patient with bilateral visual loss. Furthermore, it is important to counsel patients preoperatively as to appropriate expectations.

43.7 Acknowledgment

Thanks to this chapter's first edition author Ghassan J. Cordahi.

Suggested Reading

[1] Isernhagen RD, Smiddy WE, Michels RG, Glaser BM, de Bustros S. Vitrectomy for nondiabetic vitreous hemorrhage. Not associated with vascular disease. Retina. 1988; 8(2):81–87

[2] Smiddy WE, Isernhagen RD, Michels RG, Glaser BM, de Bustros SN. Vitrectomy for nondiabetic vitreous hemorrhage. Retinal and choroidal vascular disorders. Retina. 1988; 8(2):88–95

[3] Butner RW, McPherson AR. Spontaneous vitreous hemorrhage. Ann Ophthalmol. 1982; 14(3):268–270

[4] Morse PH, Aminlari A, Scheie HG. Spontaneous vitreous hemorrhage. Arch Ophthalmol. 1974; 92(4):297–298

[5] Jaffe NS. Complications of acute posterior vitreous detachment. Arch Ophthalmol. 1968; 79(5):568–571

[6] Spraul CW, Grossniklaus HE. Vitreous hemorrhage. Surv Ophthalmol. 1997; 42(1):3–39

44 Retinitis Pigmentosa

Byron L. Lam

Abstract

Retinitis pigmentosa (RP) is a group of genetically heterogeneous inherited retinal degenerative disorders characterized by progressive rod and cone photoreceptor dysfunction and death. The prevalence of RP is approximately 1 per 3,000 to 4,000 persons. Gradual progressive nyctalopia and progressive loss of peripheral vision are common early symptoms. Early gray retinal degenerative changes typically start in the midperipheral retina and advances with formation of pigment clumping and vascular attenuation toward the macula. Other potential features include posterior subcapsular cataract and cystoid macular edema, both of which are treatable. Most patients retain good central vision until advanced stages of the disease. Rate of progressive visual loss is highly variable, and total visual loss in both eyes occurs in a minority of patients. Over 150 genes are found to cause RP with autosomal recessive, autosomal dominant, or X-linked inheritance. Approximately 50% of RP cases are sporadic without family history. Commercialized genetic testing is available although, not all genotypes of RP are yet known. Benefits of genetic testing include determining hereditary pattern, ruling out syndromic RP, and participating in available clinical trials. Some evidence suggests the benefit of oral vitamin A palmitate, DHA (docosahexaenoic acid), and lutein, but given the diversity of genotypes and the lack of consistent beneficial laboratory data, there is a lack of general agreement among RP specialist to recommend these supplements. Retinal implant providing rudimentary vision is approved for treatment of very advanced RP with light perception or worse in both eyes. Numerous clinical trials are under way to test a wide range of treatment strategies.

Keywords: retinitis pigmentosa, retinal dystrophy, hereditary retinal degeneration

44.1 History

A 24-year-old woman with progressive visual difficulties at night was evaluated. Since the age of 10, the patient has had trouble performing outdoor activities after dusk. A year ago, the patient stopped driving at night, because she no longer felt safe. For many years, the patient has been "clumsy" and often walked into surrounding objects she could not see well. The patient was otherwise healthy. Family history was negative for ocular problems, and there was no consanguinity.

Best-corrected visual acuity was 20/25 in each eye, with no relative afferent pupillary defect. Goldmann visual fields revealed large midperipheral ring-shaped scotomas (▶ Fig. 44.1). Funduscopic examination showed atrophy of the midperipheral and peripheral retina with areas of pigment clumping ("bone spicules"; ▶ Fig. 44.2). Attenuation of the retinal vasculature in the area of retinal atrophy was evident. Full-field electroretinography (ERG) showed nondetectable rod and cone responses.

Differential Diagnosis—Key Points

1. In a young patient with progressive night visual difficulties or nyctalopia and decreased peripheral vision, a diagnosis of hereditary retinal degeneration should be considered. Among this group of disorders, retinitis pigmentosa (RP) is the most common and has a prevalence of approximately 1 per 3,000 to 4,000 persons in the general population. RP is a group of genetically heterogeneous inherited retinal degenerative disorders characterized by early rod photoreceptor dysfunction followed by progressive rod and cone photoreceptor dysfunction and death. Nyctalopia and progressive loss of peripheral vision are common early symptoms. Visual acuity and macular function, in contrast, are usually relatively spared in most but not all affected persons until late in the disease. Symptoms typically start insidiously between the second and fifth decades of life and continue to progress gradually. The primary retinal finding is retinal atrophy with vascular attenuation and pigmentary clumping (traditionally referred to as "bone spicules") that typically begins in the midperipheral regions of the retina, where there is the highest density of rod photoreceptors. With time, the areas of retinal degenerations spread peripherally as well as centrally. Other ophthalmoscopic signs may include cystoid macular edema (CME), atrophic macular lesions, optic nerve atrophy, vitreous syneresis, and mild vitritis. Central posterior subcapsular cataract is also common in RP and often acquires a stellate shape with progression. Approximately 50% of RP patients have no family history of RP and are designated as having sporadic RP, with most having autosomal recessive RP. The remaining 50% of RP patients have pedigrees consistent with autosomal dominant (20–25%), X-linked (10–15%), and autosomal recessive (15%) inheritance.

2. Aside from RP, other conditions which may produce progressive nyctalopia in healthy individuals with no other associated systemic symptoms include choroideremia, gyrate atrophy, and vitamin A deficiency. Choroideremia is an X-linked recessive chorioretinal dystrophy characterized by a progressive degeneration of the choroid and the retinal pigment epithelium. Choroideremia results from defects in the human Rab escort protein-1 (REP-1) gene that encodes for a component of rab geranylgeranyl transferase, an enzyme involved in cellular transport. Affected males with choroideremia usually start to have onset of poor night vision and decreased peripheral vision starting in the first two decades of life. The central vision is the last to be affected but is invariably affected in all affected males by the fourth and fifth decades of life. Female carriers are asymptomatic but have a diffuse or localized "moth-eaten" appearance of the retinal pigment epithelium. Gyrate atrophy is an autosomal recessive chorioretinal dystrophy due to a generalized deficiency of the mitochondrial matrix enzyme ornithine aminotransferase. Many patients are first

diagnosed with the disease when poor night vision becomes noticeable between the age of 20 and 40 years. Multiple, discrete scallop-shaped areas of chorioretinal atrophy occur initially in the peripheral and midperipheral regions of the fundus. Over time, the lesions coalesce and progress toward the macula with corresponding, progressive impairment of peripheral vision and night vision. Worldwide, dietary vitamin A deficiency is a considerable cause of progressive nyctalopia. The prevalence is higher in less developed countries, and nyctalopia is often the earliest symptom. With progression, dryness of the conjunctiva and cornea as well as metaplastic keratinization of areas of the conjunctiva may occur.

3. Several retinal degenerative disorders associated with pigmentary retinal atrophy have been traditionally listed under the broad category of syndromic or secondary RP.

The disorders include Usher's syndrome, Bardet–Biedl syndrome, Refsum's syndrome, Bassen–Kornzweig syndrome, and neuronal ceroid lipofuscinosis (Batten's disease). These conditions are associated with other systemic findings and are not likely in our healthy adult patient. Of interest, toxic retinopathies such as thioridazine-induced retinopathy may also produce a RP-like clinical picture. Of interest, Leber's congenital amaurosis refers to a group of genetically heterogeneous inherited retinal degenerative disorders characterized by severe congenital diffuse retinal dysfunction with severe visual loss and the development of nystagmus noted within the first year life. The retinal appearance is usually normal initially but diffuse retinal degenerative RP-like changes develop over time.

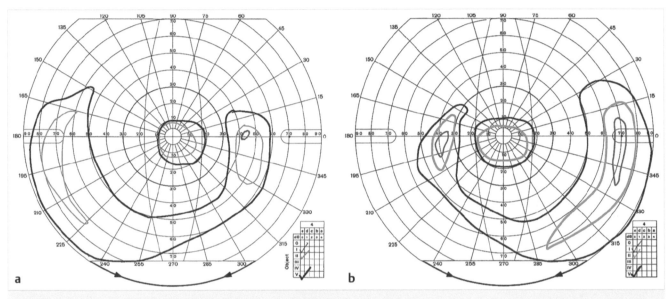

Fig. 44.1 Goldmann visual fields showed midperipheral ring-shaped scotomas in each eye.

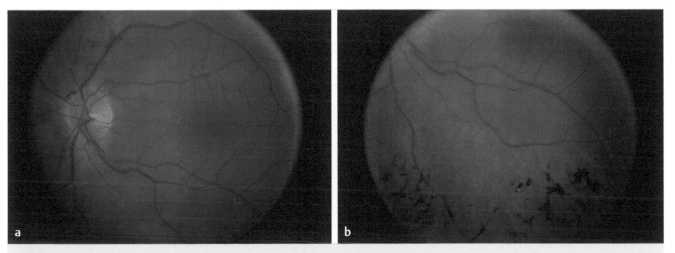

Fig. 44.2 Funduscopic findings were similar for both eyes. A view of the left fundus showing retinal atrophy midperipherally near the vascular arcades. The retinal atrophy is more apparent in a view of the inferior quadrant of the retina. Prominent choroidal vasculature appearance and retinal vascular attenuation is evident in the area of the retinal atrophy, and areas of pigmentary clumping ("bone spicules") are visible.

44.2 Test Interpretation

Commonly used clinical automated 30-degree visual fields show variable amount of constriction depending on disease stage. Automated kinetic and Goldmann visual field testing often reveal midperipheral ring-shaped scotoma in patients with early RP. As the disease progresses, the scotoma expands and the visual field becomes more constricted.

Optical coherence tomography (OCT) is very useful in identifying CME as well as foveal atrophy associated with RP. Given some RP patients respond to medical treatments for RP-related CME, OCT is of diagnostic value in RP patients with decreased visual acuity.

Full-field ERG is an extremely valuable tool in diagnosing patients in early stages of RP, who may have no or mild symptoms and the retinal atrophy may or may not be clinically apparent. The ERG responses are dramatically reduced in early stages in RP. Patients with early stages of RP have significantly reduced and prolonged dark-adapted rod ERG responses and reduced but less affected light-adapted cone responses. With further progression of the disease, the rod and cone ERG responses diminish and become nondetectable. Therefore, the ERG responses of most RP patients are often small or nondetectable. In fact, it is not unusual for ERG responses to be nondetectable on initial evaluation in some RP patients.

Genetic testing has become an increasingly useful tool in determining the specific RP genotype and thus the hereditary pattern. The genotypes of RP are numerous and extremely diverse. In a given affected individual, the RP is associated with specific change in a specific gene. The alteration may occur in one allele in cases of dominant RP and X-linked RP or the changes may occur in a homozygous or heterozygous fashion in both alleles in cases of recessive RP. A vast number of specific codon mutations in over 100 genes are found to be associated with RP, with recessive RP being the most genetically diverse. The protein alterations from the RP genotypes ultimately cause photoreceptor dysfunction and eventual death through different biochemical mechanisms such as the renewal and shedding of photoreceptor outer segments, the visual transduction cascade, the retinol (vitamin A) metabolism, etc.

44.3 Diagnosis

Retinitis pigmentosa, sporadic, moderately advanced.

44.4 Medical Management

For severe RP resulting in bare light perception or no light perception vision, retinal implants are approved for treatment under humanitarian or conventional approval in the United States or in European countries. The basic premise involves the utilization of a video camera that transmits visual signals to an electrode array implanted to the retina. The vision provided is artificial, primitive, and pixilated and allows the possibility of improvement in mobility.

In a previous prospective study, oral vitamin A palmitate (15,000 IU) daily may help to delay the progression of RP, while oral vitamin E daily may hasten progression. Oral lutein and DHA (docosahexaenoic acid) may have some modest beneficial effect to delay progression or RP. Given the diversity of genotypes in RP and that vitamin A treatment is found to be harmful for some genotypes that could cause RP (e.g., ABCA4), there is a lack of general agreement among RP specialists with respect to recommending these supplements.

Of interest, oral acetazolamide has been found to be more effective than topical agents such as dorzolamide in treating CME in RP. Reducing retinal exposure to damaging solar ultraviolet light with sunglasses is recommended in RP patients. For those RP patients with reduced visual acuity, low vision aids may be helpful.

Counseling of patients and their families regarding visual prognosis and disease susceptibility should be provided. However, the clinical expression of a known genotype may have some interindividual variability even for affected individuals of the same family.

44.5 Rehabilitation and Follow-up

If cataract or CME develops, treatment should be considered. Cataract extraction may be challenging in some cases because of weakened zonular lens support in eyes with RP. Multiple laser posterior capsulotomies after cataract extraction are often necessary in RP patients because postoperative fibrotic reaction of the posterior capsule is common. Periodic yearly liver function tests may be helpful in RP patients placed on vitamin A therapy. However, the risk of toxicity from the recommended dosage is low, and whether repeated liver function testing is necessary in all patients is uncertain.

Suggested Readings

[1] Hartong DT, Berson EL, Dryja TP. Retinitis pigmentosa. Lancet. 2006; 368 (9549):1795–1809

[2] Jacobson SG, Cideciyan AV. Treatment possibilities for retinitis pigmentosa. N Engl J Med. 2010; 363(17):1669–1671

[3] Ho AC, Humayun MS, Dorn JD, et al. Argus II Study Group. Long-Term results from an epiretinal prosthesis to restore sight to the blind. Ophthalmology. 2015; 122(8):1547–1554

Part V

Uveitis

V

45 Choroiditis

Sarah P. Read

Abstract

There are a variety of features allowing categorization of choroiditis entities, which may facilitate their accurate diagnosis, such as unilateral versus bilateral, granulomatous versus nongranulomatous, extent of involvement (panuveitis vs. anterior or intermediate), and systemic versus nonsystemic associated signs. The clinical course and other specifically characteristic features may confirm or allow more definitive diagnoses of specific entities. The principal entities presenting with choroiditis include Behçet's disease, Vogt–Koyanagi–Harada (VKH) syndrome, sympathetic ophthalmia, a variety of infectious causes (e.g., toxoplasmosis, Lyme borreliosis, tuberculosis, and syphilis), sarcoidosis, various white dot syndromes, and postsurgical inflammation. Some entities have characteristic appearances with various imaging modalities (e.g., pinpoint areas of hyperfluorescence and posterior scleritis by ultrasound examination with VKH syndrome). A multiplicity of laboratory tests may be helpful in corroborating a clinical diagnosis, but must be interpreted carefully in context of the clinical presentation and course.

Keywords: inflammation, infection, endophthalmitis, uveitis

45.1 History

A 24-year-old Hispanic woman complained of constant pain in the right eye for 3 weeks, blurred vision, redness, and tearing for 1 week, and a 1-month history of headache and neck stiffness. Computed tomography (CT) of the brain was normal. A lumbar puncture showed a mild pleocytosis. She noted flulike symptoms for 2 days previously. She denied any history of trauma.

On examination, visual acuity was 20/20 in both eyes. Intraocular pressure was 18 mm Hg in the right eye and 16 mm Hg in the left eye. Slit-lamp examination disclosed moderate anterior chamber cell and flare in the right eye with granulomatous keratic precipitates on the corneal endothelium. A mild anterior chamber inflammatory reaction was noted in the left eye. Vitreous cells were present in the right eye. Funduscopic examination of the right eye showed optic disc edema with focal areas of serous retinal detachment and folding of the retina within the macular region. The left eye was unremarkable. B-scan ultrasonography of the right eye showed diffuse choroidal thickening with low reflectivity and a shallow serous macular detachment. Treatment with topical prednisolone acetate 1% and cycloplegics was initiated.

The patient returned 1 week later with persistent pain and markedly decreased visual acuity in the right eye to 3/200 vision. Although the anterior chamber reaction had decreased slightly in the right eye, the left eye had increased cell and flare with a few keratic precipitates. The funduscopic examination showed increased optic disc edema, subretinal fluid and retinal folds, and focal yellow-white lesions at the level of the retinal pigment epithelium (RPE) in the macula (▶ Fig. 45.1). Although the vision was 20/25 in the left eye, a new focal area of subretinal fluid in the nasal macula was noted. Fluorescein angiography of the right eye demonstrated multiple areas of pinpoint hyperfluorescence in the juxtapapillary region and macula that leaked in the later frames (▶ Fig. 45.2). The area of thickening in the left eye adjacent to the optic disc had a similar appearance on fluorescein angiography.

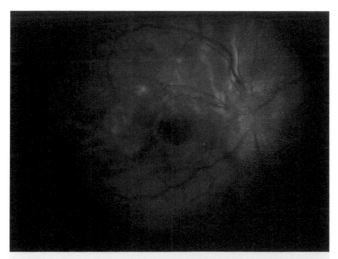

Fig. 45.1 Funduscopic appearance of the patient's right eye showing focal yellow-white lesions at the level of the RPE superior and temporal to the macula. Note the optic nerve had swelling.

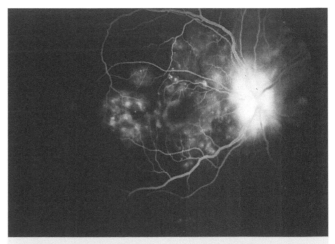

Fig. 45.2 Fluorescein angiography of the same eye at the same time showing prominent disc edema, but also end-point hyperfluorescence corresponding to RPE lesions.

Differential Diagnosis—Key Points

1. One of the first steps in evaluating patients with intraocular inflammation is defining the location and extent of tissue involvement. Panuveitis involves inflammation of all segments of the eye: anterior segment, vitreous, and the retina and/or choroid. Causes of panuveitis include Behçet's disease, sympathetic ophthalmia, tuberculosis, sarcoidosis, Vogt–Koyanagi–Harada (VKH) syndrome, and infectious endophthalmitis. Additionally, it is important to determine the primary tissue layer involved (e.g., retina or choroid) and whether the lesions are unifocal or multifocal. Causes of multifocal choroiditis, as in the presented case, include autoimmune disorders (sympathetic ophthalmia, VKH syndrome, and sarcoidosis), infectious diseases (histoplasmosis), or other inflammatory causes (white dot syndromes).

2. A second potentially distinguishing feature of patients with uveitis is the onset of symptoms. Acute causes of uveitis include postsurgical infection, trauma, toxoplasmosis, the white dot syndromes (acute posterior placoid pigment epitheliopathy and multiple evanescent white dot syndrome), VKH syndrome, acute retinal necrosis, and most causes of anterior uveitis.

3. Most causes of posterior uveitis are bilateral in presentation. Cases that remain unilateral upon follow-up examination may include sarcoidosis, trauma, parasitic disease (such as toxoplasmosis), retained intraocular foreign body, and postsurgical uveitis. Bilateral involvement may indicate a systemic cause of inflammation, such as autoimmune disorders and endogenous infectious etiologies. Some cases may present with unilateral inflammation, but manifest bilaterality only on subsequent follow-up examination, as was the case with the patient presented here.

4. Careful examination of the anterior chamber reaction with identification of granulomatous versus nongranulomatous type of inflammation is helpful in narrowing the differential diagnosis. Causes of granulomatous inflammation include sarcoidosis, VKH syndrome, sympathetic ophthalmia, toxoplasmosis, ocular Lyme borreliosis, tuberculosis, and syphilis.

5. Neurologic signs and symptoms warrant further investigation to rule out meningeal infection or central nervous system (CNS) disorder. A CT scan with and without contrast or magnetic resonance imaging (MRI) of the brain may be diagnostic. Lumbar puncture with cerebrospinal fluid (CSF) sent for cell count and differential, protein, glucose, VDRL, bacterial stains, and culture may aid in establishing the diagnosis. Primary intraocular B-cell lymphoma can masquerade as chronic uveitis with associated neurologic abnormalities. Appropriate blood tests to evaluate for malignancy or systemic infection may include a complete blood count with differential, ANA, RPR, FTA-ABS, Lyme titer, ACE, and PPD with anergy panel and a chest X-ray when the diagnosis is uncertain.

6. Several associated signs and symptoms along with patient demographics are important in the diagnosis of posterior uveitis, and may eliminate the need for extensive laboratory and ancillary testing. VKH syndrome is thought to be a primary inflammatory condition directed at melanin-containing cells. Patients with VKH syndrome are typically found in groups with greater skin pigmentation (Hispanic, Asian, Native American, and African American), females, and ages 20 to 40 years old. A link has been found between VKH syndrome and HLA-DR4 and DQ4, though the prognostic significance is unclear. VKH syndrome is associated with a number of systemic manifestations including auditory symptoms (tinnitus, hearing loss) or cutaneous findings (vitiligo, alopecia, poliosis). Neurologic symptoms (nausea, headache, vertigo, stiff neck) or signs (CSF pleocytosis) are frequent findings. Criteria for the diagnosis of VKH syndrome were set forth by the American Uveitis Society in 1978 (**see list below**).

7. The clinical course of the disease is important in confirming the diagnosis. VKH syndrome, for example, generally follows three phases. The initial prodromal stage mimics a viral illness with neurologic signs and symptoms (fever, vertigo, tinnitus, meningism). This is followed by a uveitic stage with rapid vision loss associated with bilateral posterior uveitis, exudative retinal detachment, hyper- and hypopigmentation of the RPE, peripapillary retinal elevation or disc edema, and thickening of the posterior choroid. Finally, in the convalescent stage, chronic changes are seen including a "sunset glow" fundus (yellow-orange retinal pigment epithelial color change), Dalen-Fuchs' nodules (yellow-white choroidal granulomatous inflammatory infiltrates), poliosis, vitiligo, and retinal pigment epithelial mottling.

8. VKH syndrome and sympathetic ophthalmia share many characteristics, including fluorescein angiographic appearance, clinical characteristics, and a strong association with HLA-DR4. Therefore, a careful history to elicit even a remote history of penetrating ocular trauma is important. Exudative retinal detachments can occur in central serous retinopathy, uveal effusion syndrome, and age-related macular degeneration; however, these diseases will lack the inflammation and systemic symptoms characteristic of VKH syndrome.

Vogt–Koyanagi–Harada Syndrome: Criteria for Diagnosis (American Uveitis Society, 1978)
1. No history of ocular trauma or surgery.
2. At least three of the following:
   a) Bilateral chronic iridocyclitis.
   b) Posterior uveitis, including exudative retinal detachment, forme fruste of retinal detachment, disc hyperemia or edema, and "sunset-glow" fundus.
   c) Neurologic signs (tinnitus, stiff neck, CNS problems, or CSF pleocytosis).
   d) Cutaneous findings (alopecia, vitiligo, poliosis).

45.2 Test Interpretation

Evaluation of the patient begins with a careful history, in this case with special emphasis on prior ocular surgery or trauma, systemic infections or inflammatory diseases, neurologic or auditory symptoms, and skin or hair depigmentation. Patient demographics are important clues to the diagnosis of intraocular inflammation, since many causes of intraocular inflammation affect characteristic patient populations. Next, a complete ocular examination must be performed to evaluate the location and type (granulomatous vs. nongranulomatous) of inflammation, the distribution and appearance of choroidal inflammatory lesions, and any associated posterior pole pathology, including disc edema and/or serous retinal detachment.

Fluorescein angiography is an important adjunct in the diagnosis of posterior uveitis, as entities with similar clinical appearance may have very different fluorescein angiographic characteristics. Fluorescein angiography in the acute phase of VKH syndrome typically shows numerous pinpoint areas of hyperfluorescence at the level of the RPE overlying areas of choroiditis with subretinal dye pooling. There is little to no retinal vessel leakage in the acute stage, which can distinguish VKH syndrome from other disorders. Optic disc edema is present in approximately 70% of patients. During the chronic phase, multiple retinal pigment epithelial window defects are seen. A similar angiographic appearance is seen in patients with sympathetic ophthalmia. Patients with lymphoma or a form of "white dot syndrome," such as acute posterior multifocal placoid pigment epitheliopathy (APMPPE) and multiple evanescent white dot syndrome (MEWDS), may have a similar clinical appearance but have distinct fluorescein angiographic characteristics.

B-scan ultrasonography can be helpful in evaluating patients with posterior uveitis in order to rule out posterior scleritis (scleral thickening present), uveal effusion syndrome (may have scleral thickening and often involve the peripheral choroid), or infiltrative lesions. Echographic features of VKH syndrome include diffuse, low-to-medium reflective choroidal thickening, mild vitreous opacities, and serous retinal detachment located in the posterior pole. In the acute phase, lumbar puncture shows a lymphocytic pleocytosis in 84% of patients with normal protein levels.

More recently, optical coherence tomography (OCT) has been used to evaluate for recurrence in these patients. Increased choroidal thickening has been associated with anterior segment inflammation in some patients.

45.3 Diagnosis

Vogt–Koyanagi–Harada syndrome.

45.4 Medical Management

Prompt treatment with systemic corticosteroids (80–200 mg per day orally), a cycloplegic agent, and topical prednisolone acetate 1% (frequency tailored to control anterior segment inflammation) may result in rapid resolution of symptoms of redness, pain, and photophobia. The sooner treatment is initiated, the more rapid the resolution of symptoms. H_2-blockers, such as ranitidine 150 mg twice daily orally, should be administered to protect against gastric ulcer formation while on high-dose systemic steroid treatment. In particularly severe cases, initial treatment with intravenous steroids may be considered. Oral prednisone should be tapered very slowly (over 4–6 months) with careful observation as nearly half of recurrences occur within this time period. If symptoms do not resolve with prednisone, other systemic immunosuppressants such as cyclosporine, cyclophosphamide, chlorambucil, and azathioprine can be used.

45.5 Surgical Management

Surgical intervention does not play a direct role in the management of most causes of posterior uveitis that are a result of a systemic inflammatory disease. Exudative retinal detachments usually resolve with resolution of intraocular inflammation. Complications associated with chronic intraocular inflammation, such as cataract formation, angle-closure glaucoma, or choroidal neovascularization, may require future surgical intervention.

45.6 Rehabilitation and Follow-up

The patient should be followed frequently in the initial stages of the disease in order to adjust treatment with corticosteroids for adequate control of inflammation and prevention of sequelae, such as posterior synechiae and angle closure. Early aggressive treatment with systemic corticosteroids can be followed by a gradual taper with less frequent ocular examination once a decrease in inflammation and exudative detachment is noted. When steroids alone do not control intraocular inflammation, the patient is intolerant of the side effects of steroids, or relapses occur while on high-dose steroid treatment, other immunosuppressive agents can be used. Once complete resolution of inflammation and serous detachment is achieved, a slow taper over 6 months decreases the risk of acute reactivation of disease. Patients should be monitored on a regular basis for evidence of cataract, choroidal neovascularization, or angle-closure glaucoma.

Suggested Readings

[1] Moorthy RS, Inomata H, Rao NA. Vogt-Koyanagi-Harada syndrome. Surv Ophthalmol. 1995; 39(4):265–292

[2] Nussenblatt RB, Whitcup SM, Palestine AG. Uveitis: Fundamentals and Clinical Practice. 2nd ed. St. Louis, MO: Mosby Year Book; 1996:312–324

[3] Tabbara KF, Nussenblatt RB. Posterior Uveitis: Diagnosis and Management. Newton, MA: Butterworth-Heinemann; 1994:89–94

46 Retinitis

Sarah P. Read

Abstract

Retinitis is caused by infectious agents, typically opportunistic agents that emerge in a compromised host. The most common setting is in eyes of human immunodeficiency virus (HIV)-positive or acquired immune deficiency syndrome (AIDS) patients. Viral, fungal, and parasitic etiologies are most common, but uncommon bacterial agents may also flourish as a cause of retinal-based inflammation. Since these are almost exclusively microbial in nature, their natural course is typically progressive and leads to severe visual loss. Toxoplasmosis and herpetic retinitis may occur in immunocompetent individuals. Secondary changes may include retinal detachment. Diagnosis is commonly established through clinical appearance and culture or detection of viral activity through techniques such as polymerase chain reaction (PCR) testing of procured samples. Association with choroiditis may allow suspicion of pneumocystis or *Cryptococcus* species. Treatment centers around delivery of the appropriate antimicrobial such as inserting ganciclovir implants or other antimicrobials. Treatment of the underlying immunodeficiency is a necessary goal and has been greatly aided in the case of AIDS by HAART (highly active antiretroviral therapy).

Keywords: immunodeficiency syndrome, cytomegalovirus, toxoplasmosis, syphilis

46.1 History

A 32-year-old woman with a 10-year history of acquired immune deficiency syndrome (AIDS) complained of new onset of multiple black spots in the visual field of the right and left eyes for 2 weeks. She had a CD4 count of 64 and was on highly active antiretroviral therapy (HAART).

Examination revealed a best corrected visual acuity of 20/30 in the right eye and 20/40 in the left eye. The intraocular pressure was 10 mm Hg in each eye. The anterior segment was unremarkable with no anterior chamber cell or flare. Funduscopic examination of the right eye showed creamy yellowish-white retinitis with prominent, associated hemorrhage within the lesion (▶ Fig. 46.1). There was active vitritis and vascular sheathing superior to the disc extending along the superotemporal arcade. The left eye had a peripheral area of retinitis temporally (▶ Fig. 46.2).

Differential Diagnosis—Key Points

1. Any complaint of floaters in a patient with a positive test for human immunodeficiency virus (HIV) and a relatively low CD4 count should prompt a complete funduscopic examination. A high index of suspicion for cytomegalovirus (CMV) retinitis exists, since 20 to 30% of HIV-positive patients will develop this opportunistic infection in their lifetimes. CMV is a DNA virus and CMV retinitis is thought to represent a systemic activation of a latent infection. The rate of CMV infection is markedly higher in those patients with CD4 counts below 100. Prior to the development of HAART, CMV retinitis was commonly seen within 1 year after diagnosis with AIDS; since the advent of HAART therapy, CMV retinitis is being diagnosed much later in the course of the disease.

2. Patients often present with floaters, photopsias, and cloudy vision. Exam can show mild inflammation, but there is often little conjunctival injection. The presentation of CMV retinitis is varied and often takes one of three forms. The classic or fulminant form includes hemorrhagic necrosis that can follow the blood vessels, as seen in ▶ Fig. 46.1. The granular form of disease shows a central area of atrophy

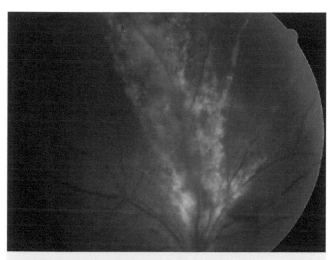

Fig. 46.1 Fundus photograph of right eye at presentation shows confluent wedge of retinitis with prominent hemorrhage extending from the superior nerve head margin anteriorly into the midperiphery.

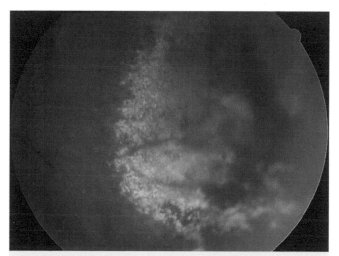

Fig. 46.2 The left eye had a large area of retinitis without hemorrhage in temporal midperiphery.

with surrounding white border of activity, seen in
► Fig. 46.2. These two forms can be seen simultaneously as in our patient. Uncommonly, CMV can present with a frosted branch angiitis in areas without retinitis.

3. The prognosis of CMV retinitis is variable and dependent on the location and extent of the lesion. Retinal detachment is estimated to complicate the disease in 50% of patients after 1 year. These detachments are due to atrophic holes that develop in the necrotic retina. The efficacy of prophylactic laser has not been proven in these patients.

4. Although CMV retinitis is the most common chorioretinal inflammatory condition in HIV-positive patients, several conditions may have similar fundus appearances. Acute retinal necrosis (ARN), which is most commonly caused by the herpes zoster virus, presents with a similar retinitis. However, ARN is much less common, often associated with prior herpes zoster dermatitis, and progresses rapidly with new disease foci, with an occlusive vasculitis. Generally, ARN tends to progress in a circumferential fashion, whereas CMV progresses along the arcades. Unlike CMV retinitis, ARN presents with prominent anterior and posterior segment inflammation.

5. Toxoplasmosis may also present with a similar appearance in HIV-positive individuals. Whereas the vast majority of toxoplasmosis seen in an immunocompetent population is unilateral and consists of small areas of retinitis often adjacent to areas of chorioretinal scarring, HIV-positive patients rarely have preexisting chorioretinal scars, develop larger lesions, and may present bilaterally in up to 40% of cases. This is because retinitis due to toxoplasmosis most commonly represents reactivation of congenital infection in immunocompetent individuals, whereas a significant proportion of immunocompromised patients have acquired new infection.

6. In patients with AIDS, syphilis may also present as a retinitis, with a vitritis and underlying large pale placoid subretinal lesions. These lesions are usually focal but may be bilateral. In addition to the opportunistic infections that cause retinitis, both *Pneumocystis carinii* and *Cryptococcus neoformans* can present with multifocal choroiditis. Neither condition typically causes a prominent retinitis.

7. Because the symptoms of CMV retinitis may initially be mild and often occur in the context of significant concurrent illness, many patients present relatively late in the course of infection. For this reason, ophthalmoscopic screening is recommended every 3 to 6 months in HIV-positive patients with a CD4 count below 100. Direct ophthalmoscopy provides only a small field of view and may be further limited in the presence of media opacities, so complete ophthalmic examination with indirect ophthalmoscopy is advised.

46.2 Test Interpretation

The diagnosis of CMV retinitis is based primarily on the ophthalmoscopic appearance. Both serologic testing and viral culture are of limited value because a large proportion of unaffected individuals show evidence of previous exposure to CMV, and many HIV-positive patients are chronic carriers of the virus in their throat, urine, and blood. A marker for CMV viral load may become available shortly and would be of use in following these patients. The use of anterior chamber paracentesis for the detection of viral DNA has proven a useful means to evaluate viral activity.

46.3 Diagnosis

CMV retinitis, OU, in a patient with AIDS.

46.4 Medical Management

The initial management of CMV is usually medical with either intravenous ganciclovir or foscarnet. After 2 to 3 weeks of high-dose induction of ganciclovir (5 mg/kg once daily) or foscarnet (60 mg/kg three times daily), patients who respond well to treatment may be switched to lower-dose daily intravenous therapy or oral therapy. Cidofovir (5 mg/kg) has been approved by the FDA for treatment of CMV. Because of its long half-life, it can be administered intravenously once per week for induction and then every 2 weeks for maintenance. Patients with progression despite induction or those with disease that imminently threatens the macula may benefit from intravitreal injection of ganciclovir (2,000 µg) or foscarnet (1.2 mg). It is important to note that intravitreal injection alone will not treat the systemic CMV infection. Since ganciclovir has myelotoxic side effects and foscarnet can result in renal toxicity, those patients who cannot tolerate systemic administration of these drugs or who progress despite it may benefit from intravitreal insertion of a ganciclovir implant that delivers adequate concentrations of the drug for 4 to 8 months.

46.5 Surgical Management

Ganciclovir implants offer a therapeutic alternative for patients with unilateral disease, especially if complications with systemic therapy are encountered.

Retinal detachment is a frequent complication of CMV retinitis, between 40 and 50% within the first year. Some small peripheral detachments may be contained by laser demarcation. However, because most of the retinal detachments seen are the result of multiple areas of necrosis and often extend to the posterior pole, pars plana vitrectomy with silicone oil tamponade is usually the procedure of choice. Often, a ganciclovir implant is inserted at the time of the procedure. Overall, approximately 90% of CMV-related retinal detachments achieve anatomic success with this approach.

46.6 Rehabilitation and Follow-up

With improvements in the care of HIV-positive patients, median survival after CMV infection has increased significantly. Therefore, issues such as cataract formation and long-term visual outcomes have become more important. Even after an initial flare-up of CMV retinitis is controlled medically or surgically, close follow-up with photographic documentation is essential.

Suggested Reading

[1] Nussenblatt RB, Lane HC. Human immunodeficiency virus disease: changing patterns of intraocular inflammation. Am J Ophthalmol. 1998; 125(3):374–382

[2] Reed JB, Schwab IR, Gordon J, Morse LS. Regression of cytomegalovirus retinitis associated with protease-inhibitor treatment in patients with AIDS. Am J Ophthalmol. 1997; 124(2):199–205

[3] Spector SA, McKinley GF, Lalezari JP, et al. Roche Cooperative Oral Ganciclovir Study Group. Oral ganciclovir for the prevention of cytomegalovirus disease in persons with AIDS. N Engl J Med. 1996; 334(23):1491–1497

[4] The Studies of Ocular Complications of AIDS (SOCA) Research Group in Collaboration with the AIDS Clinical Trials Group (ACTG). Rhegmatogenous retinal detachment in patients with cytomegalovirus retinitis: the Foscarnet-Ganciclovir Cytomegalovirus Retinitis Trial. Am J Ophthalmol. 1997; 124(1):61–70

47 The White Dot Syndromes

Tayyeba K. Ali, Blake A. Isernhagen, and Thomas Albini

Abstract

Several conditions may present with what appears to be white spots due to inflammatory foci at the level of the choroid. While there is some overlap with other causes of choroiditis, the white dot syndromes are characteristically less fulminant, but in some entities may result in severe levels of visual loss. Many of these are known to be caused by infectious etiologies, but most are only presumed to be due to viral infections. Most are self-limited, with some resulting in little or no residual visual deficit (e.g., acute retinal pigment epitheliitis, multiple evanescent white dot syndrome, and acute posterior multifocal placoid pigment epitheliopathy [APMPPE]). Diagnostic investigations almost exclusively consist of imaging modalities—fluorescein angiography and optical coherence tomography—as some entities have characteristic features (e.g., leakage with serpiginous choroiditis; early hypofluorescence followed by late staining in APMPPE). Other entities might have associated vitritis (e.g., birdshot chorioretinopathy or multifocal choroiditis). Still others might be secondarily compromised by choroidal neovascularization (e.g., punctate inner choroidopathy).

Keywords: chorioretinopathy, panuveitis, epitheliopathy

47.1 History

A 26-year-old healthy Caucasian man had a 1-week history of decreased vision and "blind spots" in both eyes. He reported recent fevers and headaches 3 weeks prior to his ocular symptoms. His best-corrected visual acuity was 20/30 in each eye. Intraocular pressures were normal, and there was no afferent pupillary defect. The anterior segment was normal, and there was no anterior or vitreous cellular inflammation. The posterior segment contained multiple, flat, deep, creamy, placoid lesions in the posterior pole of both eyes (▶ Fig. 47.1).

Fluorescein angiography (FA), indocyanine green angiography (ICG), and optical coherence tomography (OCT) were performed. The FA revealed multiple separate areas of early hypofluorescence with late staining that corresponded to areas of decreased fluorescence on ICG (▶ Fig. 47.2 and ▶ Fig. 47.3). The OCT showed areas of increased reflectivity in the outer retina, disruption of the outer segments, and retinal pigment epithelium (RPE) abnormalities that corresponded to the lesions on fundus examination (▶ Fig. 47.4).

> **Differential Diagnosis-Key Points**
>
> 1. Acute posterior multifocal placoid pigment epitheliopathy (APMPPE).
> 2. Serpiginous choroiditis (SC).
> 3. Multiple evanescent white dot syndrome (MEWDS).
> 4. Birdshot chorioretinopathy (BSCR).
> 5. Multifocal choroiditis and panuveitis (MCP).
> 6. Punctate inner choroidopathy (PIC).
> 7. Acute retinal pigment epitheliitis (ARPE).
>
> Anyone presenting with decreased vision, central scotoma, photopsias, photophobia, or floaters should undergo a thorough history and full eye examination, including a dilated fundus exam.

47.2 Case Description (APMPPE)

Presenting ocular symptoms: decreased central vision, photopsias.

Systemic symptoms: viral prodrome, headaches.

Ocular signs: multiple, deep, creamy, placoid lesions. Lesions are larger than in MEWDS and are at the level of the outer retina and RPE.

Systemic signs: rarely may be associated with neurological abnormalities, including CNS vasculitis.

47.3 Acute Posterior Multifocal Placoid Pigment Epitheliopathy

47.3.1 Epidemiology

APMPPE typically occurs in younger patients between the ages of 20 and 30 years but has also been reported in older patients up to the seventh decade of life. It is equally prevalent in men and women and is more common in Caucasian patients.

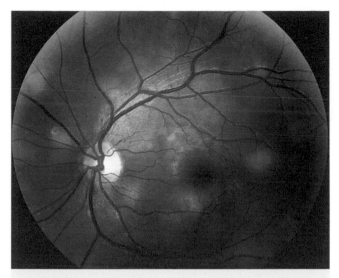

Fig. 47.1 Fundus photograph of numerous deep cream-colored placoid lesions in the posterior pole.

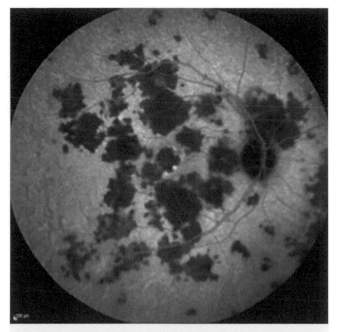

Fig. 47.3 Indocyanine green angiography of the same eye in ▶ Fig. 47.2 that shows decreased fluorescence of the same lesions.

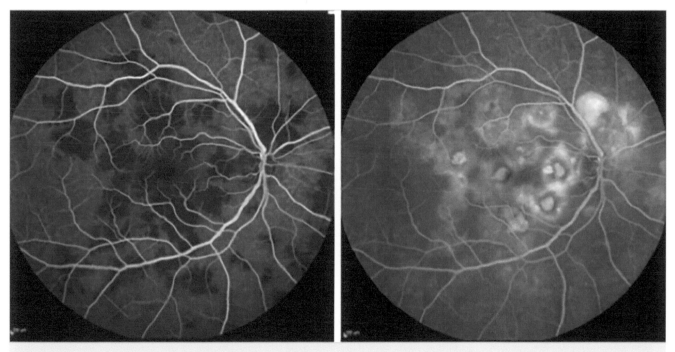

Fig. 47.2 Fluorescein angiogram with early hypofluorescence (blockage) of the lesions on the left and late staining of the same lesions on the right.

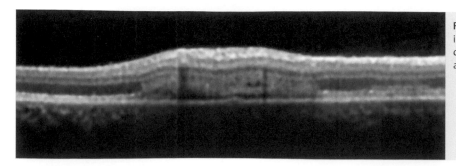

Fig. 47.4 OCT of a single lesion that reveals increased reflectivity in the outer retina, disruption of the outer segments, and RPE abnormalities.

47.3.2 History

Patients with APMPPE are typically healthy and present with complaints of sudden painless vision loss in one or both eyes. A preceding viral illness has been associated with the development of APMPPE, and many patients will report recent fevers, headache, and/or other symptoms indicating a recent upper respiratory infection. It is important to obtain a thorough history and review of systems on all patients. There are reported cases of concurrent cerebral vasculitis in some patients, and neuroimaging with appropriate referral may be indicated.

47.3.3 Clinical Findings

APMPPE is most commonly bilateral, but it can present unilaterally or asymmetrically. There is minimal anterior and vitreous cellular inflammation on clinical exam. The primary clinical findings include bilateral multiple deep, creamy-yellow lesions involving the RPE. Many times, these lesions are discrete and small to medium in size, but the lesions may also become large and confluent in more severe cases. As the acute lesions heal, they become depigmented with RPE migration and pigment clumping. Mild retinal vasculitis and optic nerve edema may also be seen on clinical exam during the acute phase.

47.3.4 Imaging

FA and ICG have characteristic findings that assist in making the diagnosis of APMPPE. The FA reveals early hypofluorescent patches representing blocking of the choroidal circulation from swollen RPE cells, followed by late staining of these same lesions due to the diffusion of dye from the choroid through the damaged RPE cells. The ICG reveals hypofluorescent choroidal lesions throughout the angiogram that correspond to the lesions seen clinically. There are frequently more lesions visible on FA/ICG than on clinical fundus examination.

OCT is another useful imaging tool to assist in the diagnosis of APMPPE. The OCT will show disruption of the outer segments with abnormal underlying RPE, and the outer nuclear layer is frequently hyperreflective in areas that correspond to the lesions on clinical exam and FA/ICG. Intraretinal fluid and subretinal fluid have also been reported in some cases of APMPPE. As the lesions heal, there is improvement in the anatomic structure of the outer segments and RPE but permanent changes usually persist.

47.3.5 Treatment and Prognosis

APMPPE is a self-limited disease that resolves without treatment over the course of several weeks to months and has a very good prognosis. Approximately 80% of patients will have a final visual acuity of 20/40 or better. Despite the observation that APMPPE is a self-limited condition, oral corticosteroids are frequently used and are recommended when the lesions involve the central macula or if there is concomitant cerebral vasculitis. Recurrences are uncommon but APMPPE can overlap with SC and become a chronic inflammatory disease. This clinical condition is now referred to as relentless placoid chorioretinitis and is treated similarly to SC.

47.4 Serpiginous Choroiditis

47.4.1 Epidemiology

SC is a rare condition that typically occurs in patients between the ages of 30 and 60 years with an equal predilection for males and females. SC tends to occur in Caucasians and patients from India.

47.4.2 History

Patients frequently present with complaints of unilateral painless decreased vision with central or paracentral visual field defects. Unlike APMPPE, it is uncommon for the patient to have had a recent viral illness. It is important to ask all patients about exposure to tuberculosis and to obtain a complete review of past medical problems and review of systems. Tuberculosis has been implicated as the cause of uveitis in some patients whose clinical presentation resembles SC.

47.4.3 Clinical Findings

Similar to APMPPE, there is rarely significant anterior chamber cell or vitritis. The primary clinical findings involve the posterior pole where confluent, deep, flat, creamy-colored lesions are seen. Classically, these lesions extend from the peripapillary region and spread centrifugally. The disease frequently becomes bilateral but is commonly asymmetric. As these lesions heal, they become atrophic and there is RPE migration with pigment clumping. SC is a chronic condition and new lesions typically occur at the edges of old healed lesions. Sometimes skip lesions develop, which represent new foci of inflammation. Many times, lesions at different stages are seen in patients who present with SC.

47.4.4 Imaging

SC is a chronic condition and it is important to document the location and size of lesions with detailed colored drawings and/or fundus photography. During the acute stage of disease, the FA closely resembles the pattern seen in APMPPE with early blocking followed by late staining of the active lesions. However, unlike APMPPE, there is frequently leakage around the active lesions in the midphase of the angiogram prior to staining of the previously hypofluorescent lesions.

ICG is also useful in diagnosing and following patients with SC. Active lesions can be either hyperfluorescent or hypofluorescent on ICG and usually have indistinct borders. All inactive lesions will be hypofluorescent with well-demarcated margins.

Another noninvasive and sensitive method to help diagnose and follow patients with SC is fundus autofluorescence (FAF). Areas of active disease will appear hyperfluorescent. In patients with previous episodes of SC, the areas of hyperfluorescence are usually at the edge of old hypofluorescent scars. The increased fluorescence of the active lesions is from the accumulation of fluorescent material due to inflamed and damaged RPE cells secondary to the underlying choroiditis. The areas of healed scars are hypofluorescent due to the severe damage of the RPE following the active phase of the disease.

OCT findings are similar to APMPPE in active lesions but inactive scarred lesions will show significant atrophy of the outer retina and RPE. OCT can help identify and follow choroidal neovascular membranes (CNVMs) that develop in areas of old chorioretinal scars.

47.4.5 Treatment and Prognosis

SC is a chronic condition that requires long-term treatment with periocular steroids and/or immunosuppression. Prior to initiating treatment, it is important to obtain laboratory evaluation to rule out infectious etiologies such as tuberculosis and syphilis. Tuberculosis has been implicated as the underlying etiology in some patients with choroiditis that resembles SC and antituberculosis therapy is indicated for initial treatment in these patients.

47.5 Multiple Evanescent White Dot Syndrome

47.5.1 Epidemiology and History

Patients who present with MEWDS are typically young, myopic females who are otherwise healthy.

Patients characteristically report an acute sudden decrease in vision in one eye. They may also have photopsias and/or a paracentral blind spot(s). They may or may not report symptoms of a preceding viral infection.

47.5.2 Clinical Findings

Findings in MEWDS are usually unilateral with mild vitritis, but without anterior chamber cellular inflammation. The principal findings on fundus examination are small, discrete, deep, white lesions in the posterior pole that can also involve the midperiphery with a granular appearance in the macula manifested by small white and orange specks (▶ Fig. 47.5). Optic nerve edema and mild retinal vasculitis may also be observed.

47.5.3 Imaging

The FA shows early hyperfluorescence with late staining of the lesions and hyperfluorescence of the optic nerve (▶ Fig. 47.6). ICG shows hypofluorescence of the corresponding lesions seen clinically, but there is usually more involvement on ICG than is seen on clinical examination and on FA.

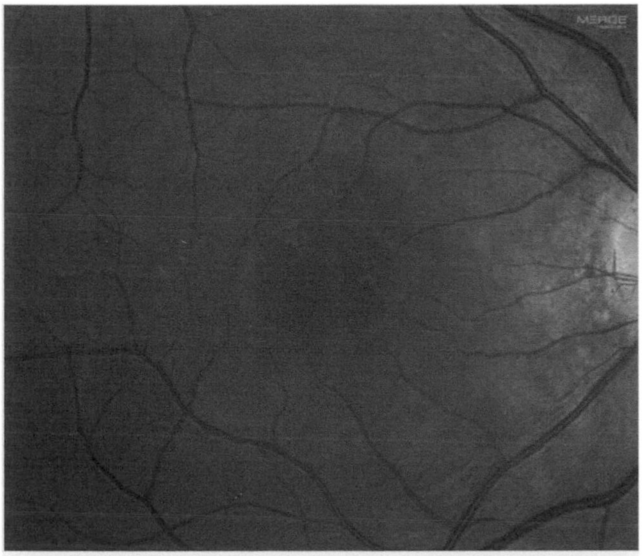

Fig. 47.5 Fundus photograph of a patient with MEWDS that demonstrates the granular appearance of the macula with small white and orange specks.

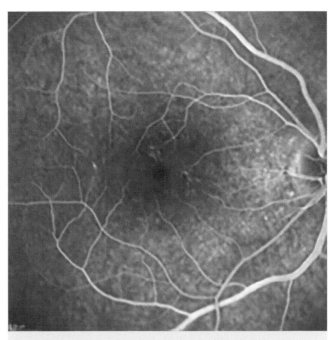

Fig. 47.6 Fluorescein angiography with hyperfluorescence of the lesions seen clinically in ▶ Fig. 47.5.

FAF can be used to help determine the extent of RPE involvement. In the acute phase of disease, the involved areas are hyperfluorescent (▶ Fig. 47.7). However, unlike other more severe chorioretinopathies, there is usually minimal permanent damage to the RPE. Follow-up studies frequently return to normal fluorescence or faint hypofluorescence in the previously involved areas.

On OCT, changes to the outer retina are seen with disruption of the outer segments (▶ Fig. 47.8). Following the acute phase, there may be a return to a more normal anatomical configuration consistent with resolution of the patient's visual symptoms.

47.5.4 Treatment and Prognosis

Patients with MEWDS usually do not require laboratory evaluation or treatment. The visual prognosis is good and most patients will have significant improvement in vision to 20/30 or better within 4 to 8 weeks. Recurrences are uncommon, but if these become frequent, immunosuppression may be used to help control the disease course.

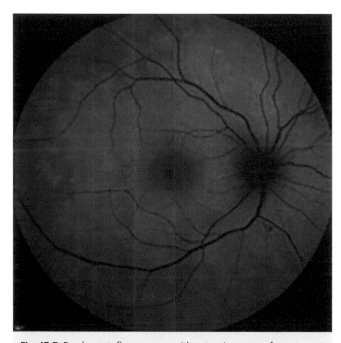

Fig. 47.7 Fundus autofluorescence with extensive areas of hyperautofluorescence that indicates more involvement of the RPE than is appreciated on clinical exam and FA.

47.6 Birdshot Chorioretinopathy

47.6.1 Epidemiology

BSCR, also known as vitiliginous chorioretinopathy, most commonly occurs among middle-aged Northern European women. However, it can occur in any Caucasian group, and patients' age ranges from 15 to 79 years.

47.6.2 History

This posterior uveitis is characterized by vitritis, retinal vasculitis, and multiple, bilateral, hypopigmented chorioretinal lesions emanating from the optic nerve in a radial pattern. Patients typically have no systemic findings, though some studies suggest a higher prevalence of cardiovascular disease. There is a strong association with HLA-A29, which can sometimes help confirm the diagnosis. The disease course is chronic, most often requiring immunomodulatory therapy (IMT).

47.6.3 Clinical Findings

BSCR is a bilateral disease, characterized by a quiet, nonpainful eye, minimal anterior cell, vitritis without pars plana exudation, retinal vasculitis (frequently with cystoid macular edema [CME] and optic nerve swelling), and distinct, deep cream-colored spots scattered throughout the fundus (▶ Fig. 47.9). Patients' visual complaints may be greatly out of proportion to the exam findings, which may be elucidated via electroretinogram (ERG) testing. The most common complication associated with BSCR is CME, followed by epiretinal membrane (ERM) formation, CNVM, and even retinal detachment.

47.6.4 Imaging

FA findings vary based on disease stage and activity. While, early in the course of the disease, FA may not correspond with the creamy lesions seen on fundus exam, typically one will see early hypofluorescence with late staining. The FA is most useful in determining the extent of the CME and other vascular leakage and also in following the clinical course of the disease. ICG depicts well-demarcated hypofluorescent choroidal lesions, often more numerous than seen clinically (▶ Fig. 47.10).

OCT shows inner segment/outer segment (IS/OS) disruption as well as RPE loss. ERG will typically show a preserved a-wave, with a reduced b-wave. Visual field testing may show generalized constriction, paracentral or central scotoma, or an enlarged blind spot. Goldmann visual field is thought to be more sensitive than Humphrey visual field testing.

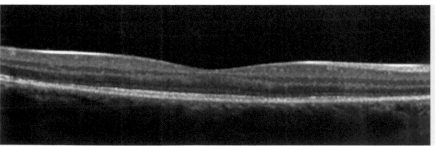

Fig. 47.8 OCT of the same patient reveals an abnormal outer retina, disruption of the outer segments, and an irregular RPE.

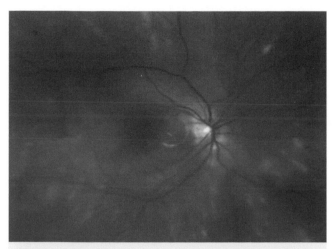

Fig. 47.9 Fundus photograph of a patient with BSCR that shows numerous distinct hypopigmented creamy lesions that are more prominent in the nasal fundus.

47.6.5 Treatment and Prognosis

Global retinal dysfunction ensues if these patients are not aggressively treated. While periocular and oral corticosteroids have been used to suppress disease activity, many patients will have progressive visual deterioration secondary to either recurrence or sequelae, such as CME. Thus, due to the waxing and waning nature of most BSCR, IMT is recommended in order to preserve maximum retinal function and vision. Monotherapy with cyclosporine or in conjunction with either low-dose steroids or an additional IMT agent is recommended. If multiple agents are to be used, cyclosporine (CSA) can be used at a lower dose (2.5–5 mg/kg/day) and mycophenolate, azathioprine, or low-dose steroids can be added. This decreases the cardiovascular side effects associated with CSA, oftentimes avoiding the need to stop the medication or add on an antihypertensive medication.

If left untreated, 80 to 90% of birdshot patients will end up with unilateral or bilateral severe vision loss with decrease in central and peripheral vision. Disease progression and control can be monitored with yearly FA/ICG and OCT imaging. Initial, aggressive treatment with multiple IMT agents for 2 years may put the disease into remission and help preserve good vision in these otherwise healthy individuals.

47.7 Multifocal Choroiditis and Panuveitis

47.7.1 Epidemiology and History

MCP most commonly occurs in young, myopic women, although it has been reported in the 6- to 69-year-old range, in hyperopes, and in men. The white dot syndrome is described as having histoplasmosislike lesions with vitritis and anterior segment inflammation. Most patients will have bilateral, though asymmetric, disease. The course is recurrent and chronic. This chronicity may lead to CME, ERM, and CNVM, which is the leading cause of vision loss in these patients.

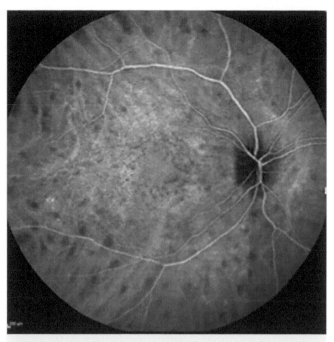

Fig. 47.10 Indocyanine green angiography with numerous small hypofluorescent spots throughout the fundus corresponding to areas of choroidal inflammation.

47.7.2 Clinical Findings

MCP is characterized by decreased or blurred vision, with less frequent complaints of photopsias and floaters. Visual acuity averages 20/50, but has been reported as poor as light perception. Mild to moderate anterior uveitis is present with nongranulomatous keratic precipitates, posterior synechiae, and cell. On dilated fundus examination, one will see oval, yellow-gray lesions at the level of the RPE in the posterior pole and midperiphery. These lesions will develop into round, punched-out chorioretinal scars. Findings may be associated with optic disc edema or peripapillary atrophy. On perimetry, there may be an enlarged blind spot, and typically, a depressed ERG is noted.

47.7.3 Imaging

MCP is a clinical diagnosis based on fundus findings and presence of vitritis and anterior segment inflammation. FA usually shows early hypofluorescence and late staining. Inactive scars will have window defects. One may also see angiographic leakage or a CNVM on FA. Acute disease will show hypofluorescent choroidal lesions on ICG that resolve with treatment. OCT will show IS/OS disruption and RPE involvement.

Autofluorescence provides an additional tool that may help differentiate acute versus chronic, as well as subclinical, disease. Larger areas of hypoautofluorescence often coincide with lesions seen on clinical exam, while smaller areas may be pre- or subclinical disease.

47.7.4 Treatment and Prognosis

Visual prognosis is guarded in patients who do not receive adequate and aggressive therapy, as the disease is chronic and recurrent in nature. Visual loss is greatly due to development of

CNVM, but also can be secondary to CME, ERM, RPE atrophy and scarring, optic neuropathy, or neovascular glaucoma. Vision can be preserved with periocular and systemic steroids in conjunction with early initiation of immunosuppression. CNVM can be treated with laser photocoagulation, intravitreal steroids, or even anti-vascular endothelial growth factor (anti-VEGF) therapy.

47.8 Punctate Inner Choroidopathy

47.8.1 Epidemiology and History

PIC is a rare disease affecting young, myopic women in their 30 s. These patients present with blurred vision and a scotoma. It is rare to see inflammation, and a fundus examination will show yellow lesions in the posterior pole. It is a self-limiting disease with a good visual outcome, though CNVM can occur and lead to visual decline.

47.8.2 Clinical Findings

PIC is diagnosed when there are multiple small deep, yellow lesions in the outer retina and inner choroid confined to the posterior pole (▶ Fig. 47.11). They may resemble POHS (presumed ocular histoplasmosis syndrome) spots, but these patients are not typically from endemic areas or have prior exposure to histoplasmosis. Also, an inflammatory reaction is absent. Development of CNVM is the leading cause of vision loss.

47.8.3 Imaging

This is primarily a clinical diagnosis; however, fundus imaging can have a classic appearance. On FA, one would see early hyperfluorescence with arteriovenous staining. Serous detachments and CNVMs may be present and can be visualized on FA. ICG typically shows hypofluorescent areas, which may correlate with choroidal hypoperfusion.

OCT will show IS/OS disruption as well as RPE elevation with a collection of sub-RPE deposits. These areas may correlate with localized fibrotic lesions during the active phase of the disease.

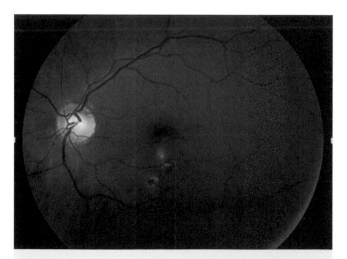

Fig. 47.11 Fundus photograph of a patient with PIC who has old chorioretinal scars in the inferior macula and small white lesions centrally representing new foci of active chorioretinal inflammation.

47.8.4 Treatment and Prognosis

Patients typically do well and do not often require treatment, with vision that is 20/40 or better. However, if there is a CNVM present or lesions are close to the fovea, treatment with systemic or local steroids is indicated. Anti-VEGF injections have also been shown to be effective for treatment of CNVMs related to PIC. Patients requiring multiple courses of systemic steroids may benefit from steroid-sparing immunosuppression, which has been shown to be effective in a small group of patients.

47.9 Acute Retinal Pigment Epitheliitis

47.9.1 Epidemiology

ARPE usually occurs in healthy patients during the second to fourth decade of life and is more common in men. The condition is rare and likely underreported due to the transient nature and mild symptoms. The etiology is hypothesized to be viral, but no studies have validated this theory.

47.9.2 History

Patients present with acute unilateral or bilateral decreased vision. They may also report a central scotoma or metamorphopsia that can be elucidated on Amsler grid testing. Unlike other conditions, such as APMPPE, patients do not endorse a recent viral illness.

47.9.3 Clinical Findings

Visual acuity may range from 20/20 to 20/100 in the affected eye(s) and there is absence of anterior and vitreous cellular inflammation. The primary area of ocular involvement is the RPE, and during the acute phase of inflammation, there are multiple, deep, small, dark spots surrounded by a yellow halo in the posterior pole. As the lesions heal, the halo disappears and there may be pigment migration around the lesions.

47.9.4 Imaging

FA will typically show early hyperfluorescent spot(s) with a hypofluorescent center that corresponds to the lesions seen clinically. During the later phases of the angiogram, there is increased fluorescence of the lesions that is more consistent with a window defect than staining or leakage. Sometimes, the FA will be normal and fail to reveal any lesions.

OCT reveals disruption of the outer and inner photoreceptor segments with an irregular RPE. As the lesion(s) heal, there is improvement in the anatomic structures.

47.9.5 Treatment and Prognosis

The visual prognosis is good in ARPE, and no treatment is routinely indicated. Most patients will have a return of vision to 20/30 or better within 3 months. There have been no significant ocular complications secondary to ARPE, and if the disease recurs or complications arise, an alternative diagnosis should be suspected.

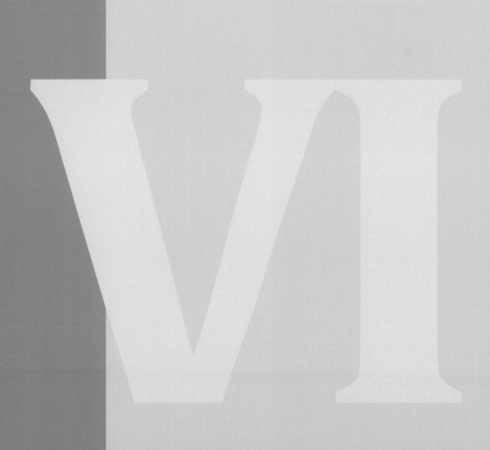

Part VI

Tumors

VI

48 Vascular Tumor

Eric D. Hansen and William E. Smiddy

Abstract

Vascular tumors are characteristic of a broad range of ocular conditions, ranging from hemangiomas associated with phacomatoses to idiopathic conditions. Distinguishing their clinical appearance as a predominantly exudative form or endophytic or vitreoretinal form may help identify the correct diagnosis. Similarly, identifying the vasoproliferation as arising from the retinal or choroidal vasculature allows distinction. In the case of phacomatoses, numerous clinical features may assist in diagnoses, such as systemic clinical associations or family history patterns. Important differential diagnostic entities include neoplasms with prominent vascular components. Careful biomicroscopy in conjunction with fluorescein angiography or echographic evaluation is important not only to distinguish the various benign proliferative entities, but also to exclude the diagnosis of malignancies with prominent vascular components.

Keywords: intraocular tumor, retinal proliferation, hemangioma, phacomatosis, ocular neoplasm

48.1 History

A 20-year-old man presents for evaluation of a peripheral retinal lesion in the left eye found on routine ophthalmic examination. The patient is asymptomatic and has no other past ocular history. He has no known systemic medical problems. A family history screening discloses his father and two siblings carry a diagnosis of von Hippel–Lindau disease. Visual acuity is 20/20 bilaterally. External examination is unremarkable. There is no afferent pupillary defect. Visual field and motility examinations are unremarkable. Slit-lamp examination is normal. The left fundus contains several dilated, tortuous arterioles and venules emanating from the optic disc and traveling nasally (▶ Fig. 48.1). These vessels lead to a collection of reddish-pink nodules surrounding a large reddish-orange lesion emanating from the surface of the retina. There is a small associated area of subretinal fluid with adjacent exudate (▶ Fig. 48.2). Funduscopic examination of the right eye is normal.

Differential Diagnosis—Key Points

- Cavernous hemangioma.
- Racemose hemangioma.
- Retinal macroaneurysm.
- Coats' disease.
- Retinal granuloma.
- Familial exudative vitreoretinopathy (FEVR).
- Retinoblastoma.
- Astrocytic hamartoma.
- Uveal melanoma.
- Vasoproliferative tumor.
1. With the family history of von Hippel–Lindau disease and the classic appearance of the lesions, the diagnosis of retinal angiomatosis is readily made in this patient. Benign retinal

hemangiomas were first described by von Hippel in 1904 and are sometimes referred to as von Hippel tumors. The appearance of retinal angiomas may vary greatly, and they are generally described according to their location, their size, and their pattern of growth. *Peripheral* retinal angiomas are associated with a dilated, tortuous feeding arteriole and draining venule, whereas *juxtapapillary* or *peripapillary* angiomas often do not feature the accompanying vessels. These associated vessels may present as twin vessels, separated by no more than a venule width. The presentation also varies greatly with size. Early lesions may be so small that they are clinically imperceptible except with imaging modalities. As the angiomas grow, they may be first noted as small yellow or red nodules with dilated vessels, and later as the typical reddish-orange mass with dilated feeding vessels. Angiomas arising from the inner retina have an endophytic appearance, while those arising from the outer retina result in an exophytic appearance. A sessile morphology is also described in the literature.

2. Retinal angiomas tend to manifest clinically in one of two forms. The exudative form is characterized by progressive vascular leakage from the angioma, resulting in accumulation of subretinal fluid and exudate. Loss of vision in these cases may result from exudative retinal detachments or from accumulation of exudative material in the central macula from a peripheral angioma. The endophytic, or vitreoretinal, form is characterized by reactive fibrosis of the overlying vitreous and gliosis, leading to epiretinal membranes and retinal traction. Vision loss occurs secondary to tractional or combined tractional–rhegmatogenous retinal detachments, or secondary to the distortion caused by epiretinal membranes. Interestingly, epiretinal membranes formation may occur centrally even in peripheral angiomas.

3. In the current case, the family history and the classic funduscopic appearance of the retinal lesions quickly narrow the differential diagnosis; however, other entities may mimic retinal angiomas. Cavernous hemangiomas present as a cluster of dilated vessels centered around a retinal vein, but these typically lack dilated feeder vessels and tend not to cause retinal exudation. Racemose hemangiomas also present with dilated tortuous arterioles and venules. Distinguishing features in this entity include the lack of a terminal lesion and the absence of exudation. Retinoblastoma and astrocytic hamartoma arise from the retina, but these lesions are typically yellowish-white as opposed to the reddish-orange appearance of an angioma, and vary in demographics and timing of presentation. An arteriolar macroaneurysm may simulate an early angioma; however, the patient's age and the lack of associated hypertensive changes of the retinal vasculature should help differentiate between the two entities. Retinal angiomas present in the second to third decade of life. A retinal granuloma, particularly papillary lesions due to a nematode, foreign body, or inflammatory disease, may be

indistinguishable from a juxtapapillary angioma. Associated findings and ancillary tests should assist in determining the correct diagnosis. In cases with exudative retinal detachment, consideration should be given to retinoblastoma, Coats' disease, and FEVR. Uveal melanomas, although commonly different in appearance and presentation, can mimic retinal angiomas and should always be considered with large endophytic lesions. Papillary or peripapillary angiomas can be particularly perplexing to the clinician and require careful attention as these can present similar to a wide variety of retinal lesions.

4. Distinguishing between von Hippel lesions and vasoproliferative retinal tumors, or acquired capillary hemangiomas, can also present unique challenges, as the appearance of these masses can be quite similar. However, the vasoproliferative tumor does not exhibit the dilated feeder vessels associated with retinal angiomas. In addition, vasoproliferative tumors often occur in the setting of an existing retinal disease and have preponderance for the inferior quadrants and the extreme periphery. Retinal angiomas, conversely, are commonly found in the midperiphery of the temporal quadrants.

5. Multiple angiomas, whether unilateral or bilateral, suggests the presence of von Hippel–Lindau disease. A careful family history and review of systems looking for features consistent with von Hippel–Lindau disease should be taken in all patients with retinal angiomas.

6. Unlike peripheral retinal hemangiomas, peripapillary and capillary hemangiomas are generally not associated with von Hippel–Lindau syndrome.

48.2 Test Interpretation

The diagnosis of a retinal angioma is usually made clinically. Slit-lamp biomicroscopy may provide a diagnostic view of posterior lesions, while indirect ophthalmoscopy provides the optimal view of more peripheral lesions. However, ancillary tests can assist in making the diagnosis in difficult cases.

Fluorescein angiography is helpful in differentiating some angiomas, particularly exophytic masses. Angiography typically reveals the dilated retinal arteriole in the early arterial phase followed by hyperfluorescence of the tumor itself due to filling of the individual capillaries. The venous phase generally reveals the prominently dilated venule as well as continued hyperfluorescence of the angioma (▶ Fig. 48.3). Late-phase angiography will exhibit continued hyperfluorescence of the angioma as well as possible leakage of fluorescein.

Although less common in practice, fluorescein angioscopy may assist detecting early angiomas. Early lesions may be very small or subtle due to the reddish coloration of the lesion, which blends into the underlying retinal pigment epithelium and choroid on indirect ophthalmoscopy. Use of angioscopy by performing indirect ophthalmoscopy with the use of an

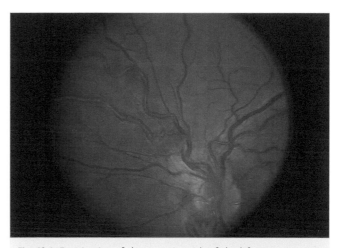

Fig. 48.1 Examination of the posterior pole of the left eye demonstrates the multiple tortuous, dilated vessels arising from the optic disc and radiating toward the nasal periphery. Note that the affected vessels include arterioles and venules.

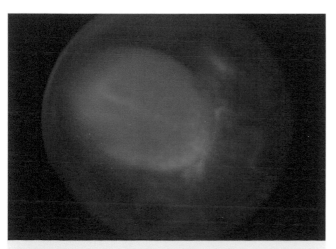

Fig. 48.2 Peripheral examination revealed a collection of reddish-orange tumors. Each had an associated dilated feeding arteriole and draining venule. There also was a small associated area of adjacent subretinal fluid and exudate.

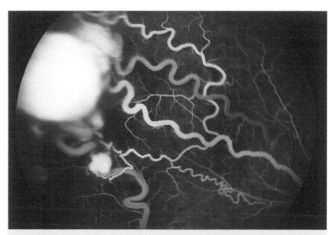

Fig. 48.3 Laminar venous phase fluorescein angiogram reveals filling of dilated arterioles and hyperfluorescence of the angiomas. Laminar filling of the venules is also seen.

excitation light during fluorescein injection can assist in locating very small angiomas.

Ultrasound examination identifies and quantitates some retinal angiomas, especially if larger than 2 mm. B-scan ultrasonography typically yields a high-density echo at the inner border of the mass with a uniform acoustic signal throughout the mass. Associated retinal detachment and subretinal fluid may be demonstrated; however, no choroidal component will be noted. A-scan ultrasonography demonstrates a high spike at the internal border of lesion and a high internal reflectivity.

Computed tomography (CT) and magnetic resonance imaging (MRI) will generally characterize only larger tumors and those with exudative retinal detachments. CT may demonstrate an enhancing intraocular mass. MRI will have a low signal intensity from a retinal angioma. This results in an isointense to hyperintense signal on Tl-weighted images and an isointense to hypointense signal on T2-weighted images with respect to the vitreous. The lesion will demonstrate moderate enhancement with gadolinium administration. Unfortunately, the MRI appearance is not diagnostic, as ocular melanomas and retinoblastomas may have similar characteristics. These imaging modalities remain important, however, as patients should undergo neuroimaging to exclude central nervous system (CNS) findings of von Hippel disease.

48.3 Diagnosis

1. Multiple retinal angiomas OS.
2. von Hippel–Lindau disease.

48.4 Surgical Management

The management of retinal angiomas first hinges on the decision whether to treat or continue observation. The treatment of asymptomatic angiomas is controversial; however, lesions causing vision loss or impending vision loss should generally be treated. Large observational studies have demonstrated that angiomas can exhibit stability, regress, or progressively enlarge and result in visual impairment. While smaller lesions (less than 2.5 disc diameters) are more easily treated and present less risk of complications, these smaller lesions are also more likely to remain stable or spontaneously regress.

Treatment modalities vary depending primarily on the size and location of the lesion. The management mainstays of retinal angiomas include observation, laser photocoagulation, and cryotherapy. More recent treatment options include antiangiogenic medications and transpupillary thermotherapy. Laser can be particularly effective against smaller lesions, but has shown effect in lesions up to 4.5 mm in size. Treatment of the feeder vessel or direct treatment of the lesion has shown similar success. Some advocate a stepwise approach, initiating feeder vessel treatment to induce closure of the vessels followed by direct treatment of the angioma. Larger and more peripheral tumors can be successfully treated with double or triple freeze-thaw cryotherapy. Plaque radiotherapy using apex dose of 1,000 to 5,000 cGy may be used with large angiomas. External beam radiotherapy is employed in the setting of an angioma associated with abundant subretinal fluid and exudate. Surgical management with pars plana vitrectomy may relieve vitreoretinal

traction, remove epiretinal membranes, and treat the angiomas directly, although such surgeries are often technically difficult and fraught with complications such as hemorrhage and recurrence.

Novel therapeutic options consisting of systemic or intravitreal antiangiogenic medicines targeting Vascular endothelial growth factor or platelet-derived growth factor have been investigated, although the early results of these studies are inconclusive. Angiogenesis, directed by such molecules, is thought to play an important role in the pathophysiology of retinal angiomas.

The response to treatment may take numerous treatments and several months; in some cases, a paradoxical response with increasing subretinal fluid, exudate, and vitreoretinal traction occurs. These untoward responses tend to occur in larger lesions and contribute to the rationale for treatment of early lesions. Importantly, epiretinal membranes may resolve spontaneously after treatment of the angioma; therefore, surgeons should wait 4 to 6 months before considering surgical correction.

48.5 Rehabilitation and Follow-up

Von Hippel–Lindau disease should be considered in any patient with retinal angiomatosis. Von Hippel–Lindau is an autosomal dominant condition affecting organ systems throughout the entire body (▶ Table 48.1). It one of the recognized phakomatoses with an incidence estimated to be 1 in 35,000 to 1 in 40,000. The von Hippel–Lindau gene is located on chromosome 3p25–26, coding for a tumor-suppressor protein. The disease requires a "two-hit" mechanism similar to retinoblastomas, and mutations causing von Hippel–Lindau disease can occur via deletion, truncating mutations, or missense mutation. Classically, the diagnosis is made in patients exhibiting two or more findings consistent with von Hippel–Lindau disease if there is no family history or in patients with one finding and an affected first-degree relative. Genetic testing is also available to assist in early diagnosis.

Retinal angiomas develop in a majority (49–85%) of patients with von Hippel–Lindau disease. They tend to be the initial findings of the disease, usually in the patient's early- to mid-20 s. However, retinal examinations should begin early in childhood, as angiomas have been described in children younger than 10 years. Because of the high risk of developing angiomas, these patients deserve periodic ophthalmic examination with

Table 48.1 Clinical manifestations of von Hippel–Lindau disease

Eye	Retinal angiomas
Central nervous system	Cerebellar hemangioblastoma
	Medullary hemangioblastoma
	Spinal cord hemangioblastoma
	Syringobulbia
	Syringomyelia
Renal	Renal cell carcinoma
	Hemangioblastoma cysts
Adrenal glands and sympathetic chain	Pheochromocytoma paraganglioma
Pancreas	Hemangioblastoma cysts
Epididymis	cysts

indirect ophthalmoscopy. Annual to biannual examination for affected individuals and first-degree relatives is recommended.

The systemic features of this disease are potentially debilitating or fatal; therefore, patients and first-degree relatives must undergo periodic systemic screenings. Systemic screenings include imaging of the CNS and the thoracic and abdominal cavities. In addition, 24-hour urine collection analysis for pheochromocytoma is warranted. As retinal angiomas are often the presenting feature of this disease, the ophthalmologist must work in concert with other specialists to ensure that patients with or at risk for von Hippel–Lindau disease receive the appropriate initial workup and subsequent follow-up.

Suggested Reading

[1] Blodi CF, Russell SR, Pulido JS, Folk JC. Direct and feeder vessel photocoagulation of retinal angiomas with dye yellow laser. Ophthalmology. 1990; 97(6): 791–795, discussion 796–797

[2] Gass JD. Stereoscopic Atlas of Macular Diseases: Diagnosis and Treatment. 4th ed. St. Louis, MO: Mosby; 1991:850–858

[3] Jennings AM, Smith C, Cole DR, et al. Von Hippel-Lindau disease in a large British family: clinicopathological features and recommendations for screening and follow-up. Q J Med. 1988; 66(251):233–249

[4] Moore AT, Maher ER, Rosen P, Gregor Z, Bird AC. Ophthalmological screening for von Hippel-Lindau disease. Eye (Lond). 1991; 5(Pt 6):723–728

[5] Shields CL, Shields JA, Barrett J, De Potter P. Vasoproliferative tumors of the ocular fundus. Classification and clinical manifestations in 103 patients. Arch Ophthalmol. 1995; 113(5):615–623

[6] Wong WT, Chew EY. Ocular von Hippel-Lindau disease: clinical update and emerging treatments. Curr Opin Ophthalmol. 2008; 19(3):213–217

[7] Singh AD, Shields CL, Shields JA. von Hippel-Lindau disease. Surv Ophthalmol. 2001; 46(2):117–142

49 Choroidal Melanoma

Basil K. Williams, Jr.

Abstract

Choroidal melanoma is the most common primary intraocular tumor in adults. These lesions are frequently pigmented, but a small percentage may be primarily amelanotic. There is a broad differential diagnosis for pigmented lesions of the choroid, but ancillary imaging studies can assist in making the diagnosis. Characteristic findings include low to medium internal reflectivity on A-scan ultrasonography and a dome- or mushroom-shaped lesion with intrinsic vascularity on B-scan ultrasonography. Fundus autofluorescence may demonstrate hyperautofluorescence representing orange-pigmented lipofuscin, and optical coherence tomography may identify subretinal fluid. Prognostic information may be attained by anatomic staging, pathologic assessment, or gene expression profiling. The most common forms of treatment are radiation, often with plaque brachytherapy, and enucleation for large melanomas. Periodic follow-up examination is required to determine response to treatment, identify recurrence, and assess for complications. These patients also require long-term systemic evaluation to monitor for metastasis, which most commonly occurs in the liver.

Keywords: choroid, eye, melanoma, pseudomelanoma, tumor, uvea

49.1 History

A 55-year-old Caucasian man presented with a 2-week history of photopsias and blurred central vision in the right eye for the previous 3 days. Past medical history was notable for hypertension, hypercholesterolemia, and skin cancer. Past ocular history was remarkable for macular degeneration.

Examination disclosed a visual acuity of 20/60 in the right eye and 20/20 in the left eye. Intraocular pressures were 15 mm Hg in both eyes. There was a 1 + right afferent pupillary defect. Slit-lamp examination was notable for mild nuclear sclerotic alterations in both eyes. Dilated funduscopic examination of the right eye revealed a dome-shaped moderately pigmented inferotemporal mass with an exudative retinal detachment located anterior to the mass (▶ Fig. 49.1). Examination of the left eye was unremarkable. The lesion had a thickness of 4.5 mm and base of 11.9 × 10.1 mm confirmed by echography. B-scan ultrasonography demonstrated a dome-shaped lesion with an exudative retinal detachment and choroidal excavation (▶ Fig. 49.2a, b). There was no evidence of extrascleral extension. A-scan ultrasonography revealed low internal reflectivity and a regular internal structure. Fluorescein angiography of the right eye demonstrated a lesion with intrinsic vascularity and progressive late leakage. The patient underwent a medical workup to rule out the presence of metastasis, including liver function tests and a chest X-ray that was unremarkable.

The patient was diagnosed with a medium-sized posterior uveal melanoma. After discussion of alternative treatment options, the patient underwent fine-needle aspiration biopsy for gene-expression profiling at the time of iodine-125 radioactive plaque placement.

Gene profiling yielded a class 1A tumor, prompting annual liver ultrasound for metastatic evaluation. Seven months following radioactive plaque therapy, visual acuity in the right eye was 20/40 and there was progressive nuclear sclerosis of the lens. The mass had decreased in size posttreatment to a height of 2.3 mm (▶ Fig. 49.3). There were significant pigmentary alterations of the lesion with resolution of the overlying neurosensory detachment. The remainder of the retina remained normal, without radiation-related changes (▶ Fig. 49.4).

49.2 Differential Diagnosis

The differential diagnosis of a choroidal lesion includes choroidal nevus, congenital hypertrophy of the retinal pigment epithelium (CHRPE), peripheral disciform lesion, melanocytoma, metastatic carcinoma, choroidal hemangioma, and choroidal detachment. Choroidal nevi are the most common pseudomelanoma. They are typically asymptomatic, lack orange pigment and subretinal fluid, are less than 2 mm thick, and rarely demonstrate growth. CHRPE lesions are flat, heavily pigmented lesions with sharp borders and a surrounding hypopigmented halo. Peripheral disciform lesions tend to show blockage on fluorescein angiography and frequently resolve spontaneously. Melanocytomas of the optic nerve are typically jet-black in color—a color rarely seen in choroidal melanomas. Metastatic melanoma lesions are more frequently bilateral and multifocal, and demonstrate higher internal reflectivity than choroidal melanomas on ultrasound. Choroidal hemangiomas demonstrate high internal reflectivity on ultrasound with widespread, diffuse leakage on fluorescein angiography. Choroidal detachment typically occurs in the setting of intraocular surgery, hypotony, or uveitis, and is often accompanied by pain.

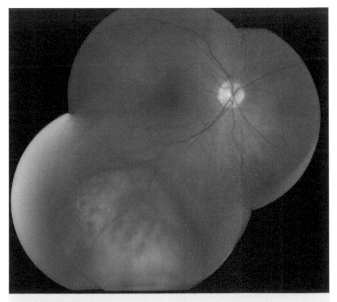

Fig. 49.1 Color photograph of the right eye demonstrating a pigmented lesion located inferotemporal to the macula with an exudative retinal detachment at the anterior portion of the lesion.

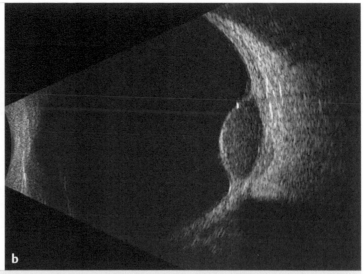

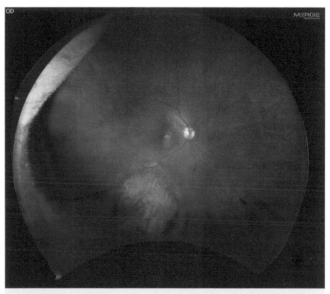

Fig. 49.2 (a) A-scan ultrasound of the mass in the right eye revealed low internal reflectivity. (b) B-scan ultrasound of the mass in the right eye revealed a dome-shaped, regularly structured mass with a shallow exudative retinal detachment choroidal excavation.

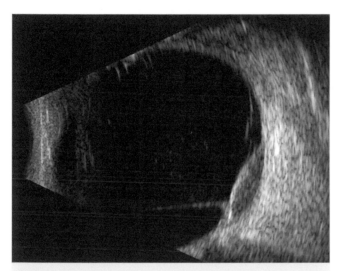

Fig. 49.3 B-scan ultrasound of the mass at 6 months follow-up revealing a decrease in tumor thickness with resolution of the anteriorly located retinal detachment.

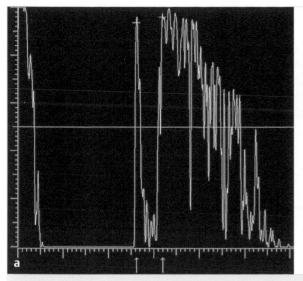

Fig. 49.4 Color photograph of the right eye posttreatment demonstrating substantial pigmentary alterations involving the original extent of the tumor and the remainder of the retina did not reveal radiation-related vasculopathy of the retina.

49.3 Test Interpretation

The diagnosis and staging of choroidal melanoma require clinical examination and local and systemic ancillary testing. The history is typically not very useful in differentiating choroidal melanomas from other simulating lesions. The most common presenting symptoms include visual acuity loss, persistent photopsias, and visual field defects. Clinical examinations including slit-lamp biomicroscopy and indirect ophthalmoscopy are the most important tools in evaluating choroidal melanomas. Lesions are pigmented in greater than 50% of cases, but may be primarily amelanotic in up to 15% of cases. They usually present with a dome configuration but may have a mushroom-shaped appearance if the lesion breaks through Bruch's membrane. The tumor appears as a mass deep to the retina often with an associated exudative retinal detachment and occasionally producing a vitreous hemorrhage. Adjacent structures may be affected causing cataract, rarely secondary glaucoma, and dilated episcleral (sentinel) vessels when affecting the ciliary body.

Combined A- and B-scan ultrasonography is the most important ancillary test in the evaluation of patients with choroidal melanomas and simulating lesions. It is useful for establishing the diagnosis, documenting the size of the lesion, and determining the therapeutic approach. A-scan ultrasonography typically reveals low to medium internal reflectivity, a regular internal structure, and intrinsic vascularity. It can also provide information on the presence or absence of scleral infiltration and extraocular extension. B-scan ultrasonography often demonstrates a dome or mushroom shape, intrinsic vascularity, solid consistency, sound attenuation, choroidal excavation, and orbital shadowing. Moreover, B-scan ultrasonography provides basal and apical dimensions that can be used to document size for periodic observation and for assessment of regression after treatment.

Fundus photography is most useful for documentation of size and location of suspicious small lesions to evaluate and monitor for growth. Additionally, this modality allows for documentation of response to therapy.

Because of improved diagnostic accuracy via clinical examination and ultrasonography, fluorescein angiography is of limited use in diagnosing choroidal melanomas, but may be extremely useful in the evaluation of simulating lesions such as peripheral disciform lesions or choroidal hemangiomas. A choroidal melanoma may demonstrate intrinsic vasculature, "hot spots," vascular leakage, and late staining within the tumor.

Fundus autofluorescence imaging is one of the newer techniques utilized in the diagnosis of melanomas. The orange-pigmented lipofuscin, helpful in the differentiation of nevi from melanomas, is brightly autofluorescent. This is especially useful in amelanotic lesions, in which the lipofuscin may appear black in color.

Optical coherence tomography (OCT) is another ancillary test that aids in diagnosis, particularly in small or potential melanomas. Enhanced depth imaging may be used to measure the thickness of small melanomas to monitor for growth, but these measurements are not interchangeable with those obtained by ultrasound. Additionally, OCT can be used to determine if there is subretinal fluid undetectable by clinical exam, as this factor makes the lesion more likely to be a melanoma than a nevus.

Fine-needle aspiration, tumor resection, or enucleation provides adequate tissue for gene expression profiling. This assay is a well-validated polymerase chain reaction–based test that measures mRNA expression of 12 discriminating genes and 3 control genes. Based on the results, choroidal melanomas are divided into two prognostic categories. Class 1 tumors have low metastatic potential and are further subdivided into class 1A and class 1B, which have 2 and 21% 5-year metastatic risk, respectively. Class 2 tumors have a high risk of metastasis, reported to be 72% at 5 years. Appropriate risk stratification allows for individualized management including metastatic screening and targeted therapy.

49.4 Diagnosis

Right eye: medium-sized choroidal melanoma.

49.5 Classification

Historically, choroidal melanomas have been divided into three categories based on tumor thickness and basal dimensions, including small, medium, and large (▶ Table 49.1). These categories were based on the Collaborative Ocular Melanoma Study (COMS), a prospective randomized multicenter clinical trial

Table 49.1 COMS classification of choroidal melanoma

Small	
• Apical height	1.0–2.4 mm
• Basal diameter	5.0–16 mm
Medium	
• Apical height	2.5–10 mm[a]
• Basal diameter	≤16 mm
Large	
• Apical height	>10 mm (8 mm for peripapillary tumors)
• Basal diameter	>16 mm

Note: As measured by ultrasound testing.
[a]Changed November 1990 from 3.1 to 8.0 mm.

designed to evaluate alternative methods of management for choroidal melanoma. More recently, the American Joint Committee on Cancer Staging updated the classification to stratify by anatomic stage for prognostication of metastatic death and disease using the universal tumor (T), node (N), and metastasis (M) (TNM) staging classification. In addition to basal diameter and tumor thickness, extraocular extension, ciliary body involvement, status of regional lymph nodes, and systemic metastasis play a role in the anatomic designation.

49.6 Management

Optimal management depends on tumor location and size, status of the fellow eye, results of metastatic workup, and patient preferences. Treatment options include transpupillary thermotherapy, plaque radiotherapy, charged particle irradiation, enucleation, and local resection.

Laser thermal therapy has been used with short-term success for small melanomas that are less than 3 mm in height and without high-risk characteristics. It is also used as adjunctive therapy for some larger melanomas depending on tumor location and radiation effect.

49.7 Surgical Management

Treatment options vary based on melanoma size using the data from the COMS and TNM classification results. Enucleation remains the treatment of choice for large choroidal melanomas in eyes with little or no vision and those with severe glaucoma. The most common alternative to enucleation is radiation therapy, which provides globe salvage. Plaque brachytherapy is the most common form of radiation currently utilized and is the method examined in the COMS for medium-sized tumors. The surgical procedure involves a conjunctival peritomy with tumor localization via any combination of direct visualization, transillumination, and echography. The plaque is positioned over the involved sclera and three or four 5–0 nylon sutures are used to secure the plaque to the sclera in a temporary fashion. Ultrasonography is used to confirm proper plaque positioning, after which the sutures are secured. The eye is then irrigated with antibiotics, and the conjunctiva is closed with 7–0 Vicryl sutures. The eye is patched with a lead shield, and the plaque remains in place from 3 to 7 days, depending on the size of the tumor and the rate of radiation delivery by the plaque (as calculated by the radiation oncologist). Postoperatively, patients may develop transient diplopia and radiation-related complications including retinopathy, optic neuropathy, and cataract.

49.8 Rehabilitation and Follow-up

Follow-up examinations are performed every 3 months during the first year, then extended to every 6 months for 2 years, and ultimately yearly after that. Clinical examination, fundus photography, and ultrasonography are performed in all patients, and autofluorescence and OCT imaging are performed in selected patients for documentation of tumor regression and for the detection of local recurrences or complications. Ultrasonography during the first 6 months following radioactive plaque therapy may demonstrate an increase in height post-treatment secondary to intratumor edema. Follow-up analysis of patients with melanomas using gene expression profiling demonstrated that class 1 tumors had 95% survival and class 2 had 31% survival at 8 years. This information led to systemic monitoring that is tiered based on risk. Annual liver imaging is recommended for low-risk class 1A patients. Intermediate-risk class 1B patients require annual liver imaging and liver enzymes staggered by 6 months. Lastly, high-risk class 2 patients require liver imaging and liver enzymes every 6 months staggered by 3 months. Complications of globe-conserving radiotherapy include radiation-vasculopathy and optic neuropathy, which occur at rates of approximately 30 to 50% at 5 years and are clearly increased for tumors adjacent to the optic nerve or fovea.

Suggested Readings

[1] Collaborative Ocular Melanoma Study Group. The Collaborative Ocular Melanoma Study (COMS) randomized trial of pre-enucleation radiation of large choroidal melanoma II: initial mortality findings. COMS report no. 10. Am J Ophthalmol. 1998; 125(6):779–796

[2] Shields CL, Kaliki S, Furuta M, Fulco E, Alarcon C, Shields JA. American Joint Committee on Cancer Classification of Uveal Melanoma (Anatomic Stage) Predicts Prognosis in 7,731 Patients: The 2013 Zimmerman Lecture. Ophthalmology. 2015; 122(6):1180–1186

[3] Singh AD, Belfort RN, Sayanagi K, Kaiser PK. Fourier domain optical coherence tomographic and auto-fluorescence findings in indeterminate choroidal melanocytic lesions. Br J Ophthalmol. 2010; 94(4):474–478

[4] Albert DM. The ocular melanoma story. LIII Edward Jackson Memorial Lecture: Part II. Am J Ophthalmol. 1997; 123(6):729–741

[5] Straatsma BR, Fine SL, Earle JD, Hawkins BS, Diener-West M, McLaughlin JA, The Collaborative Ocular Melanoma Study Research Group. Enucleation versus plaque irradiation for choroidal melanoma. Ophthalmology. 1988; 95(7):1000–1004

[6] McLean IW, Foster WD, Zimmerman LE, Gamel JW. Modifications of Callender's classification of uveal melanoma at the Armed Forces Institute of Pathology. Am J Ophthalmol. 1983; 96(4):502–509

[7] Onken MD, Worley LA, Char DH, et al. Collaborative Ocular Oncology Group report number 1: prospective validation of a multi-gene prognostic assay in uveal melanoma. Ophthalmology. 2012; 119(8):1596–1603

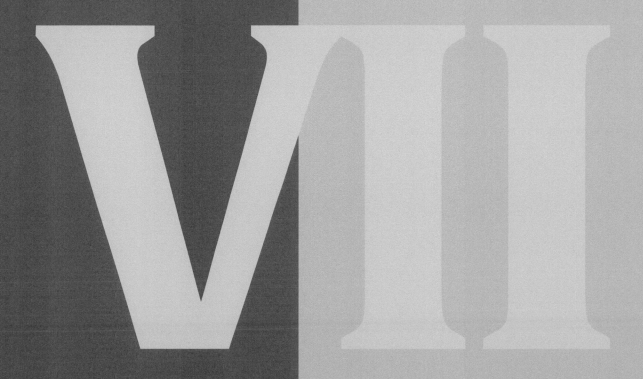

Part VII

Posterior Segment Complications

50 Dislocated Posterior Chamber Intraocular Lens

Thalmon R. Campagnoli, Mozart de O. Mello Jr., and William E. Smiddy

Abstract

A dislocated posterior chamber intraocular lens (PCIOL) is still not an uncommon complication of cataract surgery, but probably is now proportionally more common as a late occurrence after the initial cataract surgery. Compromise of zonular integrity, whether from initial surgical trauma, nonsurgical trauma, or what might be a higher prevalence of pseudoexfoliation syndrome, has increased the frequency of endocapsular dislocation. Thus, it seems less common for there to be residual capsular elements to assist in simply repositioning the IOL into the sulcus. Accordingly, scleral fixation techniques or IOL exchange is more common. Scleral fixation may be effected with various suturing techniques, or with the more recently reported haptic externalization maneuvers. Certain IOL designs do not permit some of these techniques, so the surgeon should be familiar with a range of options for surgical management.

Keywords: intraocular lens, scleral suture, cataract surgery complication, vitrectomy, repositioning IOL

50.1 History

A 64-year-old woman presented with a sudden decreased vision in the left eye 2 days after an uncomplicated extracapsular cataract extraction surgery with posterior chamber intraocular lens (PCIOL) insertion. During the procedure, a central posterior capsular rupture was noted, but the IOL was placed anterior to the remaining anterior capsule into the ciliary sulcus.

Her vision was 20/30 in the left eye with an aphakic correction. Slit-lamp examination showed a 2+ microbullous corneal edema superiorly and moderate cells in the anterior chamber. The pupil was round, but there was vitreous incarceration in the wound. The pupillary space was clear. Residual capsule was not noted. Funduscopic examination disclosed a freely mobile PCIOL within the vitreous cavity inferiorly. The retina was attached.

Surgery was recommended and performed with repositioning of the dislocated PCIOL into the ciliary sulcus using a scleral suturing technique to fixate the haptics. The scleral fixation sutures were placed through two partial-thickness superotemporal and inferonasal scleral flaps to cover the suture knots.

The IOL was in good position 1 month postoperatively with vision at 20/60. The vision returned to 20/20 within 6 months and remained so 6 years after the surgical repair. The IOL remained centered and well positioned, with no sign of complication.

In the right eye, the vision was 20/400 due to nuclear sclerosis.

Differential Diagnosis—Key Points

1. This patient developed the PCIOL dislocation following a complicated cataract extraction (posterior capsular rupture), the most common scenario for dislocated IOLs. The specific details of the cause of the dislocation are frequently not evident, although suboptimal posterior capsule support following posterior capsular rupture during cataract extraction is known to be a common element. When dislocation occurs a few days or weeks after surgery, the cause is less apparent and may be the result of spontaneous IOL haptic rotation out of a zone of posterior capsule remnant, asymmetric haptic placement, or zonular dehiscence. Dislocation months or years after placement is rare and may be due to traumatic or spontaneous loss of zonular support, as in eyes with pseudoexfoliation syndrome.

2. Visual symptoms such as decreased vision, glare, monocular diplopia, or pain, and associated ocular complications (inflammation, increased intraocular pressure, cystoid macular edema, and coexisting retinal detachment [RD]) are the main indications for surgery. A mobile IOL in the absence of other complications is surprisingly well tolerated, but may be removed if symptomatic.

3. The optimal timing for intervention for intraoperative IOL dislocation is probably during the initial cataract extraction. The logistics are easier for the patient, but may be impracticable for the surgeon. If this is not feasible, surgery within 2 weeks for acute dislocation allows initial inflammation to subside or to determine the visual or refractive severity of the dislocation. Most cases do not manifest dislocation intraoperatively, however. Thus, for other cases, surgery is usually performed within a couple of weeks unless other complications coexist or intervene.

4. A pars plana approach is generally preferred because it allows optimal treatment of complications, but a limbal approach may be suitable for decentered and subluxated IOLs, which are readily accessible and not enveloped by prolapsed vitreous. Regardless of the approach used, all accessible vitreous should be removed to avoid subsequent inflammatory and tractional complications.

50.2 Test Interpretation

Clinical examination at the slit lamp and with indirect ophthalmoscopy using a + 20D lens is the standard diagnostic method.

Echography may be helpful to rule out associated complications when the anterior and posterior segments cannot be visualized due to opaque ocular media (hyphema, inflammation, or vitreous hemorrhage). A posteriorly dislocated PCIOL appears as a large foreign body–like structure within the vitreous cavity. Gonioscopy may be helpful to evaluate how much of the peripheral lens capsule remains and to assess for unrecognized vitreous incarceration in the cataract wound.

Since IOL exchange may become necessary, IOL power calculations should be available if lens exchange is performed.

50.3 Diagnosis

Dislocated posterior chamber IOL, OS.

50.4 Medical Management

Topical miotics may satisfactorily reduce glare, eliminate monocular diplopia, and improve visual function in selected patients with decentration of the lens optic. Supportive treatment with topical anti-inflammatory or ocular hypotensive agents is the mainstay of medical treatment.

Observation only is pursued for PCIOLs with simple decentration, if other superseding medical or ocular problems prohibit further surgery, if aphakic contact lens correction is satisfactory, or if the patient chooses not to pursue further surgery.

50.5 Surgical Management

The surgical management options available for dislocated PCIOLs include IOL repositioning with or without sutures, or IOL removal with or without exchange. Vitrectomy affords the most options for control of complications, but in selected cases a limbal approach allows effective achievement of necessary objectives. The timing may be modified by associated complications, but surgery is usually pursued within 2 weeks of acute symptomatic dislocation.

Nonsutured repositioning of dislocated PCIOL in the ciliary sulcus is the least traumatic surgical alternative. It is the preferred approach in eyes with at least 6 clock hours of residual peripheral capsular support. More extensive capsular support is necessary, however, when the inferior capsule is absent or if the residual capsule is questionable in extent.

Repositioning with transscleral suture (9–0 polypropylene) fixation is elected in eyes without adequate capsular support (▶ Fig. 50.1). In some cases, it is unnecessary to suture both haptics. Components common to all scleral suture fixation techniques include (1) retrieving of the IOL; (2) introducing a suture loop through the ciliary sulcus; (3) passing the suture loop around the IOL haptic; (4) securing the suture to the sclera; and (5) covering or burying the scleral suture knot. Many techniques have been described to achieve these goals, and the method chosen may be based on surgeon preference and experience, IOL design, and associated circumstances. Transscleral suturing techniques are vulnerable to a variety of complications

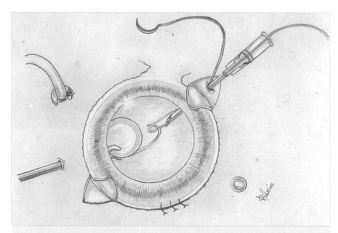

Fig. 50.1 A schematic representation (surgeon's view) depicts preferred technique for scleral suture fixation of dislocated posterior chamber lens implant. After doing a core vitrectomy, the eye wall is mobilized and ultimately grasped with the forceps through the left-hand sclerotomy site. Care is taken to grasp the optic rather than the haptic. A 25-gauge needle prethreaded with a 9–0 Prolene suture is introduced 1 mm posterior to the limbus through the bed of a partial-thickness scleral flap at the 7:00 meridian. The IOL haptic is then guided through the resultant loop with the left hand. The needle is passed through the bed of the flap, securing the inferior haptic. A similar maneuver is performed for the superior haptic.

such as suture knot erosion, endophthalmitis, hemorrhage, IOL torsion or malposition, and recurrent dislocation due to suture breakage.

IOL removal with or without exchange is usually performed for small optics implants, damaged haptics, for highly flexible haptics unsuitable for suture support, when available instrumentation is lacking, and in eyes with coexisting complex RD. Avoiding IOL removal or exchange avoids endothelial trauma and postsurgical astigmatism from reopening a limbal wound. IOL removal rates have decreased, probably because of improved repositioning techniques.

Special considerations are necessary with silicone plate IOLs. After successful placement into the capsular bag, YAG capsulotomy may allow posterior prolapse of the IOL. Also, insertion without complete posterior capsular support may result in dislocation (▶ Fig. 50.2). Silicone plate IOLs can usually be repositioned into the ciliary sulcus anterior to the residual anterior capsule (▶ Fig. 50.3). However, removal may be necessary.

The most frequent surgical complications in eyes with dislocated PCIOL include cystoid macular edema (usually low grade), elevated intraocular pressure, and RD. Although the incidence of RD is relatively low (2%), careful intraoperative and postoperative examinations of the retinal periphery to look for retinal tears or detachment are necessary.

50.6 Rehabilitation and Follow-up

Although visual acuity outcomes after surgical management of dislocated PCIOLs are usually good, the final visual acuity depends on preoperative macular function, and complications from the original cataract surgery. In a majority of cases, visual

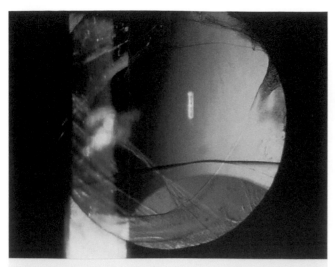

Fig. 50.2 Clinical appearance of patient 2 weeks following YAG capsulotomy. A dislocated silicone plate IOL is visible behind the capsular remnants.

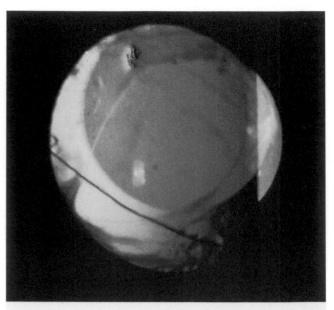

Fig. 50.3 Postoperative appearance shows the silicone plate haptic IOL well positioned in the ciliary sulcus (anterior to the anterior capsular remnants).

acuity is 20/40 or better. In this patient, after initial visual improvement to 20/60, the final visual acuity reached 20/20 6 years postoperatively. The relatively low rates of RD and cystoid macular edema limit the vision in only a minority of cases.

Suggested Reading

[1] Smiddy WE, Flynn HW, Jr. Managing retained lens fragments and dislocated posterior chamber intraocular lenses after cataract surgery. Focal Points (Clinical Module). Am Acad Ophthalmol. 1996; 14(7):1–14

[2] Smiddy WE, Ibanez GV, Alfonso E, Flynn HW, Jr. Surgical management of dislocated intraocular lenses. J Cataract Refract Surg. 1995; 21(1):64–69

[3] Flynn HW, Jr, Buus D, Culbertson WW. Management of subluxated and posteriorly dislocated intraocular lenses using pars plana vitrectomy instrumentation. J Cataract Refract Surg. 1990; 16(1):51–56

[4] Ruiz-Moreno JM. Repositioning dislocated posterior chamber intraocular lenses. Retina. 1998; 18(4):330–334

[5] Price FW, Jr, Whitson WE, Collins K, Johns S. Explantation of posterior chamber lenses. J Cataract Refract Surg. 1992; 18(5):475–479

[6] Smiddy WE, Flynn HW, Jr, Kim JE. Retinal detachment in patients with retained lens fragments or dislocated posterior chamber intraocular lenses. Ophthalmic Surg Lasers. 1996; 27(10):856–861

[7] Scheiderman TE, Johnson MW, Smiddy WE, et al. Surgical management of dislocated plate haptic silicone posterior chamber intraocular lenses. Am J Ophthalmol. 1997; 123:629–635

51 Cystoid Macular Edema

Andrew S. Camp and William E. Smiddy

Abstract

Cystoid macular edema (CME) is a common finding following intraocular surgery. Identification of cystoid macular edema by careful exam or retinal imaging is crucial to guide clinical management. CME can often be treated medically, although surgical intervention is occasionally necessary. CME was first described when the technique of fluorescein angiography was developed. It was classically associated with the post–cataract surgery eye, particularly if there had been a ruptured capsule and/or vitreous prolapse into the anterior chamber or wound. Ocular coherence tomography is now the mainstay of diagnosis. Improved surgical technique has surely decreased the incidence of this, but expanded indications for cataract surgery have still rendered the prevalence to be substantial. Topical treatment with corticosteroids and nonsteroidal agents is the first-line treatment, but surgical removal of prolapsed or incarcerated vitreous when present is still an important option. Still, this seems to occur more frequently with complicated cataract surgery, especially with iris trauma intra- or even postoperatively, or retained lens fragments, so being alert to preventing, detecting, and correcting these is important. Sub-Tenon's or intravitreal corticosteroid injections are viable modalities if first-line topical treatments have failed. Of course, CME may follow any kind of ocular surgery, or be secondary to a host of inflammatory disease entities. When CME is associated with other retinovascular diseases, the therapeutic strategy should be directed accordingly.

Keywords: cystoid macular edema, Irvine–Gass syndrome, pseudophakic macular edema, cystoid, macula, edema, cataract surgery, surgical complications, fluorescein angiography

51.1 History

A 66-year-old woman presented 8 weeks after phacoemulsification complaining of decreased visual acuity in the right eye. An acrylic intraocular lens was inserted into the ciliary sulcus at the time of surgery due to a central posterior capsular rupture. The patient reported that the visual acuity was excellent postoperatively but declined substantially after the first 4 weeks. The patient reported no other contributory medical or ophthalmic history including diabetes mellitus or hypertension.

Examination disclosed best corrected visual acuity of 20/80 in the right eye. The pupil exam was normal and visual fields were full to confrontation. The cornea was clear and of normal thickness with a well-healed corneal incision temporally. The iris appeared normal without peaking, the anterior chamber was deep and quiet, and the intraocular lens was well centered and appeared stable. Examination of the posterior pole revealed a posterior vitreous detachment. The optic nerve head was normal with a cup-to-disc ratio of 0.2. The retinal vessels were normal. The macula was thickened with cystic spaces apparent in the fovea upon examination with a Goldmann contact lens. The peripheral retina was normal without holes, breaks, or tears.

Ocular coherence tomography demonstrated macular thickening and cysts in the inner nuclear layer (▶ Fig. 51.1). Fluorescein angiography demonstrated late leakage of dye from perifoveal vessels with a symmetric, petaloid pooling pattern (▶ Fig. 51.2).

Differential Diagnosis—Key Points

1. Thickening of the macula is a clinical finding that defines macular edema. Various patterns and associations of macular edema may occur with different etiologic disease processes. Visualization of cystoid spaces within the fovea is diagnostic of cystoid macular edema (CME), but often requires examination with a Hruby or fundus contact lens for clinical detection. CME represents accumulation of intraretinal fluid (thought to be from retinal vascular leakage) in the inner nuclear and outer plexiform layers. In more exuberant cases, there may be focal subretinal fluid.

2. While postoperative inflammation is the most common cause of CME, numerous conditions may present with CME. These include any ocular surgical procedures (e.g., trabeculectomy, scleral buckling, strabismus surgery, and vitrectomy), almost any cause of intraocular inflammation (e.g., uveitis, choroiditis, or retinitis), retinal vascular disease, retinal degenerations, epiretinal membranes, and drugs (e.g., topical epinephrine, dipivefrin, betaxolol, or oral niacin or tamoxifen). The use of prostaglandin analogs may be an additional risk factor for development of CME following cataract extraction. Drug-induced CME often does not show leakage on fluorescein dye.

3. The incidence of pseudophakic CME varies according to the definition used. Visually significant CME is loosely defined as CME with a characteristic ophthalmoscopic appearance and visual acuity worse than 20/40. Visually significant CME occurs in 2 to 10% of patients after extracapsular cataract surgery, but only in 0.1 to 2.35% of patients after phacoemulsification. Angiographic CME, defined as the presence of fluorescein leakage in a petaloid pattern in the fovea, is quite frequent (20–30% of uncomplicated cataract extractions), but may not be associated with visual loss. Ocular coherence tomography identifies increased retinal thickness in up to 41% of patients after uneventful phacoemulsification. Posterior capsular rupture, vitreous loss, and retained nuclear or cortical material increase the incidence of CME and risk of visual loss.

4. The presence of vitreous incarceration into the limbal wound, iridovitreal synechiae, or iridocapsular synechiae may represent a mechanical stimulus for inflammation (thought to be a consequence of mechanical iris irritation) and may improve with surgical lysis.

5. The exact mechanism of CME is unclear. It has been postulated that inflammatory mediators cause breakdown of the blood–retinal barrier resulting in intraretinal fluid accumulation. The mediators may be released as a result of ultraviolet light exposure during and after cataract surgery,

traction from vitreomacular adhesions directly stimulating inflammation of the Müller's cells, or more generalized intraocular inflammation. Most research has focused on components of the arachidonic acid pathway, but no specific mediator has yet been identified.

6. The macular edema of CME is ophthalmoscopically distinct in appearance from that of diabetic macular edema, but overlap may exist. Distinguishing exacerbation of diabetic macular edema and primary CME may be difficult, but ocular coherence tomography or fluorescein angiography may offer insights by defining the distribution pattern of leakage. Pseudophakic CME may be expected to improve with time, whereas macular edema from other causes will likely worsen.

51.2 Test Interpretation

Fluorescein angiography is a useful adjunct to the clinical examination in the diagnosis of CME. The characteristic angiographic appearance consists of parafoveal capillary leakage with a petaloid pattern of intraretinal pooling of dye. The optic disc may demonstrate staining or leakage (especially in severe cases).

Ocular coherence tomography and retinal thickness analysis have largely supplanted angiography since they allow for rapid, quantitative, and noninvasive diagnosis and monitoring of CME. CME appears as macular thickening and cystic spaces in the outer plexiform layer on ocular coherence tomography imaging. CME identified by ocular coherence tomography or fluorescein angiography is much more common than clinically significant disease.

51.3 Diagnosis

Postoperative (pseudophakic) cystoid macular edema, OD.

51.4 Medical Management

Medical management of CME consists of both prophylaxis and treatment. Some clinicians advocate preoperative nonsteroidal anti-inflammatory drugs (NSAIDs) or steroids to suppress the arachidonic acid pathway. Typically, topical flurbiprofen or suprofen is applied before the procedure, but this practice is not consistently effective for prophylaxis.

The treatment of CME is controversial and often frustrating. The majority of patients will resolve spontaneously within 3 to 4 months without treatment; many others will improve partially. However, a substantial minority of patients may have persistent, clinically significant CME. Initial treatment usually consists of topical NSAIDs such as 0.5% ketorolac four times per day, for 4 to 6 weeks. Studies of NSAID use in the treatment of CME have yielded mixed results, and meta-analysis of the benefits has not been conclusive. Topical corticosteroids, such as 1% prednisolone four to eight times per day, are also used frequently, but their efficacy is reduced in chronic CME. Combination therapy of topical NSAIDs and corticosteroids appears to have synergistic effects with improved outcomes compared to use of either agent alone.

Periocular or intravitreal steroid injections may be beneficial in cases failing topical treatment. However, the risk of increased intraocular pressure following steroid injection must be considered. Intravitreal injection of anti-vascular endothelial growth factor (anti-VEGF) medications, such as ranibizumab, bevacizumab, or aflibercept, has also been reported in cases of chronic, intractable CME, but with lackluster results. Although studies of intravitreal anti-VEGF agents have demonstrated clinical improvement in patients with chronic CME, these studies are hampered by small sample size, variable dosing and injection schedules, and lack of randomization.

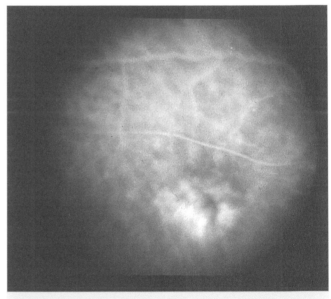

Fig. 51.2 Ocular coherence tomography macula cross-section demonstrating macular thickening and cysts.

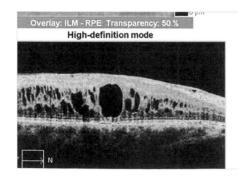

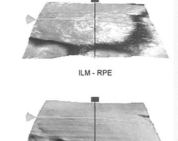

ILM - RPE

Fig. 51.1 Fluorescein angiogram frame from the midvenous phase shows pooling of extravasated dye in the macula.

51.5 Surgical Management

Surgical management of CME is usually reserved for cases in which the anterior segment manifests vitreomacular traction or adhesion or for inflammation associated with retained lens particles. Classically, vitreous prolapse to a limbal wound with peaking of the pupil is recognized as a surgically treatable cause of CME. In selected cases, Nd:YAG laser lysis of thin vitreous stands extending to the wound or sweeping via a paracentesis site at the slit lamp has been used with success. Pars plana vitrectomy may be indicated in cases of vitreomacular traction or inflammation due to retained lens material. Interestingly, pars plana vitrectomy has also successfully improved chronic CME in patients without clear vitreomacular traction or retained lens material.

51.6 Rehabilitation and Follow-up

After initiation of medical treatment for CME, the patient should be observed within 4 to 6 weeks. If no improvement is noted, further treatment may be warranted. A sizeable proportion of patients may develop recurrent CME after cessation of a successful medical regimen; therefore, even patients who experience improvement or resolution of their symptoms should be followed carefully. Chronic CME is often associated with underlying retinal pigment epithelium atrophy and attendant visual loss even after the CME resolves.

Suggested Reading

[1] Gass JDM, Norton EWD. Cystoid macular edema and papilledema following cataract extraction. A fluorescein fundoscopic and angiographic study. Arch Ophthalmol. 1966; 76(5):646–661

[2] Harbour JW, Smiddy WE, Rubsamen PE, Murray TG, Davis JL, Flynn HW, Jr. Pars plana vitrectomy for chronic pseudophakic cystoid macular edema. Am J Ophthalmol. 1995; 120(3):302–307

[3] Pendergast SD, Margherio RR, Williams GA, Cox MS, Jr. Vitrectomy for chronic pseudophakic cystoid macular edema. Am J Ophthalmol. 1999; 128(3):317–323

[4] Heier JS, Topping TM, Baumann W, Dirks MS, Chern S. Ketorolac versus prednisolone versus combination therapy in the treatment of acute pseudophakic cystoid macular edema. Ophthalmology. 2000; 107(11):2034–2038, discussion 2039

[5] Rossetti L, Autelitano A. Cystoid macular edema following cataract surgery. Curr Opin Ophthalmol. 2000; 11(1):65–72

[6] Rossetti A, Doro D. Retained intravitreal lens fragments after phacoemulsification: complications and visual outcome in vitrectomized and nonvitrectomized eyes. J Cataract Refract Surg. 2002; 28(2):310–315

[7] Kim SJ, Belair ML, Bressler NM, et al. A method of reporting macular edema after cataract surgery using optical coherence tomography. Retina. 2008; 28(6):870–876

[8] Arevalo JF, Maia M, Garcia-Amaris RA, et al. Pan-American Collaborative Retina Study Group. Intravitreal bevacizumab for refractory pseudophakic cystoid macular edema: the Pan-American Collaborative Retina Study Group results. Ophthalmology. 2009; 116(8):1481–1487, 1487.e1

[9] Sivaprasad S, Bunce C, Crosby-Nwaobi R. Non-steroidal anti-inflammatory agents for treating cystoid macular oedema following cataract surgery. Cochrane Database Syst Rev. 2012; 2(2):CD004239

[10] Guo S, Patel S, Baumrind B, et al. Management of pseudophakic cystoid macular edema. Surv Ophthalmol. 2015; 60(2):123–137

52 Endophthalmitis

Brian E. Goldhagen and William E. Smiddy

Abstract

Endophthalmitis is most commonly encountered following intraocular surgery, especially after cataract surgery, but may occur in several other settings—endogenous, late-onset bleb-associated, trauma-associated, or after intravitreal injections. While the incidence is low (generally less than 0.1% of respective cases), the especially high frequency of cataract surgery and intravitreal injections keeps endophthalmitis from being a rarely encountered entity. Generally, treatment is based on the Endophthalmitis Vitrectomy Study findings despite those results being derived only from acute postoperative pseudophakic endophthalmitis cases. Hence, unless the visual loss is severe (light perception or bare hand motions might prompt vitrectomy), a vitreous tap and injection of antibiotics (these authors prefer vancomycin and ceftazidime) and possibly corticosteroids is promptly performed and the patient is followed clinically. Exceptional cases may be suspected when there are atypical presentations. For example, late-onset, characteristically painless inflammation that appears to be associated with capsular plaques suggest *Propionibacterium acnes* and a more aggressive surgical approach with maximal removal of remnant lens cortex and capsule (and possibly even the entire intraocular lens/capsule unit) is necessary. Atypical bacterial and fungal endophthalmitis should be suspected with late- or delayed-onset presentations, especially with indolent inflammation and fluffy cortexlike accumulation. Prophylaxis of endophthalmitis is still controversial in the settings of cataract surgery, intravitreal injections, and trauma.

Keywords: infection, antibiotics, surgical complication, intraocular lens complication, microbiology

52.1 History

This 59-year-old woman awoke with 10/10 eye pain and decreased vision in her left eye. An uneventful combined cataract and LASIK procedure had been performed 5 days previously with a hitherto standard postoperative course. Her vision was hand motion, and there was pronounced conjunctival hyperemia, corneal edema, and anterior chamber reaction with hypopyon, as well as fibrin present on the intraocular lens (IOL) (▶ Fig. 52.1). There was no view to the posterior pole and B-scan ultrasonography demonstrated moderately dense membranous vitreous opacities (▶ Fig. 52.2).

The patient underwent a vitreous tap and injection of intravitreal vancomycin, ceftazidime, and dexamethasone followed by hourly treatment with topical fortified vancomycin and ceftazidime, prednisolone four times per day, and cyclopentolate three times per day. Vitreous cultures grew methicillin-resistant *Staphylococcus epidermidis*. As she improved clinically, topical medications were gradually tapered. Her vision had improved to 20/40 by 1 week; the final visual acuity was 20/20 several months later after a laser capsulotomy was performed.

Differential Diagnosis-Key Points

Endophthalmitis is a vision-threatening inflammatory reaction of the intraocular fluids or tissues that can be categorized into one of the following categories based on the clinical setting and time of onset:

1. **Acute postoperative endophthalmitis** may occur after any surgery including cataract surgery, glaucoma filtering surgery, corneal transplantation, pars plana vitrectomy (PPV), scleral buckling, and strabismus surgery. Classically developing within a week of surgery, it typically presents with rapid onset of vision loss, pain, and intraocular inflammation. The most common causative organism is *S. epidermidis*, followed by *Staphylococcus aureus* and other *Streptococcus* species.

   Acute postoperative endophthalmitis risk factors include diabetes, posterior capsular rupture, and wound leaks. Risk can be significantly reduced through the use of preoperative povidone-iodine. The efficacy of preoperative topical antibiotics, intraoperative subconjunctival antibiotics, or postoperative topical antibiotics in reducing endophthalmitis is unclear. The European Society of Cataract and Refractive Surgeons reported results supporting the use of intracameral cefuroxime during cataract surgery; however, there has been controversy due to the study's high rate of endophthalmitis in its control group as well as potential safety concerns regarding intracameral antibiotic use.

2. **Chronic postoperative endophthalmitis** is defined as presenting more than 6 weeks after surgery, although its average time of onset is about 1 year. In contrast with acute postoperative, it characteristically presents with low-grade inflammation, a white intracapsular plaque, and with or without associated pain. The most common causative organism is *Propionibacterium acnes*, followed by fungal species.

3. **Posttraumatic endophthalmitis** is an uncommon, yet severe, complication of open-globe injury. Symptoms include pain out of proportion to the degree of injury and hypopyon, but can greatly vary. Time of onset is also variable. Risk factors include intraocular foreign body, lens rupture, dirty wound, and delayed primary repair. Gram-positive organisms, particularly *S. epidermidis*, are the most common isolates. *Bacillus* species have also been reported.

4. **Bleb-associated endophthalmitis** is a vision-threatening complication of trabeculectomy surgery, which, in contrast to blebitis, has vitreous involvement. Other symptoms include eye pain, decreased vision, and hypopyon. Its onset is usually delayed (wide variability, average about 5 years) but may present acutely as well. Risk factors include bleb leakage, use of antimetabolites, and inferior surgical location. *Streptococcus* and coagulase-negative *Staphylococcus* species are the major causative organisms.

5. **Post–intravitreal injection endophthalmitis** is rare but has become more commonly encountered since the increased usage of intravitreal injection therapies. It typically presents within the first few days after injection. Use of povidone-iodine as well as a sterile lid speculum is recommended to reduce risk of endophthalmitis, although there appears to be no benefit of topical antibiotics usage. *Streptococcus* and coagulase-negative *Staphylococcus* species are the most common causative organisms. Aflibercept-associated sterile inflammation may be challenging to distinguish from endophthalmitis but frequently presents without pain, hypopyon, or conjunctival hyperemia. Preservative-containing triamcinolone may also cause painless hypopyon without infection.

6. **Endogenous endophthalmitis**, in contrast to the different types of exogenous endophthalmitis discussed above, is caused by a hematogenous spread of infectious organisms. In addition to ocular findings, which may be unilateral or bilateral, systemic signs and symptoms of infection are common. Risk factors include immunodeficiency, diabetes, intravenous drug use, indwelling catheters, and malignancy. Fungal pathogens, particularly *Candida albicans* and *Aspergillus* species, are more common than bacterial.

52.2 Differential Diagnosis

Painful loss of vision with prominent inflammation in the immediate postoperative period should be considered to be infectious endophthalmitis until proven otherwise. Other non-infectious processes that may present similarly include toxic anterior segment syndrome, retained lens material, exacerbation of preexisting uveitis, and vitreous hemorrhage (with dehemoglobinized red blood cells). Important distinguishing features include patient history, timing of presentation, and presenting symptoms.

52.3 Diagnosis

Acute infectious postoperative endophthalmitis, left eye.

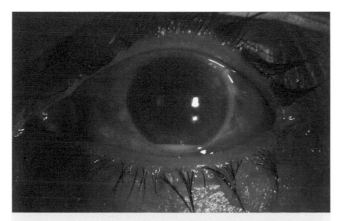

Fig. 52.1 Slit-lamp examination showing conjunctival hyperemia, hypopyon within the anterior chamber, and fibrin on the intraocular lens.

52.4 Management

Although vitreous sampling with cultures (blood, chocolate, Sabouraud, thioglycolate) and smears (Gram and Giemsa stains) is important in the diagnosis and management of endophthalmitis, empirical treatment is initially instituted with board-spectrum antibiotics. Ultrasonography is useful to assess the severity of vitreous opacities in cases of suspected endophthalmitis and look for retinal detachments, particularly in cases with a limited view to the posterior pole.

52.4.1 Acute Postoperative Endophthalmitis

Acute postoperative endophthalmitis management has historically been guided by the Endophthalmitis Vitrectomy Study (EVS), which enrolled patients with endophthalmitis following cataract surgery. Based on results of this study, PPV is recommended in patients presenting with light perception-only (LP) vision, while tap and injection is recommended for those presenting with a visual acuity better than LP. This study additionally found no benefit to the use of systemic antibiotics (amikacin and ceftazidime) on final visual acuity. The limitations of this study, now conducted approximately 20 years ago, include the following:

1. The study may not be applicable to forms of endophthalmitis other than postoperative cataract or secondary lens implantation.
2. Fourth-generation fluoroquinolones were not evaluated.
3. Patients with no light perception vision or significant opacification of the anterior chamber were excluded from the study.

Intravitreal antibiotics, most commonly vancomycin (1.0 mg/0.1 mL) and either ceftazidime (2.25 mg/0.1 mL) or amikacin (0.4 mg/0.1 mL), are recommended for all patients with post-operative endophthalmitis. Dexamethasone may or may not be added depending on the extent of inflammation and suspicion for fungal involvement. Topical vancomycin (50 mg/mL) in combination with an aminoglycoside or ceftazidime (50 mg/mL) is also usually recommended.

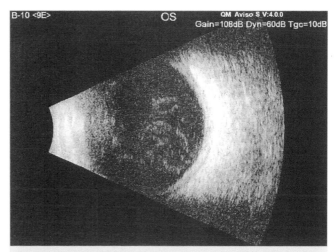

Fig. 52.2 B-scan ultrasonography showing moderately dense membranous vitreous opacities without evidence of retinal detachment.

52.4.2 Chronic Postoperative Endophthalmitis

Chronic postoperative endophthalmitis is managed typically with PPV with either a partial capsulectomy or total capsulectomy with IOL exchange/removal.

52.4.3 Posttraumatic Endophthalmitis

Posttraumatic endophthalmitis is usually managed aggressively with PPV given the high virulence of bacteria typically involved.

52.4.4 Bleb-Associated Endophthalmitis

Bleb-associated endophthalmitis, like posttraumatic endophthalmitis, is typically aggressive and is managed accordingly with prompt PPV.

52.4.5 Post–Intravitreal Injection Endophthalmitis

Post–intravitreal injection endophthalmitis is typically managed by vitreous tap and injection of intravitreal antibiotics (vancomycin and ceftazidime or amikacin) with or without dexamethasone. Cases with suspected noninfectious inflammation, particularly aflibercept-associated sterile inflammation, are treated with topical steroids and close observation without intraocular cultures.

52.4.6 Endogenous Endophthalmitis

Endogenous endophthalmitis management generally necessitates systemic antibiotic or antifungal therapy given the extraocular source of infection, with involvement of either an infectious disease or medical specialist. Severe intravitreal involvement may require intravitreal antibiotics or antifungals with or without PPV.

52.5 Prognosis

Endophthalmitis has the potential for severe visual loss, and prognosis is dependent on the type of endophthalmitis and virulence of the involved organism.

According to the EVS, more than half of the *acute postoperative endophthalmitis* patients achieved 20/40 vision. *Chronic postoperative endophthalmitis* tends to have a more favorable visual outcome, while *posttraumatic* and *bleb-associated endophthalmitis* tend to be associated with poorest endophthalmitis outcomes. *Post–intravitreal injection endophthalmitis* also tends to have worse outcomes than acute postoperative endophthalmitis due to a higher frequency of more virulent bacteria. The visual prognosis of endogenous endophthalmitis appears to be most closely linked to the promptness of treatment and causative organism.

Selected Reading

[1] Endophthalmitis Vitrectomy Study Group. Results of the Endophthalmitis Vitrectomy Study. A randomized trial of immediate vitrectomy and of intravenous antibiotics for the treatment of postoperative bacterial endophthalmitis. Arch Ophthalmol. 1995; 113(12):1479–1496

[2] Bhagat N, Nagori S, Zarbin M. Post-traumatic infectious endophthalmitis. Surv Ophthalmol. 2011; 56(3):214–251

[3] Gregori NZ, Flynn HW, Jr, Schwartz SG, et al. Current infectious endophthalmitis rates after intravitreal injections of anti-vascular endothelial growth factor agents and outcomes of treatment. Ophthalmic Surg Lasers Imaging Retina. 2015; 46(6):643–648

[4] Pathengay A, Khera M, Das T, Sharma S, Miller D, Flynn HW, Jr. Acute postoperative endophthalmitis following cataract surgery: a review. Asia Pac J Ophthalmol (Phila). 2012; 1(1):35–42

[5] Romero-Aroca P, Méndez-Marin I, Salvat-Serra M, Fernández-Ballart J, Almena-Garcia M, Reyes-Torres J. Results at seven years after the use of intracamerular cefazolin as an endophthalmitis prophylaxis in cataract surgery. BMC Ophthalmol. 2012; 12:2

[6] Shirodkar AR, Pathengay A, Flynn HW, Jr, et al. Delayed- versus acute-onset endophthalmitis after cataract surgery. Am J Ophthalmol. 2012; 153(3):391–398.e2

[7] Vaziri K, Schwartz SG, Kishor K, Flynn HW, Jr. Endophthalmitis: state of the art. Clin Ophthalmol. 2015; 9:95–108

53 Suprachoroidal Hemorrhage

Carlos A. Medina Mendez, Ingrid U. Scott, and William E. Smiddy

Abstract

This chapter utilizes a typical clinical scenario to present and discuss the history and examination findings of suprachoroidal hemorrhage. Ancillary testing, medical management, surgical management, rehabilitation, and follow-up are also discussed. Emphasis is placed on comparing and contrasting suprachoroidal hemorrhage to etiologies included in the differential diagnosis, which includes rhegmatogenous retinal detachment, exudative retinal detachment, and serous choroidal effusion.

Keywords: suprachoroidal hemorrhage, choroidal hemorrhage

53.1 History

A 78-year-old woman presented 4 days after a complicated cataract surgery in her left eye, complaining of acute-onset severe pain and loss of vision in the left eye. Past medical history was notable for cardiac bypass surgery 2 years previously and systemic hypertension. Past ocular history was significant for myopia (−9.00 sphere) and primary open-angle glaucoma. Ocular medications included timolol 0.5% in both eyes twice daily, dorzolamide 2% in both eyes three times per day, and prednisolone acetate 1% in the left eye four times per day.

Vision was 20/60 in the right eye and hand motion in the left eye. Intraocular pressure was 12 mm Hg on the right and 39 mm Hg on the left. Slit-lamp examination of the right eye disclosed nuclear sclerotic lens changes. Slit-lamp examination of the left eye was notable for 2 + conjunctival injection, a temporal clear cornea incision reapproximated with interrupted nylon sutures, a shallow anterior chamber, aphakia, and the appearance of a bullous appositional retinal detachment posterior to the iris plane (▶ Fig. 53.1). An ultrasound examination demonstrated appositional ("kissing") suprachoroidal hemorrhages (▶ Fig. 53.2a). Because of the clotted nature of the suprachoroidal blood on echography, observation including serial echography was recommended (▶ Fig. 53.2b). The patient's elevated intraocular pressure in the left eye was managed medically.

Eight days after presentation, echography demonstrated persistent retinal apposition with liquefaction of the suprachoroidal blood. A pars plana vitrectomy with drainage of the suprachoroidal hemorrhage and fluid–gas exchange was performed. A draining retinotomy was not performed since no retinal breaks were identified, so the retinal elevation was deduced to be exudative, secondary to the choroidal hemorrhage. At the 3-month follow-up visit, vision in the left eye was 20/400.

Differential Diagnosis—Key Points

1. The differential diagnosis of the bullous retinal detachment seen on the presenting examination includes rhegmatogenous retinal detachment, exudative retinal detachment, serous choroidal effusion, and suprachoroidal hemorrhage (▶ Fig. 53.3). Severe pain is not consistent with a rhegmatogenous retinal detachment, but may accompany exudative retinal detachments when due to scleritis or uveitis. Tumor lysis syndrome from a tumor which has undergone massive hemorrhage or regression may also cause inflammation and pain, and mimic otherwise typical suprachoroidal hemorrhage. Acute-onset severe pain, often seen in the context of suprachoroidal hemorrhage, is not typical of primary serous choroidal effusion.

2. The differential diagnosis of acute ocular pain accompanied by a shallow anterior chamber after cataract surgery includes aqueous misdirection, pupillary block, serous choroidal detachment, and suprachoroidal hemorrhage. Intraocular pressure is typically normal or elevated in all of these conditions, except for serous choroidal detachment, which is generally accompanied by a low intraocular pressure. The retina and choroid are flat in aqueous misdirection and pupillary block. If funduscopic evaluation is not prohibited by appositional retinal detachment, the differentiation between serous and hemorrhagic choroidal detachments may be made on the basis of the color of the choroidal elevations; serous choroidal detachments appear as light-brown choroidal elevations, while hemorrhagic choroidal detachments appear as dark-brown or dark-red choroidal elevations. In some instances, transillumination will allow or corroborate the distinction between hemorrhagic and serous choroidal detachment.

3. The history of acute-onset severe ocular pain and vision loss in a perioperative period is most consistent with suprachoroidal hemorrhage. The patient described in this case has several risk factors for the development of suprachoroidal hemorrhage, including advanced age, atherosclerotic cardiovascular disease, systemic anticoagulation, hypertension, myopia, glaucoma, aphakia, and recent intraocular surgery.

4. The nylon sutures reapproximating the temporal clear cornea incision and the lack of an intraocular lens suggest that a suprachoroidal hemorrhage (perhaps limited) may have developed intraoperatively, leading the cataract surgeon to end the case and close the cataract incision as quickly as possible.

5. The first clue of an intraoperative suprachoroidal hemorrhage may be an alteration of the light reflex (red-reflex) through the pupil or a tensing or anterior bowing of the lens–iris diaphragm. A rapid increase in the firmness of the eye to palpation is another indication of suprachoroidal hemorrhage.

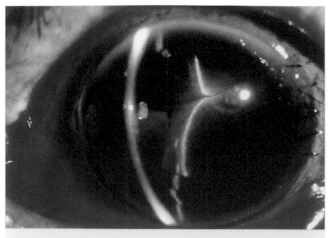

Fig. 53.1 Initial presentation of left eye. Vision is hand motion. Note temporal clear cornea cataract incision reapproximated with nylon sutures, aphakia, and dark-brown appositional choroidal detachments (hemorrhagic) posterior to the iris plane.

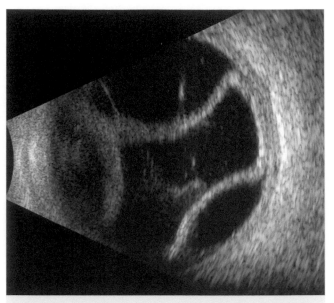

Fig. 53.3 Echography demonstrating serous choroidal detachments. Note the absence of echoic fluid in the suprachoroidal space. The choroid is attached anteriorly to the ciliary body (scleral spur) and posteriorly at the exit foramina of the vortex veins.

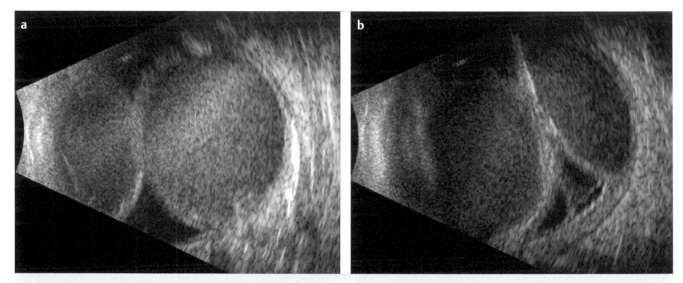

Fig. 53.2 (a) Echography at initial presentation demonstrating appositional suprachoroidal hemorrhage (kissing choroidal detachment). (b) Echography 8 days after presentation demonstrating liquefaction and decreased reflectivity of the suprachoroidal material. On dynamic ultrasonography, the liquefied clot was noted to move with eye movements.

53.2 Test Interpretation

A combination of the history and physical findings is the most definitive way to diagnose a suprachoroidal hemorrhage. Patients with suprachoroidal hemorrhage generally give a classic history of sudden-onset severe ocular pain, usually during or following intraocular surgery or ocular trauma. Intraocular pressure may be normal or elevated, and examination typically demonstrates a shallow or flat anterior chamber. Ophthalmoscopy demonstrates dark-brown or dark-red choroidal elevations.

In cases with overlying exudative appositional retinal detachment, echography may be necessary to confirm the presence of suprachoroidal hemorrhage and exclude such entities as choroidal tumor with hemorrhage or age-related macular degeneration disciform lesion with hemorrhage.

53.3 Diagnosis

Appositional ("kissing") suprachoroidal hemorrhage, right eye.

53.4 Medical Management

Given the often-guarded prognosis of eyes with suprachoroidal hemorrhage, the preferred management of this potentially devastating condition is prevention. Knowledge of risk factors permits the employment of prophylactic measures to decrease the likelihood of suprachoroidal hemorrhage. The surgical plan may even be altered in high-risk patients. Preoperative intraocular pressure should be normalized via medical therapy or anterior chamber paracentesis prior to surgery. A Flieringa ring in myopic eyes may minimize intraoperative hypotony and, thus, decrease the risk of suprachoroidal hemorrhage. In "high-risk" eyes, preplacement of sutures will permit rapid wound closure. Intraoperative hypotony should be avoided, and intraoperative blood pressure and tachycardia should be controlled.

If surgical intervention is not indicated (see below for a discussion of indications for surgical management of suprachoroidal hemorrhage) or if the suprachoroidal hemorrhage has not become sufficiently liquefied to permit surgical intervention, medications to control ocular hypertension and alleviate eye pain are employed. While systemic and topical steroids may stabilize blood vessel permeability (i.e., help prevent further bleeding) and decrease ocular discomfort, their benefit in the management of suprachoroidal hemorrhage remains unproven.

53.5 Surgical Management

For intraoperative suprachoroidal hemorrhage, all ocular incisions should be sutured closed immediately. Vitreous prolapse into the wound should be removed if possible. If the hemorrhage is massive and threatens to extrude the retina and lens-iris diaphragm, or if elevated intraocular pressure persists, a sclerotomy could be considered in the meridian of maximal elevation, ideally anterior to the ora serrata (approximately 7 mm posterior to the limbus), but these efforts are often ineffective. It may be necessary to refill the globe with sterile balanced salt solution or air/gas tamponade. The draining sclerotomy should be left open to permit continued drainage postoperatively. Although primary intraoperative suprachoroidal hemorrhage drainage is almost never complete, it is usually successful in controlling the intraocular pressure.

There are no randomized prospective controlled clinical trials addressing the optimal timing of secondary surgical intervention for intraoperative or postoperative suprachoroidal hemorrhage. Most surgeons recommend waiting 7 to 14 days to allow liquefaction of the hemorrhage to facilitate drainage of the blood. Serial echography is useful for following the extent of suprachoroidal hemorrhage liquefaction (▶ Fig. 53.2).

Indications for surgery in eyes with suprachoroidal hemorrhage include markedly increased intraocular pressure uncontrolled with medical therapy, severe intractable eye pain, "kissing choroidals" with retinal apposition, macular involvement with anterior retinal displacement and iris touch, and associated retinal detachment. Briefly, the surgical procedure consists of a 360-degree conjunctival limbal peritomy, isolation of each rectus muscle on a 2–0 cotton suture, and careful examination with indirect ophthalmoscopy to determine the areas of greatest suprachoroidal hemorrhage (if there is inadequate visualization of the fundus, this information may be obtained with echography). In eyes with massive suprachoroidal hemorrhage, the placement of a pars plana infusion cannula may be associated with iatrogenic retinal breaks or cannula placement in the suprachoroidal space; thus, in aphakic or pseudophakic eyes, a 1.5-mm infusion cannula or an infusing #23 gauge butterfly needle may be placed via the limbus; phakic eyes may require a lensectomy. A drainage sclerotomy is made radially with a 64 Beaver blade in the area of greatest hemorrhage approximately 7 mm posterior to the limbus, but a more posterior incision can be considered if the more anterior sclerotomy fails to drain. A limited anterior vitrectomy may be performed, with or without injection of perfluorocarbon liquid to facilitate drainage. Some surgeons advocate the use of perfluorocarbon liquid over air, as perfluorocarbon liquids force the blood anteriorly, while air may cause an anterior tamponading force with posterior displacement of the hemorrhage, thereby necessitating more posterior drainage sites. Perfluorocarbon liquids may also assist in the management of coexisting retinal detachment. After drainage of as much of the liquefied portion of the hemorrhage as possible, a 4- or 6-mm infusion cannula may be placed through the pars plana into the vitreous cavity and a standard pars plana vitrectomy is performed. Coexisting retinal detachment is managed with a scleral buckle and/or intraocular gas tamponade.

53.6 Rehabilitation and Follow-up

Risk factors for poor visual outcome include concurrent or delayed retinal detachment, more than two quadrants of suprachoroidal hemorrhage, vitreous incarceration in the wound/bleb, afferent pupillary defect on presentation, poor presenting visual acuity, and retinal apposition for > 14 days. Patients with postoperative suprachoroidal hemorrhage generally achieve better final visual acuities than do patients who develop suprachoroidal hemorrhage intraoperatively or following trauma.

Suggested Reading

[1] Welch JC, Spaeth GL, Benson WE. Massive suprachoroidal hemorrhage. Follow-up and outcome of 30 cases. Ophthalmology. 1988; 95(9):1202–1206

[2] The Fluorouracil Filtering Surgery Study Group. Risk factors for suprachoroidal hemorrhage after filtering surgery. Am J Ophthalmol. 1992; 113(5):501–507

[3] McMeel JW. Uveal tract circulatory problems. In: Albert DM, Jakobiec FA, eds. Principles and Practice of Ophthalmology. Vol. 1. Philadelphia, PA: W.B. Saunders Company; 1994:391–396

[4] Scott IU, Flynn HW, Jr, Schiffman J, Smiddy WE, Murray TG, Ehlies F. Visual acuity outcomes among patients with appositional suprachoroidal hemorrhage. Ophthalmology. 1997; 104(12):2039–2046

[5] Smiddy WE, Flynn HW Jr. Posterior segment complications of anterior segment surgery. In: Regillo CD, Brown GC, Flynn HW Jr, eds. Vitreoretinal Disease: The Essentials. New York, NY: Thieme; 1999:559–579

[6] Townsend-Pico WA, Lewis H. Vitreoretinal surgery for ocular trauma. In: Guyer DR, Yannuzzi LA, Chang S, Shields JA, Green WR, eds. Retina-Vitreous-Macula. Philadelphia, PA: W.B. Saunders Company; 1999:1370–1394

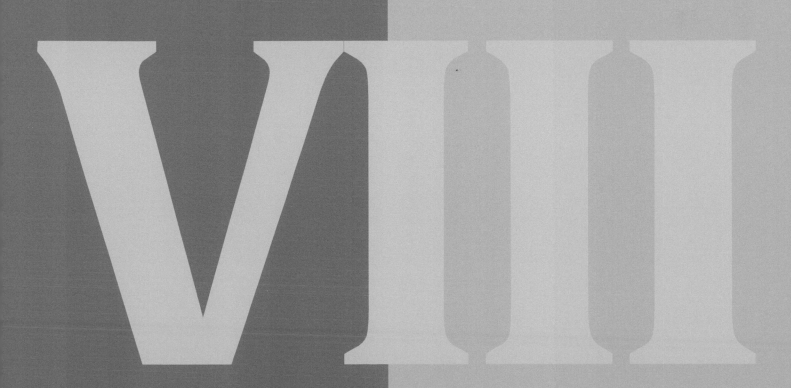

Part VIII

Trauma

54 Ruptured Globe

Jonathan H. Tzu and William E. Smiddy

Abstract

Ruptured globe encompasses a wide spectrum of ocular involvement; hence, the prognosis and management depend on the involved structures. Usually, the rupture is obvious from clinical examination and history, but may present occultly and hence certain signs must be heeded and pursued when present —chemosis or extensive subconjunctival hemorrhage, vitreous striae radiating to a possible occult defect, or afferent pupillary defect. Commonly, the rupture may occur along a previous incision, for example, after previous cataract surgery, but may occur anywhere—limbus, in association with muscle insertions, or more posteriorly as a result of coup or contra coup force. The primary objective is to restore the integrity of the globe, but most far posterior rupture sites are probably best left to heal spontaneously. Secondary objectives include removal of vitreous or lenticular opacities and addressing vitreous base traction to prevent or treat retinal detachment. The timing for secondary intervention has been debated since vitrectomy was introduced 40 years ago, but these authors favor secondary intervention in the 1- to 2-week time frame after primary closure; good results with early or even concurrent posterior segment intervention have also been reported. Concurrent intervention is especially effective when the rupture is anterior, such as a limbal wound dehiscence. Magnetic resonance imaging (MRI; when metallic foreign body is not present) or computed tomography (CT) scan may be helpful diagnostically and to assess occult ruptures.

Keywords: ocular trauma, scleral rupture, retinal detachment, vitrectomy, scleral buckling

54.1 History

An 80-year-old woman presented the morning after falling at her nursing home. Although the exact history was unclear, periocular ecchymoses suggested direct ocular trauma on a piece of furniture. Initially, the patient had not noticed pain or visual loss, but upon waking the next morning she realized poor vision and sought consultation. Cataract surgery with a nuclear expression extracapsular technique had been performed 3 years previously. Before the injury, the vision had been documented as 20/30, limited by some atrophic macular degeneration changes.

Upon presentation, visual acuity was hand motions and the intraocular pressure was 10 mm Hg. The cornea appeared relatively clear with a formed anterior chamber (▶ Fig. 54.1). However, there was conjunctival chemosis temporally and superiorly (▶ Fig. 54.2). While raising the upper lid, there was no conjunctival laceration, but a scleral dehiscence was evident, apparently at the previous cataract wound; upon examination of the superotemporal quadrant, the posterior chamber implant was seen in the subconjunctival space. The view posteriorly was limited by a dense vitreous hemorrhage. The pupil was not peaked, and there was no vitreous anterior to the iris.

The patient underwent vitrectomy that afternoon with placement of an encircling scleral band. The intraocular lens was removed. There was a sheet of vitreous streaming to the wound from behind the dehisced iris. There was no retinal detachment, but a focal subretinal hemorrhage limited to the superotemporal midperiphery was present.

Three months postoperatively, the retina was attached posteriorly with a minimal epiretinal membrane (▶ Fig. 54.3). Temporally, at the base of the buckle, the subretinal hemorrhage had organized; this traction was self-limited, counteracted by the scleral buckling effect (▶ Fig. 54.4). Visual acuity was 20/100 (with aphakic correction).

54.2 Diagnosis

Ruptured globe, OS.

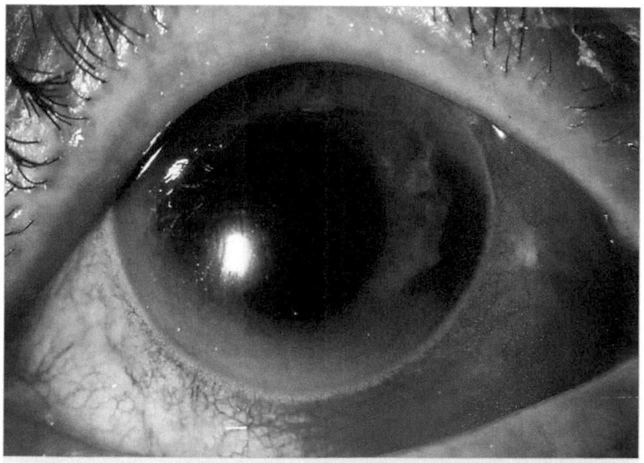

![Figure 54.1 and 54.2]

Fig. 54.1 Clinical appearance of patient 2 days after blunt trauma. Vision was hand motions and pressure was 10 mm Hg. There is subconjunctival hemorrhage and temporal and superior chemosis. The anterior chamber is deep and the patient has an aphakic pupillary space where a dense vitreous hemorrhage posteriorly.

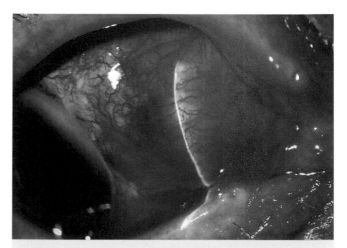

Fig. 54.2 The chemosis is much more evident and a dehiscence of the cataract wound is in evidence. The intraocular lens (as evidenced by the blue-colored haptic visible toward the bottom part of the slit) is in the subconjunctival space.

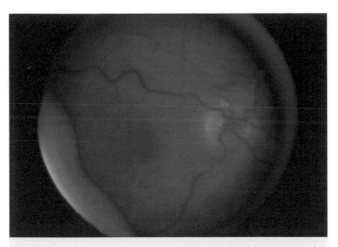

Fig. 54.3 Three months postoperatively the view to the posterior pole is clear. There is mild residual intraretinal hemorrhage superiorly, but no sign of epiretinal membrane or retinal detachment. The vision is 20/100.

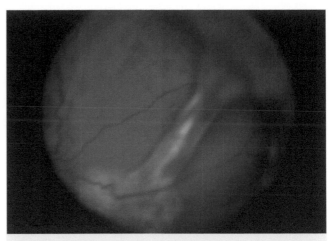

Fig. 54.4 Superiorly and nasally there is evidence of subretinal traction leading to the posterior aspect of the scleral buckle. There is no rhegmatogenous retinal detachment and this was nonprogressive.

Differential Diagnosis—Key Points

1. The most important key point is to be suspicious of what might be an occult rupture from the clinical history, and to detect the defect. In this case, the referring physician had not been aware of the anterior rupture. A valuable clinical sign in detecting occult rupture is chemosis. Another clinical sign is substantial subconjunctival hemorrhage which may obscure the rupture site. In an eye with previous cataract surgery, the previous incision line is a common site of dehiscence and should be carefully inspected. In eyes without previous surgery, more variable patterns of corneal and scleral laceration occur (whether they be from sharp or blunt objects). The sclera is thinnest behind the insertion site of the rectus muscles, and should be evaluated for an occult rupture location. Since prognosis is related to the most posterior extent and size of the rupture, there is some value in attempting to assess this extent preoperatively but balancing this against avoiding extensive diagnostic manipulations. Another important clinical sign of occult scleral rupture may be visible by slit-lamp transillumination to blood-highlighted vitreous streaming to the rupture site.

2. Another important prognostic factor is the presence or absence of an afferent pupillary defect (APD). This patient did not have an APD, and accordingly, even without being able to visualize the posterior pole, the prognosis was better since substantial retinal trauma or detachment was less likely. An APD can also be a sign of traumatic optic neuropathy which could limit the final outcome.

3. Because of the nature of the circumstances and patient population involved in ocular trauma, a clear history of the events leading to the trauma is frequently not forthcoming. While a majority of trauma occurs in a relatively young male population, it occurs in substantial numbers of elderly patients, as epitomized by this patient. A high index of suspicion must be maintained for a rupture in such cases.

54.3 Test Interpretation

The clinical history (as available) and clinical examination typically yield the most important information determining the necessary management of the patient, especially given the time constraints that the need for prompt repair usually dictates. Based on the clinical findings, the general extent of the dehiscence can often be determined (i.e., anterior to the limbus or posterior to the limbus, or large and likely posterior to the ora serrata). The integrity of the lens should also be established. Rhegmatogenous retinal detachment is uncommon in the acute phase, but hemorrhagic retinal detachment is not uncommon.

Often, the first examination offers the best view to assess extent of injury; corneal edema, hemorrhage, and inflammation often deteriorate the view subsequently.

Care must be taken not to generate additional forces on an open globe that might prolapse vitreous or other intraocular contents, compounding the injury. Still, gentle, screening B-scan ultrasonography (through the lids) may yield valuable information regarding the presence of vitreous, subretinal, or choroidal hemorrhages and estimating the posterior extent of the corneoscleral laceration.

A computed tomography (CT) scan may be useful in further delineating the integrity of the globe. However, these scans are most valuable when there is suspicion of periorbital trauma, optic nerve damage, or intraocular foreign body. Magnetic resonance imaging (MRI) scan is contraindicated if there is any suspicion of a metallic intraocular foreign body.

54.4 Medical Management

Primary medical management involves parenteral administration of broad-spectrum antibiotics to lessen the chance of endophthalmitis. Endophthalmitis occurs in up to 10% of globe injuries (a higher percentage in rural, farm settings), although many culture-positive cases are not clinically significant.

The acute management of the patient usually involves placing a protective shield over the eye to protect it from further trauma and pressure.

The patient's vaccination history should be taken; if a tetanus shot has not been delivered within the last 5 years, then it should be administered.

54.5 Surgical Management

The single most important feature directing initial management may be the patient's visual acuity. If there is no light perception (NLP) in the context of extreme ocular trauma (such as extensive, posterior, or multiple chorioretinal rupture sites with obvious major compromise of the globe integrity), primary enucleation should be considered to avoid the risk of sympathetic ophthalmia. This option is reserved only for the most exceptional and unequivocal cases since determination of visual function can be notoriously inaccurate in the acute phase of severe trauma. Also, rare trauma cases have been reported in which vision returned despite initial presentation with NLP. If there is any question, primary repair with careful follow-up monitoring is recommended.

Most commonly, cases with a ruptured globe are repaired under general anesthesia, but some cases with limited and anterior injuries only might be considered for monitored anesthesia care and peribulbar anesthesia. Except in cases of retained intraocular foreign body, the most common strategy is to perform a primary closure of the corneoscleral laceration, although some advocate simultaneous or early vitreoretinal repair. Primary closure alone is generally performed regardless of the presence of severe vitreous hemorrhage, retinal detachment, or disruption of the lens capsule. Surgical repair includes closure of the corneal portion of the rupture site. Typically, 10–0 nylon should be used for the cornea, with shorter suture bites in the central cornea and longer suture bites more peripherally to minimize irregular astigmatism. Slightly larger nylon or polyglactin sutures are recommended for the scleral wound. The suture that is placed at the limbus is critical to effect proper lateral realignment of the wound edges. After placing the limbal suture, the wound is usually best closed in the cornea and then front-to-back in the sclera. Consecutively placing adjacent sutures is recommended for best closure and to avoid making adjacent, intervening sutures too loose (and having to replace them). A viscoelastic substance may help to maintain the anterior chamber, to exclude iris or vitreous elements from the internal aspect of the wound, and to facilitate intraoperative visibility of anterior structures. The conjunctiva should be opened as necessary to allow exploration of the complete extent of the scleral rupture. A common location for scleral rupture is through the muscle insertion, since this is where the sclera is thinnest. In such cases, it may be necessary to disinsert the rectus muscle temporarily to close the scleral wound. Generally, the posterior extent of the laceration should be identified and closed. This may not be possible in lacerations extending extremely posteriorly, such as those approaching the optic nerve head.

Intravenous antibiotics are typically continued for approximately 36 hours after initial presentation. If there is no sign of infection, and clinical progress is evident, these are discontinued and the patient is discharged and followed as an outpatient.

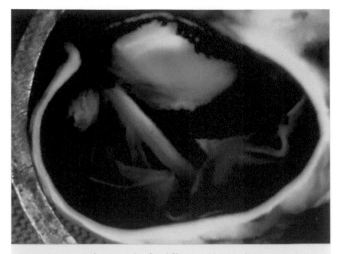

Fig. 54.5 Gross photograph of a different patient whose eye was enucleated because of trauma. Internalized retinal detachment can be seen, but most prominent is the posterior to anterior band of organized vitreous and fibrous proliferation streaming to the more interior rupture site.

The patient is monitored for the following week or 10 days. If light perception is maintained, then a secondary (vitreoretinal) repair is considered. At this point, the posterior vitreous is usually separated and may be removed more readily. However, it may be incarcerated or adherent at the area of the laceration site. It should be amputated there as effectively as possible. In cases with rupture involving the vitreous base or substantial vitreous loss, prophylactic scleral buckling may be combined with vitrectomy and, as necessary, lensectomy. Typically, endolaser photocoagulation is applied around the edges of the laceration, since subsequent contraction may cause retinal tears and traction at this site. Primary silicone oil infusion may be considered in cases with extreme traction or numerous, large retinal breaks.

Delaying the secondary repair longer than 2 weeks after the injury may allow formation of aggressive fibrous proliferation such that subsequent surgical efforts are less likely to be effective (▶ Fig. 54.5). This is especially important to consider in cases with what may appear to have vitreous hemorrhage; not infrequently, other ocular injuries coexist that result in vitreous base contracture leading to retinal detachment.

54.6 Rehabilitation and Follow-up

As long as anatomic and visual stabilization is observed, follow-up intervals are lengthened following surgical repair. Usually, the cicatricial response determining anatomic success is completed by 6 weeks following surgery. Occasionally, additional surgery such as removal of an epiretinal membrane or implantation of an intraocular lens is considered approximately 3 months following surgery for visual rehabilitation. Rigid contact lenses may be effective to neutralize aphakia or residual irregular corneal astigmatism, and may obviate the need for a secondary intraocular lens. However, a large fraction of patients are unable to tolerate aphakic contact lenses.

Shatter-proof safety glasses are strongly recommended, even if the other eye is emmetropic, to lessen the risk of a similar process occurring in the other eye.

Vocational rehabilitation may be necessary in patients with limited vision in this one eye, since unilateral visual loss may disqualify the patient from certain occupations. These efforts must be coordinated with social workers and vocational rehabilitation specialists.

Suggested Reading

[1] Cleary PE, Ryan SJ. Vitrectomy in penetrating eye injury. Results of a controlled trial of vitrectomy in an experimental posterior penetrating eye injury in the rhesus monkey. Arch Ophthalmol. 1981; 99(2):287–292

[2] Coleman DJ. Early vitrectomy in the management of the severely traumatized eye. Am J Ophthalmol. 1982; 93(5):543–551

[3] Michels RG. Vitrectomy methods in penetrating ocular trauma. Ophthalmology. 1980; 87(7):629–645

[4] Thompson WS, Rubsamen PE, Flynn HW, Jr, Schiffman J, Cousins SW. Endophthalmitis after penetrating trauma. Risk factors and visual acuity outcomes. Ophthalmology. 1995; 102(11):1696–1701

[5] Chaudhry NA, Belfort A, Flynn HW, Jr, Tabandeh H, Smiddy WE, Murray TG. Combined lensectomy, vitrectomy and scleral fixation of intraocular lens implant after closed-globe injury. Ophthalmic Surg Lasers. 1999; 30 (5):375–381

[6] Mittra RA, Mieler WF. Controversies in the management of open-globe injuries involving the posterior segment. Surv Ophthalmol. 1999; 44(3): 215–225

55 Intraocular Foreign Body

Jonathan H. Tzu and William E. Smiddy

Abstract

Intraocular foreign body (IOFB) is most commonly encountered in the context of industrial trauma, classically a consequence of metal-to-metal impact in a workplace with the victim not wearing appropriate protective eyewear. However, other unusual or traumatic circumstances may result in the same. Important aspects that determine management include the location and nature of the IOFB, and the extent of ocular tissue involvement. Certain substances are toxic to ocular structures and require timely removal, for example, metallic IOFBs. Others are not toxic and may be retained, as long as they have not induced or are in the context of other damaged structures, for example glass. Diagnosis is optimized when the clinical historical context is well understood, with a healthy dose of proper suspicion and awareness of the clinician. Clinical features include looking for entrance sites or extrapolating from patterns of injury. Because of concern about movement of magnetic IOFB during MRI study, this should be avoided unless or until it can be established to be nonmagnetic. Plane film X-rays with multiple angles or, when available in a timely fashion, computed tomography (CT) scanning are preferred. Echography can be an important modality in circumstances with good globe integrity and certain centers. IOFBs also carry substantial risk of endophthalmitis, so prophylactic antibiotics and prompt removal are recommended in the acute phase.

Keywords: intraocular foreign body, vitrectomy, ocular trauma, siderosis, magnetic, retinal detachment

55.1 History

A 32-year-old man was working aboard a docked marine biology research ship repairing a metal banister. While striking the metal rail with a metal hammer, he experienced a minor pain in his left eye. Over the ensuing 2 hours, he noticed a subtle but definite decrease in vision. On presentation, his visual acuity was 20/30. Slit-lamp examination showed a deep anterior chamber with minimal cell and flare. There was a defect in the temporal iris approximately 1 mm from the limbus. Corresponding to this site was a slitlike corneal defect that was not leaking aqueous fluid by Seidel testing. Posterior to the iris, there was a sectoral, white opacity in the peripheral lens (▶ Fig. 55.1). Examination of the posterior pole disclosed a small intraocular foreign body (IOFB) embedded in the retinal midperiphery. There was a collar of retinal edema surrounding it, but no hemorrhage (▶ Fig. 55.2).

The patient was taken to the operating room where, under a local anesthesia, vitrectomy with lensectomy and intraocular lens (IOL) implantation was combined with magnetic extraction of the IOFB. A low, encircling scleral buckle was also placed. The IOL power was estimated using measurements of the fellow eye. Laser photocoagulation was applied surrounding the retinal defect after removal of the foreign body; there was mild bleeding at the site of removal from the retina. There was not a previous posterior vitreous detachment, but one was introduced intraoperatively with the vitrectomy instrument using controlled aspiration. Postoperatively, the retina remained attached and the patient regained vision of 20/20 which has maintained throughout 25 years of follow-up examinations.

Differential Diagnosis—Key Points

1. The history in a patient sustaining an IOFB is commonly less remarkable than one might expect. If the patient was aware of the foreign body entry incident at all, it is usually perceived to be something like a piece of dust going onto the eye. Commonly, a few hours pass before pain or decreased vision from inflammatory components prompt the patient to seek consultation.

2. The most commonly encountered IOFBs are metallic and magnetic, classically occurring in the context of metal being hammered upon metal in the absence of protective eye wear.

3. The time-honored teaching that the heat generated by the launching of the small metallic IOFB sterilizes the foreign body and eliminates the risk of endophthalmitis is not true; studies have documented a 7% incidence of endophthalmitis with metallic IOFBs. Also, a more rapidly progressive and aggressive organism, *Bacillus cereus*, has been described in such cases. Catastrophic visual results, especially with delayed treatment, may result in irreversible blindness.

4. It is easier to make the diagnosis when the history is clear-cut and clear media allow direct visualization of the IOFB in the anterior or posterior segment. When the media are not clear, but the history is suspicious, other imaging studies may be necessary.

5. The clinician may need to deduce the IOFB location based on the history of the nature of the injury and the angle of entry site. Usually, the track of a posterior segment foreign body is apparent in the cornea, iris, and lens, or there is a superficial tract visible in the conjunctiva and sclera. In the latter cases, the foreign body may come to rest at the ora serrata and indirect ophthalmoscopy with careful scleral indentation may allow or even be necessary to visualize the foreign body. An apparent oblique corneal entry site may suggest that the possibility of IOFB retained in the anterior chamber angle must be considered. This would be readily apparent with gonioscopic evaluation (▶ Fig. 55.3).

6. Self-sealing, small-entry wounds usually allow sufficient globe integrity to permit surgical repair without the need for general anesthesia. However, if the wound is large or leaking, general anesthesia must be considered to lessen the risk of expulsing intraocular contents in the event of a retrobulbar hemorrhage during the block.

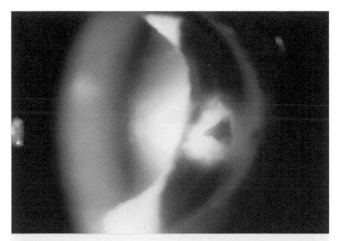

Fig. 55.1 External appearance approximately 6 hours after a metallic IOFB traversed the temporal peripheral cornea, iris, and lens.

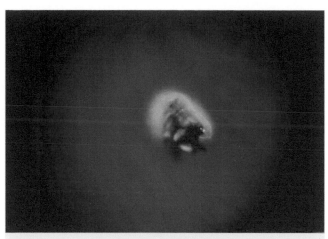

Fig. 55.2 The IOFB is embedded in the midperipheral retina temporally. It appears to be metallic and is likely magnetic. There is a collarette of retinal edema at the impact site.

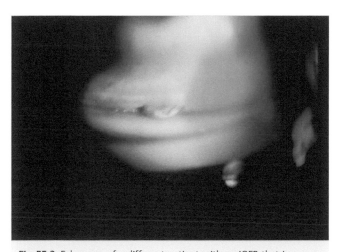

Fig. 55.3 Echogram of a different patient with an IOFB that is suspended approximately 2 mm anterior to the retinal surface. Other echograms demonstrate vitreous blood above, suggesting the possibility that the foreign body bounced off the retina and came to rest in the posterior vitreous.

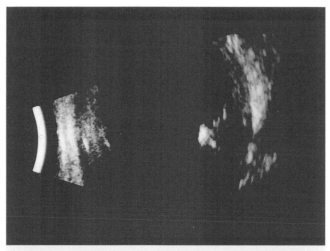

Fig. 55.4 CT image of a patient with IOFB. The radiopacity at the posterior and temporal eye wall of the patient's right eye depicts the IOFB.

55.2 Diagnosis

Retained magnetic intraocular foreign body, OS.

55.3 Test Interpretation

When direct visualization is possible, no further diagnostic testing is indicated. When the history suggests the possibility of multiple IOFBs, more comprehensive imaging might be indicated, but this is usually apparent from the nature of the injury. In eyes with opaque media or suspected occult IOFB, a screening test is the plain film X-ray. Frequently, a combination of anteroposterior and lateral views allows localization to the eye or orbit. Of critical importance is detecting whether the foreign body is intraocular or extraocular. Nonmetallic intraocular foreign bodies may not appear on plain film. Frequently, glass foreign bodies do appear, since drinking glasses or bottles usually have a high lead content.

The second test that usually allows detection of an IOFB is the combined A- and B-scan ultrasound (▶ Fig. 55.4). This is feasible for foreign bodies of all compositions and is most effective when done with probe contact on the cornea. This may be contraindicated depending on the condition of the entry site.

A third, useful diagnostic test is a computed tomography (CT) scan (▶ Fig. 55.5). For metallic and usually for glass foreign bodies, this is usually definitive. However, foreign bodies of vegetable matter will usually not manifest on radiologic evaluation. Also, the CT scan in suspected cases may localize the foreign body anteriorly, prompting reexamination using maneuvers such as gonioscopy (▶ Fig. 55.6).

Magnetic resonance imaging (MRI) is contraindicated when magnetic IOFBs are suspected.

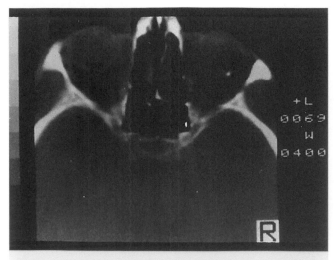

Fig. 55.5 Gonioscopic appearance of a metallic foreign body resting in the inferior anterior chamber angle. An oblique corneal entry site led to the suspicion of the foreign body being in the anterior segment.

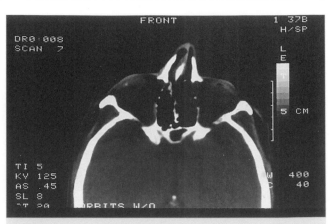

Fig. 55.6 CT scan shows a radiopacity in an anterior location. This foreign body was not clinically visible due to its peripheral location. Intraoperatively, it was ultimately detected in the vitreous base of the left eye temporally.

55.4 Medical Management

Medical management is confined initially to an efficient and prompt diagnostic evaluation. Prompt institution of prophylactic antibiotics is probably indicated in most cases and may be tailored depending on the nature of the IOFB or the setting of the injury. Although a metallic IOFB causes endophthalmitis with only a 7% incidence, the devastating consequences merit broad-spectrum antibiotic use. One study has shown a much higher incidence of infection in rural injuries. Accordingly, farm- or field-related injuries, which are at increased risk of harboring *B. cereus* organisms, should receive antibiotic coverage for anaerobic organisms. Usually, the patient is treated with systemic antibiotics while being readied for surgical repair; intravitreal antibiotics may be administered in especially suspicious cases. If surgery can commence promptly systemic antibiotics may be deferred until after surgery, allowing a culture that would not be potentially falsely negative. The initial examination may be of critical importance since subsequent corneal edema commonly hinders the view to the posterior pole. This should not be truncated in the interest of arranging ancillary evaluations.

Patients presenting with a chronic IOFB may be managed more electively if there is no sign of infection. Such cases are not treated with prophylactic antibiotics since the risk of endophthalmitis occurring more than a couple of days after the injury is minimal.

55.5 Surgical Management

Occasionally, intraocular foreign bodies confined to the anterior segment may be managed from a limbal incision. Most IOFBs present in the posterior segment and a pars plana approach is preferable. Foreign bodies lodged under the retina may be approached with an external magnet and removed via a sclerotomy, but most are approached internally.

The first surgical objective is to reestablish the tectonic integrity of the eye. Often, the entry site is small enough that few or no 10–0 nylon sutures are necessary. The second objective is to remove media opacities, which may include lens opacity, disrupted lens material, or hemorrhage. Accordingly, a lensectomy and vitrectomy are often necessary. Frequently, enough capsular support may be preserved to allow simultaneous or subsequent implantation of a posterior chamber IOL in the ciliary sulcus (as was done in the described case). The third objective is to identify, mobilize, and remove the foreign body. A pick, forceps, or intraocular magnet may be used to release embedded foreign bodies. Nonmetallic foreign bodies usually require intraocular forceps. A variety of forceps designs including the basket-like Wilson forceps may be useful for grasping and removing the IOFB once it is mobilized. A foreign body can be removed through either a sclerotomy or the entry wound, although it may be necessary to enlarge the site. An extremely large foreign body may be brought into the anterior chamber and removed via a separate limbal incision. Commonly, the foreign body is mobilized, brought anteriorly with the magnet, and transferred to forceps for extraction, since it often disengages from the magnet if withdrawn through the sclerotomy.

The final surgical objectives involve closure of retinal holes and prophylaxis against future retinal breaks. As a general rule, a low encircling scleral buckling band is considered if the foreign body traverses the vitreous base. Cases with IOFBs that traverse the lens without passing through vitreous base usually do not require scleral buckling. Endolaser photocoagulation at the impact site may not be necessary since the inflammatory reaction initiated by the impact may create an adequate adhesion; however, one row of light laser surrounding the site with fluid-gas exchange (air only) is usually performed.

Certain glass intraocular foreign bodies may be safely retained since they are inert and do not carry the risk of siderosis as for metallic intraocular foreign bodies. This option is especially attractive for glass IOFBs that are deeply embedded, especially if perforating the posterior sclera.

The timing of surgery for cases of suspected retained intraocular foreign bodies is of critical importance. IOFB removal within 6 to 12 hours is generally recommended when possible because of the substantial risk of aggressive endophthalmitis.

55.6 Rehabilitation and Follow-up

The patient is monitored postoperatively with intravenous antibiotics and topical corticosteroids, antibiotics, and/or cycloplegic agents, as indicated. If there is no sign of endophthalmitis within 24 to 48 hours and good clinical progress is in evidence, systemic antibiotics are discontinued.

Patients are observed at approximately 1- to 2-week intervals in the first month following surgery and less frequently thereafter. The patient is monitored for recurrent retinal detachment and/or epiretinal membrane formation that is of visual significance. If the patient has been rendered aphakic, then a second IOL implantation or aphakic contact lens is considered.

Suggested Reading

[1] Rubsamen PE, Irvin WD, McCuen BW, II, Smiddy WE, Bowman CB. Primary intraocular lens implantation in the setting of penetrating ocular trauma. Ophthalmology. 1995; 102(1):101–107

[2] Mieler WF, Ellis MK, Williams DF, Han DP. Retained intraocular foreign bodies and endophthalmitis. Ophthalmology. 1990; 97(11):1532–1538

[3] Thompson JT, Parver LM, Enger CL, Mieler WF, Liggett PE, National Eye Trauma System. Infectious endophthalmitis after penetrating injuries with retained intraocular foreign bodies. Ophthalmology. 1993; 100(10):1468–1474

[4] Boldt HC, Pulido JS, Blodi CF, Folk JC, Weingeist TA. Rural endophthalmitis. Ophthalmology. 1989; 96(12):1722–1726

[5] Jonas JB, Budde WM. Early versus late removal of retained intraocular foreign bodies. Retina. 1999; 19(3):193–197

[6] Arroyo JG, Postel EA, Stone T, McCuen BW, Egan KM. A matched study of primary scleral buckle placement during repair of posterior segment open globe injuries. Br J Ophthalmol. 2003; 87(1):75–78

56 Optic Neuritis

Sushma Yalamanchili and Andrew G. Lee

Abstract

Sudden vision loss in a young patient with an afferent pupillary defect, decreased color vision, no disc edema, and pain on eye movement consistent with retrobulbar optic neuritis confirmed on magnetic resonance imaging (MRI) to check for demyelinating lesions and treated as per the optic neuritis treatment trial with intravenous steroids. Optic neuritis refers optic neuropathy due to inflammation, demyelination, or infection. Typical cases generally only need an MRI to evaluate for demyelinating disease but atypical cases might require further evaluation for infectious and inflammatory etiologies including neuromyelitis optica (NMO) and myelin oligodendrocytic glycoprotein (MOG) antibodies.

Keywords: optic neuritis, eye pain on movement, multiple sclerosis, neuromyelitis optica, vision loss in the young, optic neuritis treatment trial

56.1 History

A 35-year-old woman noted the acute onset of blurred vision in her right eye 12 days ago. She complained of moderately severe retro-orbital pain on the right that was made worse by eye movements. The vision had deteriorated over the first 3 or 4 days but had since stabilized. She noted that when she attempted to perform aerobic exercises, her vision became worse. She denied any precipitating factors for her visual loss or any history of neurologic symptoms, except for rare diffuse headaches for many years. She has been otherwise healthy and denies any family history of visual impairment.

Examination revealed the visual acuity to be 20/80 on the right and 20/20 on the left. The patient identified 3 of 10 Hardy–Rand–Rittler pseudoisochromatic plates on the right and 10 of 10 plates on the left. Visual field examination revealed a superior arcuate field defect on the right and the visual field was normal on the left. The pupils were 5 mm bilaterally and reacted well to light and near, but there was a significant relative afferent pupillary defect (RAPD) on the right. Examination of the efferent system was normal. Slit-lamp examination was normal. The right optic disc was hyperemic without hemorrhages or exudates (▶ Fig. 56.1). There were no vitreous cells. The left fundus was normal.

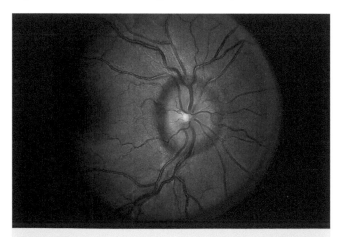

Fig. 56.1 Fundus photograph of the right eye reveals a moderately swollen and hyperemic optic disc without hemorrhages or exudates.

Differential Diagnosis—Key Points

1. The differential diagnosis in this case includes demyelinating, infectious, inflammatory, ischemic, infiltrative, compressive, and heredofamilial (e.g., Leber's disease) optic neuropathy. The patient's young age, lack of atherosclerotic risk factors, retro-orbital pain, and lack of pallid disc swelling make ischemic optic neuropathy less likely. The acute, painful onset makes a compressive or infiltrative lesion unlikely. Leber's hereditary optic neuropathy is usually painless, not common in women (although it can occur in either gender), and associated with a dense central scotoma, and patients may have a family history of optic neuropathy. The most likely diagnosis in this case is optic neuritis (ON), a general term for an optic neuropathy resulting from idiopathic, inflammatory, infectious, or demyelinating etiology. As the optic nerve is swollen, the term papillitis or anterior ON is used (if the optic nerve is normal, then it is called retrobulbar ON). Most cases of idiopathic or demyelinating ON are retrobulbar.

2. Idiopathic or demyelinating ON usually presents with a "typical" profile as outlined in **the list below**.

3. The deterioration of vision with exercise or heat exposure (e.g., a hot shower, sauna, exercise) is referred to as Uhthoff's symptom. Although this symptom is characteristically seen with demyelinating ON, it is not specific, and may occur with other optic neuropathies (e.g., Leber's hereditary optic neuropathy).

The disc swelling that occurs in approximately 35% of typical ON patients is usually of mild to moderate degree and may be associated with minimal (but usually no hemorrhages) and no or only trace vitreous cells. Demyelinating ON is not associated with marked disc edema, subretinal fluid, retinal exudates, cotton wool patches, macular edema, or macular star. Demyelinating ON is typically unilateral, retrobulbar, and resolves over time spontaneously. Thus, consider an alternate diagnosis to "typical" demyelinating ON if bilateral, nonrecovering, progressive, or in cases of ON with severe disc edema, marked hemorrhages, cotton wool spots, lipid maculopathy more than trace vitreous cells, pallid disc edema, or retinal arteriolar narrowing is present. Neuromyelitis optica (NMO) can present with a clinical picture of ON and NMO should especially be considered in cases which present bilaterally, with optic disc edema, or without improvement over time. NMO is an inflammatory central nervous system syndrome that is distinct from multiple sclerosis (MS). NMO is associated with serum aquaporin-4 immunoglobulin G antibodies (AQP4-IgG). A recent International Panel for NMO Diagnosis developed revised diagnostic criteria for NMO. The new nomenclature defines a unifying term "NMO spectrum disorder" (NMOSD) and can occur with or without positive AQP4-IgG. The core clinical characteristics, however, are clinical syndromes or magnetic resonance imaging (MRI) findings related to optic nerve, spinal cord, area postrema, other brainstem, diencephalic, or cerebral presentations. In addition, in contrast to MS where immunomodulatory therapy is used (e.g., interferons), NMO often requires immunosuppressive therapy and immunomodulatory MS treatments may in fact worsen NMO.

4. The Optic Neuritis Treatment Trial (ONTT), a randomized, controlled trial that enrolled 457 patients with ON at 15 centers in the United States between the years 1988 and 1991, has generated significant useful data concerning the treatment and natural history of demyelinating ON.

56.1.1 Features of Typical Optic Neuritis

- Acute, usually unilateral loss of visual acuity and/or visual field.
- An RAPD in unilateral or bilateral but asymmetric cases.
- Periocular pain (90%), especially with eye movement.
- Normal (65%) or swollen (35%) optic nerve head.
- Young adult (< 40 years).
- Eventual visual improvement.
- 88% improve at least one line by day 15.
- 95% improve by at least one line by day 30.
- Visual improvement may continue for months.

(Adapted from Lee AG, Brazis PW. Clinical Pathways in Neuro-Ophthalmology: An Evidence-Based Approach. New York, NY: Thieme; 1998:25, with permission.)

56.2 Test Interpretation

The ONTT determined that chest radiograph, laboratory studies (e.g., syphilis serology, antinuclear antibody [ANA] titers, serum chemistries, and complete blood count), and lumbar puncture are not necessary for typical ON but should be considered in atypical cases. See **list below**. Serologic testing for Lyme disease should be considered in patients with ON, especially with a history of the typical rash of erythema migrans, who live in or have visited Lyme-endemic areas. Testing should be performed, including consideration for NMO IgG aquaporin-4 antibody in atypical cases of ON.

MRI of the brain is of limited value in disclosing an alternate diagnosis in patients with typical ON. In the ONTT, an alternate etiology for visual loss was noted in only two patients: one with a pituitary tumor and one with an ophthalmic artery aneurysm. MRI is, however, a valuable predictor of the future development of MS. In the ONTT, the 15-year overall cumulative probability for the development of clinically definite MS was 50%, but this probability was 72% for patients who had one or more lesions suggesting demyelination on MRI. Patients with longitudinally extensive enhancement of one or both optic nerves or chiasm on MRI should be considered for additional evaluation for inflammatory ON and NMO.

In patients with clinical features of atypical ON (**see list below**), further studies are indicated. These include MRI, blood studies (e.g., syphilis serology, Lyme titers, ANA, *Bartonella henselae* titers, angiotensin converting enzyme (ACE), anti-neutrophilic cytoplasmic antibody (ANCA), NMO), or lumbar puncture to investigate for other infectious, inflammatory, and infiltrative processes.

56.2.1 Features of Atypical Optic Neuritis

- Bilateral simultaneous onset of ON in an adult patient.
- Lack of pain.
- Ocular findings suggestive of an inflammatory process.
- Anterior uveitis.
- Posterior chamber inflammation more than a trace.
- Macular exudate or star figure.
- Retinal infiltrate or retinal inflammation.
- Severe disc swelling.
- Lack of improvement of visual functioning or worsening of visual function after 30 days.
- Lack of at least one line of visual acuity improvement within the first 3 weeks after onset of symptoms.
- Age more than 50 years.
- Diagnosis or evidence of other systemic condition (e.g., inflammatory or infectious diseases, including AIDS) other than MS that might cause optic neuropathy.
- Exquisitely steroid-sensitive or steroid-dependent optic neuropathy.

(Adapted from Lee AG, Brazis PW. Clinical Pathways in Neuro-Ophthalmology: An Evidence-Based Approach. New York, NY: Thieme; 1998:26, with permission.)

56.3 Diagnosis

Typical optic neuritis (idiopathic or demyelinating)—papillitis.

56.4 Medical Management

The ONTT randomly assigned patients to one of three treatment arms: (1) intravenous (IV) methylprednisolone sodium succinate (250 mg every 6 hours for 3 days) followed by oral prednisone (1 mg/kg per day for 11 days); (2) oral prednisone (1 mg/kg per day for 14 days); (3) oral placebo for 14 days followed by a short oral taper.

Treatment with high-dose IV steroids followed by oral steroids accelerated visual recovery but provided no long-term benefit to vision. Treatment with "standard-dose" oral prednisone alone did not improve the visual outcome and was associated with an increased rate of new attacks of ON. Treatment with the IV followed by oral steroid regimen reduced the rate of development of clinically definite MS during the first 2 years, particularly in patients with three or more lesions consistent with demyelination on MRI at time of study entry. By 3 years, however, this treatment effect had subsided.

Based on the ONTT results, it is recommended that treatment with oral prednisone in standard doses be avoided in ON.

Treatment with IV methylprednisolone should be considered in patients with an abnormal MRI (may possibly reduce the subsequent risk of development of MS) or a particular need (e.g., monocular patient or occupational requirement) to recover visual function more rapidly. High-dose oral steroids (e.g., 500 mg methylprednisolone), however, have not been associated with the same risks as standard dose (e.g., oral prednisone 1 mg/kg) for ON and may be considered as an acceptable alternative for the treatment of typical ON.

However, in the past, the results of the ONTT suggested that either no treatment or IV steroids could be used for ON. The possibility of NMO, which has a much worse prognosis and often requires longer term corticosteroid and other immunosuppressive treatment, might tip the balance toward IV steroid treatment in some cases of ON. As noted in the ONTT, the risk of MS was less in patients with ON who had a negative MRI for demyelinating white matter lesions of MS. Unfortunately, patients with NMO often have brain MR studies that do not show typical demyelinating white matter lesions of MS or are normal. Thus, there might be a rationale for considering IV steroids in patients with ON and negative or atypical MRI scans for MS until the NMO titer returns. In addition, some patients with atypical optic neuritis (e.g., bilateral, optic disc edema) may harbor myeling oligodendrocytic glycoprotein (MOG) antibodies. The role of MOG antibody testing in optic neuritis remains to be determined.

56.5 Surgical Management

No surgical management is indicated.

56.6 Rehabilitation and Follow-up

In the ONTT, 88% of patients improved at least one Snellen line by day 15 after study entry and 96% improved at least one Snellen line by 30 days. For most patients, recovery of visual acuity was nearly complete by 30 days after study entry. Among the patients with incomplete recovery by 30 days, most showed slow gradual improvement for up to 1 year. The only predictor of poor visual outcome in patients enrolled in the ONTT was poor visual acuity at time of study entry. Even so, of 160 patients starting with visual acuity 20/200 or worse, all had at least some improvement and only 8 (5%) had visual acuities that were still 20/200 or worse at 6 months. In contrast to demyelinating ON, NMO does not have as good a visual prognosis and patients who do not recover vision should be evaluated for NMO as well as other etiologies for ON.

As noted above, there is significant risk of developing MS in patients with isolated ON. This risk is greater in patients with an abnormal MRI (three or more lesions), with a history of nonspecific neurologic symptoms, with a history of previous ON, or with increased cerebrospinal fluid IgG. Factors that decrease the subsequent risk of MS include a normal MRI, bilateral simultaneous ON, childhood onset, or marked disc edema. NMO should be considered in these settings.

Suggested Reading

[1] Beck RW, Cleary PA, Anderson MM, Jr, et al. The Optic Neuritis Study Group. A randomized, controlled trial of corticosteroids in the treatment of acute optic neuritis. N Engl J Med. 1992; 326(9):581–588

[2] Beck RW, Cleary PA, Trobe JD, et al. The Optic Neuritis Study Group. The effect of corticosteroids for acute optic neuritis on the subsequent development of multiple sclerosis. N Engl J Med. 1993; 329(24):1764–1769

[3] Beck RW, Trobe JD. What we have learned from the Optic Neuritis Treatment Trial. Ophthalmology. 1995; 102(10):1504–1508

[4] Lee AG, Brazis PW. Clinical Pathways in Neuro-Ophthalmology: An Evidence-Based Approach. New York, NY: Thieme; 1998:25–17

[5] Optic Neuritis Study Group. The 5-year risk of MS after optic neuritis. Experience of the optic neuritis treatment trial. Neurology. 1997; 49(5):1404–1413

[6] Optic Neuritis Study Group. Multiple sclerosis risk after optic neuritis: final optic neuritis treatment trial follow-up. Arch Neurol. 2008; 65(6):727–732

[7] Wingerchuk DM, Banwell B, Bennett JL, et al. International Panel for NMO Diagnosis. International consensus diagnostic criteria for neuromyelitis optica spectrum disorders. Neurology. 2015; 85(2):177–189

57 Optic Disc Edema with Macular Star (Neuroretinitis)

Sushma Yalamanchili and Andrew G. Lee

Abstract

Vision loss in a young adult with three cats at home and a preceding flulike illness found to have disc edema, a macular star, and positive lab work for *Bartonella* immunoglobulin G (IgG) and IgM treated with antibiotics. Other causes for optic disc edema with a macular star (ODEMS) should be considered including papilledema (in bilateral cases) as well as other infectious (e.g., Lyme disease, toxoplasmosis, tuberculosis, syphilis) or inflammatory disease (e.g., sarcoid).

Keywords: neuroretinitis, cat scratch disease, disc edema, macular star, vision loss, Bartonella henselae

57.1 History

A 22-year-old woman noted the onset of blurred vision in her right eye 3 weeks ago. She noted minimal right periorbital pain. She denied any history of previous medical, ophthalmologic, or neurologic illnesses, but she did complain of recent occasional headaches of mild and diffuse nature and noted that the visual blurring seemed to have started a week or so after a nonspecific "flulike" illness. She has three cats at home.

Examination revealed visual acuity to be 20/60 on the right and 20/15 on the left. She identified 4 of 10 pseudoisochromatic plates on the right and 10 of 10 on the left. Visual field examination revealed a cecocentral scotoma on the right and was normal on the left. Pupils were 5 mm bilaterally and equally reactive to light and near, but there was a right relative afferent pupillary defect. Motility examination was normal. The right fundus exam revealed significant optic disc edema with peripapillary and macular exudates, the latter in a star configuration (▶ Fig. 57.1). There were 1 + vitreous cells on the right. The left fundus examination was normal.

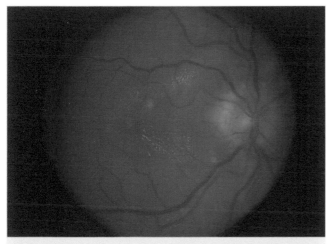

Fig. 57.1 Fundus photograph of the right eye reveals significant optic disc edema with peripapillary and macular exudates, the latter finding in a star configuration. There were 1 + vitreous cells in the right eye.

57.2 Test Interpretation

It is important to look for funduscopic changes of toxoplasmosis as a clue to this etiology as a cause for ODEMS. Syphilis serology, *Bartonella henselae* (the infectious agent of cat-scratch disease;

positive in this case) titers, toxoplasmosis titers, tuberculosis testing, and Lyme serology should be considered. Syphilis serology requires both treponemal (e.g., fluorescent treponemal antibody (FTA), microhemagglutination for treponema pallidum (MHA-TP)) and nontreponemal testing (e.g., rapid plasma reagin (RPR), veneral disease research laboratory (VDRL)) in order to reduce false-positive nontreponemal testing which has less specificity than the treponemal testing. Tuberculin skin testing (e.g., Mantoux's test) or more recently QuantiFERON gamma assays for TB can be considered especially in endemic populations (e.g., immigrants, prisoners, homeless, health care workers, HIV positive, or immunosuppressed patients). The skin testing and QuantiFERON testing for TB, however, do not differentiate between latent TB and active TB and additional history, exam, and testing (e.g., chest radiography) are necessary to confirm the diagnosis. Lyme testing is a two-tiered strategy involving a screening enzyme-linked immunosorbent assay (ELISA) followed by a confirmatory western blot for Lyme disease. *B. henselae* immunoglobulin M (IgM) and IgG testing should be performed for both the acute and convalescent period especially in cases where the initial acute titer is indeterminate. In this case, the *B. henselae* IgM and IgG were both markedly positive at high titers.

57.3 Diagnosis

ODEMS or neuroretinitis secondary to cat-scratch disease.

57.4 Medical Management

ODEMS is usually a benign disorder that resolves spontaneously over a period of months without treatment. Steroids have been used in some cases with unclear effect. If a specific infectious agent is discovered, appropriate antibiotics should be instituted.

57.5 Surgical Management

No surgical management is indicated.

57.6 Rehabilitation and Follow-up

The prognosis for visual recovery is usually good, but significant residual visual disability may occasionally occur. Optic atrophy and macular retinal pigment epithelial changes may be residuals. Recurrences of ODEMS in the same or fellow eye have been described in idiopathic as well as infectious cases, especially in patients with toxoplasmosis.

Although optic neuritis is a risk factor for the development of multiple sclerosis, ODEMS is not. Because a macular exudate may not develop in cases of ODEMS until 2 weeks after presentation, patients who demonstrate acute papillitis with a normal macula should be reevaluated within 2 weeks for the development of a macular star. The finding of ODEMS makes the subsequent development of multiple sclerosis extremely unlikely.

Suggested Reading

[1] Brazis PW, Lee AG. Optic disk edema with a macular star. Mayo Clin Proc. 1996; 71(12):1162–1166
[2] Lee AG, Brazis PW. Clinical Pathways in Neuro-Ophthalmology: An Evidence-Based Approach. New York, NY: Thieme; 1998:41–47
[3] Parmley VC, Schiffman JS, Maitland CG, Miller NR, Dreyer RF, Hoyt WF. Does neuroretinitis rule out multiple sclerosis? Arch Neurol. 1987; 44(10):1045–1048
[4] Purvin VA, Chioran G. Recurrent neuroretinitis. Arch Ophthalmol. 1994; 112 (3):365–371

58 Anterior Ischemic Optic Neuropathy—Nonarteritic

Sushma Yalamanchili and Andrew G. Lee

Abstract

Sudden painless vision loss upon awakening in an elderly patient with hypertension, diabetes mellitus, and hyperlipidemia with sectoral disc edema, a contralateral small cup-to-disc ratio, afferent pupillary defect, color dyschromatopsia, and altitudinal visual field defect is consistent with nonarteritic anterior ischemic optic neuropathy. (NAION). The differential diagnosis should include arteritic (i.e., giant cell arteritis) AION and in atypical cases (e.g., younger patient, lacking vasculopathic risk factors, bilateral) evaluation for alternative etiologies should be considered.

Keywords: NAION, sudden vision loss, altitudinal visual field defect, small cup-to-disc ratio, contralateral eye, sectoral disc edema

58.1 History

A 65-year-old woman states that on awakening from sleep 3 days ago she noted severe visual loss in the left eye. She denied any headache, eye pain, jaw claudications, episodes of transient visual loss, or any other neurologic or ophthalmologic complaints. She related a past history of hypertension, increased cholesterol, and diabetes mellitus.

Examination revealed visual acuity to be 20/20 on the right and 20/200 on the left. She identified 10 of 10 pseudoisochromatic plates on the right but only 2 of 10 plates on the left. Visual fields were normal on the right but revealed a dense inferior altitudinal defect on the left. Pupils were 3 mm bilaterally, reacted well to light on the right and poorly to light on the left, and there was a left relative afferent pupillary defect. Extraocular motility was normal. Fundus examination was normal on the right with the cup-to-disc ratio of 0.1 (▶ Fig. 58.1). The left optic disc was diffusely swollen and there were peripapillary hemorrhages (▶ Fig. 58.2).

58.1.1 Clinical Features Atypical for Nonarteritic Anterior Ischemic Optic Neuropathy

- Age younger than 40 years.
- Bilateral simultaneous onset.
- Visual field defect not consistent with an optic neuropathy (e.g., bitemporal hemianopia).
- Lack of optic disc edema in acute phase.
- Lack of relative afferent pupillary defect in unilateral cases.
- Large cup-to-disc ratio in the fellow eye.
- Lack of vasculopathic risk factors.
- Presence of premonitory symptoms of transient visual loss.
- Progression of visual loss beyond 2 to 4 weeks.
- Recurrent episodes in the same eye.
- Anterior or posterior segment inflammation (e.g., vitreous cells).

Differential Diagnosis—Key Points

1. The patient has a left optic neuropathy that may be ischemic, compressive, infectious, inflammatory, or infiltrative. The older age of the patient, lack of pain, and presence of optic disc edema argue strongly against optic neuritis. The acute onset makes a compressive lesion unlikely. The acute onset, lack of pain, altitudinal visual field defect, optic disc swelling, and vascular risk factors are all compatible with anterior ischemic optic neuropathy (AION).

2. AION is characterized clinically by the acute onset of usually painless (pain may occur in up to 8–30% in some series) unilateral visual loss in a middle age or older patient (usually greater than age 50 years); an ipsilateral relative afferent pupillary defect (if unilateral or bilateral and asymmetric); and edema of the optic nerve head with or without peripapillary hemorrhages. Later, the optic disc often develops sector or diffuse pallor.

3. A small cup-to-disc ratio (less than 0.2) is an important predisposing structural factor for the development of AION ("disc at risk"). If a patient with AION has a large cup-to-disc ratio, giant cell arteritis should be strongly considered. The most important risk factors for nonarteritic AION (NAION) are hypertension, hypotension, and diabetes mellitus.

4. Giant cell arteritis should be considered in all patients presenting with AION. This patient had no symptoms suggestive of this disease but a sedimentation rate and C-reactive protein should be considered in patients with this presentation.

5. Findings atypical for NAION are outlined in **the list below.** If any of these findings are present, other etiologies for the optic neuropathy should be considered.

6. Visual loss with AION often is noted on awakening from sleep in the morning, perhaps due to nocturnal hypotension (although unproven) contributing to optic nerve ischemia. The visual loss in AION is usually acute but some worsening of vision may occur for 2 to 4 weeks after onset. Other important predisposing factors to AION include hypotension or anemia due to surgery, severe hypotension or blood loss, and collagen vascular diseases.

(Adapted from Lee AG, Brazis PW. Clinical Pathways in Neuro-Ophthalmology: An Evidence-Based Approach. New York, NY: Thieme; 1998:53, with permission.)

58.2 Test Interpretation

A sedimentation rate and C-reactive protein should be obtained to investigate the possibility of giant cell arteritis (i.e., arteritic AION). If the sedimentation rate and C-reactive protein are elevated, if there are other clinical symptoms of giant cell arteritis (e.g., headache, jaw claudications), or if there are atypical features for NAION (e.g., a large cup-to-disc ratio), temporal artery

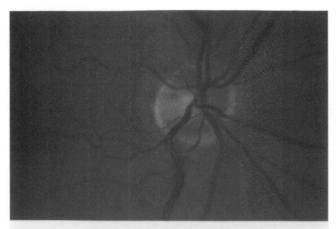

Fig. 58.1 Fundus photograph of the right optic nerve shows a cup-to-disc ratio of 0.1 (the "disc at risk") consistent with NAION.

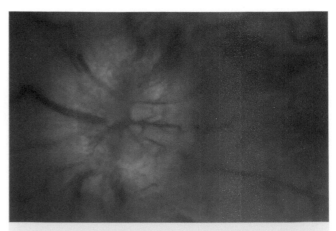

Fig. 58.2 Fundus photograph reveals a left optic disc that is diffusely swollen and pale with surrounding peripapillary hemorrhages. The retinal arterioles were attenuated somewhat on the left suggestive more of arteritic AION.

biopsy should be considered. Otherwise, laboratory studies are mainly aimed at control of vascular risk factors (e.g., hypertension, avoiding iatrogenic hypotension, diabetes, increased cholesterol, discontinue smoking). Carotid Doppler flow studies and cardiac investigations for embolic disease are not warranted in typical AION because NAION is very rarely an embolic disease.

58.3 Diagnosis

Nonarteritic AION, OS.

58.4 Medical Management

Vascular risk factors must be controlled. Although many agents have been tried (e.g., phenytoin, erythropoietin, intravitreal anti-vascular endothelial growth factor therapies, topical brimonidine, levodopa), there is no proven therapy for NAION. Aspirin therapy may reduce the risk of AION in the fellow eye and may decrease the risk of stroke and myocardial infarction. Corticosteroids for NAION remain controversial but could be considered.

58.5 Surgical Management

Initial reports of visual improvement following optic nerve sheath fenestration for NAION were encouraging but anecdotal. A well-designed, masked, prospective, randomized study at 25 clinical centers (Ischemic Optic Neuropathy Decompression Trial Research Group or IONDT) showed that optic nerve sheath fenestration is not effective and may be harmful in NAION.

58.6 Rehabilitation and Follow-up

The risk of AION in the fellow eye is approximately 12% in the patient's lifetime. Aspirin and control of stroke risk factors may decrease this risk but is unproven. According to the IONDT study, 42.7% of patients will experience spontaneous (three or more lines of Snellen acuity) improvement from baseline at 6 months.

Suggested Reading

[1] Beck RW, Hayreh SS, Podhajsky PA, Tan E-S, Moke PS. Aspirin therapy in nonarteritic anterior ischemic optic neuropathy. Am J Ophthalmol. 1997; 123(2): 212–217

[2] Ischemic Optic Neuropathy Decompression Trial Research Group (IONDT). Characteristics of patients with nonarteritic anterior ischemic optic neuropathy eligible for the Ischemic Optic Neuropathy Decompression Trial. Arch Ophthalmol. 1996; 114(11):1366–1374

[3] The Ischemic Optic Neuropathy Decompression Trial Research Group. Optic nerve decompression surgery for nonarteritic anterior ischemic optic neuropathy (NAION) is not effective and may be harmful. JAMA. 1995; 273(8):625–632

[4] Lee AG, Brazis PW. Clinical Pathways in Neuro-Ophthalmology: An Evidence-Based Approach. New York, NY: Thieme; 1998:49–66

[5] Hayreh SS, Podhajsky PA, Raman R, Zimmerman B. Giant cell arteritis: validity and reliability of various diagnostic criteria. Am J Ophthalmol. 1997; 123(3): 285–296

[6] Hayreh SS, Zimmerman MB. Non-arteritic anterior ischemic optic neuropathy: role of systemic corticosteroid therapy. Graefes Arch Clin Exp Ophthalmol. 2008; 246(7):1029–1046

59 Anterior Ischemic Optic Neuropathy—Arteritic

Sushma Yalamanchili and Andrew G. Lee

Abstract

Sudden vision loss, headaches, jaw claudication, history of poly-myalgia rheumatica, and pallid disc edema in an elderly woman with anterior ischemic optic neuropathy found to have an elevated sedimentation rate and C-reactive protein and treated with steroids. Giant cell arteritis, a medium to large vessel vasculitis of elderly patients can present with visual loss due to arteritic anterior ischemic optic neuropathy. Prompt evaluation (e.g., laboratory studies and a temporal artery biopsy) and treatment with high dose corticosteroids can be vision saving.

Keywords: AION, ischemic optic neuropathy, sudden vision loss, giant cell arteritis, pallid disc edema

59.1 History

A 68-year-old woman complained of severe visual loss in the left eye. Over a period of hours, the vision became markedly blurry. Over the last 2 weeks, she had noted two or three episodes of painless, transient visual loss lasting minutes in the left eye. She denied any periocular or orbital pain, but noted that over the last several months she had diffuse, dull headaches with occasional superimposed "ice pick–like" pains affecting her left or right temples. She had a past history of hypertension. She reported jaw claudication and polymyalgia rheumatica (PMR)-like symptoms.

Examination revealed visual acuity to be 20/20 on the right and 20/400 on the left. She could identify 10 of 10 pseudoisochromatic plates on the right but identified 0 of 10 on the left and could not name colors grossly on the left. The right visual field was normal and the left visual acuity was diffusely depressed more inferiorly than superiorly. The pupils were 5 mm bilaterally; the right pupil reacted well to light but the left pupil was minimally reactive. There was a left relative afferent pupillary defect. Motility was normal. Fundus exam was normal on the right. The cup-to-disc ratio on the right was 0.5. The left optic disc was swollen and pale, and there were several peripapillary hemorrhages (▸ Fig. 59.1).

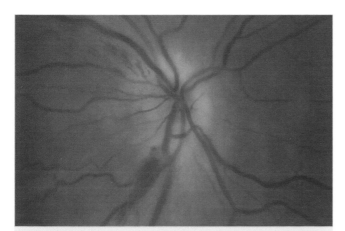

Fig. 59.1 Fundus photograph reveals that the left optic disc is swollen and pale and there were several peripapillary hemorrhages.

Differential Diagnosis—Key Points

1. The acute onset of visual loss in an elderly individual with evidence of pale optic disc swelling strongly suggests a diagnosis of anterior ischemic optic neuropathy (AION). The major question to be addressed is whether this is nonarteritic AION or arteritic AION (secondary to giant cell arteritis [GCA]).

2. Features that are suggestive of arteritic AION instead of nonarteritic AION are given in **the list below**. In this patient, the episodes of transient visual loss preceding the onset of AION, the recent onset of headache, the jaw pain, the cup-to-disc ratio greater than 0.2 (i.e., not the structural "disc at risk" for nonarteritic AION), and the chalky white, pallid disc swelling are all strongly suggestive of a diagnosis of arteritic rather than nonarteritic AION.

3. Arteritic AION occurs in patients older than 50 years and presents with acute, often severe, visual loss that may be unilateral or bilateral (bilateral visual loss more common with arteritic AION than nonarteritic AION). Constitutional symptoms are common and may include headache, scalp or temporal artery tenderness, weight loss, jaw claudication, anorexia, fever, malaise, and PMR.

4. Approximately 20% of patients with GCA present with only ophthalmic changes ("occult" GCA).

5. Causes of visual loss in GCAs include AION, posterior ischemic optic neuropathy (PION), central retinal artery occlusion (CRAO), branch retinal artery occlusion, the ocular ischemic syndrome, choroidal ischemia, and, rarely, intracranial (e.g., occipital lobe) ischemia. GCA should be strongly considered in a patient over the age of 50 who presents with a bilateral AION, pallid disc edema, PION, or CRAO with no visible emboli, or with prior transient visual loss episodes before the permanent visual loss.

59.1.1 Features Suggestive of Arteritic AION Instead of Nonarteritic AION

- Elderly patient with constitutional symptoms (especially scalp tenderness or jaw claudication).
- PMR.
- Elevated sedimentation rate (ESR) or C-reactive protein.
- Transient visual loss (amaurosis fugax) preceding constant visual loss.
- Ocular findings.
- PION (retrobulbar optic neuropathy).
- Cup-to-disc ratio greater than 0.2 in fellow eye.
- Early massive (no light perception to count fingers) or bilateral simultaneous visual loss.
- Markedly pallid optic disc edema (chalk white).
- Fluorescein angiogram or clinical findings of simultaneous choroidal nonperfusion and AION.

- AION associated with choroidal nonfilling.
- Simultaneous nonembolic CRAO or cilioretinal artery occlusion and AION.
- Simultaneous choroidal or retinal infarction and AION.

(Adapted from Lee AG, Brazis PW. Clinical Pathways in Neuro-Ophthalmology: An Evidence-Based Approach. New York: Thieme; 1998:70, with permission.)

59.2 Test Interpretation

An ESR and/or CRP occurs in most cases of GCA but a normal ESR or CRP does not rule out GCA.

The CRP is more sensitive (up to 100%) than the ESR (92%) for detection of GCA but the combination of tests gives the best specificity (97%). Temporal artery biopsy should be considered in all patients who are suspected of having GCA to confirm the diagnosis and provide rationale for continued high-dose corticosteroid treatment especially when side effects of treatment occur.

59.3 Diagnosis

Arteritic AION. The ESR was elevated at 70 mm/h, the CRP was elevated at 20 mg/dL, and the temporal artery biopsy showed transmural lymphocytic infiltration, multinucleated giant cells, and disruption of the internal elastic lamina consistent with GCA.

59.4 Medical Management

When a diagnosis of GCA s is considered, the patient should be started immediately on high-dose corticosteroids in order to prevent further visual loss. Treatment should not be delayed until after temporal artery biopsy as corticosteroids do not alter the histopathological findings acutely. Most authors recommend an initial dose of oral prednisone of 1.0 to 1.5 mg/kg per day. Some authors favor intravenous steroids (e.g., methylpred-

nisolone 1,000 mg/day) in patients with severe visual loss of less than 48 hours duration due to GCA, especially if there is bilateral involvement, if the patient is monocular, or if the patient has lost vision during oral steroid therapy. Every other day steroid therapy does not seem to sufficiently control disease activity. Most patients can be tapered off steroids within 1 year, but some patients may require prolonged or even indefinite therapy.

59.5 Surgical Management

No surgical management is indicated but histopathologic confirmation of the diagnosis of GCA with a temporal artery biopsy is recommended

59.6 Rehabilitation and Follow-up

Untreated, there is a high risk of further visual loss in the involved or fellow eye in patients with GCA. Patients must be carefully monitored for visual impairment, constitutional symptoms, and ill effects of the steroid therapy, with some guidance provided by serial ESR/CRP studies. Consultation with an internist and/or rheumatologist is recommended and some patients require consideration for steroid sparing regimens (e.g., methotrexate) if serious dose limiting side effects occur.

Suggested Reading

[1] Hayreh SS, Podhajsky PA, Raman R, Zimmerman B. Giant cell arteritis: validity and reliability of various diagnostic criteria. Am J Ophthalmol. 1997; 123(3): 285–296

[2] Hayreh SS, Podhajsky PA, Zimmerman B. Occult giant cell arteritis: ocular manifestations. Am J Ophthalmol. 1998; 125(4):521–526

[3] Hayreh SS, Podhajsky PA, Zimmerman B. Ocular manifestations of giant cell arteritis. Am J Ophthalmol. 1998; 125(4):509–520

[4] Lee AG, Brazis PW. Clinical Pathways in Neuro-Ophthalmology: An Evidence-Based Approach. New York, NY: Thieme; 1998:67–91

[5] Hayreh SS, Podhajsky PA, Raman R, Zimmerman B. Giant cell arteritis: validity and reliability of various diagnostic criteria. Am J Ophthalmol. 1997; 123(3): 285–296

60 Progressive Optic Neuropathy—Tumor

Sushma Yalamanchili and Andrew G. Lee

Abstract

A patient with painless progressive visual loss over years with an afferent pupillary defect, decreased color vision, and optic atrophy is found to have an optic nerve sheath meningioma on magnetic resonance imaging (MRI). Compressive optic neuropathy (CON) should be suspected in any unexplained optic neuropathy but especially in progressive cases. MRI of the head and orbit with gadolinium is the preferred initial imaging modality for CON. Common etiologies for CON include meningioma, pituitary adenoma, craniopharyngioma, and glioma.

Keywords: progressive optic neuropathy, tumor, optic atrophy, progressive vision loss, compressive optic neuropathy, optic nerve sheath meningioma

60.1 History

A 64-year-old woman complained of painless progressive visual loss in her right eye. Three years previously, she had noted mild visual blurring in her right eye and visual acuity had been found to be 20/40 on the right and 20/20 on the left. Her visual difficulty had been attributed to "nuclear sclerotic cataract" and observation was recommended. One year later, however, her vision continued to deteriorate to 20/60 on the right and 20/20 on the left, and right cataract surgery was performed. She felt that her "vision was no better after the surgery" and she continued to worsen. She denied any headache or eye pain.

Examination revealed visual acuity to be 20/100 on the right and 20/20 on the left. She was able to identify 2 of 10 pseudoisochromatic plates on the right and 9 of 10 on the left. Visual field exam revealed diffuse depression of the visual field on the right with a normal visual field on the left. The pupils were 5 mm bilaterally poorly reactive to light on the right and briskly reactive on the left, and there was a right relative afferent pupillary defect. Motility was normal. Hertel measurements at

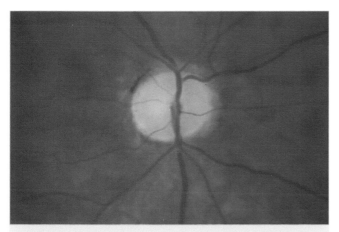

Fig. 60.1 Fundus photograph revealing a pale, atrophic optic nerve on the right.

a base of 95 were 22 mm on the right and 19 mm on the left. Slit-lamp exam revealed a posterior chamber intraocular lens on the right and a mild nuclear sclerotic cataract on the left. Fundus exam revealed a pale, atrophic nerve on the right (▶ Fig. 60.1). The left optic disc was normal.

Differential Diagnosis—Key Points

1. The patient's history of painless progressive visual loss is not consistent with typical optic neuritis or anterior ischemic optic neuropathy. Compressive or infiltrative optic neuropathies cause painless, progressive, gradual loss of visual function (e.g., loss of visual acuity, visual field, and color vision), a relative afferent pupillary defect (in unilateral or asymmetric cases), and optic disc edema or atrophy (the disc may be normal initially). Mild proptosis in this case raises the possibility of an orbital process causing her ipsilateral progressive optic neuropathy.

2. Compressive optic neuropathy that is due to an orbital or intracanalicular lesions may result in ipsilateral optic disc edema followed by atrophy and may also be associated with the development of abnormal blood vessels on the disc head called "optociliary shunt vessels." These vessels probably represent collateral circulation between the retinal and choroidal venous circulation that allows blood to bypass the compression at the level of the optic nerve and thus are probably more accurately termed retinochoroidal venous collateral vessels.

3. The presence of an unexplained relative afferent pupillary defect or unexplained optic atrophy should prompt evaluation including consideration for appropriate neuroimaging studies. Lesions causing compressive optic neuropathy include benign and malignant tumors (e.g., meningioma, glioma, craniopharyngioma, lymphoma, metastasis), orbital fracture (traumatic optic neuropathy), inflammatory or infectious diseases (e.g., syphilis, tuberculosis, Lyme disease, sinus mucocele), primary bone diseases (e.g., osteopetrosis, fibrous dysplasia), vascular masses (e.g., orbital hemorrhage, aneurysms, orbital venous anomalies), thyroid ophthalmopathy (compressive orbital apex optic neuropathy), and iatrogenic causes (e.g., intracranial catheters, intraorbital or intracranial postoperative changes).

60.2 Test Interpretation

Perimetry and color vision testing are helpful in differentiating visual loss due to optic neuropathy from media problems. All patients should have neuroimaging studies, preferably magnetic resonance imaging (MRI), of the brain and orbit with and without gadolinium contrast material to investigate the cause of the optic nerve compression. In patients who cannot undergo

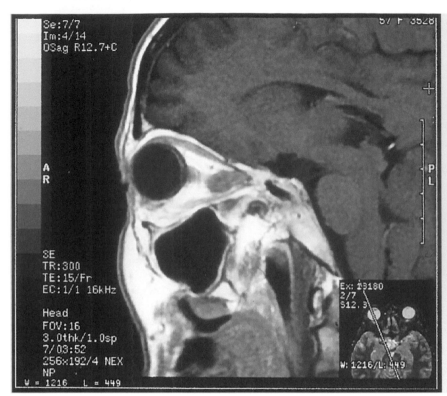

Fig. 60.2 MRI (sagittal image) revealed an optic nerve sheath meningioma on the right.

an MRI, computed tomography (CT) scan of the brain and orbit with and without contrast may be necessary.

60.3 Diagnosis

Compressive optic neuropathy on the right. MRI revealed optic nerve sheath enhancement on T1 postcontrast images consistent with an optic nerve sheath meningioma on the right (▶ Fig. 60.2).

60.4 Medical Management

The management of lesions causing optic nerve compression depends on the nature of the lesion. For optic nerve sheath meningiomas, close observation may be all that is necessary. If progressive visual deterioration occurs, stereotactic, conformal, radiation therapy may be appropriate.

60.5 Surgical Management

Surgical intervention for primary sheath meningiomas is usually not recommended. Some authors consider surgery for debulking exophytic lesions or if there is progressive intracranial extension of the lesion through the optic canal, which might have theoretic risk to the fellow eye. Most authors, however, recommend observation or radiation therapy over surgery for primary optic nerve sheath meningiomas. In contrast, intracranial meningiomas with secondary optic nerve sheath involvement causing optic nerve compression may require surgical treatment with a gross total resection if feasible or subtotal excision if the tumor surrounds vital structures. Postoperative radiation therapy for a nonresectable tumor should be considered, although some authors reserve postoperative radiation for cases in which there is clinical progression or in higher grade or atypical meningiomas.

60.6 Rehabilitation and Follow-up

Patients with tumors such as meningiomas should have serial clinical reevaluation (e.g., every 6 months) including visual fields and repeat MRIs (e.g., every 6 months for 2 years, and then yearly if no growth is indicated clinically or by imaging). More malignant processes require more frequent follow-up and more aggressive treatment measures.

Suggested Reading

[1] Dutton JJ. Gliomas of the anterior visual pathway. Surv Ophthalmol. 1994; 38 (5):427–452

[2] Dutton JJ. Optic nerve gliomas and meningiomas. Neurol Clin. 1992; 37:167–177

[3] Dutton JJ. Optic nerve sheath meningiomas. Surv Ophthalmol. 1992; 37(3): 167–183

[4] Lee AG, Brazis PW. Clinical Pathways in Neuro-Ophthalmology: An Evidence-Based Approach. New York, NY: Thieme; 1998:4–6

61 Papilledema–Pseudotumor Cerebri

Sushma Yalamanchili and Andrew G. Lee

Abstract

A young obese woman with headaches, tinnitus, transient visual obscurations, and bilateral disc edema was found to have normal neuroimaging studies (magnetic resonance imaging/magnetic resonance venography [MRI/MRV]) and an elevated opening pressure on lumbar puncture with normal cerebral spinal fluid consistent with pseudotumor cerebri (idiopathic intracranial hypertension).

Keywords: papilledema, pseudotumor cerebri, idiopathic intracranial hypertension, disc edema, obesity, headaches, elevated opening pressure, transient visual obscurations

61.1 History

A 22-year-old woman had an 8-month history of headache. The headaches occurred almost daily, were diffuse, and were rarely associated with nausea. Over the last 2 months, she had noted a "pulsating sound" in her head (i.e., pulse synchronous tinnitus). It was most noticeable when changing posture, especially when going from a lying to a standing posture. Over the last 2 weeks, she had noted episodes lasting seconds at a time of transient visual loss in the left or right eye. She denied any other neurologic complaints or diplopia. She was not pregnant and was not taking any medications that cause increased intracranial pressure.

Examination revealed an obese woman weighing 250 pounds. Blood pressure was 135/85 mm Hg. Visual acuity was 20/20 bilaterally, color vision was normal, and visual fields were normal except for enlarged blind spots bilaterally. Pupils were 5 mm bilaterally, reacted well to light, and there was no relative afferent pupillary defect (RAPD). Motility was normal. Fundus examination revealed bilateral severe optic disc swelling (▶ Fig. 61.1).

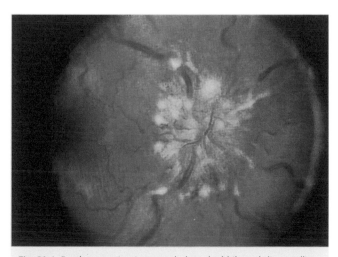

Fig. 61.1 Fundus examination revealed marked bilateral disc swelling with diffuse exudates, hemorrhages, and dilated vessels.

Differential Diagnosis—Key Points

1. Although bilateral disc swelling can be seen in a number of different bilateral optic neuropathies, the patient has no visual loss, color impairment, or visual field defects suggestive of an optic neuropathy. Bilateral disc edema with normal visual function may be seen with hypertension, but her blood pressure was normal and there were no other signs of hypertensive retinopathy. Thus, the patient's disc swelling is likely due to increased intracranial pressure (i.e., papilledema).

2. Patients with papilledema should have measurement of their blood pressure and then be assessed for space-occupying lesions of the brain, such as hydrocephalus, masses (e.g., tumor, hemorrhage, abscess), encephalitis/meningitis, and subarachnoid hemorrhage. If the patient has no cause for increased intracranial pressure, neuroimaging studies (e.g., magnetic resonance imaging [MRI] head and MR venography [MRV] with contrast) are normal, cerebrospinal fluid (CSF) contents are normal, and the lumbar puncture opening pressure is elevated (> 25 cm of water), the patient, by definition, has idiopathic intracranial hypertension (IIH) or pseudotumor cerebri (PTC).

3. PTC is often idiopathic but may occur in association with certain systemic conditions (e.g., drugs, pregnancy [weight gain], and intracranial or extracranial venous thrombosis or obstruction). Obstruction or impairment of intracranial cerebral venous sinus drainage may result in cerebral edema with increased intracranial pressure and papilledema. Tumors that occlude the posterior portion of the superior sagittal sinus or other cerebral venous sinuses may cause increased intracranial pressure as may septic or aseptic thrombosis or ligation of the cavernous sinus, lateral sinus, sigmoid sinus, or superior sagittal sinus. Venous sinus thrombosis may be the mechanism of PTC reported with systemic lupus erythematosus, protein S deficiency, antithrombin III deficiency, the antiphospholipid antibody syndrome, and other blood dyscrasias. In fact, elevated intracranial venous pressure is thought by some authors to be the "universal mechanism" of PTC of varying etiologies.

4. Many systemic diseases, drugs, vitamin deficiencies and excesses, pregnancy (weight gain), and hereditary conditions have been associated with PTC. The drugs most firmly associated with PTC include hypervitaminosis A, steroid withdrawal, anabolic steroids, lithium, nalidixic acid, all-trans-retinoic acid (ATRA) or tretinoin, cyclosporine, exogenous growth hormone, and tetracyclines (especially minocycline). Other cases have been reported including the insecticide chlordecone (Kepone), isotretinoin, ketoprofen (Orudis) or indomethacin in Bartter's syndrome, thyroid replacement in hypothyroid children, and danazol. The systemic diseases most closely linked to PTC include Behçet's syndrome, renal failure, Addison's disease, hypoparathyroidism, systemic lupus erythematosus, and sarcoidosis. Although sometimes implicated in IIH, oral and

other contraceptives have not been shown to be causal in case–control studies.

5. Idiopathic PTC (IIH) is typically a disease of obese women in the childbearing years. The occurrence of PTC in a man, the elderly, or thin patients should raise the possibility of venous occlusive disease or a secondary cause. The diagnostic criteria for PTC **are listed below**. The most common symptoms of PTC include headache, transient visual obscurations, pulsatile tinnitus, and diplopia. The headaches in patients with PTC may be constant or intermittent. Transient visual obscurations last seconds, may be unilateral or bilateral, may be related to changes in posture, do not correlate with the degree of intracranial hypertension or the extent of disc swelling, and are not considered to be harbingers of permanent visual loss. Intracranial noises are common with PTC and are perhaps due to transmission of intensified vascular pulsations via CSF under high pressure to the walls of the venous sinuses.

6. Visual field and, eventually, visual acuity loss are the major causes of morbidity in PTC. Complete blindness and permanent optic atrophy may occur. Often, the patient is initially unaware of peripheral visual field dysfunction and Snellen acuity testing is a poor indicator of early visual deficit in PTC. The papilledema causes optic nerve fiber attrition, which results in field constriction and nerve fiber bundle defects. Blind spot enlargement is commonly encountered but is more a reflection of the disc swelling itself, rather than optic nerve damage, and is improved with refraction.

61.1.1 Criteria for the Diagnosis of Idiopathic Pseudotumor Cerebri

1. Increased intracranial pressure must be documented in an alert and oriented patient without localizing neurologic findings (except for cranial nerve VI palsy). It should be noted that spinal fluid pressures between 200 and 250 mm H_2O may occur normally in obese patients, and that when elevated spinal fluid pressure is suspected, confirmation requires values greater than 250 mm H_2O.

2. The CSF should have normal contents (including protein and glucose) with no cytologic abnormalities. Occasionally, the CSF protein level may be low.

3. Neuroimaging (preferably MRI with and without contrast, and possibly MRV) should be normal with no evidence of hydrocephalus, mass lesion, meningeal enhancement, or venous occlusive disease. Neuroimaging may show enlarged optic nerve sheaths, empty sellae, and reversal of the optic nerve head in some patients with PTC.

4. No secondary cause should be present.

61.2 Test Interpretation

In all patients with bilateral optic disc swelling, blood pressure should be checked to evaluate for possible hypertensive emergency (i.e., malignant hypertension). Neuroimaging is recommended for all patients. Cranial computed tomography (CT)

imaging with CT venography may be the study of choice in the acute setting (e.g., emergency room) in evaluating the patient with possible acute vascular processes (e.g., subarachnoid, epidural, subdural, or intracerebral hemorrhage, acute infarction, cerebral venous thrombosis) or after head trauma. Otherwise, MRI, with and without contrast, is the imaging modality of choice. Most authors also recommend that MRV be obtained at the same time to evaluate the patient for venous sinus thrombosis. If neuroimaging shows no structural lesion or hydrocephalus, then a lumbar puncture is generally recommended. Studies should include an accurate opening pressure, to evaluate for intracranial hypertension, as well as CSF cell count and differential, glucose, protein, cytology, and appropriate cultures.

61.3 Diagnosis

Papilledema. The MRI showed only radiographic findings suggestive of increased intracranial pressure (i.e., CSF fluid signal in the optic nerve sheaths bilaterally and an empty sella) and MRV findings were normal in this patient. Spinal tap revealed an opening pressure of 350 mm H_2O and normal CSF contents consistent with the diagnosis of IIH.

61.4 Medical Management

Some patients require no treatment as long as symptoms are minimal and visual function is normal, but all require serial monitoring of visual function, especially visual fields, to observe closely for signs of visual impairment. Weight reduction, including surgically induced weight reduction in morbidly obese patients, may improve the papilledema and reduce intracranial pressure. Medical treatments for PTC include carbonic anhydrase inhibitors, loop diuretics, corticosteroids, and repeat lumbar punctures. Acetazolamide in doses of 1 to 2 grams per day has proven effective in most patients with PTC. A recent randomized, controlled clinical trial supports the efficacy and safety of diet and acetazolamide in patients with IIH and mild visual loss. Acetazolamide (prior FDA category C) should probably be avoided during pregnancy but may still be used if needed. The decision for medical treatment, however, requires consultation with the obstetrician and the patient. In general, we recommend avoiding acetazolamide during the first 20 weeks, because of potential teratogenic effects. The use of caloric restriction and other diuretics (e.g., furosemide) may also be relatively contraindicated during pregnancy.

Other carbonic anhydrase inhibitors, such as methazolamide (Neptazane), can be used in acetazolamide-intolerant patients but their efficacy has not been proven. Furosemide (Lasix) inhibits CSF production and may have an additive effect with acetazolamide, but the use of this agent alone has not been systematically studied. Corticosteroids may be efficacious in the short run, but the complications of this medication, especially in the chronic treatment of an already obese individual, have resulted in most clinicians suggesting that their use probably should be avoided.

Repeated lumbar punctures have never been systematically studied for the treatment of PTC. As these procedures are uncomfortable, are of questionable benefit, and are potentially associated with complications (e.g., infection, intraspinal epidermoid tumors), they should not be performed as a primary therapy. Finally, if acetazolamide does not control the headache associated with PTC, symptomatic headache treatments are warranted.

61.5 Surgical Management

When medical therapy fails for headache or visual dysfunction, surgical therapies for PTC should be considered.

The two main procedures performed include CSF shunting (e.g., ventriculoperitoneal (VP) or lumboperitoneal shunt) and optic nerve sheath fenestration (ONSF). Stenting for cerebral venous sinus stenosis remains controversial.

Various authorities have vehemently advocated one or the other procedure. There has been no prospective study comparing the efficacy of the two procedures. Both ONSF and VP shunt may improve vision and prevent deterioration of vision in patients with PTC. Both procedures have their advantages and disadvantages and either may fail with time. Patients who fail VP shunt may benefit from ONSF and vice versa. Until a prospective, randomized study comparing ONSF with VP shunt for PTC is performed, the question of which surgical procedure is best for the treatment of PTC remains unanswered.

61.6 Rehabilitation and Follow-up

Patients should generally return monthly for 6 to 12 months with careful evaluation of formal visual fields, stereo-optic disc photos, OCT nerves, visual acuity, color vision, and RAPD testing. The time between visits can be lengthened depending on the stability of the ophthalmologic findings. Regression of symptoms and papilledema are the end point. However, patients should continue to be closely followed, even after successful surgery, because of the possibility of late recurrences, failed shunts, etc.

Suggested Reading

[1] Corbett JJ, Thompson HS. The rational management of idiopathic intracranial hypertension. Arch Neurol. 1989; 46(10):1049–1051

[2] Giuseffi V, Wall M, Siegel PZ, Rojas PB. Symptoms and disease associations in idiopathic intracranial hypertension (pseudotumor cerebri): a case-control study. Neurology. 1991; 41(2, Pt 1):239–244

[3] Lee AG, Brazis PW. Clinical Pathways in Neuro-Ophthalmology: An Evidence-Based Approach. New York, NY: Thieme; 1998:103–134

[4] Wall M, George D. Idiopathic intracranial hypertension. A prospective study of 50 patients. Brain. 1991; 114 Pt 1A:155–180

[5] Menger RP, Connor DE, Jr, Thakur JD, et al. A comparison of lumboperitoneal and ventriculoperitoneal shunting for idiopathic intracranial hypertension: an analysis of economic impact and complications using the Nationwide Inpatient Sample. Neurosurg Focus. 2014; 37(5):E4

[6] Beck RW. The idiopathic intracranial hypertension treatment trial: a long-time coming but worth the wait. J Neuroophthalmol. 2016; 36(1):1–3

62 Visual Field Defect—Junctional Scotoma

Sushma Yalamanchili and Andrew G. Lee

Abstract

A patient presented with painless progressive vision loss in the right eye, a right afferent pupillary defect, a right central scotoma, right optic atrophy, and a contralateral superior temporal defect (junctional scotoma). The findings suggested a lesion in the junction between the optic nerve and the chiasm on the side with the central scotoma, and magnetic resonance imaging showed a pituitary adenoma.

Keywords: junctional scotoma, visual field defect, tumor, compressive optic neuropathy, optic atrophy

62.1 History

A 55-year-old man complained of progressive painless visual impairment in his right eye over a period of 1 and 1/2 years. He denied any visual difficulty in his left eye and denied any other history of neurologic or ophthalmologic impairment.

Examination revealed visual acuity of 20/80 on the right and 20/20 on the left. He could identify 4 of 10 pseudoisochromatic plates on the right and 10 of 10 on the left. Pupils were 4 mm bilaterally and both reacted well to light and near, but there was a right relative afferent pupillary defect. Visual fields revealed generalized diffuse depression on the right (▶ Fig. 62.1) and a superotemporal field defect respecting the vertical meridian on the left (▶ Fig. 62.2). Motility exam was normal. Slit-lamp examination was normal. The right optic disc was diffusely pale. The left optic disc, vessels, and macula were normal.

62.2 Test Interpretation

Patients with junctional scotoma of Traquair or junctional scotoma should be considered to have a compressive lesion at the junction of the optic nerve and chiasm until proven otherwise. Neuroimaging studies (preferably magnetic resonance imaging [MRI]) should be directed to this location. Patients with junctional scotomas (as the described patient) may be unaware of a small superotemporal visual field defect. Therefore, in any patient with presumed unilateral visual loss, careful testing should be performed even in the contralateral asymptomatic eye (▶ Fig. 62.1).

62.3 Diagnosis

Right optic neuropathy with junctional scotoma secondary to compressive lesion of the junction of the right optic nerve with the chiasm (pituitary adenoma) (▶ Fig. 62.3).

62.4 Medical Management

Hormone replacement for pituitary and chiasmal lesions is recommended. Prolactin-secreting pituitary tumors are

sometimes treated with dopamine agonists. In general, surgical decompression is recommended for suprasellar compressive lesions.

62.5 Surgical Management

The treatment is surgical removal, if possible, of the underlying structural lesion responsible for the visual field defect. In this case, the patient underwent decompressive surgery. Depending on the final histopathology, chemotherapy or radiation therapy might be necessary for subtotal resection.

Differential Diagnosis—Key Points

1. The visual acuity, color vision, and field impairment on the right, with a relative afferent pupillary defect and optic atrophy, all suggest a right optic neuropathy but the superotemporal visual field loss in the fellow eye places the lesion at the junction of the optic nerve and chiasm. The progressive, painless visual loss raises the possibility of a compressive optic nerve lesion.

2. Lesions at the junction of the optic nerve and chiasm may produce specific types of visual field defects that allow topographical localization. Selective compression of the crossed or uncrossed visual fibers at the junction may result in a unilateral temporal or nasal hemianopic defect, respectively (junctional scotoma of Traquair). In addition, involvement of the inferonasal fibers of the anterior knee (the supposed Wilbrand's knee) results in a superotemporal visual field defect contralateral to the lesion (junctional scotoma).

3. The patient therefore has a lesion of the optic nerve at the junction of the right nerve with the chiasm causing an ipsilateral optic neuropathy and a contralateral superior temporal defect (junctional scotoma).

4. Recently, the existence of Wilbrand's knee has come into question. It has been hypothesized that Wilbrand's knee may be an artifact of enucleation caused by atrophy of the optic nerve and not a normal anatomic finding. Nevertheless, whether Wilbrand's knee exists anatomically, the localizing value of junctional visual field loss to the junction of the optic nerve and chiasm remains undiminished since chiasmal compression alone may result in a contralateral superotemporal visual field defect.

5. Junctional field loss is usually due to a mass lesion, with a differential diagnosis including pituitary tumors, suprasellar meningiomas, supraclinoid aneurysms, craniopharyngiomas, and gliomas. Chiasmal neuritis (e.g., due to multiple sclerosis), pachymeningitis, and trauma are rare etiologies of the junctional syndrome.

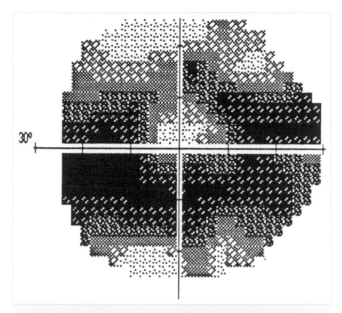

Fig. 62.1 Static perimetry showing diffuse visual field impairment on the right.

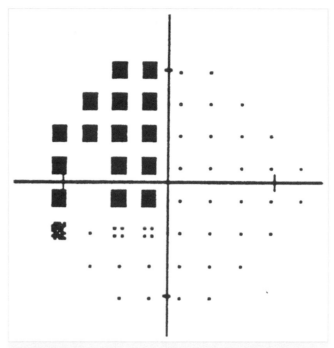

Fig. 62.2 In the left eye, perimetry revealed a superotemporal field defect respecting the vertical meridian.

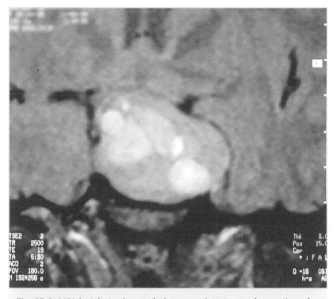

Fig. 62.3 MRI (axial view) revealed a mass (pituitary adenoma) at the junction of the right optic nerve with the chiasm.

62.6 Rehabilitation and Follow-up

Follow-up of this patient's ophthalmologic examination, including visual field testing, was performed every 4 months for 1 year, and every 6 months thereafter, with periodic MRIs to monitor for tumor growth.

Suggested Reading

[1] Lee AG, Brazis PW. Clinical Pathways in Neuro-Ophthalmology: An Evidence-Based Approach. New York, NY: Thieme; 1998:154–155

[2] Trobe JD, Glaser JS. The Visual Fields Manual: A Practical Guide to Testing and Interpretation. Gainesville, FL: Triad; 1983:176

[3] Trobe JD, Tao AH, Schuster JJ. Perichiasmal tumors: diagnostic and prognostic features. Neurosurgery. 1984; 15(3):391–399

63 Visual Field Defect—Pituitary Lesion

Sushma Yalamanchili and Andrew G. Lee

Abstract

A patient with vision loss, multiple car accidents, and headaches is found to have a bitemporal hemianopia on visual field testing, and magnetic resonance imaging revealed a pituitary adenoma in the chiasm. Painless and progressive bitemporal visual field loss should be suspected to be a chiasmal lesion until proven otherwise. Neuroimaging (preferably MRI of the sella) is recommended. Common etiologies include pituitary adenoma, craniopharyngioma, meningioma, and glioma.

Keywords: pituitary tumor, visual field defect, bitemporal hemianopia, vision loss, chiasmal lesion

63.1 History

A 45-year-old woman complained of blurred vision bilaterally and a poor driving performance with multiple accidents due to "poor vision." The visual difficulty had been present for the last year and was slowly deteriorating. She also complained of occasional frontal headaches over the last 6 months. She denied any past history of neurologic or ophthalmologic illnesses and took no medicines except acetaminophen for her headaches.

Examination revealed visual acuity to be 20/25 on the right and 20/20 on the left. She identified 10 of 10 pseudoisochromatic color plates bilaterally. The pupils were 4 mm bilaterally and were equally reactive to light and near, and there was no relative afferent pupillary defect. Motility examination was normal. Slit-lamp examination and fundus exam were normal. Visual field testing showed bitemporal hemianopic defects (▶ Fig. 63.1a, b).

63.2 Test Interpretation

Visual field testing characteristically reveals a bitemporal visual field impairment with chiasmal compression due to pituitary lesions. Because a mass lesion is likely, magnetic resonance imaging (MRI) with and without gadolinium with attention to the sellar region is warranted. If a pituitary adenoma is found, endocrinologic evaluation is warranted. Computed tomography (CT) scan may be the initial study in the acute or emergent setting (e.g., suspected pituitary apoplexy) or in cases where an MRI cannot be performed.

63.3 Diagnosis

Bitemporal visual field defect secondary to pituitary macroadenoma (▶ Fig. 63.2).

63.4 Medical Management

Prolactinomas may respond to therapy with medications, such as bromocriptine.

Differential Diagnosis—Key Points

1. The visual field exam reveals a bitemporal field defect indicating a lesion of the optic chiasm. Bitemporal hemianopias may be peripheral, paracentral, or central and are most often due to a compressive lesion of the optic chiasm.
2. Clinically, three optic chiasm syndromes may be recognized: (1) the anterior chiasm or junctional syndrome, in which a unilateral optic nerve defect is associated with a superior defect in the other eye; (2) the body of the chiasm syndrome, in which patients demonstrate bitemporal field abnormalities; visual acuity is often normal and the optic discs may be normal or pale; (3) the posterior chiasm syndrome, in which visual field testing reveals bitemporal paracentral scotomas from the crossing macular fibers. Visual acuity and the optic discs are normal.
3. Superior bitemporal field defects may also occur with tilted discs, but in these cases the field defects do not respect the vertical meridian.
4. The most common cause of bitemporal visual field impairment is a parasellar mass, most often pituitary adenomas, meningiomas, or craniopharyngiomas. Other mass lesions include dysgerminomas, chiasmal gliomas, metastases, and suprasellar aneurysms. Nonmass lesions that may cause a chiasmal syndrome include demyelinating disease (multiple sclerosis), ischemia, meningitis or encephalitis, syphilis, inflammatory diseases (e.g., neuromyelitis optica, collagen vascular disease, sarcoidosis), radiation necrosis, trauma, and some toxins (e.g., Placidyl).
5. Pituitary masses may occasionally cause an optic neuropathy without evidence for chiasmal damage, especially if the chiasm is postfixed, or may cause an optic tract syndrome (homonymous hemianopsia) if the chiasm is prefixed.

63.5 Surgical Management

Pituitary adenomas or other masses causing chiasmal compression usually are treated surgically. Postoperatively, endocrinologic follow-up and hormonal replacement may be required. Some patients may require postoperative radiation therapy.

63.6 Rehabilitation and Follow-up

Postoperatively, visual field and ophthalmologic examination should be performed as soon as the patient is able to tolerate the procedure. Visual fields and serial ophthalmologic examination should then be performed (e.g., in 3 months, then at 6-month intervals for 2 years, yearly for 5 years, and every 2 years thereafter) to monitor for recurrence. MRI studies should be repeated at regular intervals (e.g., 6 months, 1 year, and then yearly for several years).

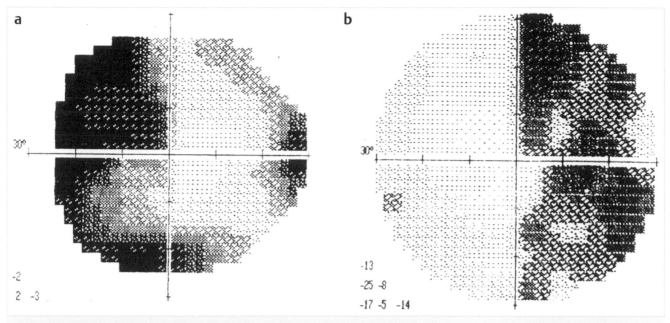

Fig. 63.1 Static perimetry revealed bitemporal hemianopic defects in the **(a)** left eye and **(b)** right eye.

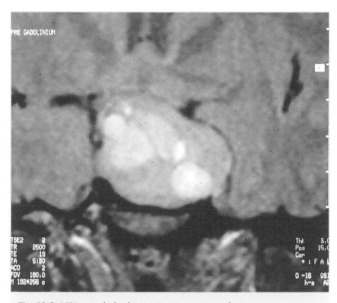

Fig. 63.2 MRI revealed a large pituitary macroadenoma.

Suggested Reading

[1] Burde RM, Savino PJ, Trobe JD. Clinical Decisions in Neuro-Ophthalmology. 2nd ed. St. Louis, MO: Mosby Yearbook; 1992:74–103

[2] Chamlin M, Davidoff LM, Feiring EH. Ophthalmologic changes produced by pituitary tumors. Am J Ophthalmol. 1955; 40(3):353–368

[3] Lee AG, Brazis PW. Clinical Pathways in Neuro-Ophthalmology: An Evidence-Based Approach. New York, NY: Thieme; 1998:155–157

64 Visual Field Defect—Homonymous Hemianopia

Sushma Yalamanchili and Andrew G. Lee

Abstract

A patient with a past history of hypertension, diabetes mellitus, and hyperlipidemia after bypass surgery notices that he is unable to read well because he "lose his place" or "miss lines" and has bumped his left front fender on several occasions when attempting to park his car in the garage. Visual field testing showed a left homonymous hemianopia indicating a retrochiasmal lesion of the visual pathways and this patient had a right occipital lobe stroke.

Keywords: homonymous hemianopia, visual field defect, stroke, vision loss, visual field cut, occipital lobe stroke, retrochiasmal lesion

64.1 History

A 57-year-old man underwent coronary bypass surgery 6 weeks prior to evaluation. His recovery was apparently uneventful, and within several weeks he returned to his usual duties. However, since surgery he noted that he would often "lose his place" or "miss lines" when reading. He had also noted that he bumped his left front fender on several occasions when attempting to park his car in the garage. He had a past history of hypertension, diabetes, and increased cholesterol. He had no other neurologic symptoms.

Examination revealed visual acuity to be 20/20 in both eyes. He identified 9 of 10 pseudoisochromatic plates bilaterally, but often had difficulty with the figures in the left part of the diagrams. The pupils were 4 mm bilaterally, reacted well to light and near, and there was no relative afferent pupillary defect. Motility exam was normal. Slit-lamp exam revealed mild bilateral nuclear sclerotic cataracts. Fundus exam revealed mild hypertensive changes (arteriovenous nicking, arteriolar sclerosis) with normal discs. There were no hemorrhages or exudates. The general neurologic examination was otherwise normal. Visual field testing showed a left homonymous hemianopia (▶ Fig. 64.1).

Differential Diagnosis—Key Points

1. The visual field exam reveals a complete left homonymous hemianopia indicating a retrochiasmal lesion of the visual pathways. In general, visual field defects with lesions affecting the optic tract or lateral geniculate body (LGB) tend to be incongruous, while more posteriorly located lesions (e.g., occipital lobe) result in more congruous field defects. In general, tumors produce sloping field defects, while vascular lesions produce sharp field defects.

2. Complete homonymous hemianopias are lateralizing and indicate a retrochiasmal lesion but are otherwise not further localizing and may occur with any lesion of the retrochiasmal visual pathways.

3. Optic tract lesions usually cause macular-splitting, incongruous homonymous hemianopia, usually without impaired visual acuity unless the lesion extends to involve the optic chiasm or nerve. Optic tract lesions may be associated with a relative afferent pupillary defect in the eye with the temporal field loss (contralateral to the side of the lesion) because within the tract there are more crossed than uncrossed fibers and the temporal visual field is larger than the nasal visual field. Chronic optic tract lesions may eventually cause bilateral optic atrophy with a characteristic "band" or "bowtie" pallor in the contralateral eye and a more generalized pallor in the ipsilateral optic nerve, with loss of nerve fiber layer in the superior and inferior arcuate regions corresponding to the bulk of temporal fibers subserving the nasal visual fields (hemianopic optic atrophy). Etiologies for optic tract lesions include space-occupying lesions, especially tumors, aneurysms, arteriovenous malformations, demyelinating disease, and trauma.

4. LGB lesions may also cause a complete macular-splitting homonymous hemianopia. LGB lesions result in an incongruous homonymous field defect. Hemianopic optic atrophy may develop and no relative afferent pupillary defect is evident. Although lesions of the LGB often cause incongruous field defects, two somewhat specific patterns of congruous homonymous field defects with abruptly sloping borders, associated with sectorial optic atrophy, have been attributed to focal lesions of the LGB caused by infarction in the territory of specific arteries. Occlusion of the anterior choroidal artery may cause a homonymous defect in the upper and lower quadrants with sparing of a horizontal sector (quadruple sectoranopia). Interruption of the posterior lateral choroidal artery, which perfuses the central portion of the lateral geniculate, causes a horizontal homonymous sector defect (wedge shaped). Etiologies for lateral geniculate damage include infarction, arteriovenous malformation, trauma, tumor, inflammatory disorders, demyelinating disease, and toxic exposure (e.g., methanol).

5. Lesions of the proximal portion of the optic radiations may result in a complete homonymous hemianopia with macular splitting. Superior homonymous quadrantic defects ("pie-in-the-sky" field defects) may result from a lesion in the temporal (Meyer's loop) lobe involving the optic radiations or in the inferior bank of the calcarine fissure. Although visual field defects may occur in isolation with temporal lobe lesions, other signs of neurologic impairment are often evident. Involvement of the optic radiations in the depth of the parietal lobe gives rise to a congruous contralateral homonymous hemianopia, denser inferiorly ("pie on the floor"). Such defects are usually more congruous than those produced by lesions of the temporal lobe and since the entire optic radiation passes through the parietal lobe, large lesions may produce complete homonymous hemianopia with macular splitting. Patients may often be unaware of their visual field defects. Visual field defects may occur in relative isolation, but often parietal lobe lesions betray themselves by other signs of neurologic dysfunction.

6. Homonymous quadrantic visual field defects may occur with unilateral occipital lesions. Superior quadrantic defects may be seen with inferior calcarine lesions and inferior quadrantic defects may occur with superior calcarine lesions. Medial occipital lesions cause highly congruous homonymous field defects. When both the upper and the lower calcarine cortices are affected, a complete homonymous hemianopia, usually with macular sparing, develops. Sparing of the central 5 degrees of vision (macular sparing) is common with occipital lesions, probably due to a large macular representation in the occipital pole. The central 10 to 15 degrees of vision fill a majority of the total surface area of the occipital cortex (as much as 50–60%). Patients with purely occipital lesions may be unaware of their deficit. The most common cause of unilateral occipital disease is infarction in the distribution of the posterior cerebral artery. Other etiologies include venous infarction, hemorrhage, arteriovenous malformations, tumors, abscess, and trauma.

64.2 Test Interpretation

The congruous nature of the visual field abnormality, the absence of a relative afferent pupillary defect, and the absence of other neurologic findings suggest an optic radiation or occipital localization for the patient's visual field impairment. In all patients with a retrochiasmal visual field defect, neuroimaging is warranted. In the acute setting, computed tomography (CT) scanning is appropriate, but in most other settings, magnetic resonance imaging (MRI) is indicated.

64.3 Diagnosis

Right occipital lobe infarction causing a dense, congruous left homonymous hemianopia (▶ Fig. 64.2).

64.4 Medical and Surgical Management

Management depends on the underlying cause of the retrochiasmal visual field impairment. In this case, there is little to offer except control of stroke risk factors and probably aspirin for stroke prophylaxis.

64.5 Rehabilitation and Follow-up

Patients should have repeat visual fields and ophthalmologic examination approximately 6 months after the onset of the defect to see if there is any improvement.

Reading problems are common in patients with homonymous field defects. Patients with right homonymous hemianopias have difficulty seeing which letters or words follow those they have already read and patients with left hemianopias often lose their place when reading, often beginning again on an unrelated line. Use of a ruler to guide the patient's vision is often useful. Hemianopic patients may also be trained to perform large saccades into the blind field and to search their entire field in various patterns resulting in some visual improvement. Optical aids such as monocular prism glasses can be used to reduce the apparent visual field loss by shifting visual stimuli from the blind field into the patient's seeing field. A computerized therapy called vision restoration therapy (VRT) also reportedly has produced subjective improvement in visual

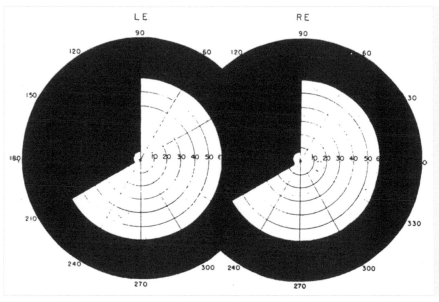

Fig. 64.1 Visual field testing revealed a dense, congruous left homonymous hemianopia indicating a retrochiasmal lesion of the visual pathways.

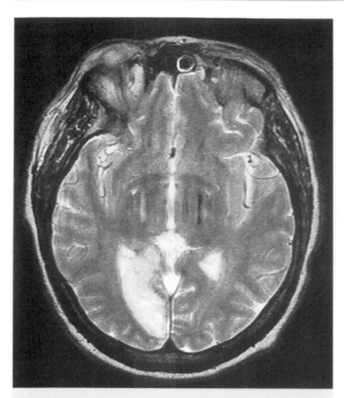

Fig. 64.2 Magnetic resonance imaging study showed a right occipital infarct.

field but independent automated perimetry studies after VRT have failed to conclusively demonstrate proven visual field improvement objectively and thus VRT remains controversial.

Suggested Reading

[1] Bell RA, Thompson HS. Relative afferent pupillary defect in optic tract hemianopias. Am J Ophthalmol. 1978; 85(4):538–540

[2] Horton JC, Hoyt WF. The representation of the visual field in human striate cortex. A revision of the classic Holmes map. Arch Ophthalmol. 1991; 109(6): 816–824

[3] Kerkhoff G, Münßinger U, Haaf E, Eberle-Strauss G, Stögerer E. Rehabilitation of homonymous scotomata in patients with postgeniculate damage of the visual system: saccadic compensation training. Restor Neurol Neurosci. 1992; 4(4):245–254

[4] Lee AG, Brazis PW. Clinical Pathways in Neuro-Ophthalmology: An Evidence-Based Approach. New York, NY: Thieme; 1998:157–163

[5] Pameijer JK. Reading problems in hemianopia. Ophthalmologica. 1970; 160 (5):322–325

[6] Pessin MS, Lathi ES, Cohen MB, Kwan ES, Hedges TR, III, Caplan LR. Clinical features and mechanism of occipital infarction. Ann Neurol. 1987; 21(3): 290–299

[7] Lane AR, Smith DT, Schenk T. Clinical treatment options for patients with homonymous visual field defects. Clin Ophthalmol. 2008; 2(1):93–102

65 Transient Monocular Visual Loss

Sushma Yalamanchili and Andrew G. Lee

Abstract

A patient with a past history of hypertension and hyperlipidemia with transient monocular vision loss and an intravascular embolic debris (Hollenhorst's plaque) in the right eye needs to be evaluated for carotid and aortic vascular disease, cardiac valvular disease, stroke, giant cell arteritis, and retinal vascular occlusion.

Keywords: transient monocular vision loss, Hollenhorst's plaque, Stroke, giant cell arteritis, retinal vascular occlusion, embolic debris

65.1 History

A 65-year-old woman noted three episodes of transient visual loss (TVL) in her right eye over the last 3 weeks. She noted no precipitating factors for the episodes but the vision would "gray-out" in the right eye for a period of 5 or 6 minutes. She denied any associated headaches, jaw claudication, persistent visual loss, or any transient neurologic dysfunction. She had a past medical history of hypertension and increased cholesterol, both being controlled by medications.

Examination revealed visual acuity of 20/25 on the right and 20/20 on the left. She identified 9 of 10 pseudoisochromatic plates bilaterally. Pupils were 4 mm bilaterally and both reacted well to light and near. There was no relative afferent pupillary defect. Visual fields were normal. Motility exam was normal. Slit-lamp exam revealed mild bilateral nuclear sclerotic cataracts. Fundus exam revealed an intravascular embolic debris (Hollenhorst's plaque) in the right eye (► Fig. 65.1).

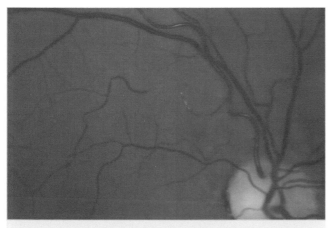

Fig. 65.1 Fundus photograph of right eye showing retinal emboli.

Differential Diagnosis—Key Points

1. The most important questions that need to be addressed in the assessment of the patient with TVL include the following:
   a) Is the visual loss monocular or binocular? Monocular TVL implies disease of the eye, retina, optic nerve, orbit, circulation to the eye (heart, aorta, carotid artery, ophthalmic artery central retinal artery, etc.), or migraine. Binocular TVL implies bilateral eye disease, disease affecting the circulation to both eyes (e.g., bilateral carotid stenosis), increased intracranial pressure with papilledema, or, most often, disease of the vertebrobasilar circulation (especially vertebrobasilar transient ischemic attacks) or migraine.
   b) What is the temporal profile of the transient loss of vision? For example, TVL in one eye lasting seconds is characteristic of transient obscurations of vision due to optic nerve ischemia or papilledema, while monocular TVL lasting 2 to 30 minutes is characteristic of TVL associated with ischemia of the retina.
   c) What are the precipitants of the visual loss? For example, patients with an intraorbital mass may develop TVL only in certain eye positions due to the mass compressing the ipsilateral optic nerve or optic nerve circulation (i.e., gaze-evoked amaurosis). Monocular or binocular TVL due to carotid disease or giant cell arteritis may occur following exposure to bright light.
   d) Are any optic nerve or retinal vessel abnormalities evident on fundus examination? For example, fundus exam may well reveal papilledema in a patient with transient obscurations of vision, retinal emboli in a patient with carotid or cardiac disease, and disc anomalies in a patient with monocular TVL.

2. Episodes of TVL lasting less than 60 seconds may occur in patients with papilledema. These transient obscurations of vision may occur in one or both eyes (individually or simultaneously) and typically last only a few seconds. Rarely, they may last for hours. The episodes may be precipitated by changes in position and are thought to be related to the effects of increased intracranial pressure on the flow of blood to the eye, perhaps where the central retinal artery penetrates the optic nerve sheath to enter the substance of the nerve. Similar monocular episodes of TVL lasting seconds may occur in patients with optic nerve sheath meningiomas and are probably unrelated to increased intracranial pressure. Transient obscurations of vision may also occur in an eye with congenital abnormalities of the optic disc, such as peripapillary staphyloma (see below) or optic disc drusen. Finally, carotid atherosclerotic disease may rarely cause very brief

episodes of TVL, but more often attacks of TVL with carotid disease last 2 to 15 minutes.

3. Monocular TVL lasting 5 to 60 minutes (usually 2–30 minutes) is strongly suggestive of thromboembolic disease. These episodes are most often due to emboli, involving the retinal arterial system, which may arise from aorta or carotid artery atherosclerotic disease or a cardiogenic source. Patients often describe a veil or shade descending or ascending (i.e., altitudinal visual field loss) over a portion or the whole of their visual field. Other patients complain of patchy visual loss ("Swiss cheese" pattern) or peripheral constriction with central visual sparing. Patients with TVL from thromboembolic disease may demonstrate emboli lodged within the retinal vessels. In general, emboli may be composed of clotted blood, fibrin, platelets, atheromatous tissue, white cells, calcium, infectious organisms (septic emboli), air, fat, tumor cells, amniotic fluid, or foreign materials (e.g., talc, artificial valve material, catheters, silicone, cornstarch, mercury, corticosteroids). The most common types of emboli seen in patients with atherosclerotic disease of the aorta/carotid arteries or cardiac disease include the following:

   a) *Cholesterol emboli* (Hollenhorst's plaques) are bright, glistening, yellow or copper-colored fragments, most often seen in peripheral arterioles in the temporal fundus. These emboli most often arise from atheromatous plaques in the aorta or carotid bifurcation.

   b) *Platelet-fibrin emboli* are dull, white, gray, often elongated, and subject to fragmentation and distal movement. These emboli most often lodge at bifurcations of retinal vessels and arise from the walls of atherosclerotic arteries or from the heart, especially from heart valves. They may also be seen in patients with coagulopathies.

   c) *Calcific emboli* tend to be large, ovoid or rectangular, and chalky-white. These emboli often occur over or adjacent to the optic disc and usually arise from cardiac (aortic or mitral) valves, less often from the aorta or carotid artery. Unlike cholesterol emboli, which often disappear in a few days, calcific emboli may remain permanently visible.

4. TVL may also occur from ocular hypoperfusion rather than embolization. In some patients, monocular TVL may occur when the patient is exposed to bright light. These patients usually have severe ipsilateral carotid occlusive disease. Venous stasis retinopathy (hypotensive retinopathy), associated with severe carotid or ophthalmic artery occlusive disease, may also be associated with TVL. This syndrome is characterized by visual loss and ischemic retinal infarction often accompanied by signs of ciliary artery obstruction, pallor of the disc, and hypotony.

5. Giant cell arteritis may produce attacks of TVL lasting minutes to hours indistinguishable from those produced by atheromatous disease. TVL probably results from intermittent inflammatory occlusion of the ophthalmic, posterior ciliary, or central retinal arteries.

6. TVL may also occur in association with increased antiphospholipid antibodies, hyperviscosity and hypercoagulable states, polycythemia vera, systemic lupus erythematosus, and arteriovenous malformations that divert blood flow from or reduce blood flow in the ophthalmic artery (ophthalmic steal syndrome).

7. Vasospasm, especially associated with migraine, may also produce TVL without any of the visual phenomena typically seen during a migraine attack. Vasospasm of the retinal vessels has been documented by ophthalmoscopy during some attacks of monocular TVL.

8. TVL lasting 15 to 20 minutes (occasionally up to 7 hours) may occur during episodes of spontaneous anterior chamber hemorrhage (hyphema). In these patients TVL may be associated with erythropsia (seeing red) and color desaturation. Such hemorrhages are most likely to occur in patients who have undergone cataract extraction and are particularly apt to occur after placement of an iris fixation lens implant. Intermittent angle-closure glaucoma may also cause brief episodes of monocular TVL that are usually, but not always, associated with ipsilateral eye pain and occasionally simultaneous dilation of the pupil. Finally, TVL may also be associated with the congenital anomalies peripapillary staphyloma and morning glory syndrome. Episodes of TVL with these anomalies may last 15 to 20 seconds (obscurations of vision) or up to 20 minutes, the latter mimicking TVL with thromboembolic disease. The episodes of TVL in patients with peripapillary staphyloma may be associated with intermittent dilation of the retinal veins and may be orthostatic.

9. Episodes of monocular TVL lasting hours are rare. However, such spells may occur with thromboembolic disease, as a postprandial phenomenon associated with critical carotid stenosis, and with migraine.

10. In the patient described, the episodes of monocular TVL lasted minutes and on examination there was evidence of plaque in the retinal arterioles. Thus, thromboembolic disease is the most likely etiology of the episodes.

65.2 Test Interpretation

All patients with monocular TVL lasting minutes should have a complete ophthalmoscopic examination to investigate for such conditions as intermittent angle-closure glaucoma, morning glory syndrome, and peripapillary staphyloma. Spontaneous anterior chamber hemorrhage (hyphema) should also be considered, especially in patients with associated erythropsia and in patients who have undergone cataract extraction (unstable intraocular lens, haptic chafing iris).

Patients with monocular TVL lasting minutes associated with visible retinal emboli need to be evaluated for carotid and aortic vascular disease and cardiac valvular disease. Stroke risk factors (smoking, hypertension, diabetes mellitus, hyperlipidemia, etc.) should be evaluated and controlled. Studies to evaluate the carotid arteries might include carotid Doppler and ultrasound, magnetic resonance (MR) angiography, and conventional angiography. Cardiac investigations might include transthoracic and transesophageal echocardiography and cardiac MR imaging.

In patients older than 55 years with a history of monocular TVL lasting minutes without visible retinal emboli, giant cell arteritis should be considered and an erythrocyte sedimentation rate (ESR) and/or C-reactive protein (CRP) should be performed. If this is significantly elevated or the patient has other symptoms of giant cell arteritis, such as recent headaches, jaw claudication, or polymyalgia rheumatica–like symptoms, the patient should probably undergo temporal artery biopsy. If the ESR and CRP are negative and there are no clinical symptoms suggestive of giant cell arteritis, then evaluation for carotid or cardiac thromboembolic disease is warranted.

Patients with evidence of monocular TVL due to ocular hypoperfusion (venous stasis retinopathy and the ocular ischemic syndrome) may have decreased retinal artery pressure documented by ophthalmodynamometry. The patient should be investigated for hemodynamically significant carotid stenosis.

If no thromboembolic source for the episodes of TVL is documented, then further studies could be performed. These include MR imaging of the brain with MR angiography to investigate for possible vascular malformation, and laboratory studies, including sedimentation rate, complete blood count, antiphospholipid antibodies, antinuclear antibodies, collagen vascular disease profile, and studies to investigate the presence of dysproteinemia. Younger patients (younger than 45 years) with monocular TVL are unlikely to have significant carotid disease. A cardiac embolic source as well as a vasculitis or coagulopathy must be sought.

65.3 Diagnosis

Retinal emboli secondary to right carotid stenosis causing transient monocular visual loss.

65.4 Medical Management

In the patient with no carotid embolic source and no hemodynamically significant carotid stenosis, a cardiac or aortic embolic source, hypercoagulable state, or vasculitic etiology should be sought and, if none is found, the treatment is aspirin or other antiplatelet therapy plus control of stroke risk factors.

65.5 Surgical Management

In patients with monocular TVL and ipsilateral carotid stenosis of 70 to 99%, carotid endarterectomy may be indicated if the patient is a suitable stenting or surgical candidate and if the perioperative morbidity and mortality rate of the surgeon is in the 2% or less range. Carotid endarterectomy in this group reduces the 2-year ipsilateral stroke rate from 26 to 9% and decreases the major or fatal ipsilateral stroke rate from 13.1 to 2.5%. Carotid stenting also is another option. In a patient with 30 to 69% stenosis, it remains to be seen whether stenting or endarterectomy would be beneficial. In patients with emboli from a cardiac valvular source, especially patients with cardiac dysrhythmias such as atrial fibrillation, anticoagulation may be warranted if the patient is an appropriate medical candidate.

65.6 Rehabilitation and Follow-up

Medical supervision of stroke risk factors is warranted. Periodic reevaluation of the carotid artery for restenosis is warranted by noninvasive studies (e.g., carotid Doppler or MR angiography).

Suggested Reading

[1] Goodwin JA, Gorelick PB, Helgason CM. Symptoms of amaurosis fugax in atherosclerotic carotid artery disease. Neurology. 1987; 37(5):829–832

[2] Hurwitz BJ, Heyman A, Wilkinson WE, Haynes CS, Utley CM. Comparison of amaurosis fugax and transient cerebral ischemia: a prospective clinical and arteriographic study. Ann Neurol. 1985; 18(6):698–704

[3] Lee AG, Brazis PW. Clinical Pathways in Neuro-Ophthalmology: An Evidence-Based Approach. New York, NY: Thieme; 1998:135–150

[4] Barnett HJM, Taylor DW, Haynes RB, et al. North American Symptomatic Carotid Endarterectomy Trial Collaborators. Beneficial effect of carotid endarterectomy in symptomatic patients with high-grade carotid stenosis. N Engl J Med. 1991; 325(7):445–453

66 Third Nerve Palsy—Ischemic

Sushma Yalamanchili and Andrew G. Lee

Abstract

A 70-year-old patient with a history of hypertension and diabetes mellitus presented with 4 weeks of binocular diplopia, normal pupils, ptosis of his right upper lid, mild bilateral diabetic nonproliferative retinopathy, and no adduction, elevation, or depression with intact abduction consistent with a pupil-sparing, complete ischemic third nerve palsy.

Keywords: ischemic third nerve palsy, ptosis, abnormal eye movement, diplopia, lid drooping, pupil-sparing third nerve palsy

66.1 History

A 70-year-old man had a 4-week history of binocular diplopia. The diplopia developed and worsened over a 5-day period, but it then "stabilized" and in fact had "improved" since his right eye "drooped." In the first 2 weeks, he had also noticed severe retro-orbital pain on the right but this pain became minimal. He had a history of bilateral cataract extraction but his vision had otherwise been "stable." He had a past history of hypertension and diabetes. He smoked one pack of cigarettes daily. He denied any facial numbness, recent headache, jaw claudications, or other neurologic deficits.

Examination revealed visual acuity of 20/30 on the right and 20/25 on the left. Pupils were 3 mm bilaterally and both reacted well to light and near. There was no relative afferent pupillary defect. Visual fields were normal. He had complete ptosis of his right lid (▶ Fig. 66.1) with markedly impaired levator function. He could not adduct (▶ Fig. 66.2), elevate, or depress (▶ Fig. 66.3) the right eye but he could fully abduct the eye. Attempts at depression of the right eye resulted in mild incyclodeviation of the eye (consistent with an intact ipsilateral fourth nerve). Motility was normal in the left eye. There was no proptosis, facial sensation was normal, and general neurologic exam was otherwise normal. Slit-lamp exam revealed bilateral posterior chamber intraocular lenses. Fundus exam revealed mild bilateral diabetic nonproliferative retinopathy without optic disc pathology.

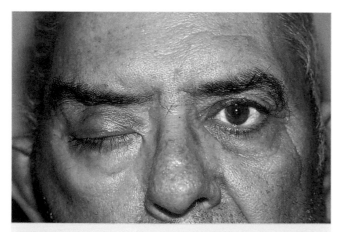

Fig. 66.1 External photography reveals a complete ptosis of the right upper eyelid with markedly impaired levator function.

Differential Diagnosis—Key Points

1. The severe ptosis and marked impairment of elevation, adduction, and depression in the right eye are compatible with a pupil-sparing, complete motor third nerve palsy (TNP). Full abduction and the incyclodeviation on downward gaze suggest that sixth nerve and fourth nerve functions, respectively, are spared.
2. TNPs are divided into nonisolated and isolated TNP. The isolated TNP were defined as TNP without associated neurologic findings (e.g., other cranial neuropathies). The types of TNPs are outlined in **the list below**.
3. Isolated TNP with a normal pupillary sphincter and completely palsied extraocular muscles is almost never due to an intracranial aneurysm. This type of TNP is most commonly caused by ischemia, especially diabetes mellitus. In patients with isolated atraumatic TNP, diabetes mellitus is the most common etiology accounting for 46% of all the cases with pupil-sparing documented in 68 to 86% of the cases. The probable explanation for pupillary sparing in diabetic TNP is the lack of damage to the periphery of the nerve where the majority of pupillomotor fibers are thought to pass. This type of TNP involvement may rarely occur with pituitary adenoma or other compressive lesions.

66.2 Definitions of the Five Types of Third Nerve Palsy

1. **Type 1**: Nonisolated TNP—TNP is considered nonisolated in the presence of the following features:
2. Other neurologic or neuro-ophthalmologic signs (e.g., other cranial nerve palsies, brainstem signs, orbital signs), evidence to suggest myasthenia gravis such as fatigability of the motility defect.
3. **Type 2**: Traumatic isolated TNP—Isolated unilateral TNPs that have a clearly established temporal relationship to significant previous head trauma and do not progress are considered traumatic in origin.
4. **Type 3**: Congenital isolated TNP—TNP that a patient is born with or is noted to have within the first 3 months of life.
5. **Type 4**: Acquired, nontraumatic isolated TNP
   a) *Type 4A*: TNP with a normal pupillary sphincter with completely palsied extraocular muscles.
   b) *Type 4B*: TNP with normal pupillary sphincter and incomplete palsied extraocular muscles.
   c) *Type 4C*: TNP with subnormal pupillary sphincter dysfunction and partial or complete extraocular muscle palsies.
6. **Type 5:** TNP with signs of aberrant regeneration.

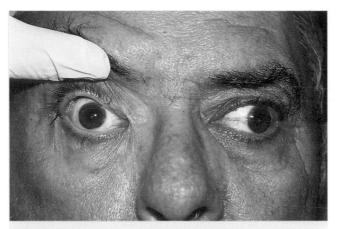

Fig. 66.2 The patient could not adduct the right eye.

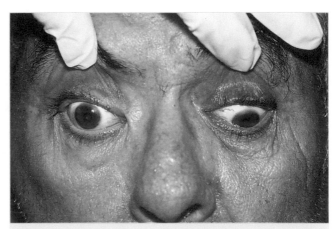

Fig. 66.3 The patient could not depress the right eye.

(Adapted from Lee AG, Brazis PW. Clinical Pathways in Neuro-Ophthalmology: An Evidence-Based Approach. New York, NY: Thieme; 1998, with permission.)

66.3 Test Interpretation

Patients who develop an isolated TNP with completely palsied extraocular muscles but with pupillary sparing do not need catheter angiography. Some authors have suggested that a neuroimaging studies (e.g., cranial computed tomography[CT]/computed tomography angiography [CTA] or magnetic resonance imaging [MRI]/magnetic resonance angiography [MRA]) in this setting need not be performed initially, as the yield for detecting a compressive lesion is very low. Other authors, however, recommend neuroimaging for all ocular motor cranial neuropathies regardless of vasculopathic risk factors because of the small but real chance of underlying treatable etiology being discovered on the imaging study. Neuroimaging should, however, be performed in patients with no vasculopathic risk factors or in patients who do not improve by 12 weeks of follow-up. Patients who are seen within 1 week of onset of this type of TNP should be observed at 24- to 48-hour intervals during the first week because some patients with aneurysms may develop delayed pupil involvement. Patients who develop pupil involvement should be reevaluated for the possibility of a compressive lesion, such as an aneurysm.

Patients older than 55 years, especially those with other symptoms suggestive of giant cell arteritis (e.g., headache, jaw or tongue claudication, polymyalgia rheumatica symptoms), should have an erythrocyte sedimentation rate (ESR) and C-reactive protein (CRP). Temporal artery biopsy should be considered if the ESR or CRP is elevated or other systemic symptoms of GCA are present.

Myasthenia gravis may rarely mimic this type of TNP, so a Tensilon test should be considered, primarily in patients with fluctuating or fatiguing ptosis or ophthalmoplegia. If the complete, pupil-spared TNP improves following a period of observation, no neuroimaging is required.

66.4 Diagnosis

Ischemic isolated TNP.

66.5 Medical Management

Vasculopathic risk factors, especially diabetes mellitus, hypertension, and increased cholesterol, should be sought and controlled.

66.6 Surgical Management

Strabismus surgery or lid surgery may be helpful in selected patients with unresolved ophthalmoplegia, diplopia, or ptosis.

66.7 Rehabilitation and Follow-up

The patient should be followed at 1- to 2-month intervals to see if the TNP improves. Complete resolution for ischemic TNP is expected to occur in 3 to 6 months. If no improvement is evident by 3 months after onset, neuroimaging for a compressive lesion is warranted.

Suggested Reading

[1] Asbury AK, Aldredge H, Hershberg R, Fisher CM. Oculomotor palsy in diabetes mellitus: a clinico-pathological study. Brain. 1970; 93(3):555–566

[2] Bondeson J, Asman P. Giant cell arteritis presenting with oculomotor nerve palsy. Scand J Rheumatol. 1997; 26(4):327–328

[3] Brazis PW. Localization of lesions of the oculomotor nerve: recent concepts. Mayo Clin Proc. 1991; 66(10):1029–1035

[4] Goldstein JE, Cogan DG. Diabetic ophthalmoplegia with special reference to the pupil. Arch Ophthalmol. 1960; 64:592–600

[5] Jacobson DM. Pupil involvement in patients with diabetes-associated oculomotor nerve palsy. Arch Ophthalmol. 1998; 116(6):723–727

[6] Lee AG, Brazis PW. Clinical Pathways in Neuro-Ophthalmology: An Evidence-Based Approach. New York, NY: Thieme; 1998;185–204

67 Third Nerve Palsy—Aneurysm

Sushma Yalamanchili and Andrew G. Lee

Abstract

A 45-year-old man presented with acute binocular diplopia, left-sided frontal-periorbital pain, left-sided lid droop, anisocoria (left pupil larger than the right), and partial paresis of elevation, adduction, and depression in the left eye consistent with a pupil involving third nerve palsy secondary to a posterior communicating artery aneurysm found on computed tomography/computed tomography angiography (CT/CTA).

Keywords: third nerve palsy, posterior communicating artery aneurysm, pupil involving third nerve palsy, diplopia, lid droop, ptosis, anisocoria

67.1 History

A 45-year-old man noted the acute onset of binocular diplopia 8 days prior to evaluation. He noted the acute onset of left-sided frontal-periorbital pain and then noted the onset of diplopia with a left-sided lid droop. He was previously well with no history of significant illnesses.

Examination revealed visual acuity of 20/20 bilaterally. He identified 10 of 10 pseudoisochromatic plates bilaterally. Pupils were 3 mm on the right and 5 mm on the left in the light and measured 4 mm on the right and 5 mm on the left in the dark. The left pupil reacted minimally to light and near, and there was no relative afferent pupillary defect. Visual fields were full to confrontation. The patient had a mild left hypotropia and a moderate exotropia. Duction testing was normal on the right but revealed partial paresis of elevation, adduction, and depression in the left eye. There were 3 mm of ptosis on the left with mildly impaired levator function. Facial sensitivity and strength were normal with normal corneal reflexes bilaterally. Slit-lamp exam and fundus exam were normal. General neurologic examination was otherwise normal.

67.2 Test Interpretation

In this patient, CT/CTA and MRI and MRA showed an ipsilateral posterior communicating artery aneurysm. Cerebral angiography confirmed the aneurysm.

67.3 Diagnosis

Partial TNP due to cerebral aneurysm of the posterior communicating artery (▶ Fig. 67.1).

67.4 Medical Management

Not applicable.

Differential Diagnosis—Key Points

1. The patient has evidence of an isolated, partial third nerve palsy (TNP) on the left with pupillary involvement.
2. Isolated TNP may occur with lesions localized anywhere along the course of the third nerve from the fascicle in the mesencephalon to the orbit.
3. Patients with a "relative pupil-sparing" TNP probably should have consideration for magnetic resonance imaging (MRI) and MR angiography (MRA), CT or CTA, and possible catheter-based cerebral digital subtraction angiography (DSA), to rule out the possibility of a compressive lesion, especially a cerebral aneurysm.
4. Because 10 to 20% of patients with ischemic TNP have pupillary dysfunction, there will be a certain percentage of normal angiograms in patients with partial TNP. In a series of 26 consecutive patients with diabetes-associated TNP, internal ophthalmoplegia occurred in 10 of 26 patients (38%), and the degree of anisocoria was 1 mm or less in most patients. None of these cases had a fully dilated, nonreactive pupil. It was concluded that anisocoria rather than pupil reactivity to light should be the defining criterion for pupil involvement.
5. Patients with an incomplete motor TNP with no pupillary involvement require an MRI and MRA to rule out a mass lesion. If the MRI is normal, cerebral angiography could be considered to investigate the presence of an aneurysm, dural-cavernous sinus fistula, or high-grade carotid stenosis. Computed tomography angiography (CTA) or MRA may eventually take the place of arteriography; however, at this time, cerebral angiography is the "gold standard" for the diagnosis of cerebral aneurysms. Although CTA/MRA may be able to detect up to 95% of cerebral aneurysms that will bleed, it cannot completely exclude aneurysm as the etiology of a pupil-involved TNP.
6. Complete TNP with pupil involvement occurring in isolation is often due to compressive lesions or meningeal infiltration; thus, a CT/CTA followed by an MRI and MRA may still be warranted. If these less invasive neuroimaging studies are negative, a cerebral DSA may still be necessary to investigate for aneurysm or less likely a dural-cavernous sinus fistula. If meningeal signs are present, spinal fluid evaluation is generally warranted. A fully dilated and nonreactive pupil occurs in up to 71% of patients with aneurysmal compression and TNP. Aneurysms impair the pupil in 96% of TNP, and the remaining 4% in which the pupil is spared have only partial TNP.

67.5 Surgical Management

Surgery or endovascular therapy to repair the aneurysm is necessary to prevent aneurysmal rupture, which carries a high morbidity and mortality.

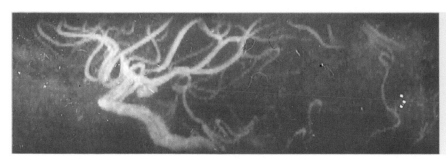

Fig. 67.1 Cerebral aneurysm of the posterior communicating artery causing a partial third nerve palsy.

67.6 Rehabilitation and Follow-up

Patching the eye to relieve the diplopia is often required.

Suggested Reading

[1] Cullom ME, Savino PJ, Sergott RC, Bosley TM. Relative pupillary sparing third nerve palsies. To arteriogram or not? J Neuroophthalmol. 1995; 15(3):136–140, discussion 140–141

[2] Jacobson DM. Pupil involvement in patients with diabetes-associated oculomotor nerve palsy. Arch Ophthalmol. 1998; 116(6):723–727

[3] Lee AG. Third nerve palsy due to a carotid cavernous fistula without external eye signs. Neuroophthalmology. 1996; 16:183–187

[4] Lee AG, Brazis PW. Clinical Pathways in Neuro-Ophthalmology: An Evidence-Based Approach. New York, NY: Thieme; 1998:185–204

[5] Trobe JD. Managing oculomotor nerve palsy. Arch Ophthalmol. 1998; 116(6): 798

68 Fourth Nerve Palsy—Congenital

Sushma Yalamanchili and Andrew G. Lee

Abstract

A 10-year-old patient experienced acute onset of vertical binocular diplopia with a right hypertropia, worse on gaze to the left and right head tilt, consistent with a right fourth cranial nerve palsy. Vertical fusional amplitudes were 10 PD characteristic of congenital cases.

Keywords: congenital fourth nerve palsy, vertical diplopia, abnormal eye movements, head tilt, large vertical fusional amplitudes, hypertropia

68.1 History

A 10-year-old boy noted the acute onset of vertical binocular diplopia for 2 weeks. He stated that one image was "below and to the side of the other" and denied any subjective torsion of the images. He denied any clear precipitants for the diplopia and denied any associated headaches, facial numbness, ptosis, or any other complaints. He had no significant past medical history.

Exam revealed visual acuity to be 20/20 bilaterally with normal color vision. Pupils were 5 mm bilaterally and equally reactive to light and near, and there was no relative afferent pupillary defect. The patient tended to tilt his head to the left (▶ Fig. 68.1). There was a 4 prism diopter (PD) right hypertropia (RHT) at distance, 8 PD RHT on left gaze, 1 PD RHT on right gaze, 2 PD RHT on upward gaze, and 7 PD RHT on downward gaze. Head tilt to the right caused an 8 PD RHT and head tilt to the left was associated with a 2 PD RHT. Double Maddox rod testing revealed 4 degrees of right excyclodeviation. Vertical fusional amplitudes were 10 PD. Ductions, versions, saccades, and pursuit eye movements were intact. There were no ptosis, facial paresis, or abnormalities of facial sensation. Slit-lamp exam and fundus exam were normal but indirect ophthalmoscopy revealed some degree of excyclotropia in the right eye.

Differential Diagnosis—Key Points

1. The RHT, worse on gaze to the left and right head tilt, is compatible with a right isolated superior oblique paresis, most often due to a fourth cranial nerve palsy. Other entities to be considered include myasthenia gravis and thyroid eye disease.

2. Fourth nerve palsies (FNPs) may cause the following:

   a) Noncomitant hypertropia demonstrated with the three-step maneuver. The hypertropia increases on head tilt toward paralyzed side (positive Bielschowsky's test). Hypotropia may occur in the normal eye if the affected eye is fixating; if the unaffected eye is fixating, hypertropia occurs in the involved eye. This hypertropia is usually most prominent in the field of gaze of the involved superior oblique muscle, especially in cases of acute or recent onset. The hypertropia may also be most prominent in the field of gaze of the ipsilateral overacting inferior oblique muscle in subacute or chronic cases or may be evident in the entire paretic field (spread of comitance).

   b) Underaction of the ipsilateral superior oblique muscle, overaction of the ipsilateral inferior oblique muscle, or overaction of the contralateral superior oblique muscle. Pseudo-overaction of the superior oblique in the uninvolved eye occurs with spread of comitance, and secondary pseudoparesis (and contracture) of the superior rectus muscle in the contralateral eye may occur. In a patient with a superior oblique muscle paralysis who habitually fixates with the paretic eye and in whom overaction of the ipsilateral inferior oblique muscle has developed, less than the normal amount of innervation will be required when the patient looks up and to the contralateral side. Since the innervation flowing to the opposite superior rectus is "determined" by the overacting ipsilateral inferior oblique (Hering's law), the opposite superior rectus muscle will seem paretic (inhibitional palsy of the contralateral antagonist). In these cases, the head tilt test will correctly determine which of the two eyes is paretic.

   c) Excyclotropia, which is usually evident on fundus exam and double Maddox rod testing. This cyclotropia is usually symptomatic only in acquired (vs. congenital) cases.

   d) A head tilt. This is present in approximately 70% of patients with FNP and is usually away from the involved side but may be paradoxical (toward the involved side) in about 3% of patients.

3. It is important to differentiate patients with decompensation of a congenital FNP from patients with an acquired FNP. In patients with congenital FNP:

   a) Old photos may show a long-standing head tilt.

   b) Patients usually are noted to have cyclotropia on examination but do not complain of cyclotropia (subjective image tilting) as do some patients with acquired FNP.

   c) Large vertical fusional amplitudes (greater than 6–8 PD) in primary gaze are characteristic of congenital cases.

   d) Facial asymmetry (hypoplasia on side of head turn) suggests a congenital FNP.

4. Bilateral FNPs are suggested by

   a) An RHT in left gaze and left hypertropia in right gaze.

   b) A positive Bielschowsky's test on tilt to either shoulder ("double Bielschowsky's test").

   c) Large excyclotropia (greater than 10 degrees).

   d) V-pattern esotropia (15 PD or more difference in esotropia between upward and downward gaze). The "V" pattern is caused by a decrease of the abducting effect of the superior oblique(s) in depression and overaction of the inferior oblique muscle(s).

   e) Underaction of both superior oblique muscles and/or overaction of both inferior oblique muscles.

   f) In general, bilateral FNPs tend to have a smaller hypertropia in primary position than do unilateral FNPs.

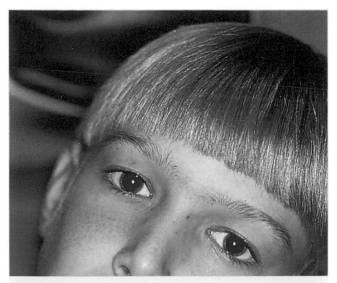

Fig. 68.1 External photograph demonstrates anomalous tilt of the patient's head to the left.

68.2 Test Interpretation

The large fusional amplitudes and lack of subjective image tilting are compatible with congenital right FNP. The recent onset of symptoms is due to decompensation of a chronic phoria. Old photographs reveal a head tilt present for years.

68.3 Diagnosis

Decompensation of old right FNP.

68.4 Medical Management

Observation or the use of prisms may be all that is required.

68.5 Surgical Management

Many patients may benefit from strabismus surgery.

68.6 Rehabilitation and Follow-up

No rehabilitation and follow-up are required if the problem is resolved.

Suggested Reading

[1] Brazis PW. Palsies of the trochlear nerve: diagnosis and localization–recent concepts. Mayo Clin Proc. 1993; 68(5):501–509

[2] Lee AG, Brazis PW. Clinical Pathways in Neuro-Ophthalmology: An Evidence-Based Approach. New York, NY: Thieme; 1998:205–216

[3] Von Noorden GK. Binocular Vision and Ocular Motility: Theory and Management of Strabismus. 5th ed. St. Louis, MO: Mosby; 1996:411–415,423–424

[4] von Noorden GK, Murray E, Wong SY. Superior oblique paralysis. A review of 270 cases. Arch Ophthalmol. 1986; 104(12):1771–1776

69 Sixth Nerve Palsy

Sushma Yalamanchili and Andrew G. Lee

Abstract

A 56-year-old patient with a history of type II diabetes mellitus with a 3-month history of binocular horizontal diplopia primarily at distance and worse on left gaze was found to have a 4 prism diopter of esotropia and limitation on abduction, consistent with a left sixth nerve palsy. A magnetic resonance imaging (MRI) showed a meningioma of the cavernous sinus.

Keywords: sixth nerve palsy, horizontal diplopia, limitation on abduction, esotropia, cavernous sinus, meningioma

69.1 History

A 56-year-old man complained of a 3-month history of binocular diplopia. The diplopia was primarily present at distance but was absent at near and was worse on gaze to the left. He had also noted some numbness and tingling in the left forehead and mild left frontotemporal headaches. He denied any recent head trauma, visual loss, or history of previous neurologic or ophthalmologic symptoms. He was a diabetic using oral agents to control his blood sugar.

Exam revealed visual acuity to be 20/20 bilaterally. He identified 10 of 10 pseudoisochromatic plates bilaterally. Pupils were 4 mm bilaterally and equally reactive to light and near, and there was no relative afferent pupillary defect. Visual fields were full to confrontation. He had a 4 prism diopter (PD) esotropia (ET) at distance, with no ET at near. The ET was nil on gaze to the right, 8 PD ET on gaze to the left, and 4 PD ET on gaze up and down. Duction testing revealed underaction of abduction in the left eye. There was no ptosis. No facial weakness was noted but sensory testing revealed decreased sensation to soft touch over the left forehead, and the left corneal reflex was slightly depressed. Slit-lamp exam and fundus exam were normal. No papilledema was evident. The rest of the general neurologic examination was normal.

69.2 Test Interpretation

Nonisolated sixth nerve palsies should undergo neuroimaging, preferably by magnetic resonance imaging (MRI) with contrast, and further evaluation, including laboratory and lumbar puncture in some cases. If a patient with a sixth nerve palsy has papilledema, neuroimaging is mandatory, as a unilateral or bilateral sixth nerve palsy may be a nonlocalizing sign of increased intracranial pressure. If the MRI is normal, a spinal tap may be warranted to investigate meningeal infectious, inflammatory, and neoplastic processes and idiopathic causes such as pseudotumor cerebri. Many authors recommend that an isolated sixth nerve palsy in a vasculopathic patient may be observed without neuroimaging, but if no improvement occurs in 3 months, neuroimaging is recommended. Other authors, however, have reported neuroimaging abnormalities in patients

> **Differential Diagnosis—Key Points**
>
> 1. Causes of acquired ET include sixth nerve palsy, orbital myositis, myasthenia gravis, thyroid eye disease, trauma, ocular neuromyotonia, cyclic ET, divergence insufficiency or paralysis, spasm of the near reflex, pseudo–sixth nerve palsies due to thalamic or midbrain lesions, acquired motor fusion deficiency, and the hemifield slide phenomena (seen with chiasmal lesions). In this patient, there is evidence of paresis of the left lateral rectus muscle, and a left sixth nerve palsy is likely. This paresis has not occurred in isolation, however, as there is also evidence of left facial numbness and sensory changes in the distribution of the ophthalmic branch (V1) of the trigeminal nerve, as well as left-sided headache. Thus, purely motor syndromes, such as myasthenia gravis, are excluded. The sixth nerve is near the ophthalmic branch of the trigeminal nerve in the cavernous sinus. A lesion in these locations must strongly be considered and neuroimaging should be performed.
> 2. Isolated, vasculopathic sixth nerve palsies are common and can be observed without neuroimaging for 4 to 12 weeks. Some authors, however, recommend neuroimaging even in these cases because of the small chance of a treatable lesion being missed. Even though the patient is diabetic, ischemic sixth nerve palsy is not a likely consideration in this case because of the trigeminal neuropathy.
> 3. Compressive lesions in the cavernous sinus may cause a sixth nerve palsy and include tumors (e.g., meningiomas, trigeminal nerve tumors, schwannomas, metastases, skull base tumors, lymphoma/leukemia, nasopharyngeal carcinoma), cavernous sinus fistulas or thrombosis, intracavernous aneurysms, and inflammatory or infectious diseases (e.g., herpes zoster, mucormycosis).

with presumed isolated and vasculopathic sixth nerve palsies and thus recommend imaging all patients. In contrast, nonvasculopathic isolated sixth nerve palsies should undergo neuroimaging (typically MRI with contrast) to rule out a treatable lesion. Younger patients and those without vascular risk factors should undergo more extensive evaluation including complete blood count, fasting blood glucose, blood pressure evaluation, and lumbar puncture. In patients with an isolated sixth nerve palsy with variable ET, fatigue of eye movements, or ptosis, myasthenia gravis should be considered. Any patient with progressive or unresolved sixth nerve palsy should undergo neuroimaging.

69.3 Diagnosis

Left sixth nerve palsy and damage to the left ophthalmic branch of the trigeminal nerve secondary to meningioma of the cavernous sinus (▶ Fig. 69.1).

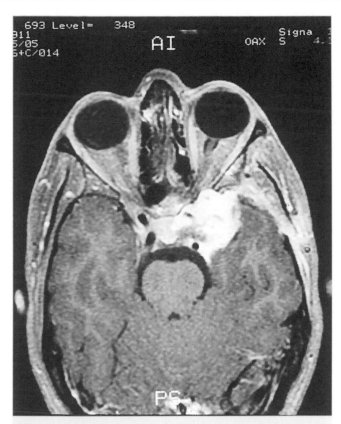

Fig. 69.1 Magnetic resonance scan shows left-sided meningioma of the cavernous sinus causing sixth nerve palsy.

69.4 Medical Management

Treatment is aimed at the responsible underlying lesion and may include surgery, radiation therapy, or even simple observation. The diplopia is controlled by patching, prisms, or, if chronic and stable and depending on the etiology, surgery. Early botulinum injection into the ipsilateral medial rectus may improve diplopia and increase the likelihood of subsequent improvement.

69.5 Surgical Management

Strabismus surgery may be necessary for residual ophthalmoplegia or diplopia.

69.6 Rehabilitation and Follow-up

Patients must be observed for recurrence of further neurologic and ophthalmologic deficits depending on the etiology of the sixth nerve palsy. Symptomatic diplopia treatment is warranted.

Suggested Reading

[1] Currie J, Lubin JH, Lessell S. Chronic isolated abducens paresis from tumors at the base of the brain. Arch Neurol. 1983; 40(4):226–229

[2] Galetta SL, Smith JL. Chronic isolated sixth nerve palsies. Arch Neurol. 1989; 46(1):79–82

[3] Keane JR. Bilateral sixth nerve palsy. Analysis of 125 cases. Arch Neurol. 1976; 33(10):681–683

[4] Lee AG, Brazis PW. Clinical Pathways in Neuro-Ophthalmology: An Evidence-Based Approach. New York, NY: Thieme; 1998:217–227

70 Internuclear Ophthalmoplegia

Sushma Yalamanchili and Andrew G. Lee

Abstract

A 27-year-old woman with a past medical history of multiple sclerosis and right optic neuritis not currently on medications presents with "difficulty focusing" her eyes. She has a mild adduction deficit in the left eye, right abducting nystagmus, slow saccades in adduction in the left eye, and intact convergence consistent with a left internuclear ophthalmoplegia.

Keywords: internuclear ophthalmoplegia, multiple sclerosis, abducting nystagmus, limitation of adduction, horizontal diplopia, intact convergence, optic neuritis, slowed saccades

70.1 History

A 27-year-old woman with a history of multiple sclerosis (MS) complained of "difficulty focusing" her eyes. Her previous MS course included a history of optic neuritis in the right eye. She did have mild gait instability, bladder disturbance, and leg numbness. Her eye difficulty started several months prior to ophthalmologic evaluation. She was taking no medications.

Ophthalmologic examination revealed visual acuity to be 20/20 bilaterally. She identified 7 of 10 pseudoisochromatic plates on the right and 10 of 10 on the left. Visual fields showed a small paracentral scotoma on the right. Pupils were 5 mm bilaterally and equally reactive to light and near, but there was a mild right afferent pupillary defect. The patient had a 2 prism diopter left hypertropia that was comitant in left, right, up, and down gaze. There was mild paresis of adduction in the left eye but otherwise ductions were full. On gaze to the right, the adducting saccade in the left eye was quite slow compared to the abducting saccade in the right eye. Saccades to the left and vertically were normal. On attempting to hold her gaze to the right, monocular dissociated horizontal nystagmus was noted in the right eye in the direction of abduction. Convergence was normal and was able to overcome the adduction deficit in the left eye. There was no ptosis. Facial sensation and movement were normal. Slit-lamp examination was normal. Fundus exam revealed mild temporal pallor in the right eye but was otherwise normal.

Differential Diagnosis—Key Points

1. The impaired color vision, relative afferent pupillary defect, and mild optic nerve pallor on the right are likely the residual of a previous episode of optic neuritis in this patient with known MS.
2. The adduction weakness in the left eye, slow saccades in adduction in the left eye, and dissociated monocular nystagmus in abduction in the right eye with preserved convergence all indicate the presence of a left internuclear

ophthalmoplegia (INO). The comitant hypertropia is likely a skew deviation due to the medial longitudinal fasciculus (MLF) lesion.
3. The abducens nucleus has two types of intermingled neurons: motor neurons and internuclear neurons. The axons of the internuclear neurons cross to the contralateral side in the lower pons and ascend in the MLF to synapse in the portion of the oculomotor nucleus that innervates the medial rectus muscle. Lesions of the MLF result in INO.
4. Clinically, INO is characterized by adduction weakness on the side of the MLF lesion and monocular nystagmus of the opposite abducting eye. Convergence may be preserved. Often, patients with INO have no visual symptoms but some complain of diplopia (due to skew deviation with the higher eye on the side of the lesion) or oscillopsia.
5. An INO can be brought out best during horizontal saccadic eye movement testing. The "adduction lag" might be seen during optokinetic testing using a rotating tape or drum. For example, with a right INO when the drum is rotated to the right, the amplitude and velocity of the adducting quick phase of the right eye is smaller and slower than that of the abducting saccades in the left eye. The pathogenesis of the nystagmus in the abducting eye is unclear but is likely a normal adaptive process that helps overcome the adducting weakness of the fellow eye. Unilateral INO may rarely be associated with exotropia (wall-eyed monocular INO, also called WEMINO syndrome).
6. Bilateral INO results in bilateral adduction paresis or lag with the eyes generally aligned in primary gaze. Occasionally, exotropia will occur, with both eyes deviated laterally (wall eyed-bilateral internuclear ophthalmoplegia, or WEBINO syndrome). These patients will often also demonstrate vertical gaze evoked nystagmus, impaired vestibular and pursuit vertical eye movements, and impaired vertical gaze holding.
7. INO is due to pathologic processes affecting the MLF in the medial pontine or midbrain parenchyma. Often, there are associated brainstem symptoms and signs although occasionally unilateral or bilateral INO may occur in isolation. The nature of the responsible pathologic process is suggested by the temporal mode of onset of the INO, the general clinical circumstances, and associated signs on neurologic and neuro-ophthalmologic examination. INO is most often due to MS or brainstem infarction. Other etiologies include brainstem infections and masses, degenerative extrapyramidal diseases, drug intoxications, and certain nutritional and metabolic disorders (e.g., Wernicke's encephalopathy and pernicious anemia). The pattern of extraocular muscle weakness with myasthenia gravis can mimic INO (pseudo-INO); myasthenic pseudo-INO is not uncommon.

70.2 Test Interpretation

In general, the investigation of a patient with INO depends on the clinical circumstances. For example, in the patient presented, MS is evident. INO in isolation or with associated unexplained brainstem signs and symptoms requires neuroimaging. If there is variability of the adduction deficit, associated fluctuating ptosis, or other variable ocular motor signs suggestive of myasthenia gravis, a myasthenic pseudo-INO should be considered.

Magnetic resonance imaging (MRI) is superior to computed tomography (CT) in evaluating patients with INO. MRI may give useful diagnostic data by also giving information about supratentorial processes likely to be involved in the etiology of the INO, such as MS and multiple cerebral infarcts. If an infarct is detected as the cause of INO in a patient greater than 50 years of age, giant cell arteritis should be considered as an etiology, especially if other stroke risk factors are not evident.

If MRI in nontraumatic cases is normal, then rarer etiologies for the INO should be considered. If the INO is bilateral, drug intoxication should be suspected. As pernicious anemia has rarely been reported to cause INO, a B_{12} level is also indicated but of low yield. Syphilis may rarely cause INO, so serology for syphilis (e.g., rapid plasma reagin (RPR), fluorescent treponemal antibody (FTA), syphilis immunoglobulin G (IgG)) is also suggested. If MRI reveals meningeal enhancement or if meningeal signs or symptoms are present, spinal fluid examination is warranted to investigate for infectious or carcinomatous meningitis.

70.3 Diagnosis

Optic neuropathy on the right and INO on the left due to MS.

70.4 Medical Management

Treatment is directed at the underlying etiology of the INO. If associated skew deviation or exotropia is symptomatic, prisms may be required to relieve diplopia.

70.5 Surgical Management

Usually, no surgical treatment is required but some patients may require strabismus surgery for residual diplopia if unresolved.

70.6 Rehabilitation and Follow-up

Follow-up for resolution of the INO is important.

Suggested Reading

[1] Atlas SW, Grossman RI, Savino PJ, et al. Internuclear ophthalmoplegia: MR-anatomic correlation. AJNR Am J Neuroradiol. 1987; 8(2):243–247

[2] Glaser JS. Myasthenic psuedo-internuclear ophthalmoplegia. Arch Ophthalmol. 1966; 75(3):363–366

[3] Hopf HC, Thömke F, Gutmann L. Midbrain vs. pontine medial longitudinal fasciculus lesions: the utilization of masseter and blink reflexes. Muscle Nerve. 1991; 14(4):326–330

[4] Lee AG, Brazis PW. Clinical Pathways in Neuro-Ophthalmology: An Evidence-Based Approach. New York, NY: Thieme; 1998:232–236

[5] Müri RM, Meienberg O. The clinical spectrum of internuclear ophthalmoplegia in multiple sclerosis. Arch Neurol. 1985; 42(9):851–855

71 Diplopia—Ocular Myasthenia Gravis

Sushma Yalamanchili and Andrew G. Lee

Abstract

A 57-year-old woman patient presented with intermittent diplopia for 6 months, which worsened "as the day goes on," and intermittent left or right eyelid droop. On exam, she had paresis of both lateral rectus muscles, bilateral ptosis, increased ptosis with elevation of the opposite eyelid (enhanced ptosis), a positive Tensilon test, and negative acetylcholine receptor antibodies, consistent with ocular myasthenia gravis.

Keywords: diplopia, myasthenia gravis, ptosis, orbicularis oculi weakness, enhanced ptosis, acetylcholine receptor antibodies, single fiber EMG, lid droop

71.1 History

A 57-year-old woman complained of intermittent diplopia over the last 6 months. The diplopia was often not present on awakening in the morning but tended to occur and worsen "as the day goes on." She especially had difficulty driving, often seeing "two lines instead of one" in the middle of the road. Her spouse also had noted that at times her left or right eyelid would droop. She denied significant past medical problems except for a history of pernicious anemia for which she takes monthly B_{12} shots. She denied any headache, facial numbness or pain, dysphagia, dysarthria, breathing difficulty, generalized muscle weakness, or extremity paresis or sensory symptoms.

Examination of the afferent visual system was normal. Pupils were 5 mm and equally reactive to light and near. No relative afferent pupillary defect was evident. She had an esotropia of 10 prism diopters (PD) in primary position that increased to 15 PD on left gaze, 18 PD on right gaze, and 12 PD on up and down gaze. When she attempted to hold her gaze to the left or the right, the separation of images worsened subjectively and her esotropia increased. Although she had no obvious vertical misalignment in primary gaze, on holding her gaze upward she eventually developed a left hypertropia. Duction testing suggested paresis of both lateral rectus muscles. She had bilateral ptosis. The ptosis worsened in each eye when the opposite lid was held upward. Levator function was mildly weak bilaterally. Facial sensation was normal but she had mild paresis of eye closure bilaterally. Slit-lamp and fundus exams were normal. General neurologic examination was otherwise normal.

A Tensilon test resulted in improvement of the patient's esotropia and ptosis. Acetylcholine receptor (AChR) antibodies were not present, thyroid-stimulating hormone (TSH) was normal, and computed tomography (CT) scan of the chest was negative for thymoma.

Differential Diagnosis—Key Points

1. Although the esotropia was worse on gaze to the left, and gaze to the right may suggest bilateral sixth nerve palsies, the patient also has bilateral ptosis. The fatigability of the esotropia on attempted lateral gaze holding, the development of a hypertropia on prolonged upward gaze (fatigue), and the increased ptosis with elevation of the opposite eyelid (enhanced ptosis) are all strongly suggestive of myasthenia gravis (MG).

2. MG is a chronic disorder of neuromuscular transmission characterized clinically by varying degrees of weakness and fatigue of voluntary muscles. MG is caused by an acquired autoimmunity to the motor end plate and is associated with antibodies that block or cause increased degradation of AChR. There is abnormal weakness in some or all voluntary muscles. The weakness increases with repeated or sustained exertion and increases over the course of the day, but is improved by rest; it also may be worsened by elevation of body temperature and is often improved by cold.

3. The levator palpebrae superioris and extraocular muscles are involved initially in approximately 50 to 70% of cases, and these muscles are eventually affected in about 90% of patients. Ocular myasthenia (OM) is a form of MG confined to the extraocular, levator palpebrae superioris, and/or orbicularis oculi muscles. Approximately 50% of patients initially present with OM, but only 12 to 50% of these remain ocular. Of the 50 to 80% of patients with purely ocular symptoms and signs at onset that go on to develop generalized MG, most, but not all, develop generalized symptoms within 2 to 3 years of onset of the disorder.

4. Ptosis in MG may occur as an isolated sign or in association with extraocular muscle involvement. The ptosis may be unilateral or bilateral and, when bilateral, is usually asymmetric. The ptosis may be absent when the patient awakens, but appears later in the day, becoming more pronounced as the day progresses. Prolonged upward gaze may increase the ptosis. Enhanced or seesaw ptosis may be demonstrated (ie, a worsening of ptosis on one side when the opposite eyelid is elevated and held in a fixed position), but this sign is not specific for MG as it may rarely be seen with age-related ptosis, ocular myopathy, Lambert-Eaton myasthenic syndrome, Fisher's syndrome, and even third nerve palsy. During refixation (a vertical saccade) from down to the primary position, the upper eyelid may either slowly begin to droop or else twitch several times before settling in a stable position (Cogan's lid-twitch sign).

5. Involvement of extraocular muscles with MG usually occurs in association with ptosis; however, cases without clinical involvement of the levator muscles occur. MG should be considered in any case of ocular motor weakness without pupil involvement because MG may mimic any pattern of neurogenic paresis. Any extraocular muscle may be selectively impaired, especially the medial rectus, and weakness characteristically increases with sustained effort. Myasthenia can mimic pupil-sparing third nerve palsies, superior division third nerve palsies, abducens nerve palsies, or trochlear nerve palsies and internuclear ophthalmoplegia.

71.2 Test Interpretation

The diagnosis of OM is based on the clinical history, the physical findings, pharmacological testing, and, in selected individuals, sleep test, electromyography (EMG) investigations including study of the decremental response, conventional needle EMG, and single-fiber recordings, and determination of the serum anti-AChR antibody titers. The diagnosis of OM should be considered in any patient with ptosis and/or ocular motor weakness without pupillary involvement. Weakness and fatigue confined to the extraocular muscles or lids combined with orbicularis oculi paresis is especially suggestive of OM. Significant clinical involvement of the pupil, eye pain or headaches, proptosis, visual loss, or involvement of trigeminal sensation essentially negate this diagnosis.

A positive Tensilon (edrophonium hydrochloride) or Prostigmin (neostigmine methyl-sulfate) test is usually, but not always, indicative of OM. The improvement of extraocular muscle function should be quantified with prisms, a Hess screen, or the Lancaster red-green test. A negative Tensilon or Prostigmin test in no way rules out MG. The "sleep test" may also be incorporated to demonstrate objective improvement in myasthenic symptoms after rest. The patient is kept in a quiet, darkened room and instructed to close the eyes and rest for 30 minutes; ptosis and ocular motility are quantified before and after the rest period. This study may be positive in some Tensilon-negative myasthenic patients but may also be negative in Tensilon-positive patients. Another noninvasive test is the ice pack test, which may be useful in the diagnosis of OM in the patient with ptosis. Ice in a surgical glove is placed over one lightly closed eye for 2 minutes or to the limit of patient tolerance. In cases of bilateral ptosis, the opposite (un-cooled) eye serves as control.

AChR antibody titers are quite useful in the diagnosis of MG. In one large and representative study, the percentages of positive tests in different clinical forms of MG were as follows: remission, 24%; ocular, 50%; mild generalized, 80%; moderately severe or acutely severe, 100%; chronic severe, 89%. Overall, AChR antibodies are positive in 80 to 95% of patients with generalized MG and 34 to 56% of patients with OM. Testing for AChR binding, blocking, and modulating antibodies increases the assay yield in patients with generalized MG and OM. In OM, the antibody titer tends to be low and the serum antibody titer correlates poorly with the severity of MG when a group of patients is studied.

As there is an increased risk of thymoma in patients with MG, all patients with the diagnosis of MG should undergo CT or magnetic resonance imaging (MRI) of the mediastinum. Thymoma occurs in 5 to 20% of myasthenic patients overall and about one-third to one-half of patients with thymoma have MG. The risk of thymoma in patients with OM is probably lower. Thymoma is more common in older patients and in patients with high AChR antibody titers. Because thyroid disease may be associated with MG, all patients should also have sensitive TSH levels measured.

71.3 Diagnosis

Ocular myasthenia gravis.

71.4 Medical Management

About 10 to 20% of patients with OM will undergo spontaneous remission, which may be temporary or permanent. Corticosteroids produce favorable response in OM in 66 to 85% of patients. At 2 years, prednisone treatment appears to reduce the incidence of generalized MG to 7% in contrast to 36% of patients who did not receive prednisone. Generalized MG may be a life-threatening disease requiring aggressive treatment with anticholinesterase drugs, corticosteroids, other immunosuppressive agents, plasmapheresis, intravenous gamma globulin, and possible thymectomy.

For patients with OM, if the diplopia or ptosis is mild, then observation or patching one eye may be sufficient. Ptosis may be eliminated in some patients by having a crutch attachment placed on a spectacle frame for one or both eyes, although this often causes irritation of the eyes from exposure.

71.5 Surgical Management

Ptosis surgery may be performed in patients with stable disease, particularly those who are refractory to medical therapy or in whom ptosis is a predominant finding. For more severe ocular motor weakness, anticholinesterase agents, such as pyridostigmine bromide (Mestinon), are warranted, although these agents often do not succeed in correcting the diplopia. Diplopia is often more refractory to treatment than is ptosis. If moderate or large doses of anticholinesterase drugs fail or cannot be tolerated and symptoms are troublesome, then corticosteroids, often at relatively low alternate-day doses, are usually effective in correcting the diplopia. Although some authors have suggested the use of azathioprine for patients who are inadequately controlled on low-dose steroids or who are experiencing steroid side effects, this agent, cyclophosphamide, cyclosporine, intravenous immunoglobulin, and plasmapheresis are not usually used in patient with purely OM because their benefit–risk ratios have not been adequately studied.

The presence of a thymoma in any patient with MG is an absolute indication for thymectomy and, thus, all patients with OM should be evaluated with mediastinal CT or MRI. Although thymectomy can be effective in ocular MG without thymoma and may prevent generalization of the disease, most clinicians are reluctant to recommend this procedure for purely ocular symptoms.

71.6 Rehabilitation and Follow-up

Patients need close supervision of medications used to control symptoms. Patients with purely OM must be warned of the possibility of generalization of the disease process and should specifically be instructed to inform their physician immediately if symptoms such as dysphagia, respiratory involvement, or extremity weakness develop.

Suggested Reading

[1] Bever CT, Jr, Aquino AV, Penn AS, Lovelace RE, Rowland LP. Prognosis of ocular myasthenia. Ann Neurol. 1983; 14(5):516–519

[2] Engel AG. Disturbances of neuromuscular transmission: acquired autoimmune myasthenia gravis. In: Engel AG, Franzini-Armstrong C, eds. Myol-

ogy: Basic and Clinical. 2nd ed. New York, NY: McGraw-Hill; 1994:1769–1797

[3] Gorelick PB, Rosenberg M, Pagano RJ. Enhanced ptosis in myasthenia gravis. Arch Neurol. 1981; 38(8):531

[4] Kupersmith MJ, Moster M, Bhuiyan S, Warren F, Weinberg H. Beneficial effects of corticosteroids on ocular myasthenia gravis. Arch Neurol. 1996; 53 (8):802–804

[5] Lee AG, Brazis PW. Clinical Pathways in Neuro-Ophthalmology: An Evidence-Based Approach. New York, NY Thieme; 1998:257–267

[6] Phillips PH, Newman NJ. Here today ... gone tomorrow. Surv Ophthalmol. 1997; 41(4):354–356

[7] Schumm F, Wiethölter H, Fateh-Moghadam A, Dichgans J. Thymectomy in myasthenia with pure ocular symptoms. J Neurol Neurosurg Psychiatry. 1985; 48(4):332–337

[8] Sommer N, Sigg B, Melms A, et al. Ocular myasthenia gravis: response to long-term immunosuppressive treatment. J Neurol Neurosurg Psychiatry. 1997; 62(2):156–162

[9] Weinberg DA, Lesser RL, Vollmer TL. Ocular myasthenia: a protean disorder. Surv Ophthalmol. 1994; 39(3):169–210

[10] Kupersmith MJ, Latkany R, Homel P. Development of generalized disease at 2 years in patients with ocular myasthenia gravis. Arch Neurol. 2003; 60(2):243–248

[11] Kupersmith MJ. Ocular myasthenia gravis: treatment successes and failures in patients with long-term follow-up. J Neurol. 2009; 256(8):1314–1320

72 Thyroid Ophthalmopathy

Sushma Yalamanchili and Andrew G. Lee

Abstract

A 35-year-old woman with a past medical history of hyperthyroidism treated with radioactive iodine 1 year ago presents with a 2-month history of mild to moderate "eye irritation" or "foreign body–type" sensation, diplopia, and eyes bulging. On exam, she has limitation of elevation and depression in both eyes, limitation of abduction in both eyes, lid retraction, lid lag, proptosis, and mild punctate keratopathy consistent with thyroid eye disease.

Keywords: thyroid ophthalmopathy, proptosis, dry eye, lid lag, lid retraction, diplopia, extraocular muscle abnormalities, scleral show

72.1 History

A 35-year-old woman complained of a 2-month history of eye discomfort and diplopia. The eye pain was a mild to moderate "eye irritation" or "foreign body–type" sensation that was constant but fluctuated in severity. She also complained of vertical diplopia that was binocular and constant. She often patched one eye in order to read or drive. Her husband noted that over the last few weeks her eyes appeared to be "bulging." She had a past medical history of hyperthyroidism treated with radioactive iodine 1 year ago. She was taking thyroid supplements. She denied any other medical problems.

Examination revealed visual acuity of 20/25 bilaterally. She identified 10 of 10 Hardy–Rand–Rittler pseudoisochromatic plates bilaterally. Pupils were 4 mm bilaterally and equally reactive to light and near, and there was no relative afferent pupillary defect. Visual fields were full on static perimetry. She had a left hypertropia of 4 prism diopters (PD) in primary gaze. This increased to 8 PD in upward gaze, 10 PD in downward gaze, and was 4 to 5 PD in left and right gaze. There was also an esotropia of 5 PD in primary gaze that was relatively comitant in up, down, left, and right gaze. Duction testing revealed limitation of elevation and depression in both eyes and limitation of abduction in both eyes, worse on the left. Adduction was relatively normal. She had no ptosis but had definite lid retraction and lid lag bilaterally. Proptosis was present with Hertel measurements at a base of 95 mm that were 22 mm on the right and 24 mm on the left, respectively (▶ Fig. 72.1). Facial sensation and movements were normal. Slit-lamp examination revealed mild punctate keratopathy bilaterally. Funduscopic examination was normal.

Differential Diagnosis—Key Points

1. The motility impairment noted could be related to myasthenia gravis, but lid lag and retraction, rather than ptosis, makes this diagnosis unlikely. Bilateral orbital pseudotumor or other infiltrative orbitopathies are also a possibility, but the pain noted is mild and superficial, rather than severe and deep, and the lid lag and retraction are not easily explained by an infiltrative process. The constellation of impaired motility, lid lag and retraction, and proptosis, especially in the light of a history of previous hyperthyroidism treated with radioactive iodine, all make thyroid orbitopathy the most likely diagnosis in this patient.

2. The ophthalmopathy of thyroid disease (thyroid eye disease, thyroid orbitopathy, or Graves' disease) is an autoimmune process with a progressive but self-limited variable course extending over 1 to 3 years. It is a common cause of acquired diplopia or exophthalmos in adults. The ophthalmopathy spans a clinical spectrum from minor eye symptoms and signs to severe, disabling, vision-threatening problems. Thyroid ophthalmopathy is considered to be present if eyelid retraction occurs in association with objective evidence of thyroid dysfunction or abnormal regulation, exophthalmos, optic nerve dysfunction, or extraocular muscle (EOM) involvement.

3. The median age at the time of diagnosis of Graves' ophthalmopathy is 43 years (range, 8–88 years). Approximately 90% of patients have Graves' hyperthyroidism, 1% have primary hypothyroidism, 3% have Hashimoto's thyroiditis, and 5% are euthyroid. Among patients with hyperthyroidism, Graves' ophthalmopathy develops in 61% within 1 year of the onset of thyrotoxicosis.

4. Eyelid retraction is the most common ophthalmic feature of autoimmune thyroid disease, present either unilaterally or bilaterally in more than 90% of patients at some point in the clinical course. Exophthalmos of one or both eyes affects approximately 60% of patients, restrictive extraocular myopathy is apparent in about 40% of patients, and optic nerve dysfunction occurs in either one or both eyes in 6% of cases. The restrictive myopathy especially affects the inferior, medial, and superior recti and rarely affects the lateral rectus muscle: therefore, exotropia in a patient with thyroid orbitopathy should raise the possibility of concomitant ocular myasthenia gravis. Only 5% of patients have a complete constellation of classic findings: eyelid retraction, exophthalmos, optic nerve dysfunction, EOM involvement, and hyperthyroidism. At the time of diagnosis of Graves' ophthalmopathy, the most frequent ocular symptom is pain or discomfort, which affects 30% of patients. Some degree of diplopia is noted by 17% of patients, lacrimation or photophobia is present in about 15 to 20%, and 7.5% of patients have blurred vision. Decreased vision attributable to optic neuropathy is present in less than 2% of patients by the time of diagnosis of Graves' disease.

5. Thyroid ophthalmopathy may be quite asymmetric between the two orbits and the disease process often undergoes spontaneous exacerbations and remissions of clinical activity. The disorder often starts with an acute, active inflammatory phase, lasting 6 to 18 months, which is mediated by lymphocytic and fibroblastic infiltration into orbital tissues.

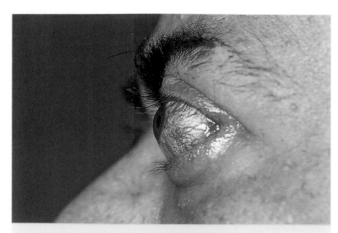

Fig. 72.1 External appearance showing proptosis.

72.2 Test Interpretation

Forced duction testing will indicate that the diplopia is due to restrictive rather than paretic disease process affecting the EOMs. Thyroid function studies need to be assessed. Computed tomography (CT) scan or magnetic resonance imaging (MRI) of the orbits is useful to document EOM enlargement.

72.3 Diagnosis

Thyroid orbitopathy.

72.4 Medical Management

The treatment of thyroid eye disease begins with adequate control of the underlying endocrinopathy, as many of the eye signs, except for proptosis, may improve with thyroid treatment. Patients should be instructed to stop smoking, as smoking has been associated with the ophthalmopathy. Ocular discomfort is usually due to corneal and conjunctival exposure and often responds to methylcellulose artificial tears during the day and ointment at night. As periorbital edema is often most prominent in the morning after a period of recumbency, elevating the head of the patient's bed and sleeping partially supine are advised. Wearing dark glasses with side protection will help photophobia.

For more severe symptoms, taping the eyelids shut at night or the use of goggles to provide a humidified chamber may be helpful. In general, patients should be observed closely throughout the period of active inflammation without more aggressive therapeutic interventions, although suppression of inflammation with systemic corticosteroids or radiation therapy may be considered for more severe symptoms. Three exceptions that require prompt and aggressive early therapy are severe exposure keratopathy, severe proptosis or globe luxation, and optic neuropathy.

Diplopia during this period is usually due to tethering of the inferior and medial rectus muscles or less often the superior rectus muscle. Patients are thus usually esotropic and have vertical ocular misalignment. The diplopia of the early inflamma-tory phase is treated with patching or prisms as outlined concerning the symptomatic management of diplopia. Botulinum toxin injection into the tight and stiff muscles may temporarily help to correct a pathologic eye position and help regain binocular single vision. Strabismus surgery is deferred until the ocular deviation has been documented as unchanged for at least a period of 6 to 12 months and the patient is in the chronic phase of thyroid ophthalmopathy.

Systemic corticosteroids have been used successfully in the treatment of congestive thyroid orbitopathy. They may improve soft-tissue involvement and compressive optic neuropathy but usually have little effect on strabismus and are not useful for chronic fibrotic thyroid ophthalmopathy. Possible indications for the use of corticosteroids include (1) acute severe signs and symptoms of orbital inflammation of recent (less than 3 months) onset; (2) optic neuropathy, especially when used in conjunction with surgical decompression of the orbit or orbital radiation therapy; (3) prevention of progressive thyroid orbitopathy during the treatment of thyroid disease with radioactive iodine; and (4) control of signs and symptoms of thyroid orbitopathy that worsen despite previous orbital radiation and/or decompression. Corticosteroids may improve the orbitopathy in approximately 50 to 60% of patients, but the orbitopathy often worsens when the dosage of medication is reduced or discontinued. Chronic corticosteroid therapy is discouraged in thyroid ophthalmopathy patients because of the multiple ill effects of the medication. In general, corticosteroids are a valuable temporizing measure for thyroid orbitopathy but rarely provide meaningful long-term benefit or resolution of the disorder.

Radiation therapy, like corticosteroids, is most effective within the first year of onset of thyroid orbitopathy before significant fibrotic changes have occurred in orbital tissues. Possible indications for orbital radiation include (1) optic neuropathy, especially if the patient is a poor surgical candidate; and (2) symptoms of active orbital inflammation and congestion.

Optic neuropathy with thyroid ophthalmopathy is usually caused by apical compression of the optic nerve by enlarged EOMs and can cause permanent visual loss. Medical treatment possibilities include high doses of oral or intravenous corticosteroids, orbital irradiation, or a combination of these procedures.

72.5 Surgical Management

In general, the major clinical problems in patients with thyroid ophthalmopathy include a congestive orbitopathy with eye irritation and inflammation, diplopia, visual loss from corneal exposure or compressive optic neuropathy, and cosmesis.

The clinical manifestations of the acute phase may be responsive, at least partially, to systemic corticosteroid treatment, other immunosuppressives, and orbital radiation therapy. Therapy during the acute period is mainly directed at local measures to protect the eyes from exposure and provide comfort while awaiting spontaneous stabilization of the disease process. The acute phase is followed by a chronic phase, characterized by hypertrophy and fibrosis of the EOMs, lacrimal glands, and orbital fat. The clinical manifestations of this late phase do not regress spontaneously, are usually unresponsive to immunotherapy or radiation, and often require surgical correction for relief.

EOM surgery in patients with thyroid ophthalmopathy should be postponed until the muscles are no longer inflamed and the deviation has remained stable for at least 6 months. Eyelid retraction in patients with thyroid ophthalmopathy may result from excessive sympathetic activity, levator fibrosis, or contracture of the inferior rectus muscle. The lid retraction may be controlled by botulinum toxin injection into the levator palpebrae superioris muscle. Surgical procedures are available to improve eyelid retraction with options including lateral tarsorrhaphy, Müller's muscle and levator muscle lengthening, lower eyelid elevation, and blepharoplasty with orbital fat excision. Orbital decompression may improve lid retraction that is due to distortion from the proptotic globe. Strabismus surgery may relieve the compensatory component of lid retraction related to restrictive EOMs but recessions of the inferior rectus muscle often worsen the eyelid retraction. Therefore, the order of surgery in a patient with thyroid ophthalmopathy requiring all three procedures should in general be orbital decompression followed by strabismus surgery followed by lid surgery. Patients who fail medical treatment of optic neuropathy in thyroid disease may require orbital decompression.

72.6 Rehabilitation and Follow-up

The patient must understand that the treatment of thyroid ophthalmopathy usually extends over several years and that often a sequence of treatments is warranted. A team approach is necessary with input from endocrinology, ophthalmology, and other clinical specialties. The patient must have close ophthalmologic supervision to monitor for corneal epithelial breakdown that would require more aggressive treatments (e.g., surgical tarsorrhaphy). Visual acuity, color vision, fields, and fundus must be observed closely for signs of optic neuropathy.

Suggested Reading

[1] Bartley GB. The epidemiologic characteristics and clinical course of ophthalmopathy associated with autoimmune thyroid disease in Olmsted County, Minnesota. Trans Am Ophthalmol Soc. 1994; 92:477–588

[2] Bartley GB, Gorman CA. Diagnostic criteria for Graves' ophthalmopathy. Am J Ophthalmol. 1995; 119(6):792–795

[3] Bartley GB, Fatourechi V, Kadrmas EF, et al. Chronology of Graves' ophthalmopathy in an incidence cohort. Am J Ophthalmol. 1996; 121(4): 426–434

[4] Bartley GB, Fatourechi V, Kadrmas EF, et al. Clinical features of Graves' ophthalmopathy in an incidence cohort. Am J Ophthalmol. 1996; 121(3):284–290

[5] Bartley GB, Fatourechi V, Kadrmas EF, et al. The incidence of Graves' ophthalmopathy in Olmsted County, Minnesota. Am J Ophthalmol. 1995; 120(4): 511–517

[6] Carter KD, Frueh BR, Hessburg TP, Musch DC. Long-term efficacy of orbital decompression for compressive optic neuropathy of Graves' eye disease. Ophthalmology. 1991; 98(9):1435–1442

[7] Char DH. Advances in thyroid orbitopathy. Neuroophthalmology. 1992; 12: 25–39

[8] Garrity JA, Fatourechi V, Bergstralh EJ, et al. Results of transantral orbital decompression in 428 patients with severe Graves' ophthalmopathy. Am J Ophthalmol. 1993; 116(5):533–547

[9] Lee AG, Brazis PW. Clinical Pathways in Neuro-Ophthalmology: An Evidence-Based Approach. New York, NY: Thieme; 1998:269–285

[10] Lee AG, Mckenzie BA, Miller NR, et al. Long-term results of orbital decompression in thyroid eye disease. Orbit. 1995; 14:59–70

[11] Prummel MF, Wiersinga WM. Medical management of Graves' ophthalmopathy. Thyroid. 1995; 5(3):231–234

[12] Vargas ME, Warren FA, Kupersmith MJ. Exotropia as a sign of myasthenia gravis in dysthyroid ophthalmopathy. Br J Ophthalmol. 1993; 77(12):822–823

73 Anisocoria—Tonic Pupil

Sushma Yalamanchili and Andrew G. Lee

Abstract

A 45-year-old woman was noted to have one pupil larger than the other by a friend. On exam, she had anisocoria greater in the light than the dark, light-near dissociation, and vermiform movements of one sector of the iris to light consistent with a tonic pupil.

Keywords: tonic pupil, Adie's pupil, anisocoria, dilated pupil, light-near dissociation, anisocoria greater in the light, vermiform movements

73.1 History

A 45-year-old woman was evaluated because of anisocoria. While at a cocktail party 2 weeks ago, a friend noted that one pupil was larger than the other, and she feared that "it could be due to a brain tumor." She complained of occasional headaches over the last several years but denied any other illnesses, significant head or eye trauma, the use of any eye drops, or any visual symptoms. She went to see a neurosurgeon who performed a magnetic resonance imaging (MRI) of the brain that was normal and stated that she may need a cerebral angiogram.

Examination revealed visual acuity to be 20/20 bilaterally. Color vision and visual fields were normal. The right pupil measured 6 mm in darkness, while the left pupil measured 3 mm. The right pupil reacted poorly and segmentally to light (▶ Fig. 73.1), while the left pupil reacted briskly and symmetrically to light. The right pupil slowly constricted to near and then slowly redilated on looking in the distance. The left pupil constricted briskly to near and quickly redilated at distance. Motility was normal and there was no ptosis. Slit-lamp exam revealed vermiform movements of one sector of the right iris to light. Fundus exam was normal.

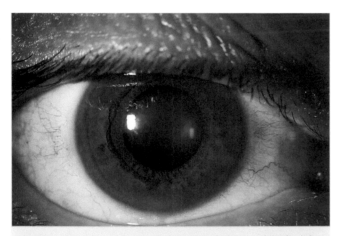

Fig. 73.1 The right pupil measured 6 mm in darkness, while the left pupil measured 3 mm. The right pupil reacted poorly and segmentally to light.

Differential Diagnosis—Key Points

1. If a large pupil is poorly reactive to light and the visual afferent system is normal, then a defect in the efferent parasympathetic innervation of the pupil is likely. The major entities causing an abnormal large pupil include third nerve palsy, iris damage, pharmacologic dilation, or tonic pupil.

2. In the absence of an extraocular motility deficit and ptosis, an isolated dilated pupil is rarely due to a third nerve palsy.

3. Careful slit-lamp biomicroscopy of the iris should be performed in all patients with anisocoria to exclude structural iris abnormalities or damage. No such damage was noted in this patient.

4. A careful history is usually all that is required in patients with inadvertent or intentional exposure to agents that may affect pupil size (e.g., scopolamine patch). The pupil size of patients with pharmacologic blockade is often quite large, of the order of 10 to 12 mm in diameter, which is much greater than the mydriasis usually noted in patients with third nerve palsy or a tonic pupil. Usually, the mydriasis of pharmacologic agents affects the pupil completely in 360 degrees, as compared to the segmental paresis of the pupil in tonic pupils. A pupil dilated from a third nerve palsy or tonic pupil will constrict to pilocarpine 1%, while a pharmacologically blocked pupil will not constrict or will constrict only partially to pilocarpine 1%.

5. The anisocoria is, thus, mostly likely due to a tonic pupil. Tonic pupils may be due to local (ocular or orbital) lesions affecting the ciliary ganglion or nerve (e.g., trauma), may be due to diffuse neuropathic processes, or may be idiopathic (Adie's tonic pupil syndrome). The clinical features of a tonic pupil are outlined in **the list below**. Pharmacologic testing with low-dose pilocarpine (0.125–0.1%) may demonstrate cholinergic supersensitivity in the tonic pupil.

73.1.1 Clinical Features of a Tonic Pupil

- Poor pupillary light reaction.
- Vermiform movements of the iris to light on slit-lamp exam.
- Segmental palsy of the sphincter.
- Tonic pupillary near response with light-near dissociation.
- Cholinergic supersensitivity of the denervated muscles (e.g., to dilute pilocarpine).
- Accommodative paresis (that tends to recover).
- Induced astigmatism at near.
- Tonicity of accommodation.
- Occasional ciliary cramp with near work.

(Adapted from Lee AG, Brazis PW. Clinical Pathways in Neuro-Ophthalmology: An Evidence-Based Approach. New York, NY: Thieme, 1998:362, with permission.)

73.2 Test Interpretation

Slit-lamp biomicroscopy revealed no iris injury but did show vermiform, segmental movements of the iris characteristic of a tonic pupil. The denervated iris sphincter is supersensitive to topical parasympathomimetic solutions. Pilocarpine drops (0.125%) can be used to demonstrate this, as the normal pupil will constrict slightly, if at all. After 60 minutes, the pupils are reexamined, and if Adie is present, the affected pupil (dilated pupil) will constrict more than the normal pupil (this supersensitivity is often not present for the first several weeks after onset). Patients with bilateral isolated tonic pupils should have serologic testing for syphilis.

73.3 Diagnosis

Isolated, idiopathic tonic pupil.

73.4 Medical and Surgical Management

There are no proven roles for medical and surgical management of this problem.

73.5 Rehabilitation and Follow-up

No treatment, except reassurance, is usually required. Unequal bifocal reading aids or a unilateral frosted bifocal segment may be used in patients with permanent accommodative paresis. The initially mydriatic pupil may become smaller over time ("little old Adie's"). Although most Adie's tonic pupils present unilaterally, bilateral involvement may develop at a rate of 4% per year. Holmes–Adie syndrome includes other features, notably diminished deep tendon reflexes and orthostatic hypotension, and should be addressed in patients with tonic pupils.

Suggested Reading

[1] Kardon RH, Corbett JJ, Thompson HS. Segmental denervation and reinnervation of the iris sphincter as shown by infrared videographic transillumination. Ophthalmology. 1998; 105(2):313–321

[2] Lee AG, Brazis PW. Clinical Pathways in Neuro-Ophthalmology: An Evidence-Based Approach. New York, NY: Thieme; 1998:357–388

[3] Loewenfeld IE, Thompson HS. The tonic pupil: a re-evaluation. Am J Ophthalmol. 1967; 63(1):46–87

[4] Thompson HS. Segmental palsy of the iris sphincter in Adie's syndrome. Arch Ophthalmol. 1978; 96(9):1615–1620

[5] Thompson S, Pilley SFJ. Unequal pupils. A flow chart for sorting out the anisocorias. Surv Ophthalmol. 1976; 21(1):45–48

74 Anisocoria—Horner's Syndrome

Sushma Yalamanchili and Andrew G. Lee

Abstract

A 50-year-old man with a past medical history of hypertension presented with left frontotemporal and periorbital headaches for the last 3 weeks and drooping of his left upper eyelid. On exam, he had anisocoria greater in the dark and 2 mm of left ptosis. Topical cocaine 10% into both eyes revealed marked dilation of the right pupil, but poor dilation of the left pupil. Four days later, hydroxyamphetamine 1% was instilled in both eyes and resulted in full dilation in the right eye but poor dilation in the left eye, consistent with a postganglionic Horner's syndrome due to spontaneous dissection of the internal carotid artery.

Keywords: Horner's syndrome, anisocoria, carotid artery dissection, miosis, anhydrosis, ptosis, anisocoria greater in the dark, cocaine, hydroxyamphetamine

74.1 History

A 50-year-old man noted the onset of left frontotemporal and periorbital headaches for the last 3 weeks. He denied any visual complaints but noted some drooping of his left upper eyelid. He denied any diplopia, trauma to his head or neck, facial numbness or weakness, or other neurologic complaints. He had a history of systemic hypertension.

Examination revealed visual acuity of 20/20 bilaterally with normal color vision. Pupils measured in bright light were 4 mm on the right and 3 mm on the left, but immediately after the lights were turned off, the pupils were noted to be 5 and 3 mm, respectively (▸ Fig. 74.1). Both pupils reacted well to light and near, and there was no relative afferent pupillary defect. Visual fields were normal. Motility was normal. There was 2 mm of left ptosis. Facial sensation and movement were normal. Slit-lamp examination and fundus exam were unremarkable.

The instillation of topical cocaine 10% into both eyes revealed marked dilation of the right pupil, but poor dilation of the left pupil (noted in darkness 45 minutes after two drops instilled in both eyes). The patient returned 4 days later and hydroxyam-phetamine 1% (Paredrine) was instilled in both eyes and resulted in full dilation in the right eye but poor dilation in the left eye.

1. In a patient with anisocoria but normal pupil reaction, the main differential is between a Horner's syndrome (HS) and physiologic anisocoria. The left ptosis strongly favors a left HS but there are many cases reported of a "pseudo-Horner's syndrome" in which physiologic anisocoria is associated with some other unrelated cause of ptosis (e.g., levator dehiscence). Simple or physiologic anisocoria has a prevalence as high as 21% in the general population and is associated with equal anisocoria in light and darkness.

2. Topical cocaine 10% will dilate both pupils equally with physiologic anisocoria but will not dilate or will poorly dilate the pupil in a patient with HS. Thus, cocaine testing is necessary to prove the existence of an HS. Cocaine inhibits the reuptake of norepinephrine at the neuromuscular junction. Therefore, topical cocaine will dilate a normal pupil but will not dilate a pupil with HS regardless of the location of the sympathetic damage.

3. HS may result from a lesion anywhere along the three-neuron pathway that arises as a first-order (central) neuron from the posterolateral hypothalamus, then descends in the brainstem and lateral columns of the spinal cord to exit at the cervical (C8) and thoracic (T1–T2) levels (ciliospinal center of Budge) of the spinal cord as a second-order neuron. This second-order (intermediate) preganglionic neuron exits the ventral root and arches over the apex of the lung to ascend in the cervical sympathetic chain. The second-order neurons synapse in the superior cervical ganglion and exit as a third-order neuron. The third-order postganglionic neuron travels with the carotid artery into the cavernous sinus, on to the sixth cranial nerve for a short course, and then travels with the ophthalmic division of the trigeminal nerve to join the nasociliary branch of the

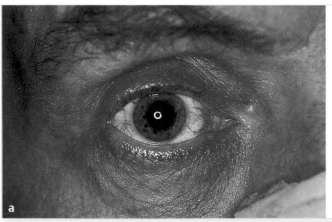 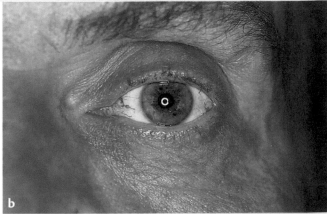

Fig. 74.1 (a) Right pupil and (b) left pupil showing anisocoria and mild left ptosis and mild upside down ptosis.

trigeminal nerve, pass through the ciliary ganglion, and reach the eye as long and short ciliary nerves. Damage anywhere along this sympathetic pathway will result in an HS.

4. Patients with central or first-order HS usually have associated signs of hypothalamic or brainstem dysfunction. Preganglionic (intermediate) HS patients may have neck or arm pain, anhidrosis involving the face and neck, brachial plexopathy, vocal cord paralysis, or phrenic nerve palsy. A second-order HS may also occur in isolation. Important etiologies of a second-order HS include neoplasms (e.g., apical lung cancer or infiltrative breast cancer), mediastinal lymphadenopathy, cervicothoracic abnormalities (e.g., disc disease), neck or shoulder trauma, thoracic aneurysm, or local infections or inflammations. Postganglionic (third-order) HS may occur in isolation but may also occur with eye pain (e.g., cluster headache) or palsies of the third, fourth, sixth, and ophthalmic division trigeminal nerves (e.g., cavernous sinus thrombosis, infection, or neoplasm). Etiologies of third-order HS include high cervical lymphadenopathy, otitis and petrositis, trauma, and vascular abnormalities of the internal carotid artery (e.g., carotid artery aneurysm or dissection). Dissection of the internal carotid artery, either spontaneous or posttraumatic, may result in a postganglionic HS. The HS in these cases may occur in isolation but is often associated with other features including ipsilateral orbital, facial, or neck pain, diplopia from cavernous sinus involvement, transient ischemic attacks (e.g., transient ipsilateral visual loss), retinal artery occlusion or ischemic optic neuropathy, neck bruit or swelling, and other cranial neuropathies.

5. Hydroxyamphetamine 1% (Paredrine) releases the stored norepinephrine from postganglionic adrenergic nerve endings at the dilator muscle of the pupil. Therefore, a preganglionic HS (with intact postganglionic third-order neuron) will dilate after administration of topical hydroxyamphetamine 1%, while a postganglionic HS pupil will not dilate (no norepinephrine stores). The Paredrine test cannot be performed on the same day as the cocaine test.

6. Cocaine drops are most commonly used (but are now difficult to obtain). Apraclonidine drops (used for glaucoma; off-label application) are now replacing cocaine for the diagnosis of HS because they are easy to obtain. Testing with apraclonidine involves instillation of two drops of 0.5 or 1% apraclonidine in both eyes. After 30 to 45 minutes, a normal pupil does not dilate, while a Horner pupil dilates and the anisocoria reverses and the palpebral fissure enlarges. Apraclonidine is a direct α-receptor agonist (strong α2 and weak α1). It has no effect in eyes with intact sympathetic innervation but causes mild pupillary dilation in eyes with sympathetic denervation regardless of the lesion location.

74.2 Test Interpretation

The response to eye drops in this patient was consistent with a postganglionic (third-order) HS, and in the setting of headache, neuroimaging was performed of the brain and cervical region and magnetic resonance (MR) angiography of the carotid artery. MR angiography revealed a dissecting aneurysm affecting the high cervical carotid artery. An etiology of all cases of HS must be aggressively sought depending on response to eye drops, associated neurologic or medical symptoms, and the clinical situation. An isolated second-order HS may, for example, be the first sign of a lung neoplasm.

74.3 Diagnosis

Postganglionic HS due to spontaneous dissection of the internal carotid artery.

74.4 Medical Management

HS per se requires no treatment. The etiology of the HS must be treated. The patient in this case was treated for 3 months with Coumadin and afterward was maintained on aspirin.

74.5 Surgical Management

No surgical treatment is indicated.

74.6 Rehabilitation and Follow-up

Cases in which no etiology is evident require close observation to investigate for the development of other neurologic or medical signs or symptoms.

Suggested Reading

[1] Biousse V, Touboul P-J, D'Anglejan-Chatillon J, Lévy C, Schaison M, Bousser MG. Ophthalmologic manifestations of internal carotid artery dissection. Am J Ophthalmol. 1998; 126(4):565–577

[2] Donahue SP, Lavin PJM, Digre K. False-negative hydroxyamphetamine (Paredrine) test in acute Horner's syndrome. Am J Ophthalmol. 1996; 122(6):900–901

[3] Keane JR. Oculosympathetic paresis. Analysis of 100 hospitalized patients. Arch Neurol. 1979; 36(1):13–15

[4] Lee AG, Brazis PW. Clinical Pathways in Neuro-Ophthalmology: An Evidence-Based Approach. New York, NY: Thieme; 1998:357–388

[5] Pilley SFJ, Thompson HS. Pupillary "dilatation lag" in Horner's syndrome. Br J Ophthalmol. 1975; 59(12):731–735

[6] Thompson BM, Corbett JJ, Kline LB, Thompson HS. Pseudo-Horner's syndrome. Arch Neurol. 1982; 39(2):108–111

[7] Kawasaki A. Disorders of pupillary function, accommodation, and lacrimation. In: Miller NR, Newman NJ, Biousse V, Kerrison JB, eds. Walsh and Hoyt's Clinical Neuro-Ophthalmology. 6th ed. Philadelphia, PA: Lippincott, Williams, and Wilkins; 2005:739–805

75 Anisocoria—Eye Drops

Sushma Yalamanchili and Andrew G. Lee

Abstract

A 24-year-old student nurse was referred for long-standing headaches, blurred vision, and anisocoria. Pupils were 8 mm on the right and 4 mm on the left. The right pupil did not react to light or near, while the left pupil reacted briskly to light and near. The pupil did not constrict to dilute pilocarpine eye drops because of pharmacologic mydriasis.

Keywords: eye drops, pharmacologic pupil, anisocoria, dilute pilocarpine, headache, blurred vision, nurse, pharmacologic mydriasis

75.1 History

A 24-year-old student nurse was referred for headaches and anisocoria. The headaches had been present for several years, but had been worse over the last few months. They occurred daily, were diffuse in nature, and were not associated with nausea or vomiting. Because of the headaches, she saw a neurologist who noted anisocoria, and she was thus sent for ophthalmologic examination. She states that her vision was always "blurry," especially with her headaches. She denied diplopia or other eye problems. She was taking medications only for her headaches.

Examination revealed visual acuity to be 20/20 bilaterally. She identified 10 of 10 Hardy–Rand–Rittler pseudoisochromatic plates bilaterally. Visual fields were full. Pupils were 8 mm on the right (▶ Fig. 75.1) and 4 mm on the left. The right pupil did not react to light or near, while the left pupil reacted briskly to light and near. No relative afferent pupillary defect was documented. Motility was normal and there was no ptosis. Facial sensation and strength were normal. Slit-lamp exam revealed both pupils to be smoothly round without irregularities, and there was no segmental contraction of the right pupil to light. Fundus exam was normal with no disc swelling noted.

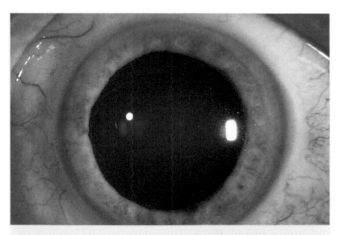

Fig. 75.1 The pupil measured 8 mm on the right and did not react to light or near.

Differential Diagnosis—Key Points

1. Presence of a unilateral large, nonreactive pupil raises several possibilities, including a right third nerve palsy, tonic pupil, iris damage, or pharmacologic mydriasis. The normal motility and absence of ptosis argue strongly against a third nerve palsy. The absence of pupillary irregularity and the absence of visible structural iris abnormality on slit-lamp examination argue against iris damage. There is no tonicity of the near response or segmental sphincter palsy suggestive of a tonic pupil. The most likely etiology of the anisocoria is thus pharmacologic mydriasis.

2. Nurses, physicians, and other health care workers are particularly prone to inadvertent or intentional exposure to pharmacologic mydriatics. The most common agents implicated in accidental exposure include sphincter blockers (such as belladonna alkaloids, scopolamine patches, anticholinergic inhalants, topical gentamicin, or lidocaine) or dilator stimulators (e.g., ocular decongestants or adrenergic inhalants used in the intensive care setting).

3. The pupil size of patients with pharmacologic blockade is often quite large, usually greater than 8 mm and often 10 to 12 mm in diameter, which is much greater than the mydriasis seen with third nerve palsy or tonic pupil syndrome. The pupil is usually smoothly dilated over the entire 360-degree circumference and no pupillary irregularities are noted.

75.2 Test Interpretation

A pharmacologic dilated pupil will not constrict to dilute pilocarpine (vs. a tonic pupil) and will constrict poorly or not at all to pilocarpine 1% (vs. third nerve palsy). Over time with observation alone, the pupil will return to normal size.

75.3 Diagnosis

Pharmacologic mydriasis.

75.4 Medical Management

No treatment is required except discussion concerning the findings, possible etiologic agents, and reassurance.

75.5 Surgical Management

No surgical treatment is indicated.

75.6 Rehabilitation and Follow-Up

Follow-up to ensure resolution of the symptoms is reasonable.

Suggested Reading

[1] Brazis PW, Lee AG. Neuro-ophthalmic problems caused by medications. American Academy Ophthalmology-Focal Points. 1998; 16(11)

[2] Goldstein JB, Biousse V, Newman NJ. Unilateral pharmacologic mydriasis in a patient with respiratory compromise. Arch Ophthalmol. 1997; 115(6):806

[3] Lee AG, Brazis PW. Clinical Pathways in Neuro-Ophthalmology: An Evidence-Based Approach. New York, NY: Thieme; 1998;357–388

[4] Thompson HS, Newsome DA, Loewenfeld IE. The fixed dilated pupil. Sudden iridoplegia or mydriatic drops? A simple diagnostic test. Arch Ophthalmol. 1971; 86(1):21–27

Part X

Pediatrics

X

76 Leukocoria

Tatyana Beketova and Dan S. Gombos

Abstract

Retinoblastoma is an ominous cause of leukocoria in young children. When a patient develops leukocoria and retinoblastoma is suspected, an exam under anesthesia followed by magnetic resonance imaging (MRI) should be performed. Genetic testing assists in prognosis and treatment strategies. Retinoblastoma management involves chemotherapy followed by focal surgical techniques, such as laser and cryotherapy. Enucleation may be preferred in advanced or relapsed cases. Frequent follow-up examinations are necessary to monitor for tumor response and recurrence. Patients with hereditary retinoblastoma should have long-term follow-up due to an increased risk of secondary malignancies, particularly soft-tissue and bony sarcomas.

Keywords: leukocoria, retinoblastoma, Coats' disease, persistent fetal vasculature, RB1 gene, Chemotherapy, Cryotherapy, laser therapy, enucleation

76.1 History

The family of a 9-month-old girl noted that her left eye has looked "funny" for the last 3 months. The girl's pediatrician detected leukocoria and immediately referred her to an ophthalmologist for evaluation and treatment. The child is an otherwise healthy 9-month-old with a negative review of systems with the exception of the white pupil. She was born 2 weeks prematurely and had a birth weight of 6 lb., 8 oz. There is no history of systemic disease or exposure to animals, and there is no family history of childhood ocular disease.

Examination reveals a normal right eye, though only the posterior pole can be seen on retinal examination. In the left eye, a white, vascular lesion is obvious with a surrounding large serous retinal detachment (▶ Fig. 76.1 and ▶ Fig. 76.2). The child fixes and follows well with her right eye, but does not fix or follow with her left eye. Strong objection to occlusion of the right eye is noted.

Differential Diagnosis—Key Points

1. When leukocoria is noted on ophthalmologic examination, an extensive differential diagnosis must be considered. Almost all of the conditions that produce leukocoria in a child are serious vision- or life-threatening problems. Leukocoria is therefore an urgent ophthalmologic problem.

2. Retinoblastoma is the most ominous cause of leukocoria. It is the most common intraocular malignancy of childhood, occurring in approximately 1 in 18,000 to 20,000 live births.[1] In the United States, there are an estimated 300 to 350 new cases per year. Most are diagnosed prior to the age of 5 years, but retinoblastoma has been reported in teenage children and adults.[2] The condition may be unilateral or bilateral, and there is no race or gender predilection.[3] The most common presenting signs include leukocoria, strabismus, poor vision, and family history of retinoblastoma.[4] Other less common presenting signs include vitreous hemorrhage, pain, microphthalmus, and orbital cellulitis.[5] Retinoblastoma is classified based on the location and extent of the tumor according to the International Classification for Intraocular Retinoblastoma (ABC or "Murphree" Classification).[6,7]

3. Coats' disease is another cause of leukocoria. It is typically unilateral and more common in boys. The condition is characterized by an exudative retinal detachment with associated telangiectatic retinal vessels and subretinal lipid exudation.[8] Coats' disease can usually, but not always, be differentiated from retinoblastoma on clinical examination alone.

4. Persistent fetal vasculature (PFV) can present with leukocoria, which on initial examination resembles an extensive retinoblastoma. The anterior portion of the lens is clear and an associated cataract, which is at the level of the posterior capsule, is stark white and vascular. Eyes with PFV tend to have a shorter axial length than normal, a feature that is uncommon in retinoblastoma.[8] The correct diagnosis can usually be made with careful ophthalmologic examination and ultrasound.

5. Numerous other conditions are included in the differential diagnosis of leukocoria, including advanced retinopathy of prematurity with cicatricial retinal detachment, toxocariasis, large chorioretinal colobomas, uveitis, extensive medullated nerve fibers, and other types of cataracts.

6. Genetics of retinoblastoma: Most patients with retinoblastoma are karyotypically normal. However, 5 to 6% of retinoblastoma patients will have a chromosome 13q14 deletion or translocation, resulting in 13q deletion syndrome.[9] Features of this syndrome include developmental delay and structural facial anomalies. Hereditary and nonhereditary cases of retinoblastoma exist. Hereditary forms present in all cases of bilateral retinoblastoma or in cases of multiple affected family members, and are confirmed with genetic testing of the *RB1* gene. Genetic testing is crucial for assessing short-term risk (additional eye tumors) and long-term prognosis (nonocular secondary malignancies) while providing cost-effective treatment and surveillance strategies. It should routinely be performed in all retinoblastoma patients.[10] Examination of siblings and parents of an affected patient is important to rule out active retinoblastoma and/or evidence of regressed disease.

76.2 Test Interpretation

The major diagnostic considerations in this child are to determine the extent of local disease, to rule out contralateral involvement, and assess if extraocular spread has occurred.

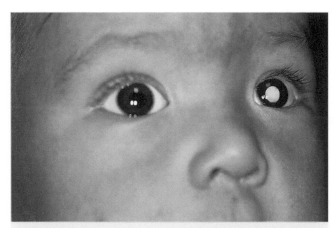

Fig. 76.1 Clinical photograph of the patient demonstrating leukocoria of the left eye.

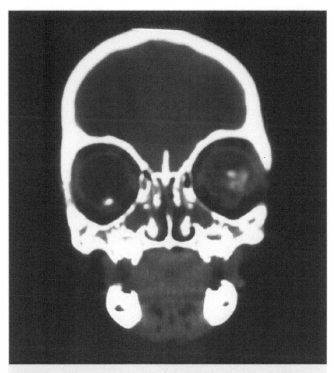

Fig. 76.2 CT scan of the of brain and orbit demonstrating bilateral involvement of retinoblastoma, left eye greater than right.

1. A magnetic resonance imaging (MRI) scan of the head and orbits is performed in all newly diagnosed retinoblastoma patients. The most important role of MRI is to assess for extraocular extension.[11] The presence of calcium in an intraocular lesion noted on exam or ultrasound in a child younger than 3 years is highly suggestive of retinoblastoma. Computed tomography (CT) was previously used primarily to confirm intraocular calcification, but ultrasound and MRI have similar sensitivity and avoid radiation exposure.[12,13] An MRI scan is also useful in detecting extraocular orbital extension, and central nervous system involvement due to either metastases or the presence of a pineal tumor (so-called trilateral retinoblastoma).

2. Ultrasound testing can offer both diagnostic and therapeutic assistance. Calcium may be detected on B-scan ultrasonography. A-scan ultrasonography is useful in determining the height of the tumor. Both are valuable in monitoring treatment response particularly if the tumor is to be treated with local measures such as plaque radiation.[14]

3. Other testing: All patients affected with retinoblastoma should undergo genetic counseling and a general physical examination. Bone marrow and cerebrospinal fluid evaluation are rarely utilized and only done in select cases when extraocular extension is suspected.[15] The enucleated eye should be submitted for pathologic examination, and genetic testing of the tumor performed.

4. Examination of the eyes under anesthesia was performed and demonstrated a massive tumor with retinal detachment in the left eye (▶ Fig. 76.3). In addition, a small tumor was noted in the inferior retina of the right eye.

76.3 Diagnosis

Bilateral retinoblastoma.

76.4 Medical Management

Chemotherapy is the most common form of medical management for retinoblastoma, and is usually used in conjunction with local surgical measures, such as laser or cryotherapy. There are four routes of chemotherapy delivery—intravenous, intra-arterial, periocular, and intravitreal. Intravenous chemotherapy is generally used for hereditary (advanced bilateral) retinoblastomas with a moderate to good prognosis and in patients at high risk of metastases. Intra-arterial chemotherapy allows for excellent control in nonhereditary cases, and is also used for recurrent disease, subretinal seeds, and vitreous seeds. Periocular chemotherapy is employed to boost local chemotherapy dose in advanced retinoblastoma. Intravitreal chemotherapy is used for recurrent or persistent vitreous seeds.[16]

76.5 Surgical Management

Examination under anesthesia is almost always required to fully evaluate infants and young children with retinoblastoma or suspected retinoblastoma.[17] This case highlights the importance of examination under anesthesia in that the tumor in the right eye was not detected on clinical office examination, where only the posterior pole could be readily examined.

While patients with retinoblastoma can be managed medically in many cases, enucleation of an eye with extensive tumor and no visual potential is still the treatment of choice.[17] This patient should undergo enucleation of the left eye using meticulous technique in an attempt to obtain a long optic nerve segment since the tumor tends to spread by direct extension into the optic nerve. ▶ Fig. 76.4 shows the gross and microscopic appearance of an eye with retinoblastoma. The right eye can be approached with both medical and surgical modalities. The potential surgical treatments include cryotherapy, laser therapy, and radioactive plaque treatment.[17]

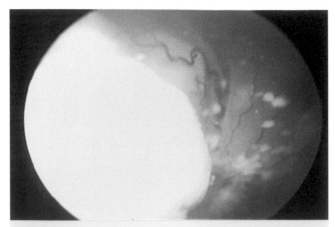

Fig. 76.3 Large retinoblastoma with vitreous seeding and exudative retinal detachment.

76.6 Rehabilitation and Follow-up

Recurrence of the tumor can occur in the orbit even if the cut margin of the optic nerve is free of disease. The physician should, therefore, examine the enucleated socket each time he or she examines the contralateral eye. Following local control of the tumor in this child's right eye, follow-up examinations under anesthesia should be conducted every 3 to 4 months until the child is 5 years of age if the genetic testing confirms an *RB1* germline mutation. Frequent examinations must continue for several more years and an annual eye examination is prudent thereafter. Long-term safety issues include protecting the remaining eye with the use of polycarbonate safety glasses and providing patient education on eye safety. These measures are important in all monocular patients. Patients with hereditary retinoblastoma have a high incidence of secondary tumors, particularly soft-tissue and bony sarcomas of the extremities, and should be followed long term with these risk factors in mind.[18]

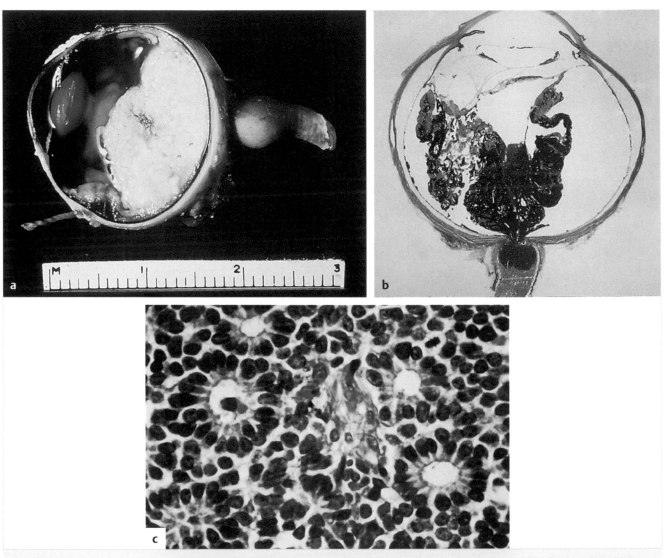

Fig. 76.4 (a) Gross appearance of retinoblastoma. Note long segment of optic nerve obtained at the time of enucleation. (b) Large retinoblastoma with invasion of the optic nerve. (c) Histologic example of retinoblastoma demonstrating Flexner–Wintersteiner rosettes. (Photos courtesy of Ramon L. Font, MD, Houston, TX.)

Suggested Reading

[1] Hurwitz RL, Shields CL, Shields JA, et al. Retinoblastoma. In: Principles and Practice of Pediatric Oncology. 6th ed. Philadelphia, PA: Lippincott Williams & Wilkins; 2010:809–837

[2] Mallipatna A, Marino M, Singh AD. Genetics of retinoblastoma. Asia Pac J Ophthalmol (Phila). 2016; 5(4):260–264

References

[1] Howlader NNA, Krapcho M, et al. SEER Cancer Statistics Review. Surveillance, epidemiology, and end results program. April 2016. Available at: https://seer.cancer.gov/csr/1975_2013/. Accessed January 15, 2017

[2] Melamud A, Palekar R, Singh A. Retinoblastoma. Am Fam Physician. 2006; 73 (6):1039–1044

[3] Broaddus E, Topham A, Singh AD. Incidence of retinoblastoma in the USA: 1975–2004. Br J Ophthalmol. 2009; 93(1):21–23

[4] Abramson DH, Beaverson K, Sangani P, et al. Screening for retinoblastoma: presenting signs as prognosticators of patient and ocular survival. Pediatrics. 2003; 112(6, Pt 1):1248–1255

[5] Abramson DH, Frank CM, Susman M, Whalen MP, Dunkel IJ, Boyd NW, III. Presenting signs of retinoblastoma. J Pediatr. 1998; 132(3, Pt 1):505–508

[6] Balmer A, Zografos L, Munier F. Diagnosis and current management of retinoblastoma. Oncogene. 2006; 25(38):5341–5349

[7] Linn Murphree A. Intraocular retinoblastoma: the case for a new group classification. Ophthalmol Clin North Am. 2005; 18(1):41–53, viii

[8] Maki JL, Marr BP, Abramson DH. Diagnosis of retinoblastoma: how good are referring physicians? Ophthalmic Genet. 2009; 30(4):199–205

[9] Bojinova RI, Schorderet DF, Addor MC, et al. Further delineation of the facial 13q14 deletion syndrome in 13 retinoblastoma patients. Ophthalmic Genet. 2001; 22(1):11–18

[10] Mallipatna A, Marino M, Singh AD. Genetics of Retinoblastoma. Asia Pac J Ophthalmol (Phila). 2016; 5(4):260–264

[11] de Jong MC, de Graaf P, Noij DP, et al. European Retinoblastoma Imaging Collaboration (ERIC). Diagnostic performance of magnetic resonance imaging and computed tomography for advanced retinoblastoma: a systematic review and meta-analysis. Ophthalmology. 2014; 121(5):1109–1118

[12] Galluzzi P, Hadjistilianou T, Cerase A, De Francesco S, Toti P, Venturi C. Is CT still useful in the study protocol of retinoblastoma? AJNR Am J Neuroradiol. 2009; 30(9):1760–1765

[13] Levy J, Frenkel S, Baras M, Neufeld M, Pe'er J. Calcification in retinoblastoma: histopathologic findings and statistical analysis of 302 cases. Br J Ophthalmol. 2011; 95(8):1145–1150

[14] Kendall CJ, Prager TC, Cheng H, Gombos D, Tang RA, Schiffman JS. Diagnostic Ophthalmic Ultrasound for Radiologists. Neuroimaging Clin N Am. 2015; 25 (3):327–365

[15] Bakhshi S, Meel R, Kashyap S, Sharma S. Bone marrow aspirations and lumbar punctures in retinoblastoma at diagnosis: correlation with IRSS staging. J Pediatr Hematol Oncol. 2011; 33(5):e182–e185

[16] Shields CL, Lally SE, Leahey AM, et al. Targeted retinoblastoma management: when to use intravenous, intra-arterial, periocular, and intravitreal chemotherapy. Curr Opin Ophthalmol. 2014; 25(5):374–385

[17] Lin P, O'Brien JM. Frontiers in the management of retinoblastoma. Am J Ophthalmol. 2009; 148(2):192–198

[18] Lohmann DR, Gallie BL. Retinoblastoma. In: Pagon RA, Adam MP, Ardinger HH, et al., eds. GeneReviews®. Seattle, WA: University of Washington, Seattle; 2015

77 The Child Who Sees Poorly Out of One Eye

David K. Coats

Abstract

A child who fails a school screening examination or is being evaluated for unexplained visual loss requires a complete history and examination to determine the etiology. Many causes are readily treatable but some may reflect underlying serious ocular pathology. Amblyopia can occur during the critical visual development period and also might be amenable to treatment if detected early.

Keywords: amblyopia, visual loss, screening

77.1 History

A 4-year-old boy failed his preschool vision screening test. The vision screening failure was confirmed by his pediatrician and he has been sent for ophthalmologic evaluation and treatment recommendations. The child is a robust 4-year-old with no history of medical or ophthalmologic problems. The review of systems is negative and, specifically there is no history of eye injury, strabismus, spectacle wear, squinting, or other ophthalmologic problems. The child has not previously had an ophthalmologic examination and there is no family history of amblyopia or childhood eye disease.

On examination, the technician found 20/40 vision in each eye with Allen figure testing. His stereoacuity is 60 seconds of ARC using the Titmus fly test. Motility evaluation reveals orthotropia at distance and an exophoria of 4 prism diopters at near with full ductions and versions. His cycloplegic refractive error following administration of 1% cyclopentolate is +3.00 in the right eye and +1.00 in the left eye. The ophthalmologist repeated the visual acuity testing using an HOTV acuity test and found a visual acuity of 20/50 in the right eye and 20/30 in the left eye.

Differential Diagnosis—Key Points

1. The majority of children who fail a school vision screening test will have a normal eye examination. However, as many as 25 to 30% of screening failures will have an ophthalmologic problem that can benefit from treatment. The differential diagnosis of poor vision in one eye includes amblyopia, uncorrected refractive error, a structural eye abnormality, and poor effort. Four causes of amblyopia must be considered including refractive, deprivational, strabismic, and idiopathic amblyopia (▶ Fig. 77.1a–c). Idiopathic amblyopia is probably amblyopia that occurred from one of the other causes, but which is now undetectable by physical examination.
2. Terminology: Before proceeding with the discussion on amblyopia, a review of some important amblyopia terminology is in order.
   a) *Occlusion amblyopia* is a term used to describe iatrogenic amblyopia that occurs in the sound eye as a result of wearing a patch to treat amblyopia in the fellow eye. This term should not be used to describe deprivational amblyopia such as that caused by a cataract or corneal opacities.
   b) *Foveal form vision deprivational amblyopia* is a term used to describe amblyopia caused by failure to produce a clear image on the fovea of the involved eye. It can be caused by media opacities and high refractive errors.
   c) *Abnormal binocular interaction* is a term used to describe a situation in which the image size or shape on the two foveas is so dissimilar that the images cannot be fused. One of the images is suppressed and amblyopia may develop. This type of amblyopia most commonly occurs due to uncorrected anisometropic refractive errors and strabismus. A combination of form vision deprivation and abnormal binocular interaction can coexist in some patients.
   d) *Anisometropic amblyopia* is amblyopia that develops on the basis of an unequal refractive error. In a hyperope, amblyopia usually develops in the most hyperopic eye. The condition is less common in children with myopia or astigmatism, but may occur when the refractive error is large.
   e) *Ametropic amblyopia* is bilateral amblyopia due to the presence of bilateral large refractive errors. It is most common with hyperopia, but may also occur with high myopia and astigmatism.
3. Refractive amblyopia is common. It most commonly occurs in one eye, but can occur in both eyes where it is called ametropic amblyopia. Because the eyes are usually straight when this condition is present and there are no other obvious abnormalities visible to the child's family, the condition is often not diagnosed until the child fails a vision screening examination either at school or in the pediatrician's office. Refractive amblyopia can occur with any type of refractive error but is more common with anisometropic hyperopia.
4. Strabismic amblyopia is also very common. It is most often seen with esotropia but can occur with any type of strabismus. It is least likely to occur with intermittent exotropia. The size of the strabismic deviation is unrelated to the presence or severity of amblyopia. Amblyopia is more likely to be detected early in children with large-angle strabismus because parents are readily able to detect large-angle strabismus prompting a visit to the ophthalmologist and subsequent diagnosis of amblyopia. Strabismic amblyopia typically responds well to treatment measures.
5. Deprivational amblyopia is the most serious form of amblyopia. It may occur in one or both eyes and is due to media opacities such as cataracts, corneal opacities, vitreous hemorrhage, and visual obstruction secondary to ptosis. Clearing of the visual axis with institution of amblyopia treatment measures such as occlusion is most likely to be successful if implemented within the first few months of life. Deprivational amblyopia can be recalcitrant to treatment.

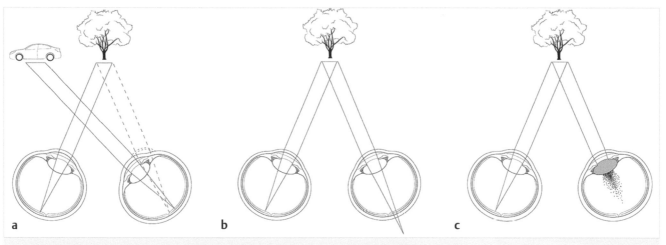

Fig. 77.1 Amblyopia can be caused by (a) strabismus; (b) refractive errors; (c) obstruction of the visual axis.

77.2 Test Interpretation

Psychophysical testing, which involves the use of recognition acuity tests such as HOTV testing and Snellen figure testing, is the most important means of detecting the presence of amblyopia and for monitoring the response to treatment. This child's examination results reveal a critically important feature of recognition acuity tests. Note that his vision was equal in the two eyes on Allen figure testing, but was reduced in the right eye on HOTV testing. Allen figure testing tends to overestimate visual acuity in children with amblyopia. Therefore, Allen figure testing should be supplemented with another test such as a fixation preference test or not used at all, and the child should be tested with a more sophisticated test such as the E game, Landolt ring test, or Snellen acuity test as soon as the child is able to cooperate. Young children are often not able to cooperate well enough to read the 20/20 line, but should have equal vision in the two eyes.

The "rule of 8's" has been proposed as a simple tool to determine if the measured screening visual acuity is typical for younger children. The premise is simple and is both verbally and graphically described as follows. For children 2 through 6 years of age, the child's age plus the first number of the denominator of the average visual acuity should equal 8. Take, for example, a 3-year-old child. Using the "rule of 8," a vision screener would subtract the child's age in years (3) from the number 8, in this case yielding 5. Thus, the expected visual acuity for a 3-year-old child is 20/**5**0. If the visual acuity is worse than 20/50, there should be a high degree of concern, and this child should be referred for further evaluation (▶ Table 77.1).

Table 77.1 The rule of 8: expected visual acuity performance by age

Age in years	Expected visual acuity	(Rule of 8)
2	20/60	(2 + 6) = 8
3	20/50	(3 + 5) = 8
4	20/40	(4 + 4) = 8
5	20/30	(5 + 3) = 8
6	20/20	(6 + 2) = 8

Used with permission from Amit R. Bhatt, MD.

Fixation behavior, fixation preference, and occlusion objection may be the only means of detecting amblyopia in small children without resorting to preferential looking tests, which are usually not necessary to diagnose amblyopia. An effort should be made to assure that each eye will readily fixate on a small target and that one eye is not preferred over the other. In children with straight eyes, the eyes can be dissociated with a vertical or horizontal prism and fixation preference tested during the period of prism dissociation.

Common among all recognition tests is a feature known as the crowding phenomenon. Patients with amblyopia are frequently able to identify much smaller optotypes if the optotypes are shown in isolation than if they are shown a line in a full chart of letters. It is, therefore, imperative that a line of letters or single letters with crowding bars be utilized to minimize the chance that amblyopia will be overlooked (▶ Fig. 77.2).

77.3 Diagnosis

Anisometropic amblyopia in the right eye due to uncorrected hyperopia.

77.4 Medical Management

The first task in management of this child with amblyopia is to correct his refractive error. The ophthalmologist may prescribe the full cycloplegic refraction or may symmetrically reduce the hyperopic correction in each eye so that the child must continue to accommodate slightly in order to see clearly. Either of these methods is reasonable provided that reduction in the spherical correction is exactly the same in both eyes, so that the same amount of accommodation is required to see with either eye.

The child should be examined several weeks to months following the initiation of spectacle correction. Often, the visual acuity on follow-up examination will have responded to glasses alone and no other treatment measures are required. If vision remains reduced on retesting, other treatment measures must be instituted. Frequently, children will not adapt to the use of

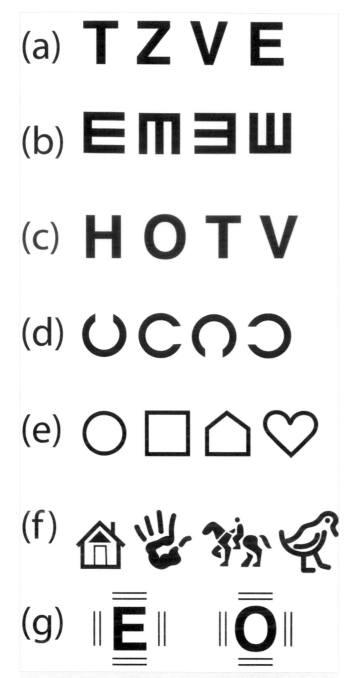

Fig. 77.2 Typical psychophysical tests of visual function: (line a) Snellen test; (line b) E game; (line c) HOTV test; (line d) Landolt test; (line e) Lea test; (line f) Allen test; (line g) single optotypes with crowding bars.

hyperopic spectacles, particularly when the hyperopic correction is moderate or high. In such cases, atropine drops may be prescribed once a day for several days. This will produce a pronounced and prolonged cycloplegia, thus encouraging the child to wear the glasses, which are needed to produce clear vision during the period of time the cycloplegia is in effect. The atropine effect will gradually wear off over several days, allowing the child to comfortably adjust to wearing spectacles.

Occlusion therapy with the use of an eye patch is a common means of treating amblyopia (▶ Fig. 77.3a, b). A patch is utilized to cover the sound eye, thus encouraging use of the amblyopic eye. Two hours of prescribed patching of the sound eye has been shown to be effective for the treatment of mild to moderate amblyopia.

Optical penalization is also a useful option in treating amblyopia. Atropine eye drops and/or spectacles are utilized for optical penalization. If atropine is used, it is placed in the sound eye. This greatly reduces the child's ability to accommodate and thus encourages utilization of the amblyopic eye. Both daily and weekend atropine have both been demonstrated to be effective in the treatment of moderate amblyopia. Atropine penalization is sometimes supplemented by temporary reduction of the spherical component of hyperopia in the sound.

77.5 Surgical Management

The role of surgery in the management of amblyopia has traditionally been limited to clearing the visual axis (i.e., correct ptosis or remove a media opacity such as a corneal leukoma or cataract). If amblyopia is caused by strabismus, many pediatric ophthalmologists believe it is best to defer strabismus surgery until amblyopia has been maximally treated. Strabismus surgery itself does not necessarily result in resolution of amblyopia.

Refractive surgery has been used successfully to improve the visual outcome in children with severe anisometropia leading to amblyopia or severe isoametropia. Photorefractive keratectomy, laser in-situ keratomileusis (LASIK), and clear lens extraction have all been studied in the treatment of amblyopia in children. While gaining acceptance, most pediatric ophthalmologists reserve these treatment modalities for children who are not responding to or resisting attempts to treat with nonsurgical modalities.

77.6 Rehabilitation and Follow-up

Ophthalmologic follow-up examinations may be needed even after amblyopia has been maximally treated. Gains from excellent amblyopia management can be lost if children are not

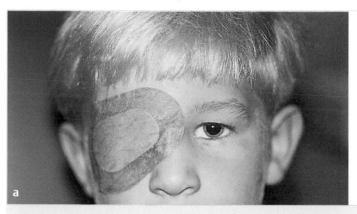
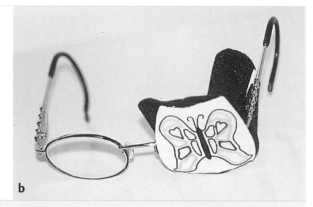

Fig. 77.3 Two commonly used methods of occlusion to treat amblyopia are (a) adhesive patch and (b) spectacle-mounted patch.

observed carefully for recurrence. Refractive error will gradually change as the child ages and updated prescriptions will be required. Strabismic amblyopia can recur even if the eyes appear aligned, due to the presence of difficult-to-detect microstrabismus. Because of the potential of recurrence, maintenance patching is often needed until the age of 7 to 8 years in some children to prevent loss of amblyopia treatment gains.

Suggested Reading

[1] American Academy of Ophthalmology. Pediatric Ophthalmology/Strabismus PPP Panel. San Francisco, CA: Hoskins Center for Quality Eye Care; 2012

[2] Von Noorden GK. Binocular Vision and Ocular Motility: Theory and Management of Strabismus. 5th ed. St. Louis, MO: Mosby; 1996

[3] Paysse EA, Tychsen L, Stahl E. Pediatric refractive surgery: corneal and intraocular techniques and beyond. J AAPOS. 2012; 16(3):291–297

[4] Repka MX, Wallace DK, Beck RW, et al. Pediatric Eye Disease Investigator Group. Two-year follow-up of a 6-month randomized trial of atropine vs patching for treatment of moderate amblyopia in children. Arch Ophthalmol. 2005; 123(2):149–157

[5] Scheiman MM, Hertle RW, Kraker RT, et al. Pediatric Eye Disease Investigator Group. Patching vs atropine to treat amblyopia in children aged 7 to 12 years: a randomized trial. Arch Ophthalmol. 2008; 126(12):1634–1642

78 Childhood Torticollis

David K. Coats

Abstract

Torticollis is a clinical symptom or sign that can manifest as a head tilt, face turn, or chin rotation. A variety of conditions may cause torticollis and the differential diagnosis in children is different than for adults. This chapter describes the differential diagnosis, evaluation, management, and treatment of torticollis. Although nonmuscular causes of torticollis should be considered, this chapter emphasizes the causes of ocular torticollis including eye muscle weakness.

Keywords: strabismus, ocular motility, torticollis, head tilt

78.1 History

A 5-year-old boy is brought to his ophthalmologist's office at the request of his pediatrician for evaluation of an anomalous head tilt. The child has undergone orthopaedic evaluation and neck muscle abnormalities are absent. The child has had a relatively constant left head tilt since he first gained head control during the first year of life. His parents note that he strongly resists any attempts to straighten his head. During the last 2 months, they have noticed that his eyes sometimes do not appear to move together. Family history is unremarkable and the review of systems is notable only for frequent eye rubbing and blinking behavior.

On examination, the patient has a constant 10- to 15-degree left head tilt (▶ Fig. 78.1a, b). He fixes and follows well with either eye, there is no objection to occlusion, and he alternates fixation on prism dissociation testing. In the primary position, an intermittent right hypertropia of 12 prism diopters is measured. The deviation increases to 18 prism diopters in left gaze and decreases to 4 prism diopters in right gaze. A 15 prism diopter right hypertropia is present on right head tilt, while a 5 prism diopter right hypertropia is present on left head tilt. Moderate overelevation of the right eye is noted in adduction (▶ Fig. 78.2a–d). Anterior segment and pupillary examination are normal. Cycloplegic refraction is +1.75 +0.75 axis 090 in both eyes. Fundus examination is normal in both eyes, though mild excyclorotation of the left fundus is noted (▶ Fig. 78.3a, b).

Differential Diagnosis—Key Points

1. The differential diagnosis of the child with a history of infantile torticollis is extensive but ocular causes can usually be easily identified on clinical examination in a cooperative child. Known causes of infantile torticollis include sternocleidomastoid abnormalities, superior oblique palsy, Brown's syndrome, dissociated vertical deviation, nystagmus, uncorrected or improperly corrected refractive errors, homonymous hemianopia, other forms of restrictive or paralytic strabismus, and even unilateral hearing loss.

2. Superior oblique palsy is a common ocular etiology of infantile torticollis seen in pediatric ophthalmology practice. Superior oblique palsy may be either congenital or acquired.

Some believe that congenital superior oblique palsy represents an anatomic laxity of the superior oblique tendon, with the muscle itself functioning normally. Superior oblique palsy, both acquired and congenital, can be bilateral or unilateral. Unilateral superior oblique palsies are much more common. It is important to make the distinction between acquired and congenital superior oblique palsy because acquired superior oblique palsy may require neurologic evaluation including neuroimaging, while congenital superior oblique palsy does not. Features that suggest the presence of a congenital or early-onset superior oblique palsy are the presence of a long-term anomalous head tilt, facial asymmetry, and absence of subjective torsion. It is theorized that a chronic head tilt results in structural musculoskeletal changes in the face due to gravity or other unknown factors resulting in permanent structural changes in the face.

3. Brown's syndrome is an interesting but uncommon cause of infantile torticollis. It is typically unilateral, but may be bilateral. Like superior oblique palsy, it can occur on a congenital or acquired basis. Brown's syndrome results from an anomaly of the superior oblique tendon/trochlea complex that prevents normal elevation of the eye. In classic Brown's syndrome, the involved eye elevates poorly or not at all in adduction, demonstrates improved elevation in supraduction, and shows normal or near-normal elevation in abduction. A Brown syndrome can typically be differentiated from a superior oblique palsy by two main factors including inability to elevate the eye in adduction, the opposite of what occurs in superior oblique palsy. In addition, the typical child with Brown's syndrome adopts a head tilt to the opposite side, but also adopts a chin-up head posture. Brown's syndrome is rarely confused with superior oblique palsy, though parents of children with Brown's syndrome often erroneously interpret the normal movements of the uninvolved eye as overelevation, not recognizing that the involved eye does not elevate fully.

4. Dissociated vertical deviation is an interesting form of strabismus characterized by elevation, abduction, and excyclotorsion of the involved eye when the eye is occluded or the patient inattentive. For largely unknown reasons, some children will adopt an anomalous head posture. The anomalous head posture may be ipsilateral or contralateral to the dissociated vertical deviation. In uncooperative children, it can be difficult to distinguish dissociated vertical deviation from superior oblique palsy. Careful evaluation and repeated examinations, when necessary, will help to make the distinction.

5. Other less common considerations in the diagnosis of infantile torticollis include congenital fibrosis syndrome, blowout fractures, orbital tumors, myasthenia gravis, thyroid disease, unilateral hearing loss, and sternocleidomastoid abnormalities.

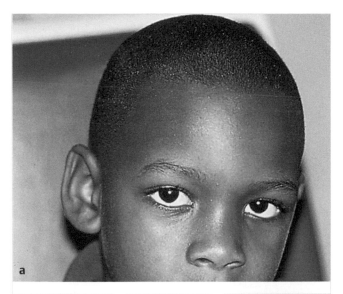
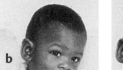

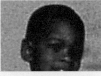

Fig. 78.1 Photographs of the patient **(a)** at examination and **(b)** during childhood, demonstrating a left head tilt.

78.2 Test Interpretation

The child should undergo a comprehensive ocular motility evaluation including a three-step test. The three-step test involves measuring the hypertropia in the primary position, right and left gaze, and on right and left head tilt. By analyzing the ocular alignment in the various positions of gaze, the examiner is able to identify the weak right superior oblique muscle.

If the timing of onset is unclear, consideration should be given to asking the family to bring in a photo album demonstrating photographs of the child in the months and years preceding the examination (▸ Fig. 78.1b). The presence of a longstanding and consistent head tilt in photos supports the diagnosis of a congenital superior oblique palsy and renders neuroimaging unnecessary.

If the examiner is not able to demonstrate features of a congenital superior oblique palsy and no other explanation is obvious, the child should undergo neuroimaging of the brain and orbit. Central nervous system structural abnormalities and orbital abnormalities can result in superior oblique palsy or a motility pattern that resembles superior oblique palsy, and these conditions should be ruled out if the palsy is thought to be acquired and the etiology is unclear.

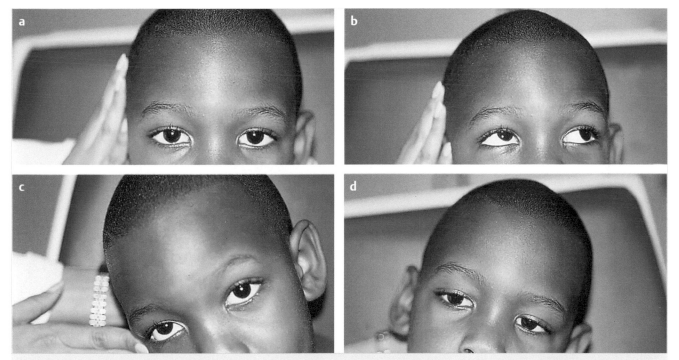

Fig. 78.2 Ocular alignment in **(a)** the primary position and **(b)** left gaze and with head tilt to **(c)** right and **(d)** left. Note secondary "overaction" of the right inferior oblique muscle with left gaze and hypertropia, which increases with right head tilt. Also note mild facial asymmetry with left side of face smaller compared to the right side of the face.

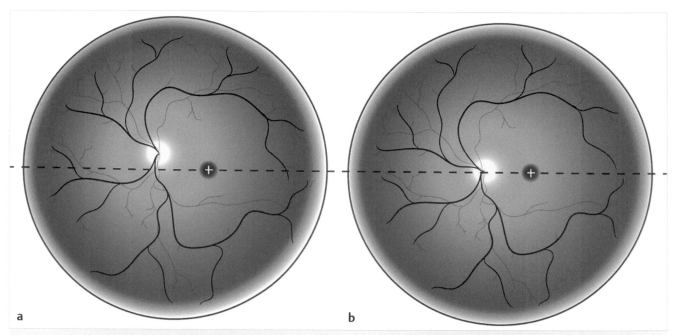

Fig. 78.3 Left fundus drawing demonstrating excyclotorsion. **(a)** The disc is rotated superiorly relative to the macula because of torsion (in reality, the optic nerve is rotated upward, while the macula maintains its central position for fixation). **(b)** Compare disc/macula orientation of the normal fundus.

78.3 Diagnosis

Right superior oblique palsy with chronic left head tilt and mild facial asymmetry.

78.4 Medical Management

Patients with asymptomatic or minimally symptomatic superior oblique palsy do not require surgical intervention. Many patients with mild superior oblique palsy are able to develop sufficient vertical fusional amplitudes to maintain comfortable single vision most or all of the time without treatment. Such patients, however, may become symptomatic later in life as control of their deviation decreases and diplopia develops. Patients with small hypertropias and a mild or absent anomalous head posture may benefit from treatment with an appropriate vertical prism. In general, patients do not tolerate prism powers greater than 4 or 5 prism diopters, though there are many exceptions to this rule. Patients with a large degree of ocular torsion are unlikely to be adequately managed with prism therapy.

78.5 Surgical Management

Indications for strabismus surgery with acquired and congenital superior oblique palsy include improvement of fusion, improvement of an anomalous head posture, and improvement of diplopia. Surgical treatment of superior oblique palsy typically involves weakening procedures of the ipsilateral inferior oblique muscle such as inferior oblique myectomy or recession. Others are treated with superior oblique strengthening

procedures such as a superior oblique tuck, while still others may undergo a combination of procedures including surgery on the superior and inferior oblique muscle of the involved eye as well as rectus muscle surgery.

78.6 Rehabilitation and Follow-up

Parents should be advised at the time of surgery of the potential for an over- or under-correction and the potential need for additional surgery in the future. Patients who have undergone a superior oblique tuck often develop a mild to moderate Brown's syndrome with limitation of elevation in adduction following surgery. This problem typically improves or resolves with time, but may persist. In children, amblyopia may have developed prior to surgery or may develop following surgery if ocular misalignment persists or later develops. Therefore, young children with superior oblique palsy should undergo periodic ophthalmologic evaluations with particular attention to fusion, stereopsis, and visual acuity testing to detect, prevent, and treat amblyopia.

Suggested Reading

[1] Helveston EW. Atlas of Strabismus. 4th ed. St. Louis, MO: Mosby; 1992

[2] Helveston EM, Krach D, Plager DA, Ellis FD. A new classification of superior oblique palsy based on congenital variations in the tendon. Ophthalmology. 1992; 99(10):1609–1615

[3] Paysee EA, Coats DK, Plager DA. Facial asymmetry and tendon laxity in superior oblique palsy. J Pediatr Ophthalmol Strabismus. 1995; 32(3):158–161

[4] Plager DA. Traction testing in superior oblique palsy. J Pediatr Ophthalmol Strabismus. 1990; 27(3):136–140

[5] Von Noorden GK. Binocular Vision and Ocular Motility: Theory and Management of Strabismus. 5th ed. St. Louis, MO: Mosby; 1980

79 Aniridia

David K. Coats

Abstract

Aniridia is a cause of visual loss and congenital nystagmus. A full history and clinical exam are required to make the diagnosis and to differentiate isolated from hereditary cases and to evaluate for potentially life threatening associations (e.g., Wilm's tumor).

Keywords: aniridia, Wilm's tumor, nystagmus

79.1 History

A 9-month-old boy is referred to his ophthalmologist with a history of "jiggling eyes" and large pupils, both noted during the first month of life. The child closes his eyes in bright sunlight and does not appear to see as well as his two older siblings. The boy was born at term, the mother received prenatal care, and there were no perinatal complications. The child's medical history is notable for a hypospadias repair 2 months earlier and for developmental delay. He has two healthy siblings and two healthy parents with no significant family history of ophthalmologic or medical problems.

On examination, the child appears to fix and follow, but the fixation behavior is abnormal. A low-amplitude/high-frequency horizontal pendular nystagmus is noted. Examination reveals peripheral corneal opacification and vascularization. The child appears to have only a very small peripheral remnant of iris and an anterior pyramidal cataract is noted in both eyes (► Fig. 79.1a, b). Retinal examination is notable for the absence of an obvious umbo or foveal pigmentation (► Fig. 79.2). The child's parents and two older siblings were examined and found to have normal ophthalmologic examinations.

Differential Diagnosis—Key Points

1. The syndrome of aniridia is a rare cause of infantile nystagmus. It is a panocular problem that occurs with a frequency of 1 in 50,000 to 100,000 live births. Multiple ophthalmological defects may be present including cataracts, glaucoma, corneal opacification and vascularization, ectopia lentis, foveal hypoplasia, colobomas, and nystagmus. It can occur as an autosomal dominant or sporadic condition.

2. The differential diagnosis of infantile nystagmus is quite extensive. Many causes of infantile-onset nystagmus can be easily detected on clinical examination. For those causes that are not obvious on clinical examination, special testing, including eye movement recordings, is required to fully evaluate and diagnose.

3. The genetics of aniridia are interesting. The condition can occur as an autosomal dominant condition with variable penetrance or as a sporadic condition. Autosomal dominant forms of the condition are due to a defect in the *PAX-6* gene.

4. Other cases of aniridia occur on a sporadic basis with no family history. As many as 25 to 40% of infants with sporadic aniridia will develop a Wilms' tumor, typically during the first few years of life. Children who are at greatest risk of developing a Wilms' tumor in association with sporadic aniridia are those with concurrent congenital genitourinary abnormalities and mental retardation. The complex of Wilms' tumor, aniridia, genitourinary abnormalities, and retardation has been referred to as the WAGR syndrome (► Fig. 79.1).

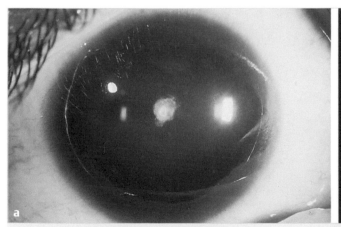
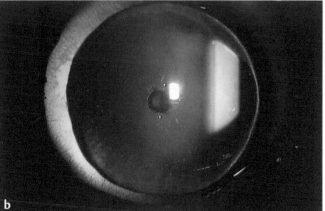

Fig. 79.1 (a) Slit-lamp photograph demonstrating multiple anterior segment abnormalities, including corneal pannus, severely hypoplastic iris, and anterior pyramidal cataract. (b) View with retroillumination. (Photographs courtesy of Jim Shigley, certified ophthalmic photographer.)

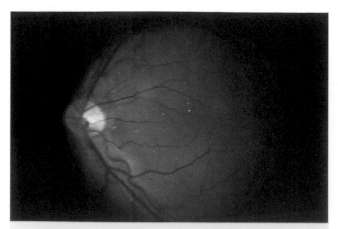

Fig. 79.2 Fundus of patient demonstrating foveal hypoplasia. (Photograph courtesy of Jim Shigley, certified ophthalmic photographer.)

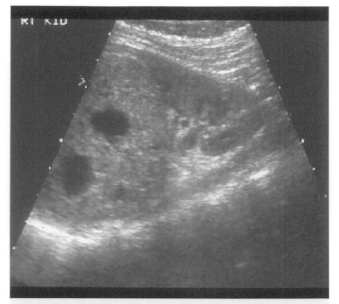

Fig. 79.3 Abdominal ultrasound demonstrating a renal mass consistent with a Wilms tumor. (Photograph courtesy of Scott R. Dorfman, MD, Houston, TX.)

79.2 Test Interpretation

Issues that must be considered in children with aniridia are the potential for development of other ophthalmologic problems and the potential development of serious systemic problems such as Wilms' tumor. Consultation with a geneticist and a pediatrician is indicated in the management of children with aniridia.

1. In autosomal dominant cases, multiple defects in the *PAX-6* gene have been identified. The parents and siblings of affected children should be evaluated for obvious and subtle signs of aniridia. Subtle signs of aniridia in affected family members include absence of the iris collarette and eccentric pupils and, on angiography, a decreased retinal foveal avascular zone and incomplete iris collarette. Deletion of a portion of the short arm of chromosome 11 (11p13 deletion) is frequently present in children with sporadic aniridia. Children with such a deletion are more likely to have the WAGR syndrome and are at high risk for Wilms' tumor. This patient has an 11p13 deletion (▶ Fig. 79.2).
2. Initial screening and periodic follow-up abdominal ultrasound evaluation and abdominal physical examination are recommended in aniridic children at risk for Wilms' tumor (▶ Fig. 79.3), and such testing is typically ordered and followed by the child's pediatrician. The frequency and duration of these examinations is controversial, but in general, most affected children will develop Wilms' tumor by the age of 3 years (▶ Fig. 79.3).

79.3 Diagnosis

Sporadic aniridia associated with developmental delay and genitourinary abnormalities. This child has three components of WAGR syndrome and is at high risk for developing Wilms' tumor. An 11p13 deletion is present.

79.4 Medical Management

The child's symptoms of photophobia can be improved by prescription of sunglasses or shaded contact lenses. Even though the child appears to have reasonable vision at this point, progressive corneal opacification and vascularization, development of progressive cataracts, and development of glaucoma can result in future vision loss. The child should undergo a careful screening ophthalmological examination including efforts to rule out glaucoma. Abdominal ultrasounds should be obtained at regular intervals until approximately 3 years of age. If a renal abnormality is noted on abdominal ultrasound, Wilms' tumor should be suspected. Further evaluation with magnetic resonance imaging (MRI) is done if an ultrasound abnormality is found, and the child should be referred for biopsy if findings consistent with Wilms' tumor are noted on MRI scan. If Wilms' tumor is confirmed on histopathologic examination, a pediatric oncologist should be consulted.

79.5 Surgical Management

While this patient does not presently demonstrate ophthalmologic abnormalities that require surgical care, the development of progressive cataracts, glaucoma, and/or progressive corneal opacification are strong possibilities in the future. Ophthalmologic surgery on patients with aniridia is difficult, and surgery should only be entertained after careful consideration of the risk/benefit ratio and after exhausting nonsurgical treatment modalities.

79.6 Rehabilitation and Follow-up

Long-term follow-up for systemic abnormalities such as Wilms' tumor has already been discussed. The child should undergo periodic ophthalmological screening examinations to detect the presence of progressive ocular disease as described above. Early childhood educational intervention and a low-vision evaluation should be done as early in the child's life as possible. Intervention in the form of preemptive education efforts and low-vision aids can prove helpful in almost any patient with vision abnormalities in childhood.

Suggested Reading

[1] Craft AW, Parker L, Stiller C, Cole M. Screening for Wilms' tumour in patients with aniridia, Beckwith syndrome, or hemihypertrophy. Med Pediatr Oncol. 1995; 24(4):231–234

[2] Gupta SK, De Becker I, Tremblay F, Guernsey DL, Neumann PE. Genotype/phenotype correlations in aniridia. Am J Ophthalmol. 1998; 126(2):203–210

[3] Mintz-Hittner HA, Ferrell RE, Lyons LA, Kretzer FL. Criteria to detect minimal expressivity within families with autosomal dominant aniridia. Am J Ophthalmol. 1992; 114(6):700–707

[4] Nelson LB, Spaeth GL, Nowinski TS, Margo CE, Jackson L. Aniridia. A review. Surv Ophthalmol. 1984; 28(6):621–642

[5] Nishida K, Kinoshita S, Ohashi Y, Kuwayama Y, Yamamoto S. Ocular surface abnormalities in aniridia. Am J Ophthalmol. 1995; 120(3):368–375

80 Retinopathy of Prematurity

David K. Coats and Evelyn A. Paysse

Abstract

Modern advances in neonatal care has resulted in the survival of smaller and more premature infants in the United States and increased the incidence for retinopathy of prematurity (ROP). Although prematurity is the major risk factor, not all premature infants develop ROP and the degree of ROP is variable. This chapter reviews the differential diagnosis, evaluation, management, treatment, and prognosis of ROP.

Keywords: retinopathy of prematurity, retinal ischemia, neovascularization, avascular

80.1 History

An 11-week-old, former 24-week estimated gestational age premature girl presented for consultation. She is due for another retinopathy of prematurity (ROP) screening examination. Her last examination occurred 1 week ago and demonstrated immature retina in zone 1, with no plus disease. Since this last examination, she has developed sepsis and respiratory compromise, requiring intravenous antibiotics and re-intubation/ventilatory support. Her birth weight was 650 g. She has anemia of prematurity and had an episode of necrotizing enterocolitis 4 weeks ago.

Examination reveals a frail-appearing infant girl who is intubated. She is receiving 50% oxygen. She blinks briskly to the light of the indirect ophthalmoscope with either eye. On fundus examination, she is found to have dilation and tortuosity of the posterior pole retinal vessels (▶ Fig. 80.1).

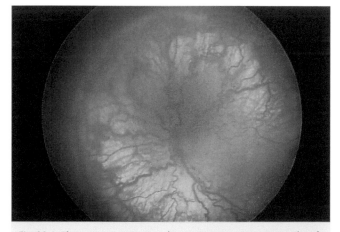

Fig. 80.1 The retina examination demonstrates zone I retinopathy of prematurity with dilation of posterior pole vessels (plus disease).

1. Differential diagnosis: The differential diagnosis of ROP is not long. It is rarely confused with other disease entities. The differential diagnosis includes familial exudative vitreoretinopathy, Eales' disease, and Norrie's disease. Though these diseases can occur in a premature infant, infants with these conditions are typically term infants; hence, there is little chance of confusion with ROP.

2. Demographics: ROP affects roughly 40,000 neonates in the United States annually. Despite significant advances in the treatment of ROP, severe visual impairment and blindness cannot be avoided in all affected infants.

3. Pathogenesis: ROP is a vasoproliferative disorder of the retina that affects premature infants. It can be mild and self-limiting or it can progress resulting in retinal detachment causing severe visual impairment or blindness. The avascular peripheral retina of a premature infant may produce vascular endothelial growth factors as a result of ischemia that lead to the development of ROP.

4. Normal retinal vascularization: Normal retinal vascularization begins at 16 weeks postconceptional age. Blood vessels grow out from the optic disc toward the periphery. The retina attains mature retinal vascularization in the nasal retina at approximately 36 weeks postconceptional age and in the temporal retina at approximately 40 weeks postconceptional age.

5. ROP risk factors: The severity of ROP is inversely proportional to birth weight and estimated gestational age. Other possible risk factors include maternal bleeding, prolonged intravenous nutrition, hypocarbia, prolonged ventilation, multiple birth status, intraventricular hemorrhage, hypotension, anemia, sepsis, and necrotizing enterocolitis. It is difficult to isolate the impact of these individual factors that tend to occur in smaller, more premature infants and therefore those most at risk of ROP.

6. Classification of ROP:
   a) ROP is most typically classified using the International Classification for ROP (ICROP), which was published in 1987 and was revised in 2005. The disease is classified based on the location, extent, and stage of the disease with an important notation made about the status of the blood vessels in the posterior pole.
   b) Location: The location of ROP is based upon three concentric rings centered on the optic nerve. Zone I is the most posterior location and involves a concentric ring the radius of which measures twice the distance from the center of the optic disc to the center of the macula. Zone II extends centrifugally from the edge of zone I to the nasal ora serrata, while zone III is the remaining crescent of temporal retina.

c) Extent: The extent of disease is recorded as the number of clock hours (30-degree sectors) of disease involvement at the leading edge of vascular development in the retina.

d) Stage: The stage of ROP describes the severity of the vascular abnormalities observed. Stage 1 signifies a demarcation line between vascular and avascular retina. Stage 2 looks similar to stage I but has height and width, therefore extending above the plain of the retina. Stage 3 represents extraretinal proliferation or neovascularization extending into the vitreous from the ridge. Stage 4 comprises a subtotal retinal detachment (stage 4A is extrafoveal and stage 4B includes the fovea). Stage 5 represents a total retinal detachment (▶ Fig. 80.2 and ▶ Table 80.1).

e) Plus disease: Plus disease is a term used to characterize pronounced venous dilation and arteriolar tortuosity. In more severe cases, it can be associated with iris vascular engorgement with poor pupillary dilation. Many ROP clinical trials have used a "standard" photograph to depict plus disease. Preplus disease represents an abnormal state of the posterior pole vessels that is insufficient to be characterize as plus disease.

f) Aggressive posterior ROP: This is a rapidly progressive form of severe ROP (designated AP–ROP) that most commonly occurs in zone I. If untreated, it can rapidly progress to retinal detachment.

g) Threshold ROP: Threshold ROP is diagnosed when there is stage 3 ROP in zone 1 or 2 for five or more contiguous clock hours or eight cumulative clock hours, in the presence of plus disease.

h) Type I ROP: Treatment is highly recommended when type I ROP is present. Type I ROP is present when any one of the following is seen:
   • Zone I ROP: Any stage with plus disease.
   • Zone I ROP: Stage 3 with no plus disease.
   • Zone II: Stage 2 or 3 with plus disease.

7. Screening criteria: The current screening guidelines for ROP are included in a consensus statement by the American Academy of Ophthalmology, the American Association for Pediatric Ophthalmology and Strabismus, and the American Academy of Pediatrics. These criteria are the following:

a) All infants with a birth weight of 1,500 g or less and/or with a gestational age of 28 weeks or less, as well as those infants over 1,500 g with an unstable clinical course felt to be at high risk by their attending pediatrician or neonatologist.

b) These examinations should be carried out by an ophthalmologist with experience in the examination of preterm infants. It should be noted that telemedicine has been successfully utilized to screen infants at risk for ROP.

c) The initial examination should be done typically between 4 and 6 weeks of chronological age, with earlier exams conducted on infants with extreme prematurity. Follow-up intervals depend upon the zone and severity of the disease.

80.2 Test Interpretation

1. Retinal examination: The most important test for an infant at risk for ROP is appropriately timed retinal examination with scleral depression when needed to visualize the peripheral retina. This patient had immature retina in zone 1 a week prior to the current examination. On the present examination, the infant has plus disease (dilation and tortuosity of the posterior pole vessels) in zone 1. This, by definition, is type I ROP.

2. Photographic screening: Photographic screening has been reported to be a successful method for diagnosing referral warranted ROP, or ROP requiring indirect ophthalmoscopic examination. Photographic screening has been proposed as having advantages over indirect ophthalmoscopy allowing remote consultation, and facilitating comparison of findings at different times, thus reducing dependence on memory and diagrams to track progress of the disease.

3. Important historical features: Factors possibly leading to higher risk in this child include the new-onset sepsis since her last examination and the worsening of her respiratory status requiring re-intubation and supplemental oxygen. The most important risk factors for ROP in this infant are her extreme prematurity and low birth weight. The overall health status of a premature infant and the postconceptional

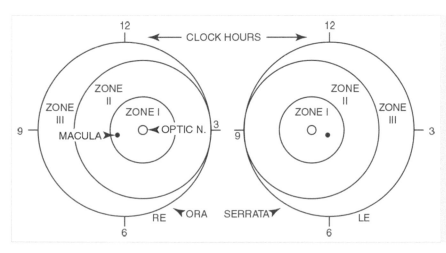

Fig. 80.2 Zone diagram for retinopathy of prematurity, from the international classification. (Reproduced with permission from Lee DA and Higginbotham EJ. Clinical Guide to Comprehensive Ophthalmology. New York, NY: Thieme, 1999:581.)

Table 80.1 International classification of retinopathy of prematurity (ROP)

Location	
Zone I	Posterior pole, concentric ring with radius twice the distance from center of disc to center of macula
Zone II	Concentric from zone I to the nasal ora serrata
Zone III	Residual crescent anterior to zone II in temporal periphery
Extent	Clock hours
Stage	
1	Demarcation line
2	Ridge
3	Ridge with extraretinal fibrovascular proliferation
4a	Partial retinal detachment excluding the macula
4b	Partial retinal detachment including the macula
5	Total retinal detachment
Plus disease	Posterior retinal vascular dilation and tortuosity May also include iris engorgement and/or vitreous haze
Preplus disease	Abnormal dilation and tortuosity of the posterior retinal vessels, but insufficient to classify as plus disease
Aggressive posterior ROP (AP-ROP)	Rapidly progressive ROP, typically occurring in zone I

age should, however, both be considered when deciding the interval for follow-up examination.

4. Prognosis: The Early Treatment for Retinopathy of Prematurity Cooperative Group reported an unfavorable structural outcome of 9.1% at 9 months for children undergoing treatment with retinal ablation for type I ROP. Recent studies have indicated an even better prognosis following intravitreal administration of bevacizumab for severe ROP.

80.3 Diagnosis

Type I, both eyes.

80.4 Medical Management

Recently, severe ROP, defined as stage 3 + ROP, has been effectively treated with monotherapy consisting of intravitreal injection of bevacizumab, an agent that inhibits vascular endothelial growth factor. Many other subsequent studies have confirmed the effectiveness of bevacizumab treatment. Monotherapy with antivascular endothelial growth factor agent is widely used. The long-term implications of bevacizumab treatment on the eye and systemically have yet to be established.

80.5 Surgical Management

The Multicenter Trial of Cryotherapy for Retinopathy of Prematurity Study in the 1980s showed an approximately 50% reduction of "poor outcome," defined as retinal detachment or posterior retinal fold, in eyes treated with cryotherapy compared with eyes that went untreated. Laser photoablation largely replaced cryotherapy in the early 1990s. Laser photocoagulation has been shown to be effective and was the most common treatment modality used in the Early Treatment for Retinopathy of Prematurity study. Potential complications of laser photoablation include cataract and subretinal, intraretinal, and vitreous hemorrhage. Severe myopia has been reported to occur more commonly and children undergoing peripheral retinal photocoagulation compared to those receiving monotherapy with bevacizumab.

80.6 Rehabilitation and Follow-up

After treatment of type I ROP with laser photocoagulation or intravitreal injection of antivascular endothelial growth factor agents, the infant should be examined frequently until the disease has regressed. Children treated with bevacizumab and related agents should undergo continuous screening until as long as 60 to 70 weeks postmenstrual age because of the potential for late disease reactivation.

Premature infants are at risk of developing other serious ophthalmologic problems, including amblyopia, strabismus, and severe refractive error including myopia, astigmatism, and anisometropia.

Suggested Reading

[1] International Committee for the Classification of, Retinopathy, of Prematurity. The international classification of Retinopathy of Prematurity revisited. Arch Ophthalmol. 2005; 123(7):991–999

[2] Cryotherapy for Retinopathy of Prematurity Cooperative Group. Multicenter trial of cryotherapy for retinopathy of prematurity: one year outcome—structure and function. Arch Ophthalmol. 1990; 108:1408–1416

[3] Palmer EA, Flynn JT, Hardy RJ, et al. The Cryotherapy for Retinopathy of Prematurity Cooperative Group. Incidence and early course of retinopathy of prematurity. Ophthalmology. 1991; 98:1628–1640

[4] Paysse EA, Lindsey JL, Coats DK, Contant CF, Jr, Steinkuller PG. Therapeutic outcomes of cryotherapy versus transpupillary diode laser photocoagulation of threshold retinopathy of prematurity. J AAPOS. 1999; 3(4):234–240

[5] Early Treatment For Retinopathy Of Prematurity Cooperative Group. Revised indications for the treatment of retinopathy of prematurity: results of the early treatment for retinopathy of prematurity randomized trial. Arch Ophthalmol. 2003; 121(12):1684–1694

[6] Mintz-Hittner HA, Kennedy KA, Chuang AZ, BEAT-ROP Cooperative Group. Efficacy of intravitreal bevacizumab for stage 3 + retinopathy of prematurity. N Engl J Med. 2011; 364(7):603–615

[7] Fierson WM, American Academy of Pediatrics Section on Ophthalmology, American Academy of Ophthalmology, American Association for Pediatric Ophthalmology and Strabismus, American Association of Certified Orthoptists. Screening examination of premature infants for retinopathy of prematurity. Pediatrics. 2013; 131(1):189–195

81 Childhood Esotropia

Evelyn A. Paysse

Abstract

This chapter presents a case of a child with esotropia. It discusses pertinent historical and examination findings of infantile esotropia, the differential diagnosis, associated ocular motility and visual abnormalities that can develop, the management approach, and long-term expectations.

Keywords: esotropia, V-pattern strabismus, amblyopia, dissociated vertical deviation, inferior oblique overaction

81.1 History

A 5-year-old girl with a history of crossed eyes since 2 months of age presents for an examination. She has a history of strabismus surgery at 8 months of age. Her mother reports that her eyes were well aligned following surgery until recently when her left eye has been noted to intermittently drift inward, especially when she is tired. She has never been treated with occlusion therapy. Her current glasses are at least 1 year old. Her past medical history is otherwise unremarkable. The family history is notable for a sister with esotropia that required surgical intervention.

On examination, the child's visual acuity, with her current spectacle correction, is 20/30 OD and 20/50 OS. Her current spectacle prescription is +2.00 OD and +2.50 OS. Motility examination with spectacle correction demonstrates an intermittent esotropia of 8 prism diopters at distance with a moderate left dissociated vertical deviation. On version testing, moderate inferior oblique muscle overaction is noted in both eyes (▶ Fig. 81.1a, b). A V-pattern is present with the esotropia in downgaze increasing to 20 prism diopters and decreasing in upgaze to 5 prism diopters. At near, an intermittent esotropia of 20 prism diopters is seen. Stereopsis testing reveals 3,000 seconds of arc stereopsis on the Titmus stereo fly test. Cycloplegic refraction is +3.00 spheres and +3.75 spheres in the right and left eyes, respectively. Optokinetic nystagmus (OKN) testing is asymmetric, demonstrating a normal response on temporal-to-nasal testing, but a poor nasal-to-temporal response in both eyes. The remainder of the ophthalmologic examination is normal.

Differential Diagnosis—Key Points

1. Differential diagnosis: Childhood esotropia can be due to many different entities. It is helpful to divide esotropia into comitant and incomitant deviations. Please see text box below for differential diagnosis of childhood esotropia.
2. History: It is important when evaluating a child with esotropia to obtain a good history. The examiner must determine the onset of the esotropia, as this will aid in defining the etiology. If the onset is before 6 months of age, the entity could be infantile esotropia; however, accommodative esotropia has also been reported as early as 3 months of age. A host of other esotropia syndromes may also have onset in the first 6 months of life, including Duane's syndrome and Moebius' syndrome.

   The quality of the esotropia is also important to elicit from the parents. Intermittent esotropia and esotropia that is greater at near than at distance are more likely to be accommodative in nature. If the deviation is larger in certain positions of gaze, all comitant etiologies will be eliminated from the differential diagnosis. An anomalous head posture with esotropia implies an incomitant (i.e., restrictive or paralytic) strabismus with fusion when using the anomalous head position, such as occurs with a sixth nerve palsy, type 1 Duane's syndrome, or Moebius' syndrome or some other advantage to using an anomalous head position such as in nystagmus blockage syndrome and early-onset homonymous hemianopia (see text box below).

   Finally, it is also important during history taking to determine if there were any preceding events to the esotropia such as a febrile illness, head trauma, or neurologic event. All of these entities can be associated with a sixth nerve palsy. Family history is also important to discuss because strabismus is often hereditary.
3. Associated ocular motility abnormalities: Inferior oblique muscle overaction, dissociated strabismus complex, A- and V-patterns, and latent nystagmus are other motility abnormalities associated with early-onset strabismus, most commonly in association with infantile esotropia. Inferior oblique muscle overaction is diagnosed from the version examination when overelevation of the eye in adduction occurs. Dissociated strabismus complex (DSC) is diagnosed with cover testing. The eye under the occluder will elevate, abduct, and excyclotort if it has all three components of DSC. Any of these components can predominate and not all components are necessary to have dissociated strabismus complex. If a vertical deviation predominates, it is called dissociated vertical deviation and if a horizontal deviation predominates, it is called dissociated horizontal deviation. Dissociated strabismus complex is often more severe in an amblyopic eye. A- and V-patterns occur when the deviation in upgaze and downgaze differ significantly. An A-pattern esotropia is present when the esotropia is greater in upgaze than downgaze by 10 or more prism diopters. A V-pattern esotropia is present when the deviation in upgaze is less than in downgaze by 15 or more prism diopters. Latent nystagmus is a nystagmus that is present only when one eye is occluded. It is most commonly associated with infantile esotropia and is usually worse in the amblyopic eye.
4. Amblyopia: Amblyopia is commonly associated with strabismus. In strabismus, amblyopia develops in children secondary to the ability to suppress the image in the deviating eye. This suppression develops in order to avoid diplopia and confusion.

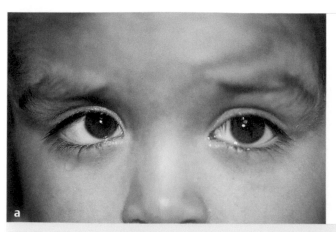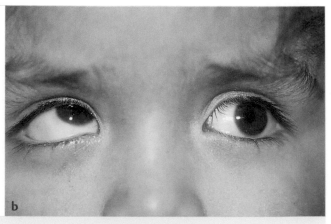

Fig. 81.1 **(a)** A 5-year-old child with esotropia. **(b)** Inferior oblique muscle overaction of the right eye is demonstrated.

Differential Diagnoses of Childhood Esotropias

Incomitant Esotropia

Neurologic
- Sixth nerve palsy:
  - Congenital.
  - Acquired (tumor, traumatic, microvascular, inflammatory).
- Duane syndrome (type 1 or 3).
- Myasthenia gravis.
- Progressive external ophthalmoplegia.
- Moebius' syndrome.

Restrictive
- Thyroid related ophthalmopathy.
- Congenital fibrosis syndrome.
- Duane's syndrome (type 1 or 3).
- Iatrogenic (e.g., postsurgical).
- Posttraumatic (e.g., medial orbital wall fracture).

Comitant Esotropias
- Infantile esotropia.
- Ciancia's syndrome.
- Nystagmus blockage syndrome.
- Accommodative esotropia:
  - Refractive.
  - Nonrefractive (high AC/A).
- Horror fusionis.
- Sensory esotropia.

81.2 Test Interpretation

Clinical examination of a strabismic patient is the key to diagnosis. This section will concentrate on the most important parts of the ophthalmologic examination for a patient with esotropia.

1. Stereopsis testing: Stereopsis testing should be the first part of any ophthalmologic examination for a strabismic patient. It will aid in determining the onset of the strabismus and in prognosticating stability of the deviation over time. Stereopsis is the highest form of binocular cooperation. It is the ability to fuse two disparate images into a single impression in depth. With good stereopsis, a patient is likely to maintain a more stable alignment. Poor stereopsis implies early-onset strabismus.

2. Ductions/versions: Ductions and versions help distinguish comitant from incomitant deviations. Versions are defined as binocular rotations of the eyes. The examiner has the patient follow a target with his eyes into the six cardinal positions of gaze to evaluate the yoke muscles and oblique muscle function. Next, the examiner has the patient follow the target into upgaze and downgaze to evaluate for an A- or V-pattern. Ductions are defined as monocular rotations of the eye. The examiner has the patient follow a target with one eye covered into the same gaze positions as for versions. If versions are normal, there is no need to test ductions. If, however, there is an incomitant deviation on version testing, ductions should be done to help differentiate a restrictive from a paralytic esotropia. Restrictive etiologies will still have a deficit of duction, whereas a paralytic etiology will often have improved ductions in comparison to versions. Our patient had full versions, inferior oblique muscle overaction, and a V-pattern. All are common findings in infantile esotropia patients as they get older.

3. Motility: Alignment at distance and near. The strabismic deviation must be measured both at distance and near in the diagnostic positions of gaze, with and without glasses using the cover test, the cover/uncover test, and either the alternate prism and cover test or the Krimsky or Hirschberg test if not cooperative for alternate prism and cover testing. If the esotropia is worse at near than at distance, especially if intermittent, an accommodative esotropia is the most likely etiology, though this does not always hold true. If the deviation is worse at distance than at near, then divergence insufficiency type esotropia is present. This is often a sign of a sixth nerve paresis, and neuroimaging is indicated in most cases to rule out hydrocephalus or an intracranial mass (tumor, arteriovenous malformation, inflammatory lesion, etc.) causing a sixth nerve paresis. During the motility examination, one evaluates for DSC. Our patient has a

constant esotropia that is minimally worse at near than at distance, with dissociated vertical deviation in the left eye. These findings are consistent with infantile esotropia or partially accommodative esotropia.

4. Cycloplegic refraction: Cycloplegic refraction should be done on every strabismus patient. If it is not performed, latent hyperopia may be overlooked. This is especially important in esotropic patients because of the association of convergence with accommodation. Cycloplegia can be accomplished using topical cyclopentolate, homatropine, scopolamine, and atropine. Most commonly, cyclopentolate is used because it is shorter acting. Atropine is the best at achieving complete cycloplegia but can last up to 2 weeks. Our child has significant hyperopia that is undercorrected in her current glasses. Her recurrent esotropia may be adequately treated with new spectacles with the full hyperopic refractive correction. Hyperopic correction can help maintain ocular alignment or treat small residual deviations.

5. OKN: Patients with early-onset esotropia, especially infantile esotropia, typically have asymmetry of optokinetic nystagmus. The temporal-to-nasal direction of this reflex is normal; however, a poor nasal-to-temporal direction nystagmus is present. OKN can be tested with an OKN drum or ribbon. The test should be performed monocularly. Our patient had OKN asymmetry signifying early-onset esotropia.

6. Neuroimaging/orbital imaging: Neuroimaging is usually indicated in patients with incomitant esotropia and divergence insufficiency esotropia to rule out causes of the sixth nerve palsy, such as hydrocephalus or intracranial mass. Orbital imaging is also often necessary to rule out a mass that could be compressing the peripheral sixth nerve. Neuroimaging should also be considered in a child with late-onset, large-angle esotropia or an atypical acquired large-angle esotropia. Our patient did not have any of these findings and, therefore, did not need an imaging study.

81.3 Diagnosis

Infantile esotropia status poststrabismus surgery, now with recurrent esotropia, dissociated vertical deviation of the left eye, bilateral inferior oblique muscle overaction, and amblyopia of the left eye.

81.4 Medical Management

Proper management of this child first involves prescription of new glasses with the full cycloplegic refraction. The examiner should follow up in the next few months to recheck the ocular alignment. Reduction or elimination of the deviation signifies the presence of a refractive accommodative component to the esotropia. Bifocal treatment can be instituted if the child on follow-up is orthotropic at distance, but still esotropic at near. Bifocals, however, should only be prescribed if fusion or stereopsis is able to be documented. If the remaining esotropia is only 10 to 12 prism diopters, most ophthalmologists believe that this deviation is small enough to develop stable monofixation syndrome, and no surgery would be indicated. Vision should be monitored at this stage for amblyopia and appropriate treatment instituted.

81.5 Surgical Management

If the deviation remains greater than 10 to 12 prism diopters at distance with the full cycloplegic refraction in spectacles, then surgical intervention can be performed. Strabismus surgery for esotropia may consist of a bilateral medial rectus recession, a medial rectus recession and ipsilateral lateral rectus resection, or a bilateral lateral rectus resection. The surgical decision depends on the patient's measurements, the previous strabismus surgery, and the surgeon preference.

81.6 Rehabilitation and Follow-up

If the eyes are aligned and stereopsis is good with the new spectacle correction, the prognosis is excellent. Regular follow-ups should be performed throughout childhood as amblyopia and/or esotropia can recur. The time interval between follow-up evaluations will vary depending on the stability of the angle, the visual acuity, and the age of the child. Strabismus surgery can be repeated if the deviation recurs or a new deviation develops. The better the stereopsis or fusion present, the more stable the ocular alignment tends to be.

Suggested Reading

[1] Ciancia AO. On infantile esotropia with nystagmus in abduction. J Pediatr Ophthalmol Strabismus. 1995; 32(5):280–288

[2] Coats DK, Avilla CW, Paysse EA, Sprunger DT, Steinkuller PG, Somaiya M. Early-onset refractive accommodative esotropia. J AAPOS. 1998; 2(5):275–278

[3] Helveston EM. 19th annual Frank Costenbader Lecture: the origins of congenital esotropia. J Pediatr Ophthalmol Strabismus. 1993; 30(4):215–232

[4] Norcia AM. Abnormal motion processing and binocularity: infantile esotropia as a model system for effects of early interruptions of binocularity. Eye (Lond). 1996; 10(Pt 2):259–265

[5] Paysse EA, Coats DK. Anomalous head posture with early-onset homonymous hemianopia. J AAPOS. 1997; 1(4):209–213

[6] Von Noorden GK. XLIV Edward Jackson Memorial Lecture: a reassessment of infantile esotropia. Am J Ophthalmol. 1988; 105:1–10

82 Childhood Exotropia

Evelyn A. Paysse

Abstract

This chapter presents a case of a child with intermittent exotropia. It discusses pertinent historical and examination findings of intermittent exotropia, the differential diagnosis, associated ocular motility and visual abnormalities that can develop, the management approach, and long-term expectations.

Keywords: exotropia, intermittent, divergence excess, pseudodivergence excess, patch test, amblyopia

82.1 History

A 4-year-old boy presents with a 2-year history of intermittent drifting out of the right eye. His mother states that the deviation is worse when the child is tired or when he is looking at distant objects. His mother initially noted this deviation approximately two to three times a day; however, it recently has been getting worse. She states that the eye is now deviated outward approximately 60% of the day. There is no history of antecedent head trauma, febrile episode, or other medical problem. There is no family history of strabismus or amblyopia. Review of systems is notable for right eye closure in sunlight.

On examination, the child's visual acuity is 20/30, OU. On stereopsis testing with the Titmus stereo fly test, the child is able to correctly identify nine of nine circles (40 seconds of arc). The pupils are 3 mm in diameter, round, with brisk response to light. No afferent pupillary defect is detected. External examination is normal, with no evidence of ptosis. An intermittent exotropia of 50 prism diopters at distance is present, with recovery of orthotropia on refixation or blinking (▶ Fig. 82.1). The deviation recurs immediately with occlusion of either eye. A 25 prism diopter poorly controlled intermittent exotropia is present at near. Ductions and versions are full. A 30-minute patch test demonstrates a 50-prism diopter intermittent exotropia at distance and a 45 prism diopter exotropia at near, after removal of the patch. Cycloplegic refraction is +0.50 OD (oculus dexter) and +0.75 OS. The remainder of the comprehensive examination is unremarkable.

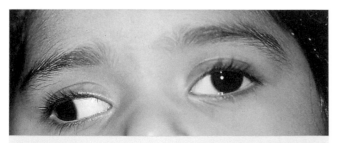

Fig. 82.1 Exotropia that is often manifest with fixation at distance.

Differential Diagnosis—Key Points

This is a 4-year-old child with an intermittent exotropia worse at distance than near. No amblyopia is noted, and stereopsis is excellent. The differential diagnosis of exotropia is extensive, but can be quickly narrowed through the use of special tests during the examination.

1. Differential diagnosis: The exotropias can be divided into comitant and incomitant deviations (see list below). Comitant exotropias include congenital exotropia, intermittent exotropia, and sensory exotropia. Incomitant exotropias can be divided into neurologic or restrictive entities. The neurologic forms of exotropia include third nerve palsy, progressive external ophthalmoplegia, synergistic divergence, and myasthenia gravis. The restrictive entities that can cause exotropia include congenital fibrosis syndrome, thyroid-related ophthalmopathy (rarely), and posttraumatic or iatrogenic exotropia. Duane's syndrome (types II and III) is unique because it can cause both a neurogenic and a restrictive strabismus. This child has a comitant deviation, so the differential diagnosis is significantly narrowed.

2. Classification of comitant exotropia: When evaluating a child with a comitant exotropia, the examiner must first classify the deviation in a number of different ways. First, he or she needs to decide if the deviation is intermittent or constant. Then the examiner must evaluate for a distance–near disparity. This allows him or her to classify the deviation either as basic exotropia, divergence excess exotropia, pseudodivergence excess exotropia, or convergence insufficiency exotropia.

3. Comitant exotropias:
   a) Intermittent exotropia occurs as a result of a cortical abnormality of fusion. The eyes are sometimes orthotropic with the patient having normal stereopsis and at other times, the eyes are exotropic and the patient has suppression. Basic exotropia occurs when the deviation is roughly the same at distance and at near. Divergence excess exotropia occurs when there is a larger deviation at distance than at near of at least 10 to 15 prism diopters. Pseudodivergence excess exotropia is an exotropia that initially presents in the same way that true divergence excess exotropia does, with a deviation worse at distance than near. True divergence excess exotropia is differentiated from pseudodivergence excess exotropia with the patch test (discussed in the next section, number 6). A patient with pseudodivergence excess exotropia will have the near deviation increase to within 10 prism diopters of the deviation at distance with the patch test, while a patient with true divergence excess will maintain the distance near disparity. Convergence insufficiency exotropia occurs when the deviation is worse at near than at distance by 10 or more prism diopters. This form of exotropia is much more common in elderly patients and is most often associated with diplopia.

b) Congenital exotropia, as the name implies, presents at birth or shortly after birth. It is rare and is often associated with intracranial structural abnormalities. Neuroimaging should be considered in these cases.

c) Sensory exotropia occurs after vision loss in one eye. An eye with poor vision tends to drift. If the vision loss occurs before the age of 3 years, the tendency is for an esotropia to develop. Conversely, if the vision loss occurs after 3 years of age, the tendency is for an exotropia to develop.

d) Myasthenia gravis is characterized by excessive fatigability of striated muscles. It is an autoimmune disease that demonstrates a reduction of available postsynaptic acetylcholine receptors in the end plates of neuromuscular junctions of skeletal muscles. Myasthenia gravis can occur in children and can cause exotropia or any other ocular motility disturbance. It can be comitant or incomitant. Typically, the deviation is variable and worse in the afternoon or when fatigued. It is often associated with ptosis and can also be associated with systemic weakness, such as difficulty swallowing, proximal limb weakness, and/or respiratory difficulty.

4. Incomitant exotropias:

a) Third nerve palsy can cause an exotropia of the affected eye. It can also be associated with hypotropia, ptosis, and mydriasis of the affected eye. A pupil-involving third nerve palsy is typically due to a compressive lesion, most commonly a posterior communicating artery aneurysm. If a total third nerve palsy is present, complete ptosis, mydriasis, exotropia, and hypotropia of the involved eye will be seen. This strabismus pattern occurs because the third nerve controls four of the six extraocular muscles. The only remaining functional extraocular muscles then are the lateral rectus and superior oblique muscles.

b) Duane's syndrome, types II and III, are conditions of miswiring of the sixth nerve to the lateral rectus muscle and/or the medial rectus muscle. In Duane's syndrome, type II, an exotropia usually occurs associated with a deficit of adduction. Duane's syndrome, type III, causes a deficit of both adduction and abduction and often leaves the eye in an exotropic position.

c) Other exotropias:

1. *Chronic progressive external ophthalmologia* is a rare hereditary condition that causes progressive deficits of ocular motility, often associated with ptosis.

2. *Congenital fibrosis syndrome* is a hereditary condition in which a child is born with fibrotic extraocular muscles and ptosis.

3. *Thyroid-related ophthalmopathy* (Graves' ophthalmopathy) can rarely lead to an exotropia due to enlargement of the lateral rectus muscles. Exotropia, however, in a patient with thyroid-related ophthalmopathy, is usually due to concomitant myasthenia gravis, which occurs in 10% of patients with Graves' disease.

4. *Iatrogenic:* Exotropia can also result as a consecutive problem after strabismus surgery for esotropia or can be iatrogenically created after surgery for retinal detachment, glaucoma, blowout fracture, or other orbital abnormality.

Types of Childhood Exotropia

Comitant Exotropia
- Essential intermittent exotropia:
  - Basic exotropia.
  - Divergence excess exotropia.
  - Pseudodivergence excess exotropia.
  - Convergence insufficiency exotropia.
- Congenital exotropia.
- Sensory exotropia.
- Myasthenia gravis. (Myasthenia can cause any type of strabismus, incomitant or comitant.)

Incomitant Exotropia
- Third nerve palsy.
- Duane's syndrome.
- Type II.
- Type III.
- Chronic progressive external ophthalmoplegia.
- Synergistic divergence.
- Myasthenia gravis. (Myasthenia can cause any type of strabismus, incomitant or comitant.)
- Congenital fibrosis syndrome.
- Thyroid-related ophthalmopathy. (Exotropia with thyroid-related ophthalmopathy is rare. It is usually due to concomitant myasthenia.)
- Iatrogenic:
  - Postsurgical.
  - Posttrauma.

82.2 Test Interpretation

1. Vision and stereopsis: Stereopsis should be tested first in a strabismic patient as other testing, such as visual acuity or motility evaluations, can be dissociative, causing the patient to temporarily lose the stereopsis and/or fusion that he normally has. Stereopsis testing is usually normal in a patient with intermittent exotropia. Vision: Visual acuity in children with intermittent exotropia is usually equal in each eye with only about 10% developing amblyopia. Amblyopia then, if present, should raise the examiner's suspicion that other entities could be the cause of the exotropia. Visual acuity should be tested with the most sensitive method possible, based on the age of a child.

2. External examination: Because a third nerve palsy can cause exotropia and ptosis, the external examination is important. Any exotropia associated with a ptosis could be a third nerve palsy and special attention should be paid during the ductions and versions examination for an adduction or vertical duction deficit.

3. Pupils: A third nerve palsy can also cause mydriasis of the involved eye, in addition to exotropia and ptosis. Therefore, the examiner needs to carefully evaluate pupil size and, if anisocoria is encountered, perform a full anisocoria workup.

4. Extraocular motility: Version should be performed first; if full, ductions do not need to be performed. If ductions are full, most of the differential diagnosis can be eliminated. A

duction deficit implies a restrictive or paralytic condition. Simultaneous prism and cover testing can be done next to assess for the tropia present when fusion is not disrupted. Alternate cover testing should be performed next, first at distance, then at near, to determine the full deviation and in order to classify the type of exotropia present (basic, divergence excess, pseudodivergence excess, or convergence insufficiency).

5. Anomalous head position: An anomalous head position should be noted. If a head turn is present, a paralytic or restrictive type of exotropia is usually present.

6. Patch test: When a deviation is found that is comitant and worse at distance than at near by 10 to 15 prism diopters or more, the examiner needs to differentiate between pseudodivergence excess exotropia and true divergence excess exotropia by performing a patch test. The patch test works by disrupting fusional convergence. With the patient wearing the correct cycloplegic refraction, an occlusion patch is placed over one eye for approximately 20 to 45 minutes. Next, the examiner carefully removes the patch, paying careful attention to continue to occlude the previously patched eye with his hand or an occlusion paddle to avoid any binocular visual stimulation. Next, the child's ocular alignment is remeasured with alternate cover testing at distance and near. Throughout the entire testing period, the child is not allowed to have binocular stimulation. If the deviation at near continues to be 10 to 15 prism diopters less than at distance, then true divergence excess exotropia is diagnosed. If the near deviation increases to within 10 prism diopters of the distance deviation, then pseudodivergence excess exotropia is diagnosed. Our patient had an increase of the near deviation to within 10 prism diopters of the distance deviation and, therefore, has pseudodivergence excess exotropia.

7. Cycloplegic refraction: It is always important to perform a cycloplegic refraction on every child with strabismus. Correction of high hyperopia (+ 4.00 diopters or more) will improve the control of an exodeviation in some children. This is counterintuitive to general understanding because accommodation (which is required with high hyperopia to see clearly) typically stimulates convergence. In the case of high hyperopia, however, some children hypoaccommodate as their brain was never exposed to a clear image and it does not realize what the world really looks like. With hypoaccommodation, the eyes then become exotropic based on a sensory etiology. By giving these children a clear visual world with the hyperopic glasses, their sensory status can improve and subsequently their motor alignment.

82.3 Diagnosis

Pseudodivergence excess type intermittent exotropia.

82.4 Medical Management

Medical management is aimed at decreasing the time that the patient is exotropic (i.e., increasing fusional control). The actual deviation will usually not change. This sort of management can be divided into either passive management or active management.

1. Passive management is utilized most in younger children (i.e., usually younger than 4 to 5 years), because they usually cannot cooperate or understand the exercises of active management. Overminused spectacles and alternate or dominant eye part-time occlusion are included in passive management options. In overminusing, a child is given glasses with a more myopic correction than he or she needs. Overminusing a spectacle correction causes an increase in accommodative demand and subsequently accommodative convergence. Overminusing is helpful in some children in order to delay surgical management or while waiting for children to mature enough for active management. It rarely cures the exotropia. Alternate eye occlusion is performed by patching alternate eyes on alternate days. Dominant eye occlusion is performed by patching the nondeviating eye daily. A daily patching period of approximately 1 to 2 hours is usually prescribed. Occlusion therapy, also known as patching therapy, is based on the theory that it weakens the suppression scotoma that has been set up in a child with intermittent exotropia and may lead to better control.

2. Active management consists of a various exercises to stimulate convergence and fusion and to increase diplopia awareness. Convergence exercises can only be accurately achieved in children who can understand how to perform them. These exercises cause asthenopia or eye fatigue, and children younger than 5 years of age are usually not able to consistently comply. An easy convergence exercise to perform at home is the "pencil pushup." This exercise is performed by having the child fixate on a small fixation target affixed to a tongue blade, popsicle stick, or pencil. Next the parent brings the object progressively closer to the child's nose while the child's eyes converge on the target until fusion breaks and one eye becomes exotropic. The fixation target is then moved back out again and the exercise is repeated. Typically, 10 repetitions are done two to three times a day. A number of other convergence exercises can be performed with a red glass or synoptophore. Computer orthoptic exercises are also available to improve convergence amplitudes. Progressively increasing base-out prism can also be used to stimulate convergence. Convergence exercises are helpful for the conditions of convergence insufficiency exotropia and basic exotropia, but are not typically helpful in patients with divergence excess exotropia.

82.5 Surgical Management

Surgery is recommended in patients when the control of the exotropic deviation becomes poor. The decision of "poor control" is based on a number of different assessments, including parental impression and clinical examination. Typically, an ophthalmologist will decide to perform strabismus surgery on a child when the deviation is present more than 40 to 50% of the time. Most pediatric ophthalmologists prefer to delay surgery in exotropic patients until the child is 4 years or older, if the control is adequate. The type of surgical procedure performed will depend on the classification of the exotropia and surgeon preference. Bilateral lateral rectus recessions can be performed for divergence excess exotropia, pseudodivergence excess exotropia, and basic exotropia. A lateral rectus recession with an ipsilateral medial rectus resection can be performed for basic exotropia, pseudodivergence excess exotropia, and convergence insufficiency exotropia. Bilateral medial rectus resections can be performed for convergence insufficiency exotropia.

82.6 Rehabilitation and Follow-up

Intermittent exotropia is a lifelong condition. Because the cause of intermittent exotropia lies with a cortical defect of fusion, the entity is never "cured." The follow-up interval depends on the level of control and age of the patient. Typically, if medical management is being used, follow-up ranges between 2 and 6 months for reevaluation. If surgery has been performed, healing occurs over approximately 6 weeks. Surgical patients must still be followed long term, because the deviation can recur. Recurrence of exotropia has been cited in the literature at a rate of 20 to 40%. Surgery can be repeated for symptomatic or cosmetically noticeable deviations. Children with exotropia should be followed for decreasing stereopsis and the onset of amblyopia, both signs of worsening control.

Suggested Reading

[1] Biglan AW, Davis JS, Cheng KP, Pettapiece MC. Infantile exotropia. J Pediatr Ophthalmol Strabismus. 1996; 33(2):79–84

[2] Campos EC, Cipolli C. Binocularity and photophobia in intermittent exotropia. Percept Mot Skills. 1992; 74(3 Pt 2):1168–1170

[3] Haldi BA. Ninth Annual Richard G. Scobee Memorial Lecture. Sensory response in exotropia. Ophthalmology. 1979; 86(12):2090–2100

[4] Ing MR, Nishimura J, Okino L. Outcome study of bilateral lateral rectus recession for intermittent exotropia in children. Ophthalmic Surg Lasers. 1999; 30 (2):110–117

[5] Kushner BJ. Selective surgery for intermittent exotropia based on distance/near differences. Arch Ophthalmol. 1998; 116(3):324–328

[6] Kushner BJ, Morton GV. Distance/near differences in intermittent exotropia. Arch Ophthalmol. 1998; 116(4):478–486

83 Childhood Ptosis

Evelyn A. Paysse

Abstract

This chapter presents a case of a child with congenital ptosis. It discusses pertinent historical and examination findings of congenital ptosis, the differential diagnosis that must be ruled out including third nerve palsy and Horner's syndrome, associated ocular motility and visual abnormalities that can develop, the management approach, and long-term expectations.

Keywords: ptosis, amblyopia, Marcus Gunn jaw wink, Horner's syndrome, third nerve palsy, congenital, anisometropia

83.1 History

A 17-month-old boy presents with a droopy right upper lid. His parents state that this right upper lid has been "lazy" since birth. They also state that he holds his chin up when he is walking or watching TV. No ocular motility disturbance has been noted. His parents also volunteer that occasionally the child lets the lid block his pupil. There is no family history of ptosis, strabismus, or hereditary muscular disorders. The child is otherwise healthy and developing normally with a negative review of systems.

The child has good fixation and following visual behavior in both eyes (without correction) without a fixation preference for either eye. The child notably has a preferred chin-up head posture of 15 degrees. External examination demonstrates a moderate to severe right upper lid ptosis (▶ Fig. 83.1). The interpalpebral fissure on the right is 6.5 mm and on the left is 10 mm. The eyelid margin-to-reflex distance with the child's head in the primary position is 0.5 and 3.5 mm in the right and left eyes, respectively. With a chin-up head posture, the eyelid margin to reflex distance is 2 mm in the right eye and 3 mm in the left eye. Levator function is 6 mm in the right eye and 12 mm in the left eye. No appreciable lid crease is noted in the right upper lid. The pupils are both 3 mm in diameter, round, and briskly reactive to light. There is no afferent pupillary defect. The eyes are orthotropic and versions are full. Cycloplegic refraction is −0.25 + 1.50 × 90 degrees in the right eye and + 0.50 sphere in the left eye. The rest of the comprehensive examination is unremarkable.

Differential Diagnosis—Key Points

1. This is a 17-month-old child who has had ptosis of the right upper lid since birth. The history is significant for the lack of variability, lack of previous trauma, lack of strabismus, and lack of anisocoria. Childhood ptosis has an extensive differential diagnosis (see list below).

2. The differential diagnosis of a child with ptosis includes the following:

   a) *Congenital ptosis* occurs from a developmental abnormality of the levator muscle. The levator muscle is hypoplastic with fibrous or fatty infiltration. The degree of the ptosis actually decreases in downgaze relative to the other eye secondary to the fibrotic nature of the levator muscle in this condition. This is helpful to the child who often assumes a chin-up posture as the ptotic lid is less ptotic when this head position is utilized and the visual axis is better exposed.

   b) *Horner's syndrome* is suspected when its classic triad of miosis, anhidrosis, and mild ptosis of the involved eye are present. Horner's syndrome occurs secondary to dysfunction of the sympathetic chain on the ipsilateral side. Acquired Horner's syndrome requires an evaluation for serious diseases such as neuroblastoma. Congenital Horner's syndrome is typically associated with heterochromia, with the lighter pigmented iris on the involved side.

   c) *Third nerve palsy* causes a moderate to severe ptosis. It may be associated with vertical strabismus, exotropia, and/or mydriasis. The severity and etiology of the third nerve palsy will determine which of these signs is present. A third nerve palsy can be congenital or it can be acquired due to tumor, trauma, vascular abnormality, or inflammatory lesions of the brainstem or orbit (see chapters 66 and 67).

   d) *Marcus Gunn jaw-wink ptosis* occurs from a synkinesis of the trigeminal (V) nerve to the oculomotor (III) nerve (trigemino-oculomotor synkinesis). Stimulation of the pterygoid branch of the trigeminal nerve, responsible for the muscles of mastication, will also stimulate the levator muscle because of the miswiring and will elevate the upper lid. Pterygoid nerve stimulation occurs most

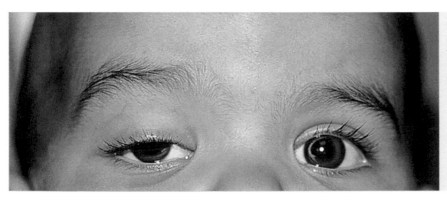

Fig. 83.1 Facial photograph of the patient demonstrating ptosis of the right upper lid. Note the absence of a lid crease on the affected lid. (Adapted from Lee DA and Higginbotham EJ. Clinical Guide to Comprehensive Ophthalmology. New York, NY: Thieme,1999:153.)

commonly with sucking, swallowing, chewing, or on lateral movement of the jaw. This entity is most commonly diagnosed in the neonatal period when a child is bottle- or breastfeeding but can occasionally be overlooked until later in life.

  e) Other causes of ptosis:

  1. *Myasthenia gravis* causes ptosis that is variable in severity and timing. It is commonly associated with other extraocular motility abnormalities that do not necessarily follow the rules of neurologic innervation. Myasthenia gravis can be purely ocular or can be ocular and systemic. Systemic findings of myasthenia gravis include respiratory compromise, weakness of proximal extremities, and dysphagia (see chapter 71).

  2. *Ptosis associated with double elevator palsy* is typically a moderate to severe congenital ptosis, associated with the inability to elevate the eye either in adduction or abduction.

  3. *Ptosis associated with chronic progressive external ophthalmoplegia* is an acquired ptosis associated with progressive extraocular motility deficits. It can also be associated with other ophthalmologic and systemic abnormalities, such as retinal pigmentary abnormalities and heart block, seen in Kearn–Sayres syndrome.

  4. *Mechanical ptosis* results from a mass lesion that restricts elevation of the lid such as a large hemangioma, lymphangioma, neurofibroma, or dermoid.

  5. *Levator dehiscence* occurs secondary to trauma or stretching of the levator muscle, usually over years as could be caused by insertion of contact lens. It is a slowly progressive, acquired ptosis. The distance between the lid crease and lid margin is increased in this entity.

  6. *Pseudoptosis* occurs secondary to a primary hypotropia on the involved side with the resultant corresponding upper lid depression. This is not a true ptosis; that is, when the hypotropic eye fixates, the apparent ptosis resolves.

3. Childhood ptosis is associated with several other important ophthalmologic abnormalities. *Amblyopia* is the most important potential problem associated with ptosis. It can occur secondary to one of several mechanisms. The most devastating amblyopia is caused by occlusion of the involved eye due to obstruction of the visual axis. This will produce severe form of vision deprivation amblyopia, such as in a child with a congenital cataract. Amblyopia due to ptosis can also occur secondary to anisometropia. The anisometropia seen in children with congenital ptosis usually occurs secondary to astigmatism, created by the upper lid compressing the flexible infant cornea. *Strabismus* can occasionally be associated with ptosis and pseudoptosis. This is frequently the case in children with double elevator palsy who have a hypotropia of the involved side and a pseudoptosis.

83.1.1 Causes of Childhood Ptosis

- Congenital ptosis.
- Horner's syndrome.
- Third nerve palsy.
- Marcus Gunn jaw-winking ptosis.
- Myasthenia gravis.
- Double elevator palsy.
- Chronic progressive external ophthalmoplegia.
- Mechanical ptosis:
  - Lid hemangioma.
  - Lid neurofibroma.
- Levator dehiscence.
- Pseudoptosis.

83.2 Test Interpretation

The major diagnostic considerations in a child with ptosis are related to careful ophthalmologic examination. The following discussion will concentrate on the most relevant parts of an examination.

1. Vision: It is imperative to obtain the best visual acuity or visual behavior (e.g., fix and follow; central, steady, maintained) possible in the child. The examiner should perform the most rigorous vision test the child is capable of. Fixation preference should be assessed in addition to visual behavior in a nonverbal or preverbal child. If the child has strabismus, it is easy to assess for fixation preference. The examiner simply covers one eye to gain fixation in the other, then removes the occluder and watches for any refixation movement to the previously covered eye. This would signify a fixation preference for the previously covered eye. Fixation preference is more difficult to ascertain when a child does not have strabismus. The vertical prism test can be useful. Several variations of this test exist. One method involves holding a 10 to 14 prism diopter hand-held prism base down in one of the examiner's hands. Next, the examiner gains the child's fixation on a small target. The examiner then places the vertical prism in front of one of the child's eyes while watching for a refixation movement. If the child refixates, the examiner will note an upward movement of both eyes as the child switches fixation to the eye looking through the prism. This test should be done several times on one eye and then repeated on the other eye. Typically, if amblyopia is not present, no refixation movement will be noted when the prism is placed in front of either eye. If there is consistent refixation movement when the prism is held before one eye but not the other, amblyopia should be suspected. Our child has normal and equal visual acuity in each eye.

2. Pupils: Anisocoria in the presence of ptosis can be due to Horner's syndrome or a third nerve palsy. If anisocoria is noted, the examiner must note whether the anisocoria is worse in lighted or dimly lit conditions, in order to discern whether the iris dilator muscle (i.e., sympathetic nervous system) or the iris sphincter (i.e., parasympathetic nervous system) is the problematic muscle. If the anisocoria is worse in dimly lit conditions, the dilator muscle is problematic and a Horner syndrome should be suspected. If the anisocoria is worse in lighted conditions, then the iris sphincter is the problem, and a third nerve palsy may be present. Further workup for each of these entities should be performed.

3. External examination: Several different measurements should be performed when evaluating a ptosis patient. The

palpebral fissure height, the margin reflex distance, and levator function are needed to evaluate ptosis to help determine etiology and to decide on the best management approach. In children, attention for an anomalous head posture is also important. A chin-up head posture is adaptive and usually signifies less risk for amblyopia than severe ptosis without a chin-up head posture. The distance between the lid crease and the lid margin is also helpful in differentiating the different types of ptosis. If this distance is higher than average, the ptosis is more likely due to a levator dehiscence. If a lid crease is completely absent or rudimentary, the ptosis is more likely congenital. One must also assess the child for a Bell phenomenon prior to surgical treatment. Ptosis caused by double-elevator palsy, congenital fibrosis syndrome, or progressive external ophthalmoplegia is often associated with a decreased or absent Bell's phenomenon. Patients with an abnormal Bell phenomenon are at increased risk of exposure keratopathy and other related problems following surgery. Finally, infants should be evaluated while sucking on a bottle and older children should be asked to move their jaw laterally from side to side to rule out trigemino-oculomotor synkinesis. Each of these maneuvers will stimulate the pterygoid branch of the trigeminal nerve and, if jaw winking is present, will stimulate the superior branch of the oculomotor nerve and elevation of the involved lid will occur. Our child has severe ptosis with moderate levator function, absent lid crease, and an increase in palpebral fissure height in down-gaze, all signs consistent with congenital ptosis.

4. Motility: Motility abnormalities can be associated with ptosis if a third nerve palsy, double-elevator palsy, congenital fibrous syndrome, or dense amblyopia (sensory strabismus) is present. A careful motility examination should be done and any abnormalities noted should be addressed.

5. Slit-lamp examination/anterior segment evaluation: If evaluating a mild ptosis for a Horner syndrome, it is helpful to look for heterochromia. Heterochromia is seen in patients who have a congenital or very early onset Horner's syndrome. The lighter pigmented iris is on the involved side.

6. Cycloplegic refraction: Significant anisometropia and astigmatism are common sequelae of long-standing ptosis. If significant anisometropia exists, spectacle correction should be prescribed. If amblyopia is detected, appropriate amblyopia treatment should also be instituted (see chapter 77.) Our child has minimal anisometropia with good vision in both eyes.

83.3 Diagnosis

Congenital ptosis of the right upper lid with anomalous chin-up head posture and absence of amblyopia.

83.4 Medical Management

Medical management is only helpful for the associations of congenital ptosis, namely, amblyopia and anisometropia. Amblyopia is typically treated either with occlusion therapy or with pharmacologic or optical penalization (see chapter 77). The type of amblyopia therapy will depend on patient compliance, cooperation, and physician preference. Anisometropia and astigmatism should be corrected if deemed significant. Vigilant follow-up throughout the childhood years must be done to insure that amblyopia, once treated, does not recur.

83.5 Surgical Management

Ptosis, if significant, is a surgical disease. Surgery also offers, in addition to an increased visual field and cosmetic benefits, improvement of an anomalous head posture, which could allow for improvement in development and coordination. Surgical treatment goals are to elevate the ptotic lid for better vision and increased visual field, and to reform the lid crease if it is absent or rudimentary for cosmesis. It is important to decrease the surgical dose if the Bell phenomenon is absent or decreased because of the risk of exposure keratopathy.

Several different surgical treatment approaches are possible. The choice of procedure depends on the severity of the ptosis and levator function. The Fasanella–Servat procedure is used for small ptosis of 2 mm or less. A small wedge of conjunctiva, superior tarsus, levator palpebrae, and Müller's muscle are resected in this procedure. This is an excellent procedure for a Horner syndrome–associated ptosis. The levator resection is the most versatile procedure and gives an excellent cosmetic result. It can be performed for mild, moderate, and severe ptosis if enough levator function is present. The frontalis suspension procedure is typically reserved only for severe ptosis without adequate levator function (typically 4 mm or less). As its name implies, it is a suspension procedure in which material is threaded through the upper lid and attached to the frontalis muscle. The material acts as a sling to hold the lid up. Different materials, including a variety of sutures (Supramid, nylon, Prolene, Gore-Tex), silicone rods, and organic materials, such as banked or autogenous fascia lata or palmaris longus tendon, have been utilized as the suspension material. The best long-term results are found with the use of an autogenous fascia lata. Results with banked fascia lata are almost as long lasting. All synthetic materials have been shown to have a shorter life span and increased risk for late complications such as granuloma formation and other inflammatory reactions. The potential complications of ptosis surgery, though infrequent, include early and late infection, suture granuloma, exposure keratopathy, retrobulbar hemorrhage, and overcorrections.

83.6 Rehabilitation and Follow-up

A child with congenital ptosis needs to be followed throughout childhood for the associated problems of amblyopia and anisometropia. Once treated, amblyopia can recur until a child is age 7 to 10 years old. Therefore, surveillance must continue. Following surgical repair of ptosis, healing will occur over approximately 1 month. It is common after surgery for the child to have some lagophthalmos when sleeping. Ocular lubrication at night helps for the first month, and can usually be abandoned thereafter, as children adapt very well to the small amount of lagophthalmos that occurs from these procedures. When the Bell reflex is absent, lubrication is usually needed permanently after surgery. Lid height should be followed over time, as ptosis can recur.

Suggested Reading

[1] Beard C. Ptosis. 2nd ed. St. Louis, MO: CV Mosby; 1976;164–169

[2] Cadera W, Orton RB, Hakim O. Changes in astigmatism after surgery for congenital ptosis. J Pediatr Ophthalmol Strabismus. 1992; 29(2):85–88

[3] Katowitz JA. Frontalis suspension in congenital ptosis using a polyfilament, cable-type suture. Arch Ophthalmol. 1979; 97(9):1659–1663

[4] Mauriello JA, Wagner RS, Caputo AR, Natale B, Lister M. Treatment of congenital ptosis by maximal levator resection. Ophthalmology. 1986; 93(4):466–469

[5] Meyer DR, Rheeman CH. Downgaze eyelid position in patients with blepharoptosis. Ophthalmology. 1995; 102(10):1517–1523

[6] Wagner RS, Mauriello JA, Jr, Nelson LB, Calhoun JH, Flanagan JC, Harley RD. Treatment of congenital ptosis with frontalis suspension: a comparison of suspensory materials. Ophthalmology. 1984; 91(3):245–248

[7] Wright KW, Walonker F, Edelman P. 10-diopter fixation test for amblyopia. Arch Ophthalmol. 1981; 99(7):1242–1246

84 The Apparently Blind Infant

David K. Coats and Evelyn A. Paysse

Abstract

The apparently blind infant may truly be blind or may simply appear to be blind. The condition may be due to prenatal, perinatal, or postnatal etiologies. Some common congenital etiologies for a blind infant include anophthalmos, microphthalmos, coloboma, congenital cataract, and infantile glaucoma. Ophthalmia neonatorum, retinopathy of prematurity, and cortical visual impairment may occur in the perinatal period. Leukocoria or white pupillary reflex (e.g., congenital cataract, persistent hyperplastic primary vitreous, or retinoblastoma) is also discussed. This chapter describes the evaluation (including possible exam under anesthesia, funduscopy, refraction, corneal diameter measurement, and measurement of intraocular pressure), management, treatment, and prognosis of specific causes of the apparently blind infant.

Keywords: blind infant, prenatal, postnatal, intrauterine, cortical visual impairment

84.1 History

A 3-month-old girl is brought to her ophthalmologist by her parents because of concerns that she may be blind. They report that she has poor eye contact, that she does not respond to parental facial expressions, and that she does not appear to respond to bright lights. The child's prenatal and birth histories are unremarkable. Her past ophthalmologic and medical histories are unremarkable. The child has two siblings, aged 2 years and 5 years, who visually responded much more at 3 months of age than the patient does and who are developmentally and visually normal at this time. The review of systems is otherwise negative. The child appears to be normal from a developmental standpoint, though the child has not been seen by her pediatrician in several weeks.

On examination, a healthy-appearing 3-month-old girl is sitting on her mother's lap. The ocular adnexal and other facial features appear normal. The child does not fixate on or follow any target and does not respond to facial gestures. She does blink when a bright light is directed into her eyes. Optokinetic nystagmus (OKN) testing demonstrates an occasional beat of nystagmus, but attention is poor and the test results are equivocal. The eyes are orthotropic with full versions to oculocephalic testing. Spontaneous nystagmus is not seen. The pupillary examination reveals pupils that are 5 mm in size and moderately reactive to light with no afferent pupillary defect, and no paradoxical pupillary reaction is present. Anterior segment and fundus examinations are normal.

Differential Diagnosis—Key Points

1. Poor vision in a child requires consideration of an extensive differential diagnosis. In general, poor vision in an infant should be divided into poor vision without nystagmus and poor vision with nystagmus. If nystagmus is present, the differential diagnosis includes bilateral structural abnormalities of the cornea lens, retina, or optic nerve leading to a bilateral severe, afferent dysfunction. Idiopathic infantile nystagmus is also a consideration if nystagmus is present. The absence of nystagmus strongly supports a cortical-based abnormality.

2. Delayed visual maturation (DVM) is an interesting and troubling problem that is not infrequently encountered in young infants. In general, the absence of fixation behavior in a child 4 to 6 weeks of age is rarely alarming to pediatricians or parents. If obvious visual fixation behavior is not present after this time, however, parents and pediatricians alike become very concerned. DVM can be classified into three major groups: (1) isolated DVM, (2) DVM with associated central nervous system (CNS) disease, and (3) DVM with associated structural eye abnormalities. In isolated DVM, the absence of obvious visual behavior is the only abnormality noted. The child is developmentally and neurologically normal and typically has normal electrophysiologic testing results. DVM can also coexist with systemic disease and/or intellectual disability or with ocular disease such as optic nerve hypoplasia and albinism. The etiology of the DVM is unknown, but some have suggested that delayed myelination of the optic nerves and/or tracts or delayed synaptogenesis in the visual pathways may be the etiology. Visual behavior in this condition eventually normalizes by 6 to 8 months of age in most cases.

3. Cortical visual impairment (CVI) is another important condition that must be considered. A child with CVI will appear clinically similar to the child with DVM. Typically the child with CVI, however, has a history of perinatal hypoxia or another serious neurological event suggesting the possibility of hypoxic brain injury and typically also has concurrent neurologic and/or systemic abnormalities.

4. Structural abnormalities of the eye must be carefully ruled out. In general, bilateral structural abnormalities that are severe enough to produce blindness typically will present with concurrent nystagmus. Affected patients may initially appear similar to the child with DVM because nystagmus may not develop until the child is several months of age. Careful ophthalmologic examination will usually eliminate the confusion.

84.2 Test Interpretation

The ophthalmologist should work in conjunction with the child's pediatrician or neurologist. The child suspected of having DVM should undergo a careful developmental assessment. If the developmental milestones are normal, isolated DVM is the likely diagnosis. Time will allow this diagnosis to be confirmed as the child begins to develop normal visual behavior with age. This child is developmentally normal.

A neurological assessment is important in this situation and can be conducted by the child's pediatrician or a neurologist. The presence of neurologic abnormalities can coexist with DVM. The prognosis, however, for DVM with neurologic abnormalities is not as good, and vision is often slower to improve compared with isolated DVM. Our patient had a normal screening neurological examination.

In general, unless neurologic and/or systemic abnormalities are found, the child with isolated DVM does not need to undergo electrophysiologic testing. If tested, however, the child's electroencephalogram (EEG) must be normal. If the EEG is abnormal, the child does *not* have isolated DVM. The visual evoked potential (VEP) test in a child with isolated DVM may be mildly delayed and attenuated or may be normal. The test is useful in predicting eventual development of good vision. The electroretinogram is also normal in children with isolated DVM. This child's parents requested a VEP test.

It is of paramount importance for the ophthalmologist to interact appropriately with parents, pediatricians, and neurologists. It is extremely important to explain carefully to the parents what DVM is and its prognosis. It is improper to declare an infant visually impaired in the first 4 to 6 months of life, as many will prove to have normal vision as the visual system matures. Alleviating parental and referring physician fear is a major role of the ophthalmologist in treating infants with this condition. An extensive workup, however, is not initially needed if the infant is developmentally and neurologically normal.

84.3 Diagnosis

Isolated DVM.

84.4 Medical Management

The child should undergo a careful initial developmental and neurologic assessment. Periodic assessments of development and neurologic function should also be undertaken by the child's pediatrician. Continued normal development is strongly suggestive of isolated DVM and the likelihood of eventual improvement of vision.

84.5 Surgical Management

No surgical treatment is indicated.

84.6 Rehabilitation and Follow-up

For the typical infant with isolated DVM, vision typically will become normal by the time the infant is 6 to 8 months old. At this point, no further evaluation or intervention is required, and such a child can be expected to do well. On the other hand, if the vision fails to improve by 6 to 8 months of age, further evaluation including electrophysiologic testing and neuroimaging is indicated. In a child with DVM associated with neurologic abnormalities, developmental delay, and/or ocular abnormalities, visual response may be delayed until as late as 1 to 2 years of age.

Suggested Reading

[1] American Academy of Ophthalmology. Vision Assessment of the Pediatric Patient Refinements. San Francisco, CA: American Academy of Ophthalmology; 1997

[2] Cole GF, Hungerford J, Jones RB. Delayed visual maturation. Arch Dis Child. 1984; 59(2):107–110

[3] Fielder AR, Russell-Eggitt IR, Dodd KL, Mellor DH. Delayed visual maturation. Trans Ophthalmol Soc U K. 1985; 104(Pt 6):653–661

[4] Hoyt CS, Jastrzebski G, Marg E. Delayed visual maturation in infancy. Br J Ophthalmol. 1983; 67(2):127–130

[5] Lambert SR, Kriss A, Taylor D. Delayed visual maturation. A longitudinal clinical and electrophysiological assessment. Ophthalmology. 1989; 96(4):524–528, discussion 529

[6] Taylor B. Delayed visual maturation. In: Taylor D, ed. Pediatric Ophthalmology: Malden, MA: Blackwell Science, Inc.; 1990:21–22

85 Optic Nerve Hypoplasia

David K. Coats and Evelyn Paysse

Abstract

Optic nerve hypoplasia (ONH) produces variable visual loss and a small optic nerve in one or both eyes. It can be associated with other intracranial defects (e.g., septo-optic dysplasia [SOD] or DeMorsier's syndrome, brain and pituitary malformations, and hypoplasia of the corpus callosum). Some children with ONH have nystagmus and vision can range from no light perception to 20/20. Hormone deficiencies should be tested and treated. Neuroimaging may be required. This chapter reviews the evaluation, management, treatment, and prognosis of ONH.

Keywords: optic nerve hypoplasia, hypothalamic pituitary axis

85.1 History

A 3-year-old boy is referred by another ophthalmologist. The child was diagnosed with esotropia and amblyopia in the right eye at age 2 years. The referring ophthalmologist prescribed full-time patching of the left eye, which was done sporadically for approximately 6 months. No improvement in the child's vision was noted, prompting referral for a second opinion and treatment recommendations.

The child's medical history is notable for a weight and height in the 15th percentile, but is otherwise unremarkable. The review of systems is completely negative with the exception of the ophthalmologic complaints and there is no family history of strabismus or amblyopia.

The patient is shown in ▶ Fig. 85.1. Best-corrected visual acuity is 20/200 in the right eye and 20/30 in the left eye. Motility evaluation reveals an esotropia of 25 prism diopters at distance and at near with full ductions and versions. Pupillary testing reveals a 1 + relative afferent pupillary defect (RAPD) in the right eye. Cycloplegic refraction is + 1.25 diopters in both eyes and initial evaluation of the posterior pole reveals a normal disc, macula, and vessels. The ophthalmologist is concerned by the presence of the RAPD and performs a more careful evaluation of the posterior pole. The disc of the right eye appears slightly pale. The vessels on the nerve are crowded. The disc diameter is small, and a double-ring sign is noted (▶ Fig. 85.2a, b). The left disc is also slightly smaller than normal.

85.2 Test Interpretation

1. When an RAPD was noted in this child, careful scrutiny of the optic discs became paramount. Several methods can be utilized to obtain a better view of the posterior pole in an uncooperative or marginally cooperative child. These measures include the use of direct ophthalmoscopy, or indirect ophthalmoscopy using a 14-diopter lens. Both of these techniques offer greater magnification compared to indirect ophthalmoscopy with a 20-diopter lens but have the disadvantage of being either difficult to perform on an uncooperative child (direct ophthalmoscopy) or not readily

Differential Diagnosis—Key Points

1. An RAPD should always be a tip-off that amblyopia is *not* the problem and a careful evaluation to determine the etiology of the afferent abnormality should be carried out. While it is true that trace RAPDs may occasionally be seen in children with amblyopia, the presence of an easily identifiable RAPD is not consistent with a diagnosis of amblyopia. The examiner must explain its presence and is advised to refer the child for a second opinion if a plausible explanation cannot be found.

2. Optic nerve hypoplasia is a relatively common congenital anomaly of the optic nerves. It may occur in one or both eyes and may be isolated or may be associated with central nervous system (CNS) and endocrine abnormalities. The condition is difficult to diagnose in an uncooperative child. Nevertheless, a detailed and magnified view of the disc must be obtained. The so-called double-ring sign may or may not be present, and when present, may be mistaken for a normal-sized optic nerve. This is especially true if indirect ophthalmoscopy, which offers only minimal magnification, is the only technique used to examine the discs. Often, an anomalous configuration of retinal vessels on the disc is the first tip-off that there is a problem with the optic nerve, prompting a more detailed look.

3. Vision can vary from 20/20 to no light perception. Many children with severe optic nerve hypoplasia appear completely blind at birth but demonstrate useful vision later in life. When severe and bilateral optic nerve hypoplasia is present, the child will also have nystagmus and presents a less formidable diagnostic challenge.

4. Optic nerve hypoplasia is commonly associated with midline CNS defects such as absence of the septum pellucidum and/ or corpus callosum and posterior pituitary ectopia. Hemispheric migrational anomalies may also be present. When optic nerve hypoplasia coexists with these midline CNS defects, the terms *septo-optic dysplasia* or *De Morsier syndrome* have been utilized.

5. Patients with septo-optic dysplasia may suffer a variety of pituitary hormone abnormalities, including abnormalities of growth hormone and of the adrenocorticosteroid axis. It is important to recognize this condition because corticotrophin deficiency has been associated with sudden death in children with septo-optic dysplasia following an otherwise uneventful febrile illness, and growth hormone deficiency can result in severe growth retardation. Endocrine abnormalities are most likely to occur in children with posterior pituitary ectopia and hemispheric migrational abnormalities.

6. Optic neuritis and optic atrophy are included in the differential diagnosis of this child with poor vision in one eye and an RAPD. These conditions can be ruled out on clinical examination.

available (14-diopter lens) in most ophthalmology practices. Modified (monocular) indirect ophthalmoscopy offers a useful imaging option. With this technique, a standard 20-diopter lens is held 5 to 6 cm in front of the child's eye. The direct ophthalmoscope is then held approximately 18 cm away. The aerial image produced by the 20-diopter lens is then focused with the direct ophthalmoscope. This technique allows adequate magnification to accurately assess the optic nerves without requiring the close proximity to the child that is required for direct ophthalmoscopy. Examination of the eyes under anesthesia is sometimes required in particularly uncooperative children. The potential for serious problems due to corticotrophin deficiency should be considered and steroids administered before anesthesia if this problem is suspected. For this reason, consultation with an endocrinologist should be completed before undergoing any surgical intervention or anesthetic.

2. Magnetic resonance imaging of the brain is the preferred neuroimaging study to rule out midline CNS defects and hemispheric migrational abnormalities. Specifically, the examiner should review the scan for absence of the corpus callosum or septum pellucidum and for pituitary abnormalities. Ectopia of the posterior pituitary bright spot is highly suggestive of current or future endocrine abnormalities. This child's MRI scan is shown in ▶ Fig. 85.3.

Endocrine testing should be conducted by an endocrinologist or the child's pediatrician. This is imperative and urgent. This patient had a markedly reduced growth hormone level. The most common endocrine abnormalities that present in septo-optic dysplasia are growth hormone and corticotrophin deficiency. These conditions should be detected early in the disease course to prevent a potential medical disaster. The child's pediatrician should be advised of the child's condition and the need to follow growth and endocrine parameters carefully and frequently.

85.3 Diagnosis

Septo-optic dysplasia, with bilateral, asymmetric optic nerve hypoplasia. The child is also suffering from a growth hormone deficiency with resulting short stature and low weight.

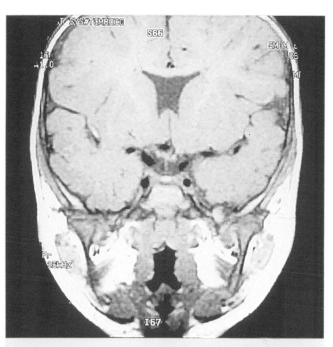

Fig. 85.3 Magnetic resonance scan demonstrating absence of the septum pellucidum. (This image is provided courtesy of Andrew G. Lee, MD, Iowa City, IA.)

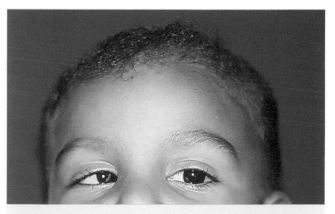

Fig. 85.1 Esotropia noted in a patient on initial examination. (This image is provided courtesy of Andrew G. Lee, MD, Iowa City, IA.)

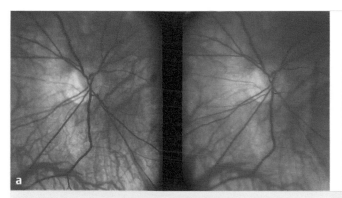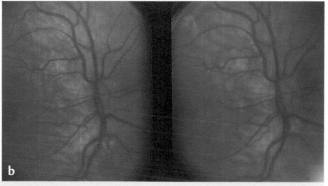

Fig. 85.2 (a) Small right optic nerve with "double ring" sign. (b) Normal left optic nerve of another patient for comparison. (These images are provided courtesy of Andrew G. Lee, MD, Iowa City, IA.)

85.4 Medical Treatment

The child should be under the care of an endocrinologist and should undergo pituitary hormone replacement as needed with close follow-up of his growth parameters. Despite the fact that the child has optic nerve hypoplasia, there is still the potential to improve the vision in his right eye if a component of functional amblyopia coexists with the anatomical defect. Such patients should receive a trial of amblyopia therapy before concluding that the visual impairment is irreversible.

85.5 Surgical Treatment

Strabismus surgery or botulinum toxin injection can be offered to repair the child's esotropia. The child's parents should be advised, however, that the strabismus has a higher likelihood to recur following surgery due to the poor vision. Surgery should be deferred until amblyopia treatment has been maximized. Typically, strabismus surgery is postponed until school age to minimize the total number of strabismus surgeries the patient will have to undergo in his lifetime.

85.6 Rehabilitation and Follow-up

As with all functionally monocular patients, polycarbonate safety spectacles should be prescribed to protect the child's better-seeing eye. In children with optic nerve hypoplasia, ongoing evaluation of growth and endocrine parameters should continue throughout early childhood, even if the child appears to be growing normally at initial diagnosis. Endocrine abnormalities have been detected and problems have been noted with delayed onset as late as 3 to 4 years of age. Stress doses of corticosteroids should be administered in patients with corticotrophin abnormalities in situations such as acute illness, surgery, or serious injury.

85.6.1 Note

The child described in this case is a composite of several children used to demonstrate common findings of optic nerve hypoplasia.

Suggested Reading

[1] Brodsky MC, Conte FA, Taylor D, Hoyt CS, Mrak RE. Sudden death in septo-optic dysplasia. Report of 5 cases. Arch Ophthalmol. 1997; 115(1):66–70
[2] Brodsky MC, Glasier CM. Optic nerve hypoplasia. Clinical significance of associated central nervous system abnormalities on magnetic resonance imaging. Arch Ophthalmol. 1993; 111(1):66–74
[3] Coats DK, Paysse EA. Modified (monocular) indirect ophthalmoscopy for examination of the pediatric retina to rule out organic amblyopia. Binocul Vis Strabismus Q. 1997; 12(1):43–46
[4] Siatkowski RM, Sanchez JC, Andrade R, Alvarez A. The clinical, neuroradiographic, and endocrinologic profile of patients with bilateral optic nerve hypoplasia. Ophthalmology. 1997; 104(3):493–496

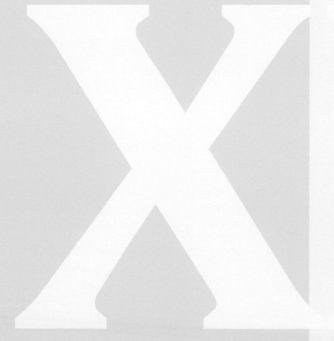

Part XI

Orbit / Oculoplastics

86 Ptosis

Amina I. Malik

Abstract

Ptosis involves droopiness of the upper eyelid and is most commonly due to levator aponeurosis dehiscence from age. Other etiologies include congenital, myogenic (myasthenia gravis or other myopathy), mechanical (mass on eyelid), or Horner's syndrome. If the ptosis is mild, it can be observed, but if it is interfering with superior peripheral vision, surgical repair can be performed.

Keywords: ptosis, eyelid droop

86.1 History

A 72-year-old woman was referred for drooping of her upper eyelids. The patient stated that the drooping had slowly progressed over the last 3 to 4 years. The drooping was now severe enough to interfere with her vision, and she often found herself manually lifting her lids to improve her visual field. There was no previous history of periocular trauma or surgery. She had undergone bilateral cataract extraction with placement of intraocular lenses 4 years previously. There was no history of muscle weakness or fatigue, and she had no known neurologic disease. She did not complain of diplopia or significant fluctuation of the lid position during the day. Inspection of old photographs did not show the presence of ptosis.

Examination showed corrected visual acuity of 20/20 OU. The patient was orthophoric with full ductions and versions on motility examination. Ptosis of both upper eyelids was present, with the right upper lid being lower than the left upper lid in both primary position and downgaze. The palpebral fissures measured 5 mm on the right and 6 mm on the left (▶ Fig. 86.1). The marginal reflex distances were 0 on the right and 1 on the left. The levator function measured 14 mm on both sides. Inspection of the tarsal conjunctiva on both sides showed no significant abnormalities and no orbital masses were palpated.

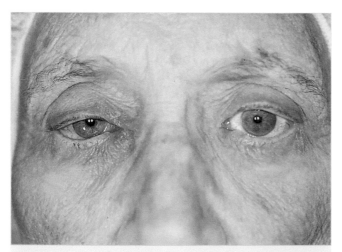

Fig. 86.1 Clinical photograph depicting bilateral ptosis of the eyelids that is more marked on the right side. Note the absent lid crease and the deep superior sulcus on both sides.

The upper eyelid creases were effaced on both sides, and the superior sulci were deepened.

Differential Diagnosis—Key Points

1. In this patient, there is bilateral ptosis, which has been slowly progressive. There is good preservation of levator function, and the absent upper eyelid crease and the deep superior sulci are consistent with an aponeurotic ptosis. The more ptotic eyelid is lower in downgaze, which contrasts with congenital ptosis. Furthermore, the opportunity to inspect previous photographs confirms the acquired nature of the lid malposition.

Aponeurotic ptosis results from a disinsertion of the levator aponeurosis from its normal attachment on the anterior tarsus. While levator disinsertion may occur following trauma or severe edema, it is most commonly an age-related change. The presence of good lid excursion (> 12 mm) indicates preservation of levator function and is important in distinguishing aponeurotic ptosis from other types of ptosis.

2. Neurogenic ptosis results from interruption of the innervation to the eyelid elevators, including levator aponeurosis (cranial nerve III) and Muller's muscle (sympathetic innervation). It may be congenital or acquired. Horner's syndrome, myasthenia gravis, or other neurologic conditions may cause neurogenic ptosis. Careful pupil examination and testing with topical cocaine and Paredrine will confirm the presence of Horner's syndrome. Ice testing, edrophonium (Tensilon) testing, or acetylcholine receptor antibodies should be performed if there is history of ptosis worsening with fatigue and myasthenia gravis is suspected.

3. Myogenic ptosis may also be congenital or acquired. Myogenic congenital ptosis results from abnormal development and fibrosis of the levator muscle and may be unilateral or bilateral. In contrast to aponeurotic ptosis, the ptotic lid will be higher in downgaze and the levator function is severely reduced, usually measuring less than 7 mm.

Acquired myogenic ptosis occurs in muscular diseases such as muscular dystrophy, chronic progressive external ophthalmoplegia (Kearns–Sayre syndrome), or oculopharyngeal dystrophy. The levator function is markedly diminished, and ocular motility is often severely impaired.

4. Mechanical ptosis results from the presence of a mass within the eyelid. The mass may be congenital or acquired and may be inflammatory or neoplastic. The ptotic lid should be everted to allow examination of the tarsal conjunctiva and fornix. Palpation of the orbit may reveal a mass superiorly. More commonly, severe blepharochalasis may produce mechanical ptosis.

5. Conditions that may mimic the presence of eyelid ptosis should be included in the differential diagnosis. The eyelid may appear ptotic if the globe is small (phthisis bulbi) or displaced posteriorly (enophthalmos). Eyelid retraction on one side may simulate ptosis of the contralateral lid.

86.2 Test Interpretation

If neurogenic or myogenic ptosis is suspected, appropriate testing as discussed earlier should be performed. It is critical to establish the correct diagnosis, not only to allow the correct management of the lid malposition, but also to ensure that any systemic disease is identified and treated appropriately.

86.3 Diagnosis

Ptosis of both upper eyelids due to levator aponeurosis disinsertion.

86.4 Medical Management

If ptosis is mild and the patient is asymptomatic, no treatment is indicated. If ptosis is severe enough to cause symptomatic visual field impairment, taping of the lid or the use of eyelid crutches attached to the patient's spectacles may be tried. In most patients, these measures are only temporizing, and surgical correction of the lid malposition is required to effect a long-term solution.

86.5 Surgical Management

Most cases of severe aponeurotic ptosis will require surgical treatment to achieve long-term satisfactory results. The anterior approach to ptosis repair allows reattachment or advancement of the dehisced levator aponeurosis to the anterior tarsus. This is accomplished through an external incision that also allows for re-establishment of the eyelid crease. Alternatively, a posterior approach can be used where Muller's muscle is resected. Complications of surgery include undercorrection or overcorrection, asymmetric or unsatisfactory lid contour, or lagophthalmos with exposure symptoms.

86.6 Rehabilitation and Follow-up

The patient underwent external levator advancement on both upper eyelids. The procedure was performed using local infiltrative anesthesia allowing for intraoperative adjustment of lid height and contour. Postoperatively, the patient noted an improvement in her visual field, and she suffered no complications from the surgical procedure.

86.6.1 Acknowledgment

Thanks to this chapter's first edition authors, Debra Shetlar and Milton Boniuk.

Suggested Reading

[1] Callahan MA, Beard C. Beard's Ptosis. 4th ed. Birmingham, AL: Aesculapius Publishing Co; 1990
[2] Dortzbach RK, Levine MR, Angrist RC. Approach to acquired ptosis. In: Smith BC, Della Rocca RC, Nesi FA, Lisman RD, eds. Ophthalmic Plastic and Reconstructive Surgery. Vol. 1. St. Louis, MO: CV Mosby; 1987;654–680
[3] Jones LT, Quickert MH, Wobig JL. The cure of ptosis by aponeurotic repair. Arch Ophthalmol. 1975; 93(8):629–634
[4] Linberg JV, Vasquez RJ, Chao GM. Aponeurotic ptosis repair under local anesthesia. Prediction of results from operative lid height. Ophthalmology. 1988; 95(8):1046–1052
[5] Waller RR, McCord CD, Tanenbaum M. Evaluation and management of the ptosis patient. In: McCord CD, Tanenbaum M, eds. Oculoplastic Surgery. 2nd ed. New York, NY: Raven Press; 1987:325–375

87 Thyroid Eye Disease

Amina I. Malik

Abstract

Thyroid eye disease is the most common etiology of proptosis, which is unilateral or bilateral. Signs include proptosis, eyelid retraction, limited extraocular motility, increased intraocular pressure in upgaze, and, in extreme cases, optic neuropathy. Diagnosis is established by exam, thyroid blood work, and imaging confirming the presence of enlarged extraocular muscle bellies. Treatment can include observation for mild cases, but surgical decompression may be indicated to reduce proptosis and for optic neuropathy. This can be followed by eye muscle surgery for diplopia and by eyelid retraction repair if present.

Keywords: thyroid eye disease, proptosis, eyelid retraction, decompression

87.1 History

A 44-year-old woman was referred for evaluation of pain around both eyes. The pain was described as dull ache, and worsened with eye movement. She had noted increasing prominence of both eyes over the past 18 months and complained that both eyes felt "gritty." She had no complaints of diplopia or blurred vision, and there was no previous ocular history of surgery or trauma. Her past medical history was unremarkable, and there was no history of thyroid dysfunction. Her review of symptoms was significant for heat and cold intolerance, but she reported no recent change in weight, body hair growth or loss, or change in the quality of her voice. There was no known cardiovascular or neurologic disease.

Examination showed corrected visual acuity of 20/20 in each eye. Normal color vision defect was detected with Hardy–Rand–Rittler color plates. Both pupils reacted normally, without relative afferent pupillary defect. The motility exam showed orthophoria with mild (–1) restriction of upgaze on both sides. Upper and lower eyelid retraction was present with palpebral fissures measuring 16 and 15 mm on the right and left sides, respectively (▶ Fig. 87.1). Temporal flaring of the upper lids was noted, and 2 mm of lagophthalmos was present bilaterally. There was increased resistance to retropulsion of both globes; no orbital masses were palpated. Exophthalmometry measurements were 22 mm on the right side and 21 mm on the left (▶ Fig. 87.2). Intraocular pressures were 21 mm Hg on the right side and 20 mm Hg on the left. Slit-lamp examination showed scattered punctate epithelial erosions of both corneas inferiorly. Mild bulbar conjunctival injection was present bilaterally, most pronounced at the insertion of horizontal rectus muscles. The anterior segments were otherwise unremarkable. Dilated fundus exam showed both optic discs to be flat without pallor. The retina appeared normal, and there were no choroidal striae.

Differential Diagnosis—Key Points

1. One of the most common causes of proptosis in middle-aged adults is thyroid eye disease (Graves' disease), and this patient demonstrates many of the salient features of this condition.

For purposes of evaluation and management, the ophthalmic findings of thyroid eye disease can be divided into three categories: optic nerve dysfunction, motility disturbance, and eyelid retraction. Vision loss in Graves' disease can be due to corneal exposure, compressive optic neuropathy from enlarged extraocular muscles and increased orbital fat, or stretch optic neuropathy from severe proptosis. Restrictive motility disturbances in Graves' disease result from inflammation and swelling of the extraocular muscles, followed by fibrosis. The inferior rectus muscle is most frequently involved, followed by the medial, superior, and lateral rectus muscles. Fibrosis of the levator and Müller's muscle in the upper eyelid and the lid retractors in the lower eyelid causes upper and lower eyelid retraction. Eyelid retraction can also be worsened by proptosis. Scleral show and lagophthalmos leading to severe corneal exposure may result from eyelid retraction.

The diagnosis of thyroid-related ophthalmopathy is made on clinical grounds, and confirmed radiographically. In addition to demonstrating the enlarged extraocular muscles, computed tomography (CT) or magnetic resonance imaging (MRI) of the orbit allows assessment of the degree of proptosis and of the optic nerve near the orbital apex. Consultation with an internist or endocrinologist should be sought to evaluate the patient's thyroid status. The ophthalmic disease and thyroid dysfunction, if present, often run independent courses, and the patients should be thoroughly educated in this regard.

2. Idiopathic orbital inflammation may also occur as a bilateral disease, though it is more common unilaterally, and may produce a localized myositis. In idiopathic orbital inflammation, the CT scan will show enlargement of the entire muscle, including the tendon. This contrasts with the tendon sparing typically seen in Graves' disease.

3. Other causes of bilateral proptosis include bilateral orbital metastasis from a distant primary malignancy and diffuse orbital infiltrative processes such as amyloidosis or sarcoidosis. A detailed clinical history and lab work radiographic evaluation of the orbits will help distinguish these entities from Graves' disease.

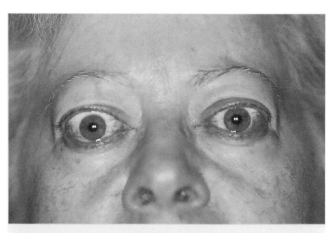

Fig. 87.1 Clinical photograph depicting marked eyelid retraction with widened palpebral fissures and scleral show.

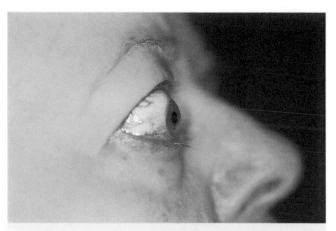

Fig. 87.2 Lateral view demonstrates proptosis of the globe.

87.2 Test Interpretation

Automated perimetry (Humphrey visual field) testing was performed and showed no significant abnormalities. A CT scan of the orbits demonstrated mild to moderate extraocular muscle enlargement of both inferior rectus muscles and the left medial rectus muscle. Tendon sparing, typical of Graves' disease, was present. Posteriorly, the optic nerves did not appear compressed.

87.3 Diagnosis

Thyroid eye disease (i.e., Graves' orbitopathy) with eyelid retraction and bilateral proptosis.

87.4 Medical Management

Corneal exposure changes may be treated with frequent instillation of artificial tears and lubricating ointment at bedtime. Punctal occlusion, either temporary or permanent, may be considered. Wearing of a moisture shield at bedtime may help ameliorate nocturnal drying due to lagophthalmos and decreased Bell's phenomenon. Elevated intraocular pressure due to orbital congestion and/or associated glaucoma may be treated with topical intraocular pressure–lowering drops.

Active orbital inflammation or the presence of optic neuropathy warrants treatment. High doses of oral corticosteroids (prednisone 80–100 mg daily) or pulsed high-dose intravenous steroids can be administered. Patients who cannot take steroids could be considered for radiation therapy to the orbits or surgical decompression.

Most patients with symptomatic restrictive strabismus will eventually require strabismus surgery. During the active inflammatory phase, wearing a patch over one eye may relieve the patient's symptoms. Prisms are usually not effective because of the noncomitant nature of the motility disturbance. Motility measurements should be stable for at least 3 to 4 months before strabismus surgery is performed.

87.5 Surgical Management

Patients with compressive optic neuropathy that is unresponsive to steroid therapy or radiation treatment or in whom the steroids cannot be successfully tapered may be considered for orbital decompression. In addition, patients with severe proptosis leading to corneal exposure may be considered for orbital decompression, even in the absence of optic neuropathy. Orbital decompression can be achieved with one-, two-, or three-wall decompression or with orbital fat removal. Surgical approach is tailored to each patient depending on degree of disease severity. Orbital decompression may cause exacerbation of existing diplopia or creation of diplopia in a patient without previous symptoms. The patient must be fully apprised of this risk and must understand that subsequent strabismus surgery may be required.

Strabismus surgery may be indicated in thyroid eye disease if symptomatic diplopia is present. Motility measurements should be stable for at least 3 to 4 months before surgery to ensure that the patient is not in an active inflammatory phase. Additionally, strabismus surgery should follow orbit decompression surgery because the motility pattern may be altered after orbit surgery.

Severe eyelid retraction is addressed only after any needed orbit or muscle surgery. Eyelid retraction can cause severe functional as well as cosmetic problems, and again, treatment must be individualized. Recession of the levator aponeurosis in the upper eyelid and of the lower lid retractors allows for improved coverage of the bulbar surface and improved cosmesis.

87.6 Rehabilitation and Follow-up

The patient maintained good visual acuity and did not develop significant diplopia. She was treated initially with frequent artificial tears and punctal occlusion to improve the corneal surface. After 4 months of stable symptoms, she underwent recession of all four eyelids. There were no intraoperative or postoperative complications, and the patient was satisfied with the cosmetic result as well as the relief of her exposure symptoms. Endocrinology evaluation revealed hypothyroidism, and the patient has been maintained on thyroid hormone replacement therapy.

87.6.1 Acknowledgment

Thanks to this chapter's first edition authors, Debra Shetlar and Milton Boniuk.

Suggested Reading

[1] Gorman CA, Waller RR, Dyer JA, eds. The Eye and Orbit in Thyroid Disease. New York, NY: Raven Press; 1984

[2] Leone CR, Jr. The management of ophthalmic Graves' disease. Ophthalmology. 1984; 91(7):770–779

[3] Rootman J. Diseases of the Orbit. Philadelphia, PA: JB Lippincott; 1998:241–280

[4] Sergott RC, Glaser JS. Graves' ophthalmopathy. A clinical and immunologic review. Surv Ophthalmol. 1981; 26(1):1–21

[5] Wilson WB, Manke WF. Orbital decompression in Graves' disease. The predictability of reduction of proptosis. Arch Ophthalmol. 1991; 109(3):343–345

88 Ectropion

Amina I. Malik

Abstract

Ectropion of the lower eyelid is usually involutional, due to increased laxity of the tarsoligamentous sling that normally supports the eyelid. This can lead to problems with tearing due to poor punctal apposition to the globe, dryness from poor tear distribution, and irritation from conjunctival hypertrophy as well as keratinization of the exposed tarsal conjunctival surface. Cicatricial ectropion can also be seen, due to chronic UV damage or other trauma to the eyelid causing anterior lamellar shortening. A mechanical ectropion is usually easily identified by the presence of a mass on the lid causing the lid margin to be displaced downward. Paralytic ectropion occurs following temporary or permanent seventh nerve palsy. The presence of other accompanying signs of seventh nerve impairment, including facial weakness and brow ptosis on the ipsilateral side, makes the diagnosis apparent. Nonsurgical treatment involves lubrication for dry eye. Surgical treatment is tailored toward the underlying etiology.

Keywords: ectropion, lid sagging, dry eye

88.1 History

A 70-year-old man presented with left eye irritation that had been present for the last year. He had bilateral cataract surgery 3 years previously, and there was no other history of ocular disease or trauma.

Examination showed a corrected vision of 20/20 OD and 20/25 OS. The external examination showed a marked "out-turning" of the left lower eyelid with associated tarsal conjunctival injection diffusely (▶ Fig. 88.1a, b). His left corneal exam showed 1 + superficial punctate keratitis inferiorly. No masses were palpated. There was mild dermatochalasis of both upper lids. Both lower lids exhibited moderate horizontal laxity with delayed snapback test. The remainder of the eye examination was within normal limits.

Differential Diagnosis—Key Points

1. The patient has an ectropion of the left lower eyelid. In this age group, the most common cause of ectropion is related to involutional (age-related) changes within the eyelid. The most prominent change relates to increased laxity of the tarsoligamentous sling that normally supports the eyelid. As the laxity of the lid progresses, the eyelid will commonly develop a medial ectropion first. At this stage, the patient may complain of epiphora due to eversion of the lower lid punctum. If untreated, the eyelid will eventually develop a generalized ectropion involving the entire lid. Prolonged eyelid eversion may then result in conjunctival hypertrophy as well as keratinization of the exposed tarsal conjunctival surface.

2. Cicatricial ectropion must be included in the differential diagnosis of an out-turning eyelid. This condition results from a vertical shortening of the anterior lamella of the lid, which may occur after surgical or accidental trauma to the lower lid or cheek area. Excision of malignant skin cancers or overaggressive skin removal during a lower lid blepharoplasty may produce a cicatricial ectropion. To determine if the anterior lamella is vertically shortened, a manual attempt to lift the lid into its normal position should be made. Inability to easily lift the lid to its normal position indicates the presence of a cicatricial component. This shortening of the anterior lamella must be addressed in any surgical correction of the lid malposition.

3. A mechanical ectropion is usually easily identified by the presence of a tumor or other mass on the lid causing the lid margin to be displaced downward. Less common causes of mechanical ectropion include edema of the lid or herniation of orbital fat.

4. Paralytic ectropion occurs following temporary or permanent seventh nerve palsy. The presence of other accompanying signs of seventh nerve impairment, including facial weakness and brow ptosis on the ipsilateral side, make the diagnosis apparent.

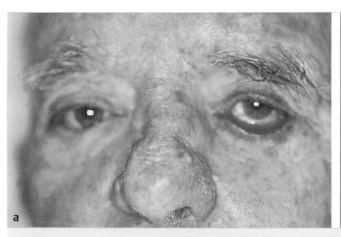
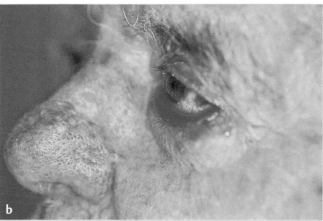

Fig. 88.1 (a) Clinical appearance of lower lid ectropion. (b) Injection of the exposed tarsal conjunctiva is best seen on lateral view.

88.2 Test Interpretation

Inability to lift the eyelid manually might suggest cicatricial or restrictive etiology.

88.3 Diagnosis

Involutional ectropion of the left lower eyelid with resultant ocular irritation.

88.4 Medical Management

Mild involutional ectropion may be treated with artificial tears or lubricating ointment. If the condition is progressive or if symptoms are not alleviated with lubrication, then surgical management is the definitive treatment.

88.5 Surgical Management

The correct type of ectropion must be diagnosed so that the appropriate surgical procedure can be chosen. If a cicatricial component exists, the anterior lamella of the lid must be vertically elongated through the use of a free, full-thickness skin graft. Paralytic ectropion is most commonly addressed using a lateral tarsorrhaphy or medial or lateral canthoplasties.

The surgical treatment for involutional ectropion most commonly employs one of several horizontal shortening procedures, such as the lateral tarsal strip procedure or a full-thickness wedge resection of the eyelid. If the ectropion is primarily medial, the "lazy-T" procedure may be efficacious. This procedure includes a full-thickness pentagonal wedge resection immediately lateral to the lower lid punctum combined with an elliptical excision of tarsal conjunctiva and retractors posterior to the punctum (medial spindle procedure). If medial canthal laxity comprises a significant contribution to the lid malposition, a medial canthal plication may be performed.

88.6 Rehabilitation and Follow-up

The patient underwent a lateral tarsal strip procedure in conjunction with a medial spindle procedure. The corrected eyelid position ameliorated the patient's symptoms of ocular irritation.

88.6.1 Acknowledgment

Thanks to this chapter's first edition authors, Debra Shetlar and Milton Boniuk.

Suggested Reading

[1] Anderson RL, Gordy DD. The tarsal strip procedure. Arch Ophthalmol. 1979; 97(11):2192–2196

[2] Frueh BR, Schoengarth LD. Evaluation and treatment of the patient with ectropion. Ophthalmology. 1982; 89(9):1049–1054

[3] Nowinski TS, Anderson RL. The medial spindle procedure for involutional medial ectropion. Arch Ophthalmol. 1985; 103(11):1750–1753

[4] Smith B. The "lazy-T" correction of ectropion of the lower punctum. Arch Ophthalmol. 1976; 94(7):1149–1150

89 Entropion

Amina I. Malik

Abstract

Entropion is most commonly involutional due to (1) horizontal laxity of the eyelid; (2) disinsertion or dehiscence of the lower eyelid retractors; (3) overriding of the preseptal orbicularis; and (4) relative enophthalmos of the globe due to atrophic changes of the orbital soft tissues. Temporizing everting sutures (Quickert-Rathbun sutures) may be used to effect immediate relief of the patient's discomfort. Surgical treatment involves reinsertion of the lower eyelid retractors with lateral horizontal eyelid-tightening surgery. Other causes of entropion include spastic (from ocular irritation or lid edema), cicatricial (due to vertical shortening of the posterior lamella of the eyelid) due to Stevens–Johnson syndrome, cicatricial pemphigoid, or post-trauma scarring after chemical or thermal burns. Treatment of cicatricial entropion includes tarsal fracture with placement of everting sutures for mild cases. More severe cases in which the tarsus is severely scarred and distorted may require tarsal and mucus membrane grafting. Available materials for grafting include hard-palate mucosa, preserved scleral grafts, and autogenous ear cartilage

Keywords: entropion, eyelid rotation

89.1 History

A 75-year-old woman presented with complaints of severe right eye pain that has been progressively worsening for 2 years. The patient has discovered that she can alleviate her pain if she manually retracts her right lower eyelid.

Examination shows "in-turning" of the right lower eyelid causing the lashes to rub against the epibulbar surface (▶ Fig. 89.1). Moderate horizontal laxity of the lower lid is present. With gentle downward traction on the right lower eyelid, the lid margin can be restored to its normal position; however, the in-turning recurs when the patient blinks.

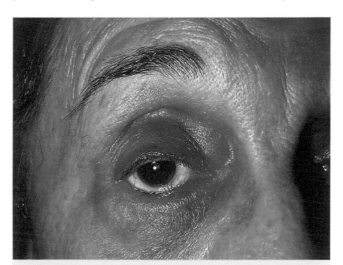

Fig. 89.1 Clinical appearance of lower lid entropion. Overriding of the preseptal orbicularis can be seen.

Differential Diagnosis—Key Points

1. The patient has an entropion of the right lower eyelid. Involutional entropion is the most common type of entropion in this clinical setting. Age-related changes that contribute to the development of the condition include the following: (1) horizontal laxity of the eyelid; (2) disinsertion or dehiscence of the lower eyelid retractors; (3) overriding of the preseptal orbicularis; and (4) relative enophthalmos of the globe due to atrophic changes of the orbital soft tissues.

2. Other causes of entropion should be considered and ruled out before proceeding with treatment. Ocular irritation or lid edema may cause a temporary spastic entropion. This condition occurs after intraocular surgery or other trauma to the lid that produces edema of the periocular soft tissues. The combination of lid edema, orbicularis spasm, and underlying involutional changes can result in a spastic entropion. The condition may improve once the underlying cause of the edema is corrected; however, it may be necessary to correct the involutional changes surgically via Quickert-Rathbun sutures to evert the lid to its normal anatomic position.

3. Cicatricial entropion occurs when there is vertical shortening of the posterior lamella of the eyelid. This condition may result from a variety of conditions including Stevens–Johnson syndrome, cicatricial pemphigoid, or posttrauma scarring after chemical or thermal burns. The digital eversion test, or the ability to easily rotate the lid margin to its normal position using downward traction on the lid, allows the examiner to determine if a cicatricial condition is present. The posterior tarsus should be inspected for evidence of scarring or loss of the inferior fornix. Treatment of cicatricial entropion includes tarsal fracture with placement of everting sutures for mild cases. More severe cases in which the tarsus is severely scarred and distorted may require tarsal and mucus membrane grafting. Available materials for grafting include hard-palate mucosa, preserved scleral grafts, and autogenous ear cartilage.

89.2 Test Interpretation

The lid was not restricted, suggesting involutional entropion.

89.3 Diagnosis

Involutional entropion of the right lower eyelid.

89.4 Medical Management

Taping the lid may provide acute relief of the patient's symptoms; however, this is rarely satisfactory over the long term. Lubricating drops and ointment should also be given to improve the ocular irritation.

89.5 Surgical Management

Temporizing everting sutures (Quickert-Rathbun sutures) may be used to effect immediate relief of the patient's discomfort. To achieve a more permanent correction, surgical management directed toward the primary cause(s) of the entropion is indicated. Horizontal tightening of the lid using a lateral tarsal strip procedure will often satisfactorily correct the entropion. The Wies procedure, in which a full-thickness horizontal incision is used to create an adhesion between the anterior and posterior lamellae of the lid, is another option. Lastly, direct repair of the lower lid retractors can be performed through a skin–orbicularis incision. This procedure may be combined with a horizontal shortening procedure.

89.6 Rehabilitation and Follow-up

The patient underwent a Wies procedure of the lower eyelid with satisfactory correction of the lid entropion. She experienced no postoperative complications.

89.6.1 Acknowledgment

Thanks to this chapter's first edition authors, Debra Shetlar and Milton Boniuk.

Suggested Reading

[1] Dortzbach RK, McGetrick JJ. Involutional entropion of the lower eyelid. In: Bosniak SL, ed. Advances in Ophthalmic Plastic and Reconstructive Surgery. New York, NY: Pergamon Press; 1983;257–267

[2] Jones LT, Reeh MJ, Wobig JL. Senile entropion. A new concept for correction. Am J Ophthalmol. 1972; 74(2):327–329

[3] Quickert MH, Rathbun E. Suture repair of entropion. Arch Ophthalmol. 1971; 85(3):304–305

[4] Wesley RE, Collins JW. Combined procedure for senile entropion. Ophthalmic Surg. 1983; 14(5):401–405

90 Trichiasis

Amina I. Malik

Abstract

Trichiasis involves rubbing of eyelashes against the cornea. Most commonly, this is due to lower eyelid entropion or aberrant lashes present posterior to the gray line (distichiasis). In the face of chronic prolonged inflammation, the meibomian glands may undergo metaplastic transformation into hair follicles. This transformation results in the presence of fine lashes emanating from the previous meibomian gland orifices. This occurs commonly when posterior lamellar scarring is present and may be diffuse or segmental. Treatment includes epilation with forceps, cryotherapy, electrolysis, or laser. Surgical options include eyelid wedge excision, lash follicle excision, or entropion repair.

Keywords: trichiasis, entropion, distichiasis

90.1 History

A 64-year-old woman presented with complaints of chronic irritation of the left eye that had been worsening over the last 2 years. There was no previous ocular history.

Ophthalmic examination was remarkable for an entropion of the left lower eyelid (▶ Fig. 90.1). The lid was easily returned to its normal position using gentle manual downward pressure. The tarsal conjunctiva showed mild erythema without evidence of cicatricial changes, and the inferior fornix was deep without symblepharon. When the lid was everted, a row of fine nonpigmented lashes was noted posterior to the gray line. These lashes were in contact with the epibulbar surface. Mild punctate corneal changes were present inferiorly. The inferior bulbar conjunctiva showed rose bengal staining in the areas associated with the abnormal lashes. Diffuse thickening of the lid margin was noted as well as the presence of fine telangiectatic vessels. Scattered debris, including collarettes, were present on the lashes of all four eyelids.

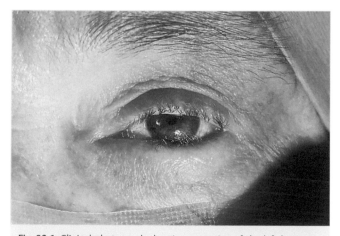

Fig. 90.1 Clinical photograph showing entropion of the left lower eyelid with trichiasis.

Differential Diagnosis—Key Points

1. This patient has ocular irritation due to two components. The first is the eyelid malposition, or entropion of the lid. The second component is the abnormal row of lashes present posterior to the gray line. In the face of chronic prolonged inflammation, the meibomian glands may undergo metaplastic transformation to hair follicles. This transformation results in the presence of fine lashes emanating from the previous meibomian gland orifices, a condition referred to as *distichiasis*. These abnormal lashes may, in turn, rub the globe and cause trichiasis with ocular irritation.

This occurs commonly when posterior lamellar scarring is present and may be diffuse or segmental.

2. Ocular irritation may be produced by ocular surface disorders such as Sjögren's syndrome, blepharitis, or meibomian gland dysfunction. Careful evaluation of the ocular tear film should be performed including assessment of the tear breakup time. Instituting a lid hygiene program, frequent use of artificial tears, and consideration of punctal occlusion may help these disorders.

90.2 Test Interpretation

Schirmer's testing may provide some quantitative measurement of tear production. The use of fluorescein and rose bengal dye aids in the identification of abnormal dry areas of the epibulbar surface.

90.3 Diagnosis

1. Trichiasis of the lower eyelid due to aberrant lashes (distichiasis) and lower lid entropion.
2. Blepharitis and meibomian gland dysfunction of all four eyelids.

90.4 Medical Management

Treatment of misdirected lashes may be challenging, and recurrence is frequent regardless of the modality used. Until surgery can be performed, lubricating drops and ointment should be prescribed. If only a few abnormal lashes are present, simple epilation may be performed. While this will effect immediate relief of the patient's symptoms, the lashes will almost always recur within 3 months, and consideration of other treatments is usually required:

- Electrolysis may be used for focal areas of trichiasis. The recurrence rate is high, and extensive use of electrolysis may result in scarring of the eyelid margin.

- Cryotherapy is one of the more effective treatments for trichiasis. It may be performed using a local infiltrative anesthetic. A nitrous oxide probe is applied to the area of aberrant lashes using a double freeze-thaw technique. The concomitant use of a thermocoupler allows for monitoring of the eyelid temperature and helps avoid overtreatment. Bringing the eyelid tissues to −20 °C will effect ablation of the hair follicle without damage to the surrounding tissues. Complications include loss of skin pigmentation and eyelid notching. If some of the aberrant lashes recur, the procedure can be repeated.
- Argon laser ablation has been used to treat focal areas of aberrant lashes. The laser is less effective than cryotherapy but does not result in the posttreatment edema produced after cryotherapy. This may be particularly important in patients with existing inflammatory lid conditions such as ocular cicatricial pemphigoid.

90.5 Surgical Management

The lower lid entropion may be surgically corrected as discussed elsewhere.

Surgical management of trichiasis may be considered if the lashes are grouped in one area of the eyelid and there is sufficient horizontal laxity of the lid. Under these circumstances, a full-thickness pentagonal wedge containing the area of aberrant lashes may be excised. The lid defect is repaired in the standard fashion, and a cantholysis can be performed to allow closure of the defect without undue tension.

A lid-splitting procedure can also be used in which the lid is split between the anterior and posterior lamella. The bulbs of the hair follicles can then be identified within the tarsus and removed, or the cryoprobe can be applied directly to the tarsal plate.

90.6 Rehabilitation and Follow-up

The patient underwent a Wies procedure to correct the lower eyelid entropion. At the same time, cryotherapy was applied to the aberrant lashes. Postoperatively, the patient did well, with only focal recurrence of the distichitic lashes. These were retreated with additional cryotherapy in the office. A lid hygiene program to address the patient's blepharitis and meibomian gland dysfunction was also instituted.

90.6.1 Acknowledgment

Thanks to this chapter's first edition authors, Debra Shetlar and Milton Boniuk.

Suggested Reading

[1] Anderson RL, Harvey JT. Lid splitting and posterior lamella cryosurgery for congenital and acquired distichiasis. Arch Ophthalmol. 1981; 99(4):631–634

[2] Bartley GB, Lowry JC. Argon laser treatment of trichiasis. Am J Ophthalmol. 1992; 113(1):71–74

[3] Bedrossian EH, Simonton JT. Management of trichiasis. In: Smith BC, ed. Ophthalmic Plastic and Reconstructive Surgery. Vol. 1. St. Louis, MO: CV Mosby; 1987:556–561

[4] Collin JRO. Entropion and trichiasis. In: Collin JRO, ed. A Manual of Systematic Eyelid Surgery. 2nd ed. New York, NY: Churchill Livingstone; 1989:7–26

[5] Sullivan JH. The use of cryotherapy for trichiasis. Trans Sect Ophthalmol Am Acad Ophthalmol Otolaryngol. 1977; 83(4)(,)(Pt 1):708–712

91 Dacryocystitis

Amina I. Malik

Abstract

Dacryocystitis is an infection of the lacrimal sac due to blockage in the nasolacrimal duct. Symptoms include tearing, pain, redness, and swelling in medial canthal area. Diagnosis is clinical. Treatment includes antibiotics and surgical drainage of lacrimal sac abscess, followed by dacryocystorhinostomy surgery.

Keywords: dacryocystitis, epiphora, nasolacrimal duct obstruction, lacrimal sac mass

91.1 History

A 44-year-old woman was referred for evaluation of tearing and pain of the right lower eyelid medially. Her past medical history was significant for lethal midline granuloma (midfacial necrotizing lesion) for which she had undergone multiple procedures, including removal of the nasal septum and frontoethmoidectomies. She reported constant epiphora of the right eye since the time of her surgeries and had more recently noted intermittent redness of the right lower eyelid, associated with tenderness and mucous discharge from the eye. She had been previously treated with an unknown ophthalmic antibiotic drop.

Examination showed erythema of the right lower lid medially with associated tenderness to palpation (▶ Fig. 91.1). No definite masses were palpated in the lacrimal sac region. There was a whitish mucoid discharge expressed from the punctum upon palpation of the lacrimal sac, and the conjunctiva was mildly injected. The puncta of the right upper and lower eyelid were present and appeared patent. There was a well-healed surgical incision over the nose with residual distortion of the nasal architecture. The remainder of the ophthalmic examination was completely normal. Nasolacrimal irrigation was performed and demonstrated complete obstruction of the distal nasal lacrimal system. The upper system was patent as demonstrated by the reflux of irrigating solution through the upper and lower puncta. Inspection of the inner nose showed a large nasal defect with an absent septum.

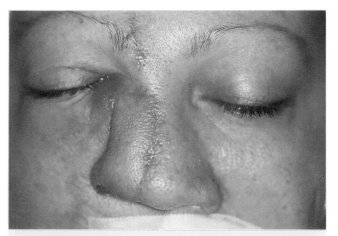

Fig. 91.1 Clinical appearance of patient with erythema and mild edema of the right lower eyelid over the region of the lacrimal sac. The previous surgical incision over the nose is visible.

Differential Diagnosis—Key Points

Dacryocystitis, or inflammation of the lacrimal sac, may be caused by a wide variety of disorders. The common denominator is obstruction of the nasal lacrimal duct (NLD) causing impaired drainage of tears from the lacrimal sac. The affected patient will complain of epiphora, and repeated episodes of dacryocystis may ensue due to the chronic stasis of tears in the lacrimal sac and resultant infection.

1. Congenital NLD obstruction occurs in approximately 5% of full-term newborns and may lead to acute dacryocystitis. The cause is usually a thin residual mucosal membrane at the lower end of the lacrimal duct causing impaired drainage of tears.

2. In adults, acquired NLD obstruction more commonly occurs at the junction of the lacrimal sac and the duct. Chronic inflammation from adjacent sinus disease, viral infections, autoimmune disorders, stones, and use of some medications such as 5-fluorouracil or Phospholine Iodide may contribute to the development of NLD obstruction. A careful history to rule out previous facial or canalicular trauma or surgery should be obtained. Rarely, tumors of the lacrimal sac may produce epiphora and dacryocystitis. A palpable mass within the lacrimal sac, particularly with extension above the level of the medial canthal tendon, should raise the suspicion of a neoplasm.

3. Preseptal cellulitis and orbital cellulitis may initially present as a dacryocystitis. The infection may extend to involve the periocular tissues both anterior and posterior to the orbital septum. Preseptal and orbital cellulitis are discussed elsewhere in the text.

91.2 Test Interpretation

Many authors recommend delaying NLD irrigation until the acute infection has resolved, although gentle irrigation may be safely performed if the infection does not appear too severe. The presence of the obstruction should be demonstrated, and the level of the obstruction (NLD, canalicular) must be determined. Passage of the Bowman probe into the canaliculus and sac will help distinguish the level of obstruction. Observation of reflux through the upper and lower puncta signifies patency of the upper lacrimal system. Failure of the irrigant to reach the nose confirms the presence of an NLD obstruction.

Other tests that may be of use in evaluating the lacrimal system include dacryocystography and scintigraphy. In dacryocystography, radiopaque dye is injected into the canaliculi, and an X-ray is subsequently obtained. If an obstruction is present, the dye will be visualized remaining within the lacrimal sac. To perform dacryoscintigraphy, a drop containing a radioactive marker is placed on the conjunctival surface, and sequential scans are obtained. The passage of the marker into the canaliculi, lacrimal sac, and duct can thus be documented. The advantage of this latter test is that it more closely mimics physiologic conditions and may demonstrate functional obstruction of the lacrimal system when other testing methods have demonstrated anatomic patency.

91.3 Diagnosis

Dacryocystitis, right side, secondary to disrupted NLD as a result of the patient's previous nasal surgery.

91.4 Medical Management

The acute infection should be treated with oral or intravenous antibiotics, depending on the severity of the infection. If a pyocele or abscess is present, aspiration may yield material for smears and cultures to guide antibiotic therapy. The patient should be instructed to apply warm compresses frequently to the inflamed site. Addition of antibiotic ophthalmic drops is of limited value and is usually not needed.

91.5 Surgical Management

Most patients with dacryocystitis will eventually require dacryocystorhinostomy (DCR) to prevent further episodes of infection. Surgery is best deferred until resolution of the infectious process. In a few patients, however, medical management will not totally resolve the infection, and a DCR will need to be performed while active inflammation is still present.

91.6 Rehabilitation and Follow-up

The patient was treated with oral antibiotics resulting in rapid resolution of the inflammation. She subsequently underwent a DCR with placement of silicone tubing, with good resolution of her epiphora. She continues under the care of her ear, nose, and throat physician and oncologist for treatment of the lethal midline disease.

91.6.1 Acknowledgment

Thanks to this chapter's first edition authors, Debra Shetlar and Milton Boniuk.

Suggested Reading

[1] Bartley GB. Acquired lacrimal drainage obstruction: an etiologic classification system, case reports, and a review of the literature. Part 1. Ophthal Plast Reconstr Surg. 1992; 8(4):237–242

[2] Linberg JV, McCormick SA. Primary acquired nasolacrimal duct obstruction. A clinicopathologic report and biopsy technique. Ophthalmology. 1986; 93(8): 1055–1063

[3] Linberg JV, Moore CA. Symptoms of canalicular obstruction. Ophthalmology. 1988; 95(8):1077–1079

[4] Meyer JH, Scharf B, Gerling J. Midline granuloma presenting as orbital cellulitis. Graefes Arch Clin Exp Ophthalmol. 1996; 234(2):137–139

[5] White WL, Glover AT, Buckner AB, Hartshorne MF. Relative canalicular tear flow as assessed by dacryoscintigraphy. Ophthalmology. 1989; 96(2): 167–169

92 Idiopathic Orbital Inflammation

Amina I. Malik

Abstract

Idiopathic orbital inflammation typically presents with acute onset of pain and orbital signs. Differential diagnosis includes infection, autoimmune diseases (sarcoidosis, rheumatoid arthritis, Wegener's granulomatosis) or thyroid-related orbitopathy. Treatment is with high-dose corticosteroids with slow taper, typically with a rapid response to the treatment.

Keywords: idiopathic orbital inflammation, orbital pseudotumor, proptosis, chemosis, eye pain

92.1 History

A 63-year-old man presented with a 2-day history of left eye pain and decreased vision. There was no previous history of ophthalmic disease, surgery, or injury. His past medical history was significant for poorly controlled hypertension. His review of systems revealed no history of rheumatoid disease or collagen vascular disease. There was no history of diabetes mellitus.

Examination showed best corrected vision of 20/20 OD and 20/400 OS. There was a 2+ relative afferent pupillary defect of the left pupil. Marked periorbital edema and erythema with 3 mm of left globe proptosis was noted. There was increased resistance to retropulsion of the left globe. There was significant motility deficit in all directions of gaze with associated pain. The slit-lamp examination was notable for 3+ left conjunctival injection with diffuse chemosis (▶ Fig. 92.1). Dilated fundus exam was notable for left diffuse choroidal thickening.

Differential Diagnosis—Key Points

1. This patient presents with signs and symptoms of diffuse orbital inflammation of acute onset. Inflammatory processes, either infectious or noninfectious, should be strongly considered. The absence of known risk factors such as history of sinus disease, diabetes mellitus, malignancy, immunosuppressive therapy, or recent trauma lowers the suspicion for an infectious process.

Idiopathic orbital inflammation may present in several forms: *acute anterior orbital inflammation* in which the inflammatory process primarily affects the globe, including the sclera, Tenon's capsule, and the immediate adjacent orbital structures. The differential diagnosis includes a ruptured dermoid cyst, acute hemorrhage into an orbital lymphangioma, orbital cellulitis, leukemic infiltrate, and collagen vascular disease. Idiopathic orbital inflammation may also present as *diffuse idiopathic orbital inflammation* in which the majority of the orbital structures are involved in the inflammatory process. On occasion, the inflammation may be confined primarily to one orbital structure; for example, an *orbital myositis* may occur when an extraocular muscle is preferentially affected, and *dacryoadenitis* may occur if the orbital inflammation is centered in the lacrimal gland. These

latter patients present with eyelid edema, and a diffusely enlarged, painful, lacrimal gland. The enlarged lacrimal gland can be readily visualized by manually lifting the lid and inspecting the superotemporal forniceal region. Other causes of lacrimal gland enlargement include bacterial infections, sarcoidosis, and lymphomatous infiltration of the gland.

2. Thyroid-related orbital inflammation must be considered in any case of orbital inflammation with proptosis. A careful medical history and review of symptoms will reveal a concurrent history of thyroid disease or symptoms suggestive of thyroid dysfunction such as heat/cold intolerance, unexplained changes in body weight, or changes in body hair or voice quality. The neck should be carefully palpated for evidence of an enlarged thyroid gland. Orbital imaging will show extraocular muscle enlargement with sparing of the tendon insertions of the muscles. While thyroid-related orbital inflammation is often asymmetric, there will usually be radiographic evidence of bilateral disease.

3. Orbital inflammation may be a manifestation of systemic collagen-vascular disease, such as polyarteritis nodosa or Wegener's granulomatosis. A review of systems will often reveal a history of renal or pulmonary disease. Systemic evaluation should include assessment of serum antineutrophil cytoplasmic antibody including both the cytoplasmic pattern and the perinuclear pattern (c-ANCA and p-ANCA), rheumatoid factor, and ANA testing.

4. Unsuspected orbital infections may result in pronounced signs of orbit inflammation. Most bacterial infections are the result of penetrating trauma to the orbit. Fungal infections may occur both in the setting of ocular trauma and in immunosuppressed individuals such as patients with diabetes mellitus or patients receiving chemotherapy. Immunosuppressed patients may be susceptible to orbital infections caused by *Mucor* or *Aspergillus*. Lastly, the possibility of a retained orbital foreign body, with or without associated infection, must be excluded. The clinical history is paramount in guiding the subsequent evaluation and workup.

92.2 Test Interpretation

A magnetic resonance imaging (MRI) of the orbit, before and after administration of gadolinium contrast material, was obtained (▶ Fig. 92.2). There was diffuse anterior orbital inflammation with diffuse scleral thickening, especially posteriorly. Inflammation of the adjacent tissues was noted. The choroidal thickening seen on the funduscopic exam was well demonstrated. There was no evidence of a discrete neoplastic process.

92.3 Diagnosis

Idiopathic orbital inflammation with associated scleritis and secondary choroidal effusion.

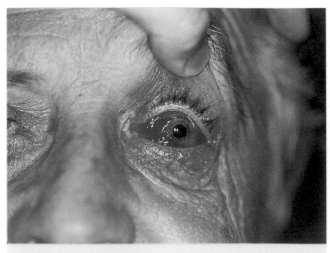

Fig. 92.1 Clinical photograph demonstrating left periorbital inflammation and conjunctival injection.

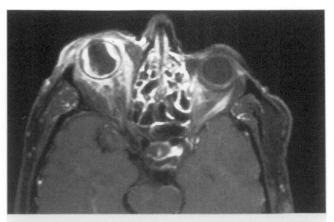

Fig. 92.2 Postgadolinium magnetic resonance imaging shows diffuse thickening of the sclera and episcleral tissues as well as the presence of choroidal thickening.

92.4 Medical Management

The patient was afebrile and the white blood cell count was normal. Systemic evaluation revealed no evidence of collagen-vascular disease. Intravenous steroid treatment (methylprednisolone, 250 mg every 6 hours) was instituted. Within 24 hours, there was marked improvement in the orbital inflammation, and the patient reported resolution of his pain. By 48 hours, the vision in the left eye was 20/40, and the relative afferent pupil defect had resolved. The patient was converted to oral prednisone and discharged from the hospital. At subsequent follow-up examination, his vision had returned to normal, and all of the orbital inflammatory signs had resolved. A follow-up MRI was obtained to rule out the possibility of inflammation masking an underlying neoplastic process. The MRI was normal.

92.5 Surgical Management

In the current case, the patient's orbital disease responded promptly and dramatically to the institution of steroid therapy, which is a hallmark of idiopathic orbital inflammation. If clinical improvement had not been seen after 48 hours of steroid treatment, orbital biopsy to obtain tissue for histopathologic and microbiologic studies would have been indicated.

92.6 Rehabilitation and Follow-up

The patient was referred for systemic evaluation for collagen-vascular disease or lymphoma. All studies were negative, and the patient did well as the oral steroid therapy was slowly tapered. He has not experienced further episodes of orbital inflammation.

92.6.1 Acknowledgment

Thanks to this chapter's first edition authors, Debra Shetlar and Milton Boniuk.

Suggested Reading

[1] Char DH, Miller T. Orbital pseudotumor. Fine-needle aspiration biopsy and response to therapy. Ophthalmology. 1993; 100(11):1702–1710

[2] Heersink B, Rodrigues MR, Flanagan JC. Inflammatory pseudotumor of the orbit. Ann Ophthalmol. 1977; 9(1):17–22, 25–29

[3] Kennerdell JS, Dresner SC. The nonspecific orbital inflammatory syndromes. Surv Ophthalmol. 1984; 29(2):93–103

[4] Leone CR, Jr, Lloyd WC, III. Treatment protocol for orbital inflammatory disease. Ophthalmology. 1985; 92(10):1325–1331

[5] Rootman J, Nugent R. The classification and management of acute orbital pseudotumors. Ophthalmology. 1982; 89(9):1040–1048

93 Orbital Cellulitis

Amina I. Malik

Abstract

Orbital cellulitis presents with eye pain, redness, chemosis, proptosis, and limited extraocular motility. The most common etiologies are ethmoid sinusitis or trauma to the eyelid. The differential diagnosis includes idiopathic orbital inflammation, preseptal cellulitis, or vascular malformation. Diagnosis is made by examination and computed tomography (CT) scanning confirming involvement beyond the orbital septum. Treatment includes intravenous antibiotics. If orbital abscess is present, surgical drainage may be indicated if vision is threatened.

Keywords: orbital cellulitis, proptosis, eye pain, chemosis

93.1 History

A 7-year-old boy was referred for evaluation and treatment of right-sided eyelid swelling, pain, and fever. His symptoms began 4 days prior to presentation. No definite complaint of decreased vision was elicited. The presumptive diagnosis of preseptal cellulitis had been made, and the patient had been placed on oral antibiotics. Two days later, the child was reevaluated and found to have progression of the right upper lid edema, now causing a complete ptosis. Because of the disease progression despite oral antibiotics, the patient was referred to a tertiary care center.

Upon his arrival, it was noted that the child was somewhat lethargic and continued to complain of pain around the right eye. The patient's temperature was 100 °F. There was marked periorbital edema and erythema with complete ptosis of the eyelid (▶ Fig. 93.1). Enlarged preauricular and submandibular lymph nodes were palpated. The eyelid was gently lifted to allow for testing of the visual acuity, which was found to be 20/25 OD and 20/20 OS. The conjunctiva appeared diffusely injected, and there was decreased motility of the right globe in all directions of gaze. No conjunctival discharge was noted. Mild proptosis of the globe appeared to be present; however, the diffuse lid edema and tenderness precluded formal exophthalmometry measurements. The pupils reacted normally with no relative afferent defect. The anterior segments were quiet, and the dilated fundus exam showed no significant abnormalities.

Differential Diagnosis—Key Points

1. Preseptal cellulitis produces inflammation and infection of the eyelids and periorbital tissues anterior to the orbital septum. The condition most commonly results from periocular trauma or a skin infection. Clinical findings include marked erythema and edema of the eyelids and periocular soft tissues. Conjunctival discharge and regional lymphadenopathy may be present. The globe is not involved, and pupillary function, visual acuity, and ocular motility remain undisturbed. Conjunctival cultures should be obtained, and treatment with oral antibiotics instituted. If an abscess is present or develops during the course of the disease, it may be surgically drained. Care must be taken to avoid violating the orbital septum as this may allow seeding of the deeper orbital structures by the infection. The most common organism causing preseptal cellulitis is *Staphylococcus aureus*, and use of a penicillinase-resistant penicillin, such as oxacillin, results in prompt resolution of the infection.

2. Orbital cellulitis results from inflammation and infection of the orbital tissues posterior to the orbital septum. Orbital cellulitis is most commonly caused by secondary extension of acute or chronic bacterial sinusitis. Less commonly, preseptal cellulitis, dacryocystitis, or dental infection may progress to an orbital cellulitis. Clinical findings include the changes associated with preseptal cellulitis including eyelid edema and erythema. In addition, there is conjunctival chemosis, ocular motility restriction, and pain with eye movement. Decreased vision and pupillary abnormalities may be present in severe cases. The patient may be febrile and lethargic. Urgent radiographic imaging, preferably computed tomography (CT) scan, is indicated to evaluate the paranasal sinuses and the extent of the orbital disease. The presence of a subperiosteal abscess may be an indication for surgical drainage. Recent reports of successful medical management of children with subperiosteal abscesses have prompted reevaluation of the best treatment protocol for these patients. It may be appropriate to institute antibiotic therapy and observe the patient carefully. Worsening of the visual acuity or ocular motility, or failure to show clinical improvement after 48 hours of treatment, is an indication to proceed with surgical drainage of the subperiosteal abscess. This should be performed in conjunction with an ear, nose, and throat (ENT) surgeon if significant sinusitis is present. In children, orbital cellulitis is commonly caused by a single microorganism (*Streptococcus sp* or *Haemophilus influenzae*), whereas, in adults, multiple organisms, including anaerobes, are often isolated. With the advent of the *H. influenzae* type-B vaccine (HiB), there has been a decreasing incidence of *H. influenzae*–associated cases of orbital cellulitis in children.

   Complications of orbital cellulitis can ensue if appropriate evaluation and management are delayed. These include orbital apex syndrome, blindness, brain abscess, cavernous sinus thrombosis, and even death.

3. Infiltration of the orbit by leukemic cells or extraocular extension of retinoblastoma may mimic an orbital cellulitis. Appropriate radiographic imaging and a complete ophthalmic examination, including dilated fundus exam, must be performed in all patients with presumed orbital cellulitis.

4. Idiopathic orbital inflammation can also present with pain, swelling, and redness similar to orbital cellulitis. However this is not associated with fever or any of the predisposing factors seen with cellulitis.

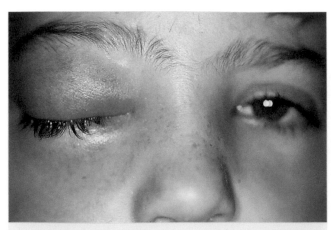

Fig. 93.1 Clinical photograph depicting marked erythema and edema of the right eyelid producing secondary ptosis of the right upper eyelid.

93.2 Test Interpretation

A CT scan of the orbits and paranasal sinuses was obtained emergently. The scan showed a large subperiosteal abscess in the superomedial aspect of the right orbit. There was extensive thickening of the ethmoid sinus mucosa consistent with sinusitis. No bony abnormalities were present.

93.3 Diagnosis

Orbital cellulitis with associated sinusitis.

93.4 Medical Management

Systemic intravenous antibiotic treatment is indicated and infectious disease consult may be helpful.

93.5 Surgical Management

Because the patient had failed to improve on previous therapy, he was taken to the operating room where the large subperiosteal orbital abscess was drained, and an ethmoidectomy was performed by an ENT surgeon. Preoperative blood cultures obtained and intraoperative cultures of the purulent material within the abscess failed to reveal a causative organism. The patient was treated with intravenous ceftriaxone and clindamycin on the recommendation of the pediatric infectious disease consultation.

93.6 Rehabilitation and Follow-up

The patient showed marked improvement of his clinical findings, and he remained afebrile. After 48 hours of intravenous antibiotics, treatment was converted to oral antibiotics, and he was discharged. Subsequent follow-up examination showed complete resolution of the periorbital swelling and motility restriction.

93.6.1 Acknowledgment

Thanks to this chapter's first edition authors, Debra Shetlar and Milton Boniuk.

Suggested Reading

[1] Donahue SP, Schwartz G. Preseptal and orbital cellulitis in childhood. A changing microbiologic spectrum. Ophthalmology. 1998; 105(10):1902–1905, discussion 1905–1906

[2] Harris GJ. Subperiosteal abscess of the orbit. Age as a factor in the bacteriology and response to treatment. Ophthalmology. 1994; 101(3):585–595

[3] Lessner A, Stern GA. Preseptal and orbital cellulitis. Infect Dis Clin North Am. 1992; 6(4):933–952

[4] Souliere CR, Jr, Antoine GA, Martin MP, Blumberg AI, Isaacson G. Selective non-surgical management of subperiosteal abscess of the orbit: computerized tomography and clinical course as indication for surgical drainage. Int J Pediatr Otorhinolaryngol. 1990; 19(2):109–119

[5] Uzcátegui N, Warman R, Smith A, Howard CW. Clinical practice guidelines for the management of orbital cellulitis. J Pediatr Ophthalmol Strabismus. 1998; 35(2):73–79, quiz 110–111

94 Dacryoadenitis

Amina I. Malik

Abstract

Dacryoadenitis involves inflammation of the lacrimal gland that typically presents with eye pain and fullness to the upper outer aspect of the eyelid in area of the lacrimal gland. Etiology can be infectious, idiopathic, or cancerous. Diagnosis involves clinical exam and computed tomography (CT) showing lacrimal gland enlargement. Treatment is with antibiotics if infectious or steroids if inflammatory.

Keywords: dacryoadenitis, lacrimal gland mass, tearing

94.1 History

A 12-year-old boy presented with a 1-week history of swelling of the left upper eyelid. The boy was otherwise healthy without known chronic medical disease. On examination, there was redness and fullness of the temporal aspect of the left upper lid that created an "**S**-shaped" deformity of the eyelid (▶ Fig. 94.1). Manual elevation of the left upper eyelid revealed marked injection and chemosis of the bulbar conjunctiva laterally with enlargement and erythema of the palpebral lobe of the lacrimal gland (▶ Fig. 94.2). There was moderate tenderness over the enlarged lacrimal gland. Mild enlargement of the regional lymph nodes was also noted. The remainder of the ocular examination, including motility, was normal. There was no evidence of intraocular inflammation.

94.2 Test Interpretation

Computed tomography (CT) or magnetic resonance (MR) scan of the orbit might show enlargement of the lacrimal gland or a mass without any surrounding bony erosion or soft-tissue invasion.

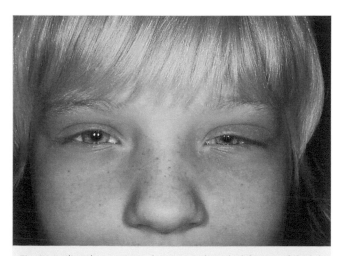

Fig. 94.1 Clinical appearance showing "**S**-shaped" deformity of the left upper eyelid. (Figure courtesy of Robert R. Waller, MD.)

Differential Diagnosis—Key Points

1. The clinical course and physical findings of inflammation centered within the lacrimal gland strongly suggest acute dacryoadenitis. Patients with acute dacryoadenitis typically present with rapid enlargement and inflammation of the lacrimal gland. The clinical examination reveals erythema and edema of the temporal aspect of the upper eyelid as well as the temporal aspect of the tarsal and bulbar conjunctiva. Palpation of the superotemporal orbit shows the lacrimal gland to be diffusely enlarged and tender. Regional lymphadenopathy is often present.

   Before the advent of widespread childhood immunization, mumps represented the leading cause of acute dacryoadenitis. More recent studies have demonstrated an association between recent Epstein–Barr virus (EBV) infection and episodes of dacryoadenitis. Up to one-third of patients with clinical acute dacryoadenitis will have serologic evidence of EBV infection. Antibodies to viral capsid antigen are detectable with the onset of clinical symptoms about 6 weeks after exposure. Viral capsid antigen IgM falls to low levels after several weeks, while viral capsid antigen IgG will persist indefinitely. Antibodies to EBV nuclear antigen increase a few weeks after the onset of clinical infection and remain detectable for years. Thus, the presence of antiviral capsid antigen antibodies with absent or rising anti-EBV nuclear antigen antibodies is diagnostic for recent EBV infection.

2. Other infectious causes of acute dacryoadenitis have been identified. These include staphylococcus, streptococcus, and gonococcus. The presence of purulent discharge should prompt cultures. Empiric antibiotic therapy, both topical and systemic, may be instituted until culture results are available to guide further therapy.

3. Idiopathic orbital inflammation may involve the lacrimal gland preferentially, producing a clinical picture of acute dacryoadenitis. While eyelid erythema and edema may occur, additional orbital signs such as orbital pain, restricted eye movement, and proptosis may also be present.

4. Primary and secondary lacrimal gland tumors may also cause enlargement of the lacrimal gland. Primary lacrimal gland tumors include both epithelial and nonepithelial lesions. The lacrimal gland may also be secondarily involved by direct extension of a tumor from an adjacent orbital site, or by hematogenous spread of a metastatic lesion. Lacrimal gland tumors are discussed in detail elsewhere.

94.3 Diagnosis

Acute dacryoadenitis, presumably secondary to EBV infection.

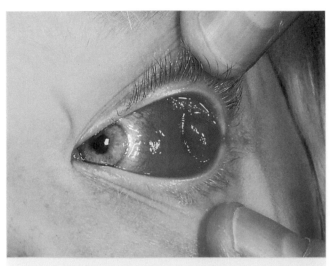

Fig. 94.2 Enlargement of the palpebral lobe of the lacrimal gland of the left eye with associated conjunctival injection and chemosis. Note the absence of purulent discharge. (Figure courtesy of Robert R. Waller, MD.)

94.4 Medical Management

In the present case, the clinical picture is highly characteristic of acute dacryoadenitis, and the patient had no accompanying orbital signs or symptoms. Serologic evaluation was positive for anti-EBV capsid antigen antibodies and negative for antiviral nuclear antigen antibodies, thereby establishing the diagnosis of acute dacryoadenitis secondary to EBV infection. Management may include anti-inflammatory therapy with topical or oral corticosteroid medication, though the disease is self-limited.

94.5 Surgical Management

There is no proven role for surgical management of this problem.

94.6 Rehabilitation and Follow-up

Follow-up for resolution of symptoms is reasonable.

94.6.1 Acknowledgment

Thanks to this chapter's first edition authors, Debra Shetlar and Milton Boniuk.

Suggested Reading

[1] Aburn NS, Sullivan TJ. Infectious mononucleosis presenting with dacryoadenitis. Ophthalmology. 1996; 103(5):776–778

[2] Fitzsimmons TD, Wilson SE, Kennedy RH. Infectious dacryoadenitis. In: Pepose JS, Holland GN, Wilhelmus DR, eds. Ocular Infection and Immunity. St. Louis, MO: CV Mosby; 1996:1341–1345

[3] Rhem MN, Wilhelmus KR, Jones DB. Epstein-Barr virus dacryoadenitis. Am J Ophthalmol. 2000; 129(3):372–375

[4] Wilhelmus KR. Mumps. In: Gold DH, Weingeist TA, eds. The Eye in Systemic Disease. Philadelphia, PA: JB Lippincott; 1990:262–265

95 Orbital Tumors of Childhood

Amina I. Malik

Abstract

The most common primary benign orbital tumors in children are dermoids, epidermoids, and cystic lesions. Vascular tumors such as capillary hemangiomas are also common tumors in children. Neural tumors including optic nerve gliomas and neurofibromas can also be seen in pediatric population. The most common primary orbital malignant tumor is rhabdomyosarcoma. Secondary tumors with orbital invasion can be seen with neuroblastoma and metastasis can see with Ewing's sarcoma or osteosarcoma. Treatment is based on type of tumor.

Keywords: orbital tumors, pediatric tumors, eyelid swelling

95.1 History

An 8-month-old healthy boy presented for evaluation of a mass over the right eye. The mass had been present since shortly after birth, and the parents reported a slow continual enlargement of the mass. The child was born at full-term after an uncomplicated pregnancy. He was otherwise healthy with no known medical problems. There was no associated change in color or size of the mass with crying or Valsalva's maneuvers.

Examination showed central fixation with following in each eye. The rest of his ophthalmic exam was only notable for a moderately firm mass over the superotemporal right eyelid (▶ Fig. 95.1). The mass measured approximately 20 mm × 10 mm × 5 mm and was fixed to the underlying tissues. The overlying skin was intact without discoloration or ulceration. Careful palpation of the superior orbital rim revealed no discernable defect. There was no measureable proptosis, and both orbits were normal to retropulsion. No other masses were palpated.

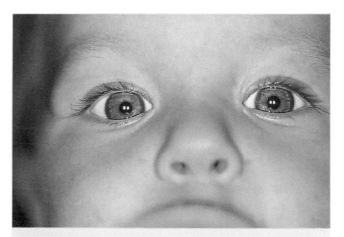

Fig. 95.1 Clinical photograph showing well-circumscribed mass in the superotemporal right orbit. The overlying skin is intact.

Differential Diagnosis—Key Points

1. Orbital tumors in children, as in adults, may be subdivided into primary tumors and secondary tumors. The most common primary orbital tumors in children are dermoids, epidermoids, and cystic lesions. These tumors are considered to be choristomas, and are congenital with variable age of presentation related to their slow growth.

Histologically, dermoids are cystic structures lined by keratinized epithelium with adnexal structures, such as hair follicles or sweat glands, contained within the cyst wall. Epidermoid cysts have a similar histologic appearance except that adnexal structures are not present. Dermoids most commonly occur at the superotemporal orbital rim at the zygomaticofrontal suture. Less commonly, they may be present at the superonasal aspect of the orbit. While these lesions are benign, they tend to slowly enlarge. They may also rupture as the result of minor trauma to the area, inciting a severe granulomatous inflammation of the surrounding tissues. Therefore, it is recommended that these lesions be excised surgically, making certain that the entire cyst wall and its contents are removed.

2. Vascular lesions of the orbit also occur commonly in children. The most common of these is the capillary hemangioma, which may involve the eyelids or orbit. There is an associated reddish discoloration of the overlying skin, and the size of the lesion may enlarge with crying or Valsalva's maneuvers. Hemangiomas may be of sufficient size as to induce visually significant astigmatism or obstruct the visual axis, with the risk of developing amblyopia. Thus, although these tumors are benign, the child should be followed carefully to check for amblyopia. The natural history of these lesions is often slow and spontaneous involution. If, however, the risk of amblyopia is imminent, treatment may be required, including surgery, systemic or intralesional steroids, and topical or systemic beta-blocker therapy. Other modalities that have been employed include radiotherapy, cryotherapy, and laser (CO_2, Nd:YAG, argon) ablation.

Lymphangioma is another vascular tumor that may involve the orbit in children. These lesions may wax and wane in size and may undergo rapid enlargement in association with upper respiratory infections. They are also prone to spontaneous hemorrhage, which can cause dramatic enlargement. If the lesion involves the anterior orbit, a dark-colored cystic lesion may be evident beneath the conjunctiva. Hemorrhage within a deep orbital lymphangioma may produce sudden proptosis of the affected globe. Lymphangiomas are typically poorly circumscribed tumors that interdigitate with the surrounding orbital structures, thereby precluding complete surgical extirpation. They can, however, be surgically reduced by excising a portion of the cyst wall and evacuating the hemorrhagic material. This material has a characteristic dark-brown color, giving rise to the clinical appearance of a "chocolate cyst."

3. Neural tumors include optic nerve glioma and neurofibroma. Both of these tumors occur with increasing frequency in children with neurofibromatosis. Optic nerve glioma may cause slowly progressive axial proptosis with variable effects on the visual acuity and visual field. Radiographically, these tumors create a characteristic fusiform enlargement of the optic nerve. The appropriate management of these tumors remains controversial. Careful monitoring of vision and the degree of proptosis is indicated. Periodic radiographic evaluation should also be performed to evaluate for extension of the glioma into the intracanalicular portion of the optic nerve. Surgical removal of an optic nerve glioma involving the intracanalicular optic nerve or threatening the optic chiasm may be indicated.

Plexiform neurofibromas of the eyelid and orbit are considered pathognomonic for neurofibromatosis type 1. These tumors may cause a mechanical ptosis of the eyelid as well as cosmetic deformity, classically described as "S-shaped." The lesion often interdigitates with other eyelid structures, including the levator aponeurosis, thereby making complete surgical extirpation unfeasible. The surgical approach involves debulking the tumor while maintaining as much function of the eyelid and eye as possible.

4. Rhabdomyosarcoma should be included in the differential diagnosis of a childhood orbital tumor. This tumor represents the most common primary orbital malignancy of childhood. Typically, these lesions will present with rapidly progressive proptosis, and prompt radiographic evaluation and surgical biopsy are indicated. Adequate tissue should be obtained to allow for special testing, including immunohistochemical studies and transmission electron microscopy to demonstrate the presence of diagnostic cross striations. Treatment must be coordinated with oncologists and radiotherapists and usually includes radiotherapy and chemotherapy.

5. Secondary tumors of the orbit include retinoblastoma with extraocular extension into the orbit. Therefore, a complete ophthalmic examination is mandatory in the evaluation of a child with a suspected orbital tumor. Malignancies may also metastasize to secondarily involve the orbit. In children, neuroblastoma is the most common metastatic orbital tumor, producing sudden proptosis, often associated with ecchymosis, which may be bilateral. A thorough physical examination may reveal a palpable abdominal mass. Treatment may include a combination of surgery chemotherapy and radiation. Despite treatment, the prognosis for metastatic neuroblastoma is poor. Other malignancies that may metastasize to the orbit in children include Ewing's sarcoma and osteosarcoma.

95.2 Test Interpretation

Computed tomography or magnetic resonance scan of the orbit will better delineate the lesion.

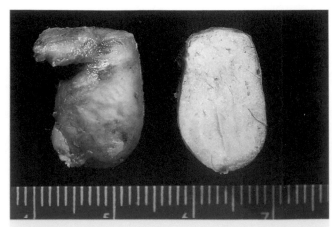

Fig. 95.2 Gross appearance of dermoid cyst showing keratinous debris with hair filling the cyst cavity.

95.3 Diagnosis

Dermoid cyst of the right orbit.

95.4 Medical Management

There is no medical treatment for this condition.

95.5 Surgical Management

As discussed previously, surgical removal of a dermoid cyst is recommended due to the risk of traumatic rupture and resultant inflammatory response. Some authors recommend delaying surgery until the infant is at least 6 months old to decrease the risk of anesthesia. In the current case, the tumor was approached through a lid crease incision to allow for a cosmetically acceptable inconspicuous scar. The lesion was dissected from the surrounding tissues and completely excised (▶ Fig. 95.2). The patient has done well without further sequelae.

95.5.1 Acknowledgment

Thanks to this chapter's first edition authors, Debra Shetlar and Milton Boniuk.

Suggested Reading

[1] Abramson DH, Ellsworth RM, Tretter P, Wolff JA, Kitchin FD. The treatment of orbital rhabdomyosarcoma with irradiation and chemotherapy. Ophthalmology. 1979; 86(7):1330–1335
[2] Kodsi SR, Shetlar DJ, Campbell RJ, Garrity JA, Bartley GB. A review of 340 orbital tumors in children during a 60-year period. Am J Ophthalmol. 1994; 117 (2):177–182
[3] Kushner BJ. Infantile orbital hemangiomas. Int Pediatr. 1990; 5:249–257
[4] Sherman RP, Rootman J, Lapointe JS. Orbital dermoids: clinical presentation and management. Br J Ophthalmol. 1984; 68(9):642–652

96 Orbital Tumors in Adults

Amina I. Malik

Abstract

The most common orbital tumor is a cavernous hemangioma. Orbital tumors typically present with painless progressive proptosis. Other orbital signs such as chemosis, limited extraocular motility, and resistance to retropulsion can be seen. Other orbital neoplasms include lymphoid tumors, neural tumors, vascular tumors, metastatic tumors, or lacrimal gland neoplasm. Imaging is indicated to determine extent of tumor involvement. Treatment depends on type of tumor and the clinical presentation ranging from observation to surgical excision with chemotherapy and/or radiation.

Keywords: orbital tumors, cancer, neoplasm, proptosis

96.1 History

A 44-year-old man was referred for evaluation of proptosis of the left eye. The patient had no previous medical history. He reported increasing painless prominence of the left eye without associated diplopia. His glasses prescription had been changed twice in the past year.

Examination showed visual acuity of 20/20 OU with a manifest refraction of –2.25 D OD and + 1.00 D OS. Motility and pupil examination were within normal limits. The palpebral fissure was widened on the left side, and Hertel exophthalmometry disclosed 4 mm relative proptosis OS (▶ Fig. 96.1). There was increased resistance of the left globe to retropulsion OS. No bony defects or definite masses were palpated. There was no regional lymphadenopathy and no bruits were auscultated over the orbits. The anterior segment was quiet by slit-lamp examination; the bulbar conjunctiva was unremarkable without evidence of abnormal vascularity. Dilated examination of the left fundus revealed choroidal striae of the posterior pole. The optic nerve was normal, and no hemorrhage or exudate was present. The right fundus was normal.

Differential Diagnosis—Key Points

1. This patient presents with evidence of a mass lesion of the left orbit, namely progressive proptosis and a decrease in his myopic refractive error. Tumors may arise within the orbit primarily, or they may involve the orbit secondarily. Secondary orbital tumors may extend directly into the orbit from adjacent structures such as paranasal sinuses, or malignancies may metastasize to the orbit hematogenously from a distant site.

The most common primary orbital tumor in adults is the cavernous hemangioma. Patients are typically middle-aged and present with painless proptosis. Radiographically, cavernous hemangiomas are well-circumscribed, retrobulbar lesions that may show irregular enhancement after injection of contrast material. Ultrasound examination reveals medium to high internal reflectivity. Because of the typical clinical and radiographic appearance, biopsy is usually not required to establish a diagnosis, and treatment is not required if the proptosis is minimal and the patient is asymptomatic. If treatment is indicated, the tumor can be removed in toto via a medial or lateral orbital approach. Because the cavernous hemangioma has limited communication with the systemic circulation, preoperative arteriography is not indicated. Histopathologically, these tumors are encapsulated and contain numerous endothelial-lined vascular channels containing red blood cells.

2. Hemangiopericytoma is another vascular orbital tumor that arises in middle-aged adults. The tumor arises from pericytes, and although it may radiographically and grossly appear well circumscribed, hemangiopericytoma is an infiltrative lesion that may produce proptosis, motility abnormalities, or conjunctival prolapse. The treatment is complete surgical extirpation. Local tumor recurrence may occur and is not predictable based on the histopathologic features of the lesion. Treatment of recurrent hemangiopericytoma is problematic, and there is a risk of malignant transformation. Surgical debulking procedures in combination with radiation treatment have been employed to treat tumor recurrences with mixed results.

3. Lymphoproliferative lesions of the orbit range from reactive lymphoid hyperplasia to orbital lymphoma. These lesions have a variety of clinical appearances, depending on the exact orbital structures that are involved. Diagnosis usually requires tissue biopsy with special studies (e.g., immunohistochemistry flow cytometry, gene rearrangement studies) to determine the presence of a clonal population of lymphocytes. Lymphoma may be limited to the orbit or may involve the orbit as part of a systemic process, so systemic workup in conjunction with oncology is indicated. Treatment involves surgical debulking with radiation.

4. Neural tumors that may involve the orbit in adults include meningioma and schwannoma. Meningiomas may arise from the optic nerve sheath and involve the orbit primarily. More commonly, the meningioma arises intracranially and extends to involve the orbit secondarily. Meningiomas typically present in middle-aged women, with the clinical findings determined by the tumor location. Primary meningiomas of the optic nerve cause early visual symptoms with axial proptosis. Computed tomography (CT) imaging shows a diffusely thickened optic nerve that may contain calcifications. Injection of contrast material may give rise to the characteristic "railroad track" appearance of the enlarged optic nerve sheath. In contrast, secondary orbital meningiomas may have little effect on the vision until the tumor has achieved significant size. If the tumor is arising from the lateral portion of the sphenoid, the patient may present with a temporal fossa mass in addition to proptosis.

Schwannomas, which are composed of proliferations of Schwann cells, often arise from the sensory nerves of cranial nerve V, but may arise from any peripheral nerve sheath. Orbital schwannomas are typically intraconal, well-circumscribed tumors, and multiple tumors may be present. Symptoms and signs are determined by the tumor location. Because of their encapsulation, schwannomas are amenable to complete surgical removal.

5. Fibrous histiocytoma is the most common primary mesenchymal orbital tumor in adults. These tumors infiltrate the surrounding orbital structures, making them difficult to remove completely. Fibrous histiocytomas may be locally aggressive leading to frequent recurrences. There are benign and malignant forms of fibrous histiocytoma, and histopathologic study of the tumor is necessary for accurate diagnosis. Cases of malignant transformation of a previous benign tumor have also been reported.

6. Lacrimal gland tumors generally fall into two categories: epithelial and nonepithelial. Within these two categories, both benign and malignant variants exist. Of the nonepithelial lesions, the vast majority are inflammatory and may be infectious or noninfectious. Noninfectious inflammatory entities include sarcoid, Wegener's granulomatosis, and orbital pseudotumor.

The most common epithelial neoplasm of the lacrimal gland is the pleomorphic adenoma. Other epithelial tumors of the lacrimal gland include adenoid cystic carcinoma, squamous carcinoma, and mucoepidermoid carcinoma. Epithelial lacrimal gland tumors present as a mass in the lacrimal fossa and produce downward displacement and proptosis of the globe. Bony erosion of the lacrimal fossa is often seen on CT scan. If an epithelial lacrimal gland tumor is suspected preoperatively, a lateral orbitotomy should be performed and the entire tumor removed en bloc. Failure to preserve the surrounding capsule results in an increased risk of recurrence and malignant transformation. Malignant epithelial lacrimal gland tumors have the capacity to metastasize widely and cause death.

7. A wide variety of visceral carcinomas as well as cutaneous melanomas may involve the orbit secondarily by metastatic spread. However, breast and lung carcinomas account for the majority of orbital metastatic tumors. A previous history of malignancy exists in 75% of patients presenting with metastatic orbit disease. Thus, in 25% of patients, the orbital tumor is the first manifestation of the patient's malignancy. In a patient with a previously established cancer diagnosis, a fine-needle aspiration biopsy may be performed to confirm the orbit diagnosis before the patient proceeds with therapy. Some orbital lesions may not be amenable to fine-needle biopsy; this is particularly true for fibrotic tumors, such as scirrhous breast carcinoma or tumors that are posteriorly located in the orbit adjacent to the optic nerve.

96.2 Test Interpretation

An orbital CT scan demonstrated a well-circumscribed retrobulbar tumor pressing on the posterior aspect of the globe (▶ Fig. 96.2). There were no associated bony changes, and the tumor showed only marginal enhancement with contrast material.

96.3 Diagnosis

Probable cavernous hemangioma of the left orbit.

96.4 Medical Management

There is no medical treatment for this condition.

96.5 Surgical Management

Because of the patient's progressive proptosis and changing refractive error, surgical excision was recommended. A lateral orbitotomy was performed and a dark-red encapsulated tumor was removed in toto (▶ Fig. 96.3). Histopathologic evaluation confirmed the diagnosis of cavernous hemangioma.

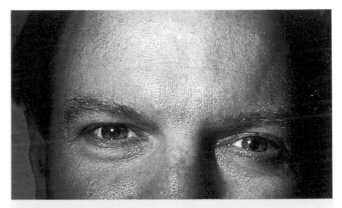

Fig. 96.1 Clinical photograph showing proptosis of the left eye.

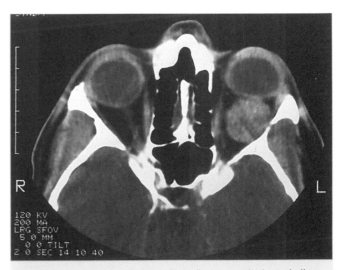

Fig. 96.2 CT scan demonstrating the well-circumscribed retrobulbar tumor in the left orbit. The mass is pressing on the posterior aspect of the left eye.

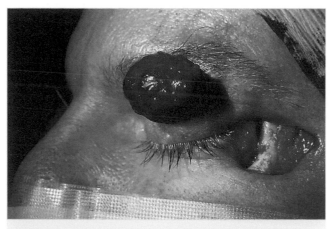

Fig. 96.3 Intraoperative photography showing the lateral orbitotomy and the excised reddish well-circumscribed tumor.

96.6 Rehabilitation and Follow-up

The patient did well postoperatively. The refractive error in his left eye stabilized at −2.00 D, and the choroidal striae in the left eye slowly resolved.

96.6.1 Acknowledgment

Thanks to this chapter's first edition authors, Debra Shetlar and Milton Boniuk.

Suggested Reading

[1] American Academy of Ophthalmology. 2017–2018 Basic and Clinical Science Course, Section 07: Orbit, Eyelids, and Lacrimal System. San Francisco, CA: American Academy of Ophthalmology; 1996:75–93

[2] Font RL, Ferry AP. Carcinoma metastatic to the eye and orbit III. A clinicopathologic study of 28 cases metastatic to the orbit. Cancer. 1976; 38(3):1326–1335

[3] Henderson JW. Orbital Tumors. 3rd ed. New York, NY: Raven Press; 1994

[4] Jakobiec FA, Depot MJ, Kennerdell JS, et al. Combined clinical and computed tomographic diagnosis of orbital glioma and meningioma. Ophthalmology. 1984; 91(2):137–155

[5] Leone CR, Jr, Lloyd WC, III. Treatment protocol for orbital inflammatory disease. Ophthalmology. 1985; 92(10):1325–1331

97 Benign Tumors of the Eyelid

Amina I. Malik

Abstract

Benign eyelid tumors are characterized by very slow growth over many years and a lack of skin ulceration, scaling, madarosis, or telangiectasia. These tumors include nevi, seborrheic keratosis, actinic keratosis, and squamous papillomas. Adnexal structures of eyelid can also give rise to benign eyelid tumors including syringoma, hidrocystoma, and pilomatrixoma. The lesion may be observed, or it may be surgically excised. In most cases, the procedure can be performed as an office procedure using a local anesthetic. The resulting small defect can be repaired primarily or allowed to heal by secondary intention.

Keywords: eyelid tumor, swelling of eyelid, eyelid neoplasm

97.1 History

A 32-year-old man presented for evaluation of a left upper eyelid lesion that had been present for several years and that had been slowly enlarging for last several months. He reported no associated redness or bleeding from the lesion and there was no history of previous skin disease or skin cancer. He was in good health and took no medications. His ophthalmic examination was within normal limits with the exception of the external exam. There was a 10 mm × 8 mm × 5 mm smooth dome-shaped skin lesion involving the preseptal eyelid skin of the left upper lid (▶ Fig. 97.1). The tumor was amelanotic, and the overlying skin was intact without ulceration or telangiectasia. There was no regional lymphadenopathy and no other skin lesions were present on the head and neck region.

Differential Diagnosis—Key Points

1. The very slow growth over many years and the lack of skin ulceration, scaling, madarosis, or telangiectasia support the benign nature of this tumor. Nevi are melanocytic lesions that may appear pigmented or amelanotic, and they are among the most common benign eyelid tumors. Histopathologically nevi are divided into three categories, depending on the depth of the nevus cells. In *junctional* nevi, the nevus cells are grouped at the epidermal–dermal junction. As some of the nevus cells drop into the deeper dermis, the lesion is categorized as a *compound nevus*. Lastly, when all of the nevus cells are present in the dermis, the term *intradermal nevus* is employed. Nevi are most likely present at birth and may acquire melanin pigment over time, particularly in association with puberty. They may also display slow growth over time. Nevi frequently occur at or near the eyelid margin, but do not cause loss of cilia or significant distortion of the eyelid architecture. Changes in pigmentation of the lesion may raise the concern of possible melanoma, or nevi may cause cosmetic concerns due to their location on the eyelid or eyelid margin. Nevi are amenable to an excisional biopsy or shave biopsy, and the specimen should be submitted for histopathologic evaluation to confirm the clinical diagnosis.

2. Benign epithelial lesions occur often on the eyelid and should be considered in the differential diagnosis. *Squamous papilloma* appears as a well-circumscribed nonpigmented lesion on the eyelid or eyelid margin. In contrast to the smooth surface of an intradermal nevus, the papilloma has an irregular frondlike surface. Examination of the lesion under magnification at the slit lamp will usually reveal small pinpoint vessels at the tip of each frond. Histopathologically, papillomas are composed of thickened, or acanthotic, epidermis, overlying numerous fibrovascular cores. The normal maturation pattern of the epidermis is not disturbed.

Seborrheic keratosis is another common benign tumor that affects sun-exposed skin including the eyelids. These lesions may be appear variably pigmented and have an oily crusty appearance. The lesions are sessile and appear to "sit" on the epidermal surface. Histopathologically, acanthosis, hyperkeratosis, and papillomatosis are present. Additionally, pseudohorn cysts, representing infoldings of the epidermis, are frequently observed.

Inverted follicular keratosis is considered by most pathologists to represent an inflamed variant of seborrheic keratosis. These lesions may display exuberant hyperkeratosis creating a cutaneous horn. At the base of the lesion, the acanthotic epithelium contains numerous whorls of keratin, referred to as squamoid eddies.

Actinic keratosis appears as reddish flat, slightly scaly lesions on sun-exposed skin of the face, including the eyelids. Histopathologically, they display hyperkeratosis and parakeratosis, or abnormal retention of squamous cell nuclei in the surface keratin. Additionally, there is disruption of the normal orderly maturation pattern of the epidermis, and increased mitotic activity is present. Actinic keratoses are considered premalignant lesions, meaning that if left untreated, they may transform to a squamous cell carcinoma. Complete surgical excision is therefore indicated.

Keratoacanthomas may display relatively rapid growth and display a keratin-filled central crater surrounded by an elevated thickened epidermal margin. These lesions are often self-limited with spontaneous involution after 4 to 6 weeks. Keratoacanthomas arise from pilosebaceous glands and closely resembles squamous cell carcinoma.[5] Some arguments support classifying keratoacanthoma as a variant of invasive squamous cell carcinoma. Surgical excision is indicated for histologic confirmation or for cosmetic concerns.

Epithelium may proliferate beneath the skin surface where it may form *epidermal inclusion cysts*. These cysts grow slowly and form a firm subcutaneous nodule, appearing whitish-yellow clinically. Epidermal inclusion cysts may arise from the infundibulum of the hair follicle or from entrapped epithelial rests that become implanted during minor trauma.

Histologically, the cysts are lined by stratified squamous epithelium and are filled with keratin debris.

3. The adnexal structures of the skin may give rise to a number of benign eyelid tumors. Of these lesions, syringomas, arising from the sweat glands, are the most common. Clinically, these tumors appear as multiple yellowish papules. Histologically, numerous proliferating ductal structures, lined by a double row of cuboidal epithelium, are present. Some of the ductal structures have a characteristic "comma" shape, and there may be extensive fibrosis of the surrounding stroma.

Hidrocystomas may arise from either eccrine or apocrine sweat glands and appear as translucent cysts beneath the skin surface. Eccrine hidrocystomas frequently appear as multiple small cysts, whereas the apocrine hidrocystoma is most often a solitary nodule. Hidrocystomas occur most commonly at the lateral canthus or are associated with the eyelid margin.

Pilomatrixoma is a tumor that occurs more frequently in children or young adults. The lesion has a reddish-blue color, and there may be a history of minor trauma to the area. Microscopically, the tumor is composed of islands of basophilic cells with interposed "shadow" cells. Areas of dystrophic calcification are scattered throughout the lesion, and associated granulomatous inflammation is often present.

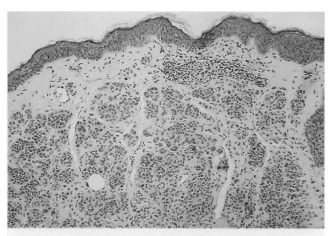

Fig. 97.2 Low-power photomicrograph showing nests of nevus cells within the superficial and deep dermis (H&E; original magnification × 13.2).

97.2 Test Interpretation

The morphologic appearance of the lesion is usually characteristic, but tissue diagnosis by pathologic examination is recommended in suspicious cases.

97.3 Diagnosis

Benign eyelid tumor, most likely intradermal nevus.

97.4 Medical Management

There is no medical treatment for this condition.

97.5 Surgical Management

Because of the apparent benign nature of the tumor, no further ancillary testing is indicated. The lesion may be observed, or it may be surgically excised. In most cases, the procedure can be performed as an office procedure using a local anesthetic. The resulting small defect can be repaired primarily or allowed to heal by secondary intention. Care must be taken not to create distortion of the eyelid margin or significant shortening of the anterior lamella of the eyelid. Any excised specimen should be sent for histopathologic confirmation.

97.6 Rehabilitation and Follow-up

The patient underwent excisional biopsy of the upper eyelid lesion, and histopathologic examination of the specimen confirmed the diagnosis of intradermal nevus (▶ Fig. 97.2). The patient has done well without evidence of recurrence.

97.6.1 Acknowledgment

Thanks to this chapter's first edition authors, Debra Shetlar and Milton Boniuk.

Suggested Reading

[1] Albert DM, Jakobiec FA, eds. Principles and Practice of Ophthalmology. 2nd ed. Philadelphia, PA: WB Saunders Co; 1994:1713–1823

[2] American Academy of Ophthalmology. Ophthalmic pathology and intraocular tumors. In: Basic and Clinical Science Course. Section 4. San Francisco, CA: American Academy of Ophthalmology; 1998:97–110

[3] Font RL. Eyelids and lacrimal drainage system. In: Spencer WH, ed. Ophthalmic Pathology: An Atlas and Textbook. 4th ed. Philadelphia, PA: WB Saunders Co; 1990:2218–2407

[4] Marines HM, Patrinely JR. Benign eyelid tumors. In: Liesegang TJ, ed. Oculodermal Disease. Philadelphia, PA: WB Saunders Co; 1992:243–260

[5] Najjar T, Meyers AD, Monroe MM. (2016, June 28). Cutaneous Squamous Cell Carcinoma. 2016. Available at: http://emedicine.medscape.com/article/1965430-overview. Accessed May 2, 2017

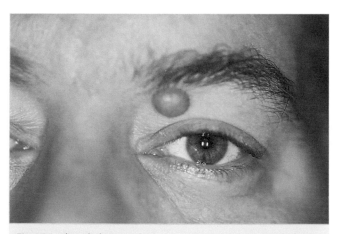

Fig. 97.1 Clinical photograph showing nonpigmented smooth dome-shaped lesion of the upper eyelid.

98 Malignant Tumors of the Eyelid

Amina I. Malik

Abstract

Malignant eyelid tumors can present with skin ulceration, telangiectasias, madarosis, and asymmetry in growth. The most common eyelid malignancy is basal cell cancer, typically on the lower eyelid. Other eyelid malignancies include squamous cell cancer, sebaceous cell cancer, and melanoma. Wide surgical excision of the tumor is indicated once the diagnosis is established. Because sebaceous gland carcinoma can metastasize widely, a complete metastatic evaluation should also be obtained. Incomplete excision will leave the patient at risk for local recurrence as well as metastatic dissemination. Radiation treatment has been employed for palliative therapy but is not effective as a primary treatment modality.

Keywords: malignant eyelid tumors, eyelid swelling, eyelid cancer, skin cancer

98.1 History

A 55-year-old man presented for evaluation of an enlarging skin nodule of his right upper eyelid. The lesion had been present for approximately 8 months and had grown fairly rapidly. The patient recalled one episode of bleeding from the area after he had picked at the lesion. While there was no previous history of skin cancer, the patient reported an extensive sun-exposure history. His ophthalmic examination was within normal limits except for the external examination. There was a large elevated nonpigmented nodule involving the skin of the right upper eyelid near the medial canthal region (▶ Fig. 98.1). The nodule measured 15 mm × 12 mm × 7 mm and showed numerous small telangiectatic vessels on its surface. The edges of the tumor had a thickened pearly appearance. There was no ulceration present. The skin underlying the lesion was freely moveable, and the tumor did not appear fixed to the underlying deep

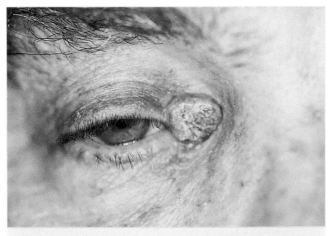

Fig. 98.1 Clinical photograph showing nonpigmented elevated lesion over the medial canthal region. There is irregular crusting over the surface of the lesion.

structures. There was no regional lymphadenopathy. The skin of the patient's face showed diffuse sun-exposure changes consisting of fine wrinkles and telangiectatic vessels and scattered areas of crusting.

Differential Diagnosis—Key Points

1. The relative rapid growth of this lesion, the history of previous bleeding, and the clinical features suggest a malignant tumor. Basal cell carcinoma is the most common malignancy of the eyelid and most commonly involves the lower eyelid and the medial canthal region. Risk factors for basal cell carcinoma include fair skin, northern European ancestry, history of extensive sun exposure, or history of previous basal cell carcinoma. Patients with a family history of skin cancer may be at an increased risk for developing basal cell carcinoma.

Clinically, basal cell carcinomas are categorized as nodular, nodular-ulcerative, or morpheaform. Microscopically, basal cell carcinomas are composed of nests and cords of proliferating epidermal basilar cells. Palisading nests of the nuclei at the periphery is a characteristic feature. In the morpheaform variant, the tumor nests invade the deep dermis and are associated with a marked stromal fibrosis.

The treatment for basal cell carcinoma is complete surgical extirpation of the tumor. The lesion should be excised with a margin of uninvolved adjacent tissue, and the free margins should be confirmed pathologically. Reconstruction should ensue only after complete removal of the malignancy is verified. On occasion, the basal cell carcinoma may be very extensive and involve deep vital structures such that complete removal is not possible. In such cases, radiation therapy and chemotherapy have been employed after surgical debulking of the tumor.

2. The second most common malignancy of the eyelid is squamous cell carcinoma. The ratio of basal cell carcinoma to squamous cell carcinoma frequency is approximately 40 to 1. In contrast to basal cell carcinoma, squamous cell carcinoma more frequently involves the upper eyelid and behaves more aggressively. The tumor may have an ulcerative appearance and may show crusting or hyperkeratosis. Squamous cell carcinoma may invade adjacent structures such as the orbit or lacrimal drainage system and may metastasize to regional lymph nodes or spread hematogenously to distant sites. Squamous cell carcinoma can also undergo perineural spread, leading to cranial nerve palsies.

As with basal cell carcinoma, the treatment for squamous cell carcinoma is complete surgical removal. A wide margin of uninvolved tissues should be obtained. There is a higher recurrence rate for squamous cell carcinoma as compared to basal cell carcinoma. If there is orbital invasion, exenteration may be required to achieve complete removal of the tumor.

3. Sebaceous carcinoma accounts for less than 0.8% of eyelid tumors; however, its protean clinical appearance causes this entity to be frequently confused with inflammatory lesions or other eyelid disorders, thereby delaying correct diagnosis and appropriate treatment. Sebaceous carcinoma arises from the meibomian glands or, less frequently, from the glands of Zeiss. It may also arise from sebaceous units within the caruncle or eyebrow. Patients are usually over 50 years old, and the tumor may masquerade as a chalazion, chronic blepharitis, ocular cicatricial pemphigoid, basal cell carcinoma, or squamous carcinoma. Therefore, the clinician should maintain a high level of suspicion for possible sebaceous carcinoma in an older patient with a recurrent chalazion or chronic unilateral blepharitis that is refractory to treatment.

Biopsies of suspicious lesions should be sent to the pathology laboratory with a request for special lipid stains. These include oil red O and Sudan black stains and must be performed on frozen tissue, because routine processing of the tissue will dissolve any lipid that is present. Good communication between the clinician and the pathologist is therefore of paramount importance. Because many general pathologists lack familiarity with this entity, the clinician should not hesitate to seek outside consultation if there is a high clinical suspicion of sebaceous gland carcinoma.

Wide surgical excision of the tumor is indicated once the diagnosis is established. Because sebaceous gland carcinoma can metastasize widely, a complete metastatic evaluation should also be obtained. Incomplete excision will leave the patient at risk for local recurrence as well as metastatic dissemination. Radiation treatment has been employed for palliative therapy but is not effective as a primary treatment modality.

4. Malignant melanoma may arise in the eyelid, just as it may occur in the skin or mucus membranes throughout the body. Cutaneous melanomas may be subclassified as lentigo maligna, superficial spreading melanoma, and nodular melanoma. The nodular melanoma is the most common type affecting the eyelid and has a more aggressive clinical course. The eyelid can be secondarily involved from primary melanoma arising in the conjunctiva or by metastasis of melanoma from other sites.

The treatment for cutaneous melanoma is wide surgical excision with microscopic verification of clear margins. The finding of lymphatic or vascular invasion on microscopic evaluation should prompt referral for possible regional lymph node dissection. As with cutaneous melanomas arising elsewhere, an invasion depth of greater than 1.5 mm portends a higher risk for recurrence and the development of metastatic disease.

98.2 Test Interpretation

Morphologic appearance is suspicious, but tissue diagnosis is required for confirmation of malignancy.

98.3 Diagnosis

Lesion of the right upper eyelid (medial canthal region); probable basal cell carcinoma.

98.4 Medical Management

Imiquimod and 5-fluorouracil are FDA-approved topical creams used for superficial basal cell carcinomas. These are applied to the lesions for up to 6 weeks or longer and have shown cure rates up to 80%. Vismodegib can be taken orally for rare cases of metastatic basal cell carcinoma or locally advanced basal cell carcinoma. This medicine works by blocking the "hedgehog" signaling pathway, which is a key step in the development of basal cell carcinoma. Vismodegib is approved only for very limited circumstances where the nature of the cancer precludes other treatment options (such as surgery or radiation). Sonidegib, a second oral hedgehog inhibitor drug, was approved by the FDA in 2015 for patients with locally advanced basal cell carcinomas, specifically patients whose tumors have recurred following surgery or radiation therapy, or who are not candidates for surgery or radiation therapy.

98.5 Surgical Management

Ancillary testing is not indicated prior to establishing the diagnosis by incisional or excisional biopsy. Once the diagnosis is known, patients with sebaceous carcinoma or cutaneous melanoma should undergo a complete metastatic evaluation. This is usually conducted under the supervision of an oncologist. If complete removal of the tumor will require extensive reconstructive procedures, an incisional biopsy can be performed first to correctly establish the diagnosis. Small lesions, however, may be removed in toto at the time of initial biopsy. Many surgeons advocate the use of cryotherapy to the margins of the resulting defect to decrease the risk of tumor recurrence. Reconstruction procedures are dictated by the size and location of the defect once clear surgical margins have been verified.

The current patient underwent excisional biopsy of the lesion due to the high clinical suspicion of basal cell carcinoma. Intraoperative frozen section analysis confirmed the diagnosis of basal cell carcinoma with free surgical margins (▶ Fig. 98.2).

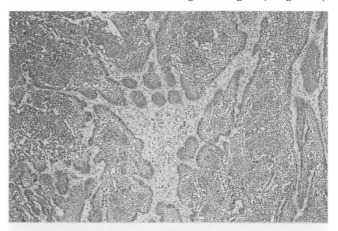

Fig. 98.2 Histopathology of the tumor showing a nodular basal cell carcinoma. The nuclear palisading around the periphery of the nests is apparent (H&E; original magnification × 13.2).

Because of the location of the defect, a full-thickness skin graft was used to repair the defect to avoid creating lagophthalmos or webbing of the medial canthal region.

98.6 Rehabilitation and Follow-up

The patient did well postoperatively with a satisfactory functional and cosmetic result. He has been educated about his increased risk for the development of new skin malignancies and is under the care of a dermatologist for continued surveillance.

98.6.1 Acknowledgment

Thanks to this chapter's first edition authors, Debra Shetlar and Milton Boniuk.

Suggested Reading

[1] Doxanas MT, Green WR. Sebaceous gland carcinoma. Review of 40 cases. Arch Ophthalmol. 1984; 102(2):245–249

[2] Lederman M. Radiation treatment of cancer of the eyelids. Br J Ophthalmol. 1976; 60(12):794–805

[3] Margo CE, Waltz K. Basal cell carcinoma of the eyelid and periocular skin. Surv Ophthalmol. 1993; 38(2):169–192

[4] Mohs FE. Micrographic surgery for the microscopically controlled excision of eyelid cancers. Arch Ophthalmol. 1986; 104(6):901–909

Index

Note: Page numbers set **bold** or *italic* indicate headings or figures, respectively.